Horizons in Medicine

number 8

Edited by
Michael J G Farthing MD FRCP
Professor of Gastroenterology
St Bartholomew's & The Royal London School of Medicine and Dentistry, London

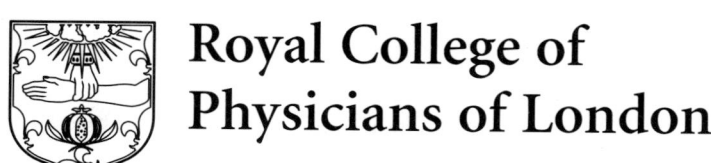

Royal College of
Physicians of London

Publisher's Acknowledgements

The Royal College of Physicians is pleased to acknowledge generous support towards the cost of production of this book from:

> Glaxo Wellcome Research and Development
>
> Hoechst Marion Roussel Ltd
>
> Napp Laboratories Ltd
>
> 3M Health Care Ltd

The Editor, Professor Michael Farthing, was responsible for compiling the programme for the conference upon which this book is based. The College is indebted to him and to the contributors to this volume for allowing their papers to be included and for taking the time to prepare them for publication.

The College greatly values the continued support and encouragement of Professor Stephen Holgate in his capacity as Series Editor.

Royal College of Physicians of London
11 St Andrews Place, London NW1 4LE

Registered Charity No. 210508

Copyright © 1997 Royal College of Physicians of London
ISBN 1 86016 0689

Typeset by Dan-Set Graphics, Telford, Shropshire
Printed in Great Britain by The Lavenham Press Ltd, Sudbury, Suffolk

British Library Cataloging in Publication Data
A catalogue record of this book is available from the British Library

Preface

During the past five decades our understanding of disease mechanisms at a molecular and cellular level has grown spectacularly and the new therapies that this knowledge has already delivered presents a formidable challenge to practising clinicians. Although medical education has always emphasised the necessity for rational, information-based therapy, this has been further emphasised by government support for evidence-based medicine. Similarly, the rapidly emerging discipline of health care economics and the pressures on industrialised nations in particular to reduce spending on health care, has given politicians, purchasers, health care managers and clinicians yet another platform from which to examine the appropriateness of all health care interventions.

There is of course no shortage of information, evidence and sound opinion. They vary in quality and quantity depending on the particular area of clinical medicine concerned, the availability of useful clinical interventions and their accessibility to formal evaluation in randomised controlled trials. The task for the general physician to evaluate this deluge of information is unprecedented in the evolution of the science and practice of clinical medicine.

The Royal College of Physicians has recognised this need since 1964 by organising an annual Advanced Medicine Conference to provide general physicians with the evidence they require to practice medicine across the specialties. In 1996, I assembled a group of experts who were renowned for their expertise as clinicians, as clinical investigators and for their skills in distilling the essence of their topic and presenting it in a succinct, lively and amusing manner. The emphasis of the conference was unashamedly 'clinical' although the contributors were encouraged to touch on molecular and cellular aspects where appropriate. It was a tall order, but I believe we achieved all of these objectives. This book is a record of this conference and each chapter summarises individual contributions in gastroenterology and hepatology, endocrinology, diabetes and metabolism, respiratory medicine, bone, joint and connective tissue disorders, neurology, infectious diseases, nephrology and cardiovascular medicine. In addition, we were honoured to incorporate Tim Cox's Bradshaw Lecture on *Lysosomal disease: a credible therapeutic target*, David Warrell's Croonian Lecture on *Pathophysiology and treatment of malignant tertian malaria*, and George Davey Smith's Lord Rayner Lecture, *Down at heart: The meaning and implications of inequalities in cardiovascular disease*.

For those who take self-education seriously, we provide multiple choice questions at the end of most chapters so that you can judge how much you have learnt. High marks will enhance your medical practice as well as increase your self-esteem.

This book should prove useful to all of us who are struggling to keep up to speed with the information highway!

MICHAEL JG FARTHING
Editor

Series Editor:
STEPHEN HOLGATE MD FRCP
MRC Clinical Professor of Immunopharmacology
University of Southampton

Contributors

DR M AHMED BSc MRCP *Senior Registrar in Gastroenterology, Liver and Hepatobiliary Unit, Queen Elizabeth Hospital, Edgbaston, Birmingham B15 2TH*

DR Q AZIZ MRCP *Clinical Lecturer and Senior Registrar, Department of Medicine, Hope Hospital, Eccles Old Road, Salford M6 8HD*

DR D BATES MA FRCP *Consultant Neurologist and Senior Lecturer in Neurology, Department of Neurology, Royal Victoria Infirmary, Queen Victoria Road, Newcastle upon Tyne NE1 4LP*

DR G D BELL MD MSc FRCP *Consultant Gastroenterologist, Department of Medicine, The Ipswich Hospital, Heath Road Wing, Ipswich, Suffolk IP4 5PD*

DR R W BILOUS MD FRCP *Consultant Physician, Diabetes Care Centre, Middlesbrough General Hospital, Middlesbrough, Cleveland TS5 5AZ*

PROFESSOR C M BLACK MD FRCP *Professor of Rheumatology, Academic Unit of Rheumatology and Connective Tissue Diseases, Royal Free Hospital School of Medicine, Rowland Hill Street, London NW3 2PF*

PROFESSOR D R BLAKE FRCP *ARC Professor of Rheumatology, Bone and Joint Research Unit, The London Hospital Medical College, London E1 2AD*

PROFESSOR P M A CALVERLEY FRCP FCCP *Professor of Medicine (Pulmonary Rehabilitation), Aintree Chest Clinic, Fazakerley Hospital, Longmoor Lane, Liverpool L9 7AL*

PROFESSOR R W F CAMPBELL BSc FRCP *Professor of Cardiology, University Department of Cardiology, Freeman Hospital, Newcastle upon Tyne NE7 7DN*

PROFESSOR D W CHADWICK DM FRCP *Professor of Neurology, Department of Neurological Science, The University of Liverpool, Walton Centre for Neurology and Neurosurgery, Rice Lane, Liverpool L9 1AE*

DR I C CHIKANZA MD MRCP *Consultant Rheumatologist, Bone and Joint Research Unit, The London Hospital Medical College, London E1 2AD*

PROFESSOR J COHEN MSc MB FRCPath *Professor and Head of Department of Infectious Diseases and Bacteriology, Hammersmith Hospital and Royal Postgraduate Medical School, Du Cane Road, London W12 0NN*

DR P COLLINS MA MD FRCP FACC *Senior Lecturer and Honorary Consultant Cardiologist, Department of Cardiac Medicine, Royal Brompton Hospital, Dovehouse Street, London SW3 6LY*

PROFESSOR D A S COMPSTON PhD FRCP *Professor of Neurology, Neurology Department, University of Cambridge, Addenbrooke's Hospital, Hills Road, Cambridge CB2 2QQ*

DR J CORDINGLEY MB MRCP FRCA *Research Fellow, Intensive Care, Charing Cross Hospital, Fulham Palace Road, London W6 8RF*

PROFESSOR T M COX MA MSc MD FRCP *Professor of Medicine, University of Cambridge, Clinical School of Medicine, Addenbrooke's Hospital, Hills Road, Cambridge CB2 2QQ*

DR D CUNNINGHAM MD FRCP *Consultant Medical Oncologist and Head of GI and Lymphoma Units, Department of Medicine, The Royal Marsden Hospital, Downs Road, Sutton, Surrey SM2 5PT*

PROFESSOR G DAVEY SMITH MA MSc MD MFPHM *Professor of Clinical Epidemiology, Department of Social Medicine, University of Bristol, Carynge Hall, Whiteladies Road, Bristol BS8 2PR*

DR D D'CRUZ MRCP *Senior Lecturer and Consultant Rheumatologist, Rheumatology Department, The Royal London Hospital, Bancroft Road, Mile End, London E1 4DG*

DR D S DYMOND MD FRCP *Consultant Cardiologist, Cardiac Clinical Group, St Bartholomew's Hospital, West Smithfield, London EC1A 7BE*

DR E ELIAS MD FRCP *Consultant Physician and Reader in Clinical Hepatology, Liver and Hepatobiliary Unit, Queen Elizabeth Hospital, Edgbaston, Birmingham B15 2TH*

DR J D FIRTH DM FRCP *Consultant Nephrologist and Physician, Addenbrooke's Hospital, Hills Road, Cambridge CB2 2QQ*

PROFESSOR K A A FOX BSc FRCP *Professor of Cardiology and Head of Department, Cardiovascular Research Unit, The Royal Infirmary of Edinburgh, Lauriston Place, Edinburgh EH3 9YW*

PROFESSOR J A FRANKLYN MD PhD FRCP *Professor of Medicine, Department of Medicine, University of Birmingham, Queen Elizabeth Hospital, Edgbaston, Birmingham B15 2TH*

PROFESSOR E A M GALE MB FRCP *Professor of Diabetes, Department of Diabetes and Metabolism, Andrew Cudworth Laboratories, St Bartholomew's Hospital, 3rd Floor Dominion House, West Smithfield, London EC1A 7BE*

DR G R V HUGHES MD FRCP *Consultant Physician, Lupus Research Unit, The Rayne Institute, St Thomas' Hospital, London SE1 7EH*

DR S JAWED MRCP *ARC Clinical Research Fellow, Bone and Joint Research Unit, The London Hospital Medical College, Whitechapel, London E1 2AD*

DR R W KEEN BSc MRCP *ARC Clinical Research Fellow, Rheumatology Department, St Thomas' Hospital, Lambeth Palace Road, London SE1 7EH*

DR W A LYNN MD MRCP *Consultant in Infectious Diseases, Cameron Centre, Ealing Hospital, Uxbridge Road, Southall, Middlesex UB1 3EW*

DR J T MACFARLANE DM FRCP *Consultant Physician in General and Respiratory Medicine, Respiratory Medicine Department, Nottingham City Hospital, Hucknall Road, Nottingham NG5 1PB*

DR J MOORE-GILLON MA MD FRCP *Consultant Physician and Co-Director, East London TB Service, Department of Respiratory Medicine, St Bartholomew's Royal London Chest Hospitals, London EC1A 7BE*

DR J G O'GRADY MD FRCPI *Consultant Hepatologist and Director of the Institute of Liver Studies, King's College Hospital, Denmark Hill, London SE5 9PJ*

DR M G A PALAZZO FRCA FRCP MD *Director, Intensive Care, Charing Cross Hospital, Fulham Palace Road, London W6 8RF*

DR M R PARTRIDGE MD FRCP *Consultant Physician, The Chest Clinic, Whipps Cross Hospital, Whipps Cross Road, Leytonstone, London E11 1NR*

PROFESSOR G PASVOL DPhil FRCP *Professor of Infectious and Tropical Medicine, Imperial College School of Medicine, Department of Infectious and Tropical Medicine, Northwick Park Hospital, Harrow HA1 3UJ*

DR P A REILLY FRCP *Consultant in Rheumatology, Frimley Park Hospital, Portsmouth Road, Camberley, Surrey GU16 5UJ*

DR P M ROTHWELL MD MRCP *Clinical Lecturer in Neurology, Department of Clinical Neurology, University of Oxford, Radcliffe Infirmary, Oxford OX2 6HE*

PROFESSOR J G P SISSONS MD FRCP *Professor of Medicine, Department of Medicine, University of Cambridge Clinical School, Addenbrooke's Hospital, Hills Road, Cambridge CB2 2QQ*

DR T D SPECTOR MSc MD MRCP *Consultant Rheumatologist, Department of Rheumatology, St Thomas' Hospital, London SE1 7EH*

DR S G SPIRO MD FRCP *Consultant Physician, Clinical Director of Medicine, Department of Thoracic Medicine, The Middlesex Hospital, Mortimer Street, London W1N 8AA*

DR D L STEVENS MD FRCP *Consultant Neurologist, Department of Neurology, Gloucestershire Royal Hospital, Great Western Road, Gloucester GL1 3NN*

DR J R STRADLING MD FRCP *Consultant and Director, Osler Chest Unit, Churchill Hospital, Headington, Oxford OX3 7LJ*

DR R H SWANTON MD FRCP *Consultant Cardiologist, Department of Cardiology, The Middlesex Hospital, Mortimer Street, London W1N 8AA*

PROFESSOR R V THAKKER MD FRCP *Professor of Medicine and Head, MRC Molecular Endocrinology Group, MRC Clinical Sciences Centre, Royal Postgraduate Medical School, Hammersmith Hospital, Du Cane Road, London W12 0NN*

DR D G THOMPSON MD FRCP *Senior Lecturer/Consultant, Department of Medicine, Hope Hospital, Eccles Old Road, Salford M6 8HD*

DR C R V TOMSON DM FRCP *Consultant Nephrologist, Renal Medicine Department, Southmead Hospital, Westbury-on-Trym, Bristol BS10 5NB*

DR R C TURNER MD FRCP *Professor of Medicine, University of Oxford, Nuffield Department of Clinical Medicine, Diabetes Research Laboratories, Radcliffe Infirmary, Woodstock Road, Oxford OX2 6HE*

PROFESSOR C P WARLOW MD FRCP *Professor of Medical Neurology, Department of Clinical Neurosciences, Western General Hospital, Crewe Road, Edinburgh EH4 2XG*

PROFESSOR D A WARRELL MA DM DSc FRCP *Professor of Tropical Medicine and Infectious Diseases, University of Oxford, and Director, Centre for Tropical Medicine, Nuffield Department of Clinical Medicine, John Radcliffe Hospital, Oxford OX3 9DU*

PROFESSOR J A H WASS MD FRCP *Consultant in Endocrinology and Metabolism, Nuffield Orthopaedic Centre, Windmill Road, Oxford OX3 7LD and Radcliffe Infirmary, Woodstock Road, Oxford OX2 6HE*

DR A WEBB BSc MRCP *Senior Registrar, Department of Medicine, The Royal Marsden Hospital, Downs Road, Sutton, Surrey SM2 5PT*

PROFESSOR G WILLIAMS MA MD FRCP *Professor of Medicine (Diabetes and Endocrinology), University Clinical Departments at Aintree, Fazakerley Hospital, Longmoor Lane, Liverpool L9 7AL*

Contents

Preface iii

List of contributors v

LECTURES

The Bradshaw Lecture
Lysosomal storage diseases: a credible therapeutic target 1
TM Cox

The Croonian Lecture
Pathophysiology and treatment of malignant tertian malaria 21
DA Warrell

The Lord Rayner Lecture
Social inequalities in cardiovascular disease – their origins
   and implications 35
George Davey Smith

GASTROENTEROLOGY AND HEPATOLOGY

Helicobacter pylori: clinical implications 49
GD Bell

Advances in gastrointestinal cancer 59
A Webb and D Cunningham

Practical aspects of the brain-gut axis 71
Q Aziz and DG Thompson

Management of acute liver failure 83
JG O'Grady

Management of chronic viral hepatitis 93
M Ahmed and E Elias

ENDOCRINOLOGY, DIABETES AND METABOLISM

Diagnosis and management of Cushing's syndrome 111
JAH Wass

The management of thyroid lumps 119
JA Franklyn

Molecular genetics of multiple endocrine neoplasia type 1 129
RV Thakker

Reappraisal of insulin therapy 143
EAM Gale

Management of non-insulin-dependent diabetes mellitus 155
RC Turner

Brain, fat and the fulfilling of prophecies 167
G Williams

RESPIRATORY MEDICINE

Delivering optimal care to patients with asthma 183
Martyn R Partridge

Practical problems in the management of chronic obstructive
   pulmonary disease 197
PMA Calverley

Tuberculosis 211
J Moore-Gillon

Guidelines and the management of community acquired pneumonia . . 221
JT Macfarlane

Practical approach to sleep disordered breathing 233
JR Stradling

New approaches to lung cancer 249
SG Spiro

BONE, JOINT AND CONNECTIVE TISSUE DISORDERS

Advances in the drug therapies of rheumatoid arthritis 259
S Jawed, IC Chikanza and DR Blake

Scleroderma spectrum disorders 271
CM Black

The antiphospholipid syndrome 291
D D'Cruz and GRV Hughes

Management of osteoporosis in the 1990s 301
RW Keen and TD Spector

Fibromyalgia revisited: the vicious cycle of chronic pain 309
PA Reilly

NEUROLOGY

Management of transient ischaemic attacks: from clinical trials
   to individual patients 315
PM Rothwell and CP Warlow

Disease modifying treatments in multiple sclerosis 333
Alastair Compston

Management of status epilepticus 351
DW Chadwick

Management of medical coma 359
D Bates

Headaches: how good are we at early management 369
David L Stevens

INFECTIOUS DISEASES

Imported infections 379
G Pasvol

Prevention and treatment of hospital acquired infection 391
J Cohen

Progress in the diagnosis and treatment of human virus infections 399
JGP Sissons

Infections in the immunocompromised host 411
WA Lynn

NEPHROLOGY

Modern management of acute tubular necrosis: prevention of oliguria . . 425
MGA Palazzo and J Cordingley

Urinary tract infection 437
CRV Tomson

Hypertension and the kidney: villains and victims 451
JD Firth

Diabetic nephropathy: detection and intervention 463
RW Bilous

CARDIOVASCULAR MEDICINE

Assessment of prognosis in patients with angina and coronary artery
   disease 479
DS Dymond

Intervention in acute coronary syndrome: unstable angina and
   non-Q wave myocardial infarction 487
KAA Fox

Modern management of arrhythmias 495
RWF Campbell

Valve disease in the 1990s 503
RH Swanton

Chest pain in women 513
P Collins

The Bradshaw Lecture
Lysosomal storage diseases: a credible therapeutic target

T M Cox

'I never think of the future: it comes soon enough.' A Einstein, 1930.

☐ INTRODUCTION

It has been observed that a long interval often elapses between the discovery of an entity that can be exploited for therapeutic purposes and its practical application for clinical use. In scientific terms, the identification of the intracellular organelle designated the lysosome in 1955 by the Belgian scientist Christian de Duve has been followed by a logical scientific development and richness of discovery that would hearten even the most cynical practitioner. Nonetheless, the emergence of the lysosome as a focus for credible therapeutic exploration has taken the better part of 40 years.

☐ DISCOVERY OF THE LYSOSOME

de Duve was a biochemist rather than a microscopist: his discovery of the lysosome was fortuitous. He was conducting experiments to investigate the action of insulin on the liver. At this stage, simple centrifugal techniques were being used to allow the chemical composition, enzyme content and other properties of different cell fractions (nuclear, mitochondrial and microsomal) to be determined. de Duve wished to localize the gluconeogenic enzyme glucose-6-phosphatase in liver cells and used a related activity, acid phosphatase, as a control. To separate populations of subcellular constituents into different populations, de Duve and colleagues introduced continuous density-gradient centrifugation techniques. To identify small differences in the density distribution of particulate components within the whole homogenate, the activities of 'marker' enzymes associated with specific organelles were determined. During the conduct of these experiments it was found that the activity of acid phosphatase increased on freezing and thawing and after disruption by mechanical or chemical means – the phenomenon of enzymic 'latency'. de Duve realized that this was related to the impermeability of enzymes in intact particles to their substrates; enzymes present together in the same native particle would not only co-sediment but would be released together on disruption of the material. By 1955, the results of this work were sufficiently advanced for de Duve and his colleagues to postulate the existence of a new group of organelles that contain a rich complement of acid hydrolases and to suggest the occurrence of another group of particles – ultimately named the peroxisomes. It must be emphasized that the initial description of these organelles was entirely biochemical. Eventually, advances in electron microscopy made it possible for the structures contained within subcellular fractions to be examined; these studies showed that the lysosomes corresponded to the so-called 'peri-canalicular dense bodies' and that the peroxisomal function contained the organelles previously described as the 'microbodies'. Fifteen years of research had thus ultimately bridged the gap between biochemistry and morphology: Christian de Duve was awarded the Nobel Prize jointly with Palade and Claude in 1974 [1]. A new science, of cell biology, had been launched and approved.

☐ STRUCTURE AND FUNCTION OF LYSOSOMES

Lysosomes are strikingly diverse in shape and size, but belong to a single class of almost ubiquitous organelles containing at least 40 acid hydrolases including proteases, nucleases, glycosidases, lipases and phospholipases, sulphatases and phosphatases with an optimum activity at about pH5 (Table 1). It has been suggested that the acidic pH optima of lysosomal enzymes normally protect intracellular components from their hydrolytic action – unless the components are engulfed and exposed to the degradative milieu of this specialized compartment. The matrix space

Table 1 Lysosomal hydrolases.

Enzyme	Substrate class
Acid phosphatases	Phosphomonoesters
Acid phosphodiesterase	Oligonucleotides
Acid ribonuclease	Ribonucleic acid (RNA)
Acid deoxyribonuclease	Deoxyribonucleic acid (DNA)
Acid sphingomyelinase	Sphingomyelin
Acid lipase	Cholesterol esters, triacylglycerols
β-Hexosaminidase A	G_{M2} ganglioside, glycosaminoglycans, glycolipids
β-Hexosaminidase B	Glycosaminoglycans, oligosaccharides, glycolipids
α-Glucosidase	Glycogen
α-Galactosidase	Galactosides, glycolipids, glycoproteins
β-Galactosidase	G_{M1} ganglioside, keratan sulphate
α-Mannosidase	Glycoproteins, mannosides
β-Glucuronidase	Mucopolysaccharides
Lysozyme	Bacterial cell walls
Hyaluronidase	Hyaluronic acids and chondroitin
Arylsulphatases	Organic sulphates and glycolipids
Cathepsins	Proteins
Collagenase	Collagen
Peptidases	Peptides
Esterases	Fatty acyl esters
Phospholipases	Phospholipids

in the lumen of these organelles is surrounded by a single unit membrane containing transport proteins that facilitate the egress of hydrolysed products of the hydrolases and a specialized component that uses ATP-derived energy to maintain the proton gradient. Enzymic latency reflects the integrity of this lysosomal membrane and its impermeability to substrates. The proteins of the lysosomal membrane are themselves highly glycosylated: this may offer protection from the activated luminal proteases with which they are in contact. Lysosomes can be identified histochemically by the release of insoluble reaction products of the hydrolases that they contain; by this definition lysosomes are observed in nearly all eukaryotic cells. Their morphological diversity appears to reflect the multiplicity of functions they fulfil as part of an intracellular digestive system. Macromolecular substrates for lysosomal digestion are delivered to the lysosome for degradation by three main pathways [2] (Fig. 1).

Receptor-mediated endocytosis

Receptor-mediated endocytosis via coated pits to the peripheral and later perinuclear endosomal, mildly acidic, compartment. Conversion of this 'endolysosome' into a mature lysosome involves loss of certain membrane components and further acidification. Unless they are specifically retrieved, the molecules that are endocytosed are delivered by fusion with mature lysosomes for degradation. If they are retrieved, they are ultimately returned to the cell surface. A classic example of this pathway is that of the low-density lipoprotein receptor-mediated uptake of low-density lipoproteins

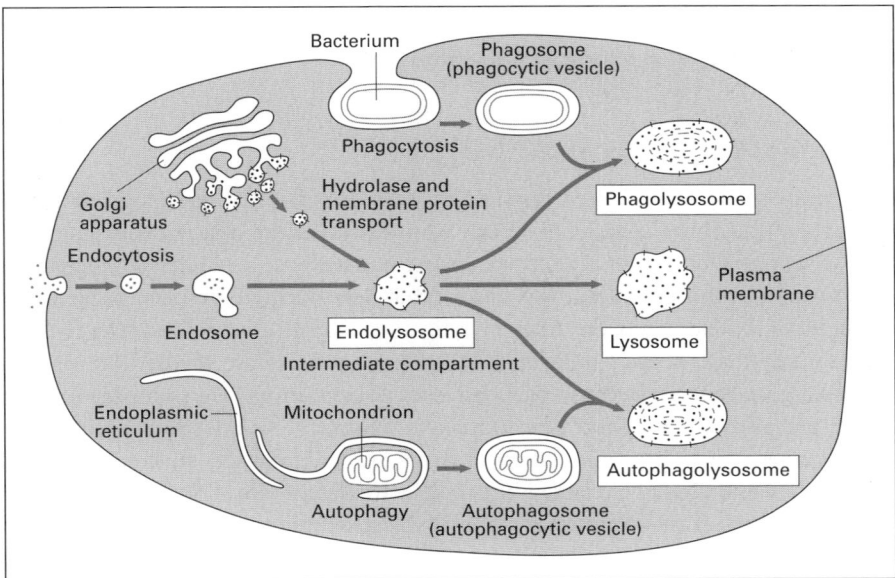

Fig. 1 The lysosome – an intracellular digestive system. The diagram shows the routes of entry for extrinsic and intrinsic delivery of proteins and materials to the lysosomal system (see text). (From Alberts et al. [3] with permission.)

(LDL). LDL receptors are returned to the plasma membrane by means of special transport vesicles, while the LDL ligand itself is degraded to release cholesterol in the lysosome.

Autophagy

Examination of lysosomes within cells shows that they frequently fuse with, engulf and degrade other organelles and membrane components – a process known as autophagy. This process is involved in the constant breakdown and renewal of intracellular components throughout the life of a cell. Entities such as peroxisomes and mitochondria are constantly synthesized *de novo* and at the same time their effete counterparts are degraded every few days within autophagocytic vesicles.

Engulfment and fusion

A pathway involving lysosomes observed equally throughout nature occurs in cells specialized for the degradation of extracellular materials and particulates. This process is active in macrophages and other phagocytes, including the related osteoclasts, whose resorptive vacuole acts as a vast exteriorized lysosomal compartment that is independently acidified. In macrophages, effete endogenous elements such as erythrocytes and neutrophils, as well as microbes and inanimate particulates, are engulfed: surface components are recognized by specific receptors at the plasma membrane to which they bind. Following surface recognition, phagocytes engulf material to form large vesicles in which acidification and proteolysis, as well as secretion of degradative molecules, eg nitric oxide or superoxide, is initiated. After membrane fusion with lysosomes, further acidification occurs and the acid hydrolases are activated to complete the breakdown of the entire ingested structure.

☐ LYSOSOMAL STORAGE DISEASES [4]

After this outline of lysosomal physiology, what of lysosomal pathology? It was a colleague of de Duve, Henri-Géry Hers, who identified the first lysosomal storage disease – originally known as Pompe's disease and now recognized as glycogenosis, Cori type II. In this disorder it was known that deposition of glycogen occurred in the heart and skeletal muscle. After investigating cellular glucosidases, Henri-Géry Hers showed that a specific deficiency of an acid α-glucosidase was deficient in this heritable glycogenosis. Because of its unusual pH optimum, Hers considered that acid α-glucosidase would have a lysosomal distribution. This was soon proved, since the enzyme activity co-sedimented in tissue subfractionation studies with acid phosphatase and could be released in parallel with 'latent' acid phosphatase activity by various physical and chemical treatments. Electron microscopy revealed glycogen aggregates surrounded by unilaminar membranes with some glycogen also freely dispersed in the cytoplasm (as occurs normally). Until the discovery of this lysosomal defect, the apparently normal metabolism of glycogen within the tissues of patients with Pompe's disease was unexplained. In Pompe's disease, the defect of acid α-glucosidase is specific and shows that, in healthy cells, fragments of endogenous glycogen are continuously being taken up by lysosomes and degraded. When α-glucosidase activity is deficient, uptake continues but degradation of the polymer is retarded so that the organelles become distended with undigested glycogen.

Investigation of glycogenosis type II thus indicated that specific deficiencies of one or another of the many acid hydrolases that occur in lysosomes could cause storage diseases, each of which would be related to a specific enzymic defect. In practice, the progressive accumulation of the particular complex macromolecule in the target cell gives rise to typical ultrastructural appearances caused by the sequestration, and sometimes aggregation, of substrate within lysosomal vacuoles. These substrates are usually intermediates in the turnover of compounds that form an integral part of cells: they are broken down sequentially by various acid hydrolases that are specific for the particular chemical bonds that occur in the parent macromolecules. Autophagy occurs in all tissues of the body and the nature and amount of material that accumulates in the lysosomal storage diseases varies considerably from one organ to another, according to the distribution and normal turnover rates of the parent macromolecules in the constituent cells. The extent of pathological storage and the severity of the condition often also relates to the amount of residual enzymic function [5]. The appearance of the diseased lysosomes varies greatly according to the physicochemical properties of the storage material. There may be crystalline deposits of water-soluble products or arrays of aggregated hydrophobic products, such as the undegraded sphingolipids that form characteristic membranous cytoplasmic bodies readily seen with the electron microscope.

Acid α-glucosidase deficiency was the first of over 30 lysosomal storage disorders now recognized. As stated above, most of these result from genetically determined deficiencies in the activity of specific acid hydrolases but in at least two disorders (cystinosis and Salla disease) defective transport of hydrolytic products out of the lysosome is responsible for lysosomal storage. The catalogue is enriched by the occurrence of rare phenocopies of single or multiple hydrolase deficiencies, such as those resulting from genetically determined deficiencies of one or more of the activator proteins (eg the sphingolipid activator proteins, saposins A-C) that are responsible for the full function of the lysosomal hydrolases. A parallel defect, multiple sulphatase deficiency, results from a unique deficiency of an enzymic system that modifies specific active-site cysteine residues to an oxo-propionate derivative that is found in the catalytic domains of all active eukaryotic sulphatases. A classification of the lysosomal storage disorders is set out in Table 2.

☐ ACCESS TO LYSOSOMES

The discovery of lysosomes, and especially the intracellular pathway for the formation of phagolysosomes, led to the prediction that the organelle would be accessible to molecules presented at the cell surface [6]. Remarkable experiments carried out by Neufeld and her colleagues at the National Institutes of Health in

Table 2 Lysosomal storage disorders.

Disease type	Defect	Substrate(s) accumulating
(i) Lysosomal targetting disorders		
I-cell/pseudo-Hurler polydystrophy	6-Phospho-N-acetylglucosamine transferase (mis-localization of many lysosomal hydrolases)	Nascent hydrolases
(ii) Disorders of membrane transport		
Cystinosis	Cystine efflux	Cystine
Salla disease	Sialate efflux	Sialic acid
(iii) Disorders of carbohydrate metabolism		
Glycogenosis II (Pompe's disease)	α-Glucosidase	Glycogen
(iv) Disorders of lipid metabolism		
Wolman's disease	Acid lipase	Cholesterol esters
Cholesterol ester storage disease	Triglycerides	
(v) Disorders of glycoprotein degradation		
Aspartylglycosaminuria	Aspartylglycosaminidase	N-Linked oligosaccharides
Fucosidosis	α-L-Fucosidase	α-L-Fuc oligosaccharides
Galactosialidosis	Protective protein/cathepsin (β-galactosidase and sialidase)	Substrates of β-Gal and sialidase
α-Mannosidosis	α-Mannosidase	α-Man oligosaccharides
β-Mannosidosis	β-Mannosidase	β-Man oligosaccharides
Sialidosis	Sialidase	Sialyl oligosaccharides
(vi) Disorders of glycosaminoglycan degradation		
Hunter's disease	Iduronate sulphatase	Dermatan sulphate, heparan sulphate
Hurler's & Scheie's disease	α-L-Iduronidase	''
Maroteaux-Lamy syndrome	GalNAc 4-sulphatase/Arylsulphatase B	Dermatan sulphate
Morquio-Brailsford disease A	Galactose 6-sulphatase	Keratan sulphate, chondroitin sulphate
Morquio-Brailsford disease B	β-Galactosidase	Keratan sulphate
Sanfilippo syndrome A	Heparan N-sulphatase	Heparan sulphate
Sanfilippo syndrome B	α-N-Acetylglucosaminidase	Heparan sulphate
Sanfilippo syndrome C	Acetyl CoA: glucosamine N-acetyltransferase	Heparan sulphate
Sanfilippo syndrome D	GlcNAc 6-sulphatase	Heparan sulphate
Sly syndrome	β-Glucuronidase	Dermatan sulphate, heparan sulphate Chondroitin 4 & 6 sulphates (Sly syndrome)
(vii) Disorders of sphingolipid degradation		
Fabry's disease	α-Galactosidase A	Trihexosyl-ceramide
Farber's disease	Acid ceramidase	Ceramide
Gaucher's disease	Glucocerebrosidase	Glucosylceramide
G_{M1} gangliosidosis	β-Galactosidase	G_{M1} ganglioside, galactosyl oligosaccharides, keratan sulphate
G_{M2} gangliosidosis:		
Tay-Sachs disease	β-Hexosaminidase A α-subunit	G_{M2} ganglioside, oligosaccharides
Sandhoff's disease	β-Hexosaminidases A & B β-subunit	''
Activator deficiency	G_{M2} activator	G_{M2} ganglioside
Krabbe's disease	Galactosylceramidase	Galactosylceramide, galactosylsphingosine
Metachromatic leucodystrophy	Arylsulphatase A	Galactosylsulphatide
Metachromatic leucodystrophy (activator-deficient form)	Sulphatide activator	Galactosylsulphatide
Mucolipidosis IV	Unknown, affects ganglioside sialidase	Gangliosides
Multiple sulphatase deficiency	Enzymic modifier system of conserved active-site cysteine residue in all sulphatases	All sulphatase substrates including dermatan; heparan; chondroitins; cerebroside sulphatide
Niemann-Pick disease	Acid sphingomyelinase	Sphingomyelin
Schindler disease	α-N-Acetylgalactosaminidase	α-GalNAc glycolipids, glycoproteins

Maryland, USA provide direct experimental support for this proposition. These workers investigated the storage of glycosaminoglycans in fibroblast cells grown in tissue culture systems – a system that has turned out to be unexpectedly informative for the investigation of lysosomal storage diseases.

☐ FUNCTIONAL COMPLEMENTATION OF LYSOSOMAL ENZYME DEFICIENCIES [7]

The original experiments used fibroblasts obtained from patients with genetically distinct but at the time enzymically uncharacterized mucopolysaccharidoses. The studies involved the addition of radioactive sulphate to the medium so that the synthesis and breakdown of intracellular glycosaminoglycans could be analysed after biosynthetic labelling. It was quickly shown that the rate of degradation, rather than the rates of secretion or synthesis of the radiolabelled glycosaminoglycans, was markedly reduced in these disorders. Indeed the turnover rates were prolonged at least tenfold. Comparable observations were made with fibroblasts cultured from patients suffering from other mucopolysaccharidoses. Particularly striking was the discovery that emerged from an experiment in which fibroblasts obtained from patients with the autosomal recessive disorder Hurler's disease (now known to be caused by deficiency of α-L-iduronidase) and the sex-linked recessive Hunter's disease (deficiency of iduronate sulphatase) were co-cultured. Co-culture prevented the progressive accumulation of glycosaminoglycans that occurred when the fibroblasts were grown separately (Fig. 2). Pulse-labelling studies of glycosaminoglycan synthesis showed that degradation of this substrate was restored to normal.

Further experiments demonstrated that each of the fibroblast cultures elaborated a specific 'corrective factor' that could be reciprocally taken up in co-culture experiments. Later studies demonstrated that these corrective factors proved to be particular high-molecular-weight forms of the enzymes that were lacking in the pathological fibroblasts [9]. The factors were secreted into medium conditioned also by the presence of normal fibroblasts. Selective uptake of this enzyme from the medium restored the normal pathway for degradation of glycosaminoglycans and was later shown to be mediated, at least in part, by a mannose-6-phosphate-containing carbohydrate component – the so-called lysosomal recognition marker. Extensive studies have now been carried out using cells deficient in particular lysosomal enzymes that can be supplied and taken up from the extracellular phase. Functional complementation has been demonstrated in metachromatic leucodystrophy, Wolman's disease, β-glucuronidase deficiency, Sandhoff's disease and fucosidosis. The particular corrective factors have, in each case, proved to be specific forms of the enzymes that are deficient in each disorder and immediately raised the possibility that agents for the functional complementation of lysosomal storage disorders can be supplied by normal cells or by administration of the individual corrective factors they elaborate.

☐ INCLUSION-CELL (I-CELL) DISEASE: A DISORDER OF LYSOSOMAL PROTEIN RECOGNITION [10]

Studies of I-cell disease, a very rare and distinctive storage disorder, recognized at about this time, proved to be crucial for understanding the intracellular sorting of

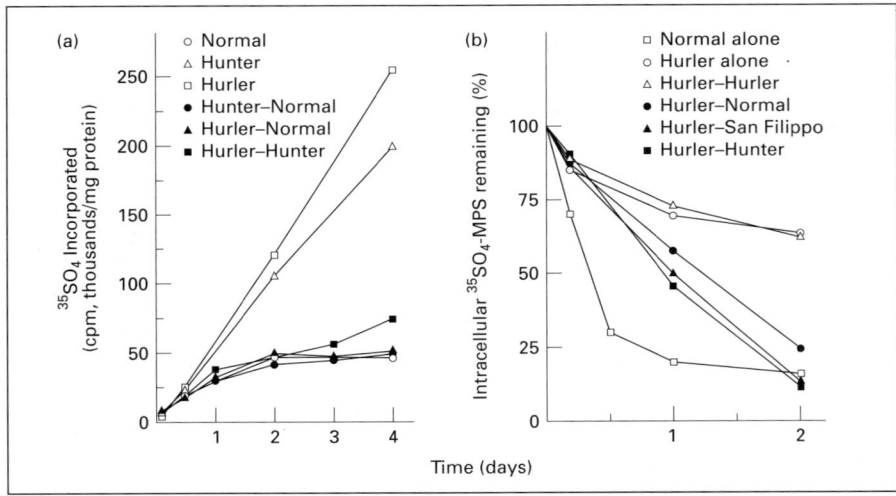

Fig. 2 Effect of mixing cells of various genotypes on accumulation (a) and chase (b) of labelled intracellular mucopolysaccharide. (a) Hurler, Hunter, or normal cells were trypsinized and replated singly or in combination at a density of about 2×10^6 cells per plate. After 2 days, 6 ml of medium containing $^{35}SO_4$ (9×10^6 counts/min per ml) was added. Ratio of cells in the mixed plates – Hurler: Hunter, 44:56; Hunter: normal, 43:57; Hurler: normal, 38:62. (b) Hurler and normal fibroblasts had been previously labelled for 3 days in medium containing $^{35}SO_4$ (8×10^6 counts/min per ml). After trypsinization they were plated in unlabelled medium; the Hurler fibroblasts were plated either alone or with an approximately equal number of unlabelled cells of the indicated genotype. Radioactive mucopolysaccharide was determined.

The original demonstration of the abnormal metabolism of biosynthetically labelled mucopolysaccharide (glycosaminoglycans) in fibroblasts cultured from patients with mucopolysaccharide storage disorders. The effects of mixing cells of distinct genotypes on the accumulation and metabolism of labelled material is shown and led Neufeld and her colleagues to demonstrate the synthesis of 'corrective factors' that correct the lysosomal storage defect and are released by human cells into culture media. (From Fratantoni et al. [8] with permission.)

nascent lysosomal enzymes and for functional complementation of lysosomal defects. Patients with I-cell disease show clinical features of both the mucopolysaccharidoses and the sphingolipidoses. Although the microscopic examination reveals characteristic membrane-limited inclusion bodies consisting of fibrogranular and lamellar material, in contrast to the mucopolysaccharidoses, the urinary secretion of glycosaminoglycans is normal. Cells cultured from patients with I-cell disease take up and retain secreted lysosomal enzymes. However, not only are the cells themselves deficient in many lysosomal enzyme activities, but the enzymes they release into culture cannot be taken up by normal fibroblasts.

It had been thought that lysosomal enzymes simply leaked through defects in the cellular membrane, but Neufeld postulated that a failure of essential modifications required for recognition by surface receptors that normally direct nascent acid hydrolases to their lysosomal destination accounted for the I-cell defect. Many years of work showed the nature of the recognition marker for lysosomal proteins to be a carbohydrate moiety. Chemical treatment under mild conditions to remove carbohydrates changed 'high-uptake' forms of lysosomal enzymes that were transported intracellularly to 'low-uptake' forms that entered by non-specific fluid-phase endocytosis. Measurements of the inhibition constants for uptake of several enzymes by normal fibroblasts using a range of simple sugars demonstrated that mannose and the phosphohexose moiety, mannose 6-phosphate, were the most potent inhibitors of receptor-mediated endocytosis of secreted lysosomal enzymes.

The use of radiophosphorus to label enzymes biosynthetically made it possible to confirm the existence of the phosphohexosyl moiety in nascent lysosomal enzymes. Phosphorylation of mannose residues took place post-translationally and was absent from fibroblasts obtained from patients with I-cell disease. Direct biochemical analysis of the phosphorylated oligosaccharide showed that it is linked covalently after translation of lysosomal polypeptides. This clarified the pathway for formation of this recognition marker and showed that sorting of intracellular lysosomal enzyme using this moiety is required for lysosomal translocation. In I-cell disease, a recessively transmitted phosphotransferase defect leads to failure of lysosomal targetting and the characteristic pattern of deficiency involving many lysosomal proteins [11]. These enzymes, however, are abundantly secreted into the plasma – thus explaining the absence of undegraded glycosaminoglycans in the urine.

☐ INTRACELLULAR SORTING OF LYSOSOMAL PROTEINS

The later identification of specific receptors for mannose 6-phosphate in the trans-Golgi network and intermediate endosomes completed the identification of the components responsible for intracellular sorting of lysosomal enzymes. Two mannose 6-phosphate receptors have been identified, of which the larger (about 205 kDa) is the calcium-independent form that is also the natural receptor for insulin-like growth factor. Insulin-like growth factor binds at a site independent of the mannose 6-phosphate domain. Nonetheless, this receptor appears to be the predominant one involved in the intracellular sorting pathway. Nascent lysosomal enzymes harbouring the mannose 6-phosphate moiety bind to the receptor on the endolysosomal component in the trans-Golgi network, allowing the nascent proteins to be segregated to the endolysosomal pathway. Mild acidification in the endosomal compartment facilitates dissociation of the processed lysosomal hydrolase from the mannose 6-phosphate receptor, thus promoting unidirectional delivery to these organelles. The membrane-bound receptor recycles to the trans-Golgi and a residual fraction of approximately 10% is expressed on the cell surface, where it participates in receptor-mediated endocytosis of secreted enzymes. This process provides the basis for cross-correction by transfer of lysosomal enzymes secreted by fibroblasts. Soluble lysosomal hydrolases appear to follow both intracellular pathways: most are delivered to the lysosomal counterpart by the intracellular route but a proportion appear to be secreted and recaptured by a mechanism involving cell-surface receptors that recognize glycoproteins harbouring the appropriate carbohydrate ligands.

It is now known that mannose 6-phosphate receptors on the cell surface do not serve as the only means by which functional restoration of lysosomal enzyme defects can be brought about. However, the identification of this mechanism provided direct evidence confirming de Duve's prediction that molecules could be delivered to a site of action in the lysosome by addition at the cell surface.

☐ GAUCHER'S DISEASE: A MODEL LYSOSOMAL DISORDER

Gaucher's disease, the most common lysosomal disorder, is an autosomal recessive condition in which defects of glucocerebrosidase (an acid β-glucosidase) lead to the accumulation of the glycosphingolipid glucosylceramide [12]. The disorder, one of the class of glycosphingolipidoses, was first identified in 1882 by the characteristic appearance of the abnormal histiocytes in the greatly enlarged spleen of a young woman.

The eponymous cells are abnormal histiocytes and it is indeed the cells of the mononuclear phagocytic series that are the pathological focus of Gaucher's disease. A defect in the final stages of the degradation of glycosphingolipids derived from effete blood cells is the primary source for the storage material and, as a consequence, the main sites affected in Gaucher's disease are the parenchymal organs, such as the liver, spleen and bone marrow, which are rich in mononuclear phagocytes. The macrophages become engorged with undegraded glycolipid giving rise to their pathognomic appearance (see Plate 1), which results from the aggregation of glucosylceramide in membranous arrays within the storage cells. The cells show signs of 'activation', and it is believed the release of cytokines and other proteins associated with such stimulation contributes to the increased metabolic rate and persistent inflammatory manifestations of the condition [13].

Chronic forms of Gaucher's disease are associated with marked hepatosplenomegaly (Fig. 3) and skeletal disease with osteopenia, avascular necrosis, focal osteolysis sometimes complicated by pathological fractures (Fig. 4). Acid β-glucosidase activity assayed in leucocytes or fibroblasts obtained from patients with Gaucher's disease is generally less than 10% of control values. Multiple mutations have been identified in the glucocerebrosidase gene on chromosome 1q that are responsible for the enzymic deficiency. Inactivating mutations tend to lead to a more serious phenotype, and occasionally the development of neuronopathic forms of the disease where storage of complex sphingolipids occurs in microglia and, occasionally, neurons.

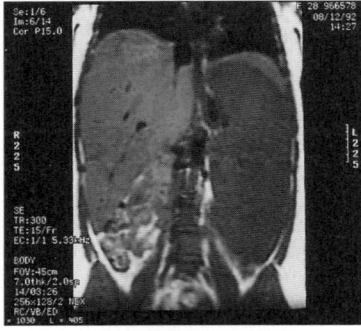

Fig. 3 Massive hepatosplenomegaly shown on an abdominal T1 weighted magnetic resonance imaging (MRI) scan. Because of severe pancytopenia, abdominal pain and pressure symptoms, splenectomy was carried out in this young woman who had succeeded in carrying two pregnancies to term. The spleen weighed almost 4 kg. Enzyme replacement therapy has subsequently led to improved wellbeing and a marked reduction in hepatic volume. (Courtesy of Dr David Lomas, Department of Radiology, Addenbrooke's Hospital, Cambridge.)

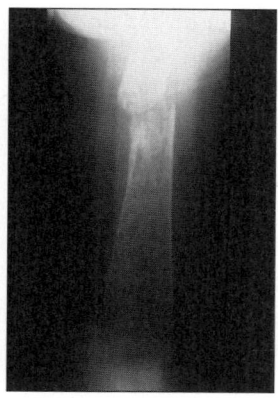

Fig. 4 X-ray of the left femur of a 30-year-old woman with adult Type I Gaucher's disease who had had a diagnostic splenectomy in childhood. A pathological fracture of the femoral shaft is shown following a minor injury: note the effects of defective bone modelling with absent tubulation leading to the characteristic conical (Erlenmeyer flask) deformity, patchy sclerosis with generalized osteopenia and foci of distinct osteolysis.

☐ DEFINITIVE TREATMENT FOR GAUCHER'S DISEASE

Marrow transplantation

Because macrophages are derived from granulocyte-monocyte progenitor cells in the bone marrow, it was likely that bone-marrow transplantation would replenish these cells and correct the defect [14]. Marrow transplantation has been successfully carried out in infants, children and young adults with Gaucher's disease who have received marrow from normal or heterozygous human leucocyte antigen (HLA)-matched sibling donors. Successful engraftment is associated with a clinical regression of the disease: there is catch-up growth in stunted children and ultimately a complete disappearance of the pathological storage cells in the tissues. Although only a minority of patients with Gaucher's disease are suitable candidates for bone-marrow transplantation, its success in eradicating the disease confirms that a complement of tissue macrophages derived from the bone marrow (with at least 50% of normal acid β-glucosidase activity) is sufficient to correct the manifestations of the non-neuronopathic forms of this condition.

Enzymic augmentation

Brady and his colleagues at the National Institutes of Health (NIH) attempted enzyme replacement therapy for glucocerebrosidase deficiency in Gaucher's disease in 1974. Glucocerebrosidase was purified by affinity chromatography from human placentae and was administered to two patients with advanced Gaucher's disease who were thereafter studied in detail. Intravenous infusions of the native protein were associated with the reduction in red cell-associated glucocerebroside in the few days following the infusion with suggestive evidence of a reduction in the amount of stored glucocerebroside in the liver as shown by repeated needle biopsy. However, this experiment and subsequent trials of native enzyme, enzyme trapped within red-cell ghosts or liposomes, failed to show convincing clinical improvement.

In view of the existence of the secretion-recapture mechanism for extracellular delivery of lysosomal enzymes and of contemporaneous studies on the uptake of glycoproteins by parenchymal and non-parenchymal hepatic cells carried out by Ashwell and his colleagues, also at the NIH, Barranger and his colleagues suggested that native human glucocerebrosidase purified from placentae may lack the critical recognition signals for uptake and delivery to the diseased macrophages of Gaucher's disease. Independent research had identified a mannose receptor on the surface of macrophages and it was shown that human alveolar macrophages would preferentially take up proteins with exposed mannose residues. Analysis of human glucocerebrosidase purified from the placenta revealed that it had a complex carbohydrate structure and only a small fraction contained exposed mannose residues. At the suggestion of Barranger, experiments to modify terminal carbohydrate residues by sequential enzymic glycosylation were undertaken. After treatment with neuraminidase, galactosidase and *N*-acetyl glucosaminidase, human placental glucocerebrosidase injected into living rats was preferentially taken up by non-parenchymal rather than parenchymal hepatic cells. These studies provided the experimental basis for further human trials of enzyme replacement therapy in Gaucher's disease.

The first recipient was a 4-year-old boy with severe hepatosplenomegaly, anaemia, thrombocytopenia and skeletal disease due to Gaucher's disease. Infusions given every 2 weeks intermittently over a period of 2 years corrected the anaemia, increased the platelet count and improved the mineralization and trabecular structure of the long bones. Since that time, he has continued to receive enzyme therapy with regression of visceral enlargement, normal somatic growth and restoration of well-being. The further remarkable commercial development of enzyme replacement therapy involved concerted activities of the medically qualified mother of this child and the North American Gaucher's Association together with the pharmaceutical and biochemical supply company Genzyme. With their support, a pivotal trial of enzyme replacement therapy using enzymically modified human placental glucocerebrosidase was undertaken in 12 patients with Type I Gaucher's disease. There was regression of symptoms and visceromegaly with accompanying improvement in blood counts [15]. Three of the original 11 patients with skeletal disease showed early restoration of bone integrity. The preparation secured approval as an orphan drug under the Food and Drug Administration (FDA) of the USA in 1990 and has subsequently been approved in the UK and Europe under the trade name Ceredase (alglucerase) (Fig. 5).

About 2000 patients with non-neuronopathic Gaucher's disease are currently receiving enzyme therapy worldwide. There is not space here to describe the many fascinating aspects of the development of alglucerase engineered for this rare disorder. However, the emergence of commercial agents for enzyme augmentation for Gaucher's disease sets an important precedent for the treatment of other 'orphan' diseases – and especially those associated with pathological lysosomal storage. At the time of writing, a recombinant preparation of human glucocerebrosidase (imiglucerase: Cerezyme), also modified by deglycosylation but purified from Chinese hamster ovary cells transduced with the human glucocerebrosidase gene, has recently received a licence under the orphan drug category from the FDA. In the

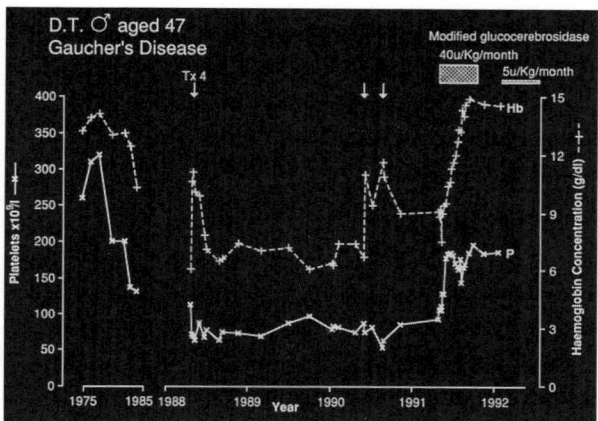

Fig. 5 Effects of enzyme replacement therapy in a man with Gaucher's disease suffering from bone marrow failure. The patient was diagnosed as having Gaucher's disease in adolescence when a splenectomy was carried out for splenic enlargement complicated by left hydronephrosis. Subsequently anaemia and thrombocytopenia developed with attendant bone pain. The patient was unable to work and became dependent on red-cell transfusion as indicated by arrows. Within 3 weeks of administration of twice weekly alglucerase at the indicated doses, the blood counts were restored to normal with an attendant alleviation in symptoms and restoration of magnetic resonance signals obtained from bones in the extremities. The patient now receives maintenance enzyme replacement therapy and continues in full-time work independent of hospital services. (From Mistry et al. [21], with permission.)

long term, this should obviate many of the intrinsic difficulties and theoretical risks associated with manufacture and administration of a product derived from pooled human tissue. There are far-reaching consequences for the costs of replacement therapy and questions have been asked as to whether or not mannose-terminated enzyme preparations are efficiently targetted to the cells and tissues of patients affected by Gaucher's disease.

Studies recently conducted at Addenbrooke's Hospital, Cambridge by my colleagues Pramood Mistry and Philip Wraight using a radiolabelled modified human placental and recombinant glucocerebrosidase to determine the distribution of the enzyme *in vivo* have ably confirmed targetting in Gaucher's disease [16]. The ligand is rapidly taken up by the affected parenchymal organs, including sites of skeletal disease where there is evidence of bone marrow localization (see Plate 2 a and b). The metabolism of the administered enzyme has been followed and a slow component accounting for most of the turnover within the tissues appears to have a half-life of between 36 and 42 h. In an experiment where Gaucher's cells were isolated from the spleen at the time of an elective splenectomy for pancytopenia in a Gaucher's patient, it was also possible to demonstrate restoration of normal macrophage acid β-glucosidase activity by prior infusion of a therapeutic dose of unlabelled enzyme.

These and related experiments using unlabelled enzyme to displace the trace-labelled protein from binding sites have confirmed selective targetting of mannose-terminated glucocerebrosidase to the cells and tissues affected by Gaucher's disease. They suggest that the frequent administration of subsaturating doses of the enzyme would in most circumstances optimally augment the enzymic deficiency that underlies this disorder; however, pharmacological dosing studies are needed to confirm this suggestion.

The success of enzyme augmentation in Gaucher's disease provides a powerful intellectual stimulus to develop comparable treatments for other lysosomal storage disorders. Clearly the identification of the appropriate ligands for delivery to the target cells, eg the endothelial cells in Fabry's disease due to deficient acid α-galactosidase A activity and to the skeletal and heart muscle in glycogenosis type II for uptake of acid α-glucosidase, is of critical importance. There can be little doubt that enzyme replacement therapy using appropriately modified lysosomal glycoproteins will soon be attempted in clinical trials. In the medium term, experimental models of lysosomal disorders in animals, eg the conehead mouse – a model of a mucopolysaccharidosis syndrome in man – due to β-glucuronidase deficiency will be used. In this model, correction of lysosomal storage in the liver and spleen following implantation of an artificial organ containing collagen-supported autologous fibroblasts that were transduced to express β-glucuronidase within the peritoneal cavity has recently been achieved.

☐ FUTURE PROSPECTS

Gene therapy

Gaucher's disease responds to transplantation of allogeneic bone marrow. The marrow provides a source of granulocyte-monocyte progenitor cells giving rise to a population of macrophages that can metabolize endogenous glucocerebroside. Thus the possibility of gene therapy directed towards the stem cells of the haematopoietic system is opened up [17]. Several trials have been approved in the USA for the genetic transduction of haematopoietic stem cells (marked by the CD34 surface antigen) therapeutically corrected by transfer of the active human glucocerebrosidase gene. This approach has already been successful in mice, where prolonged expression of human glucocerebrosidase at a high level has been achieved in the macrophages of recipients at primary and secondary marrow transplantation. Although at the time of writing trials are underway to transduce appropriate stem cells in human bone marrow from patients with Gaucher's disease (Table 3), it is not clear that the transfected cells would carry a sufficient selective advantage for survival in the presence of diseased bone marrow to provide long-term remission of glycolipid storage. Thus high-efficiency transfection of

Table 3 Development of gene therapy for Gaucher's disease.

1985	Cloning of glucocerebrosidase gene
1986	Transfer and expression in fibroblasts
1989	Transfer and expression in haematopoietic colony forming units (CFUs)
1990	Transfer to mouse haematopoietic stem cells
1992	Long-term expression in macrophages of irradiated mice after infusion of transduced stem cells
1993	Approval of first clinical trials (RAC)
1995–6	First human gene therapy recipients

the engrafted autologous cells would be needed to secure corrective expression with the wild-type glucocerebrosidase gene and myeloablative therapy or selective procedures may be required to secure their preferential survival.

Novel biochemical approaches to the therapy of sphingolipid disorders: substrate depletion

Recently, the concept of substrate depletion to prevent the accumulation of glycosphingolipids by inhibiting their biosynthesis has been developed by colleagues in Oxford, Drs Platt and Butters [18]. This proposal followed their discovery that the imino sugar derivatives *N*-butyldeoxynojirimycin (NB-DNJ) and *N*-butyldeoxygalactonojirimycin (NB-DGJ) selectively inhibit the glucosyl transfer step in the biosynthesis of glycosphingolipids without affecting glucocerebrosidase and other acid glucosidases. Studies in cultured cells with pathological storage of glycolipids in lysosomes demonstrated regression of the accumulated material after exposure to low concentrations of these natural product derivatives and comparably encouraging findings have been observed in genetically modified animals that represent experimental models of debilitating human glycosphingolipidoses, such as Tay-Sachs disease.

Although further studies in the differential effects of particular analogues of these imino sugars may indicate those with the greatest potential for selectivity towards the biosynthetic pathway for glycolipid formation rather than α-glucosidases involved in processing or intestinal digestion of oligosaccharides, both NB-DNJ and NB-DGJ have differential effects on these pathways that may be exploited. In fact, the NB-DNJ analogue, with potentially useful selectivity towards the glycosyl transferase enzyme involved in glycolipid biosynthesis, is already under clinical evaluation as an antiviral agent to inhibit the replication of human immunodeficiency virus in infected humans. The drug is relatively non-toxic in such subjects, who only experience mild gastrointestinal symptoms – probably related to intestinal α-glucosidase inhibition. The NB-DGJ analogue is more specific for the glycosphingolipid pathway but has yet to be tested in humans. Clearly *partial* inhibition of glycosphingolipid biosynthesis, with or without augmentation by exogenous enzyme, would shift the substrate/product equilibrium in favour of degradation and permit regression of the pathological storage of accumulated substrate in the lysosomes. Thus the introduction of these analogues with selectivity towards inhibition of glycolipid function, other than α-glucosidases, offers additional promise for intractable disorders of lysosomal glycosphingolipid storage either where enzyme therapy is unavailable or ineffective or where the clinical condition is beyond other means of correction. For many glycolipid disorders, the potential benefits of such therapy probably exceed the theoretical risks; at present few better options appear to be available for exploration by carefully conducted trials in selected patients who might otherwise be without hope.

☐ FUTURE CHALLENGES

Although individually uncommon, lysosomal storage disorders collectively represent a heavy burden to the patients, families and communities affected; this is reflected in their high costs for medical services. The diseases are usually incurable and often severely disabling. They appear to occur with an overall frequency of about 1 in 5–10 000 live births in the general population. Despite much experimental work, enzyme replacement therapy has so far only been successful in Gaucher's disease; early trials of enzyme augmentation in the mucopolysaccharidoses and Fabry's disease have hitherto given, at best, equivocal results. Because of earlier difficulties in supplying sufficient enzyme and in the appropriate glycoforms for therapeutic effects, with the advent of recombinant methods for expressing large amounts of glycoproteins secreted by eukaryotic cells, there are grounds for renewed optimism that this approach will alleviate other lysosomal diseases [19]. Those lysosomal disorders that are associated with neuronopathic features (Table 4), either due to

Table 4 Lysosomal storage disorders with neurological features.

Mucopolysaccharidoses
    eg Hunter, Hurler, Sanfilippo A–D, Morquio

Disorders of glycoprotein degradation
    eg mannosidosis, fucosidosis, sialidosis,
    aspartylglucosaminuria, Salla, Schindler's disease

Glycosphingolipidoses
    eg Farber, Niemann-Pick A, C, Tay-Sachs, Gaucher,
    Krabbe, metachromatic leucodystrophy, GM_1 gangliosidosis

Miscellaneous
    Deficiency of GM_2 activator
    Deficiency of saposins A, B or C
    I-cell disease

neuronal storage or to glial disease, often (with attendant demyelination and inflammatory effects throughout the nervous system) present particular challenges. Diseases such as Tay-Sachs disease, Sanfilippo's disease, Krabbe's globoid leucodystrophy, metachromatic leucodystrophy, G_{M1} gangliosidosis and fucosidosis are vivid examples of these potentially devastating disorders. The personal tragedy is often heightened by onset of ineluctable mental and neurological deterioration in late infancy and childhood. Preliminary evidence suggests that in metachromatic leucodystrophy identified in the presymptomatic period early marrow transplantation, which provides a source of lymphocytes and microglia with a complement of normal lysosomes, may arrest or prevent the development of brain disease. This opens up the future possibility of using substrate depletion and enzyme replacement directed to the nervous system, possibly combined with infusion of genetically transduced cells to correct the neuronopathic defect before nervous damage is established (Table 5). It must be admitted, however, that much

Table 5 Possible approaches to therapy of neuronopathic lysosomal diseases.

Cell complementation to supply enzymically competent microglia
  Validity established by effects of marrow transplantation in metachromatic leucodystrophy, Type III Gaucher's disease and Twitcher mouse.

Enzyme replacement
  Receptor-mediated endocytosis pathway of delivery based on success of mannose-terminated glucocerebrosidase in Type I and Type III systemic disease.
  Little evidence of neurological benefit; intrathecal route has potential.
  Other receptor systems can be explored for delivery (transferrin, tetanus toxin receptor)

Gene therapy
  Adenovirus or herpes simplex-based vectors for long-term expression in non-mitotic cells
  Could be used to transduce cultured glial cells (oligodendrocytes, microglia) before injection into brain to complement activity *and* induce repair.

Substrate deprivation
  Derivatives of deoxynorijimycin *selectively* inhibit terminal step of glucosylceramide biosynthesis and penetrate cerebrospinal fluid.
  This depends on the presence of residual enzyme activity; method could synergize with enzyme therapy.

---

experimental work is currently needed to establish the means of repairing the nervous system. Nonetheless, for genetic transduction of cells within the field of potential neural cell injury, the use of modified herpes simplex virus vectors is already yielding results of therapeutic promise. The recent modification of HSV I vectors that allow abundant and stable expression of genes in the nervous system of living mice by my colleagues Robin Lachmann and Stacey Efstathiou in Cambridge represents a significant advance in this direction [20].

☐ SUMMARY

After the recognition of lysosomes as a focus for genetically determined defects of the breakdown of endogenous macromolecules, developments in cell replacement, gene therapy, substrate deprivation and the delivery of exogenous proteins to correct the storage diseases have been initiated. On the basis of the secretion-recapture mechanism related to the intracellular pathway for the sorting of nascent lysosomal proteins, experimental correction of lysosomal defects has been established. In Gaucher's disease, the identification of a novel receptor system for the uptake of proteins by macrophages that are the focus for pathological storage has led to the development of a successful drug preparation. Although not based strictly on the normal secretion-recapture mechanism for lysosomal proteins, the use of mannose-terminated human glucocerebrosidase in Gaucher's disease has provided a decisive stimulus towards the design of specific treatment for other lysosomal storage disorders and for general commercial exploration of agents engineered to treat rare diseases. Given the striking progress that has been made in this apparently intractable area of medicine, one can only concur with Einstein's relativistic view of the future and marvel at Shaw's prescient dictum: 'There is at bottom only one genuinely scientific treatment for all diseases, and that is to stimulate the phagocytes' (*The Doctor's Dilemma*, 1911, Act I).

REFERENCES

1. de Duve C. Exploring cells with a centrifuge. *Science* 1975; **189**: 186–94.
2. Steinmann RM, Mellman I, Muller WA, Cohn ZA. Endocytosis and the recycling of plasma membrane. *J Cell Biol* 1983; **96**: 1–27.
3. Alberts B, Bray D, Lewis J, Raff M, Roberts K, Watson JD (eds). Intracellular sorting and the maintenance of cellular compartments. In: *Molecular Biology of the Cell*, 2nd edn. New York: Garland Publishing, 1989: 461.
4. Neufeld EF, Lim TW, Shapiro LJ. Inherited disorders of lysosomal metabolism. *Ann Rev Biochem* 1975; **44**: 357–76.
5. Conzelmann E, Sandhoff K. Partial enzyme deficiencies: residual activities and the development of neurologic disorders. *Dev Neurosci* 1983–84; **6**: 58–71.
6. de Duve C. From cytoses to lysosomes. *Fed Proc Fed Am Soc Exp Med* 1964; **23**: 1045–9.
7. Cantz M. Corrective factors for inborn errors of mucopolysaccharide metabolism. *Methods Enzymol* 1972; **28**: 884–97.
8. Fratantoni JC, Hall CW, Neufeld EF. Hunter and Hurler syndromes: mutual correction of the defect in cultured fibroblasts. *Science* 1968; **162**: 571.
9. Cox TM. Therapeutic advances in Gaucher's disease: a model for the treatment of lysosomal storage diseases. *Trends Exp Clin Med* 1994; **4**: 144–57.
10. Nolan CM, Sly WS. I-cell disease and pseudo-Hurler polydystrophy: disorders of lysosomal enzyme phosphorylation and localization. In: Scriver CS, Beaudet AL, Sly WS, Valle DA (eds). *The Metabolic Basis of Inherited Disease*. New York: McGraw-Hill, 1989: 1677–98.
11. Kornfeld S. Trafficking of lysosomal enzymes in normal and disease states. *J Clin Invest* 1986; **77**: 1–6.
12. Mistry PK, Cox TM. The glucocerebrosidase locus in Gaucher's disease: molecular analysis of a lysosomal enzyme. *J Med Genet* 1993; **30**: 889–94.
13. Allen MJ, Myer BJ, Khoker AM, Rushton N, Cox TM. Pro-inflammatory cytokines and the pathogenesis of Gaucher's disease: increased release of IL-6 and IL-10. *Quart J Med* 1997; **90**: 19–25.
14. Hoogerbrugge PM, Brouwer OF, Bordigoni P, *et al*. Allogenic bone marrow transplantation for lysosomal storage diseases. *Lancet* 1995; **345**: 1398–402.
15. Barton NW, Brady RO, Dambrosia JM, *et al*. Replacement therapy for inherited enzyme deficiency – macrophage-targeted glucocerebrosidase for Gaucher disease. *New Engl J Med* 1991; **324**: 1464–70.
16. Mistry PK, Wraight EP, Cox TM. Delivery of proteins to macrophages: implications for treatment of Gaucher's disease. *Lancet* 1996; **348**: 1555–9.
17. Correll PH, Karlsson S. Towards therapy of Gaucher's disease by gene transfer into haematopoietic cells. *Eur J Haematol* 1994; **53**: 253–64.
18. Platt FM, Neises GR, Reinkensmeier G, *et al*. Prevention of lysosomal storage in Tay-Sachs mice treated with N-Butyldeoxynojirimycin. *Science* 1997; **276**: 428–31.
19. Neufeld EF. Lysosomal storage diseases. *Ann Rev Biochem* 1991; **60**: 257–80.
20. Lachmann RH, Efstathiou S. Utilization of the herpes simplex virus I latency-associated regulatory region to drive stable reporter gene expression in the nervous system. *J Virol* 1997; **71**: 3197–207.
21. Mistry PK, Davies S, Corfield A, Dixon AK, Cox TM. Successful treatment of bone marrow failure in Gaucher's disease with low-dose modified glucocerebrosidase. *Quart J Med* 1992; **303**: 541–6.

☐ MULTIPLE CHOICE QUESTIONS

1. Lysosomes:
   (a) Contain oxidative enzymes for cell respiration
   (b) Are restricted to red blood cells and their precursors
   (c) Are soluble, bactericidal enzymes found in tears and other external secretions
   (d) Contain acid hydrolases that digest intracellular macromolecules

2. Lysosomal storage diseases:
   (a) Are inherited as X-linked dominant traits
   (b) Usually become apparent in early middle life
   (c) Are common in populations where nutritional deficiencies have historically been frequent
   (d) Are caused by inherited defects of acid hydrolases normally present in most cells of the body
   (e) May affect the brain

3. Gaucher's disease:
   (a) Is an inherited disorder affecting the mononuclear phagocytes
   (b) Is associated with hepatosplenomegaly
   (c) Is a severe lysosomal storage disorder for which no treatment is available
   (d) Is associated with fatty deposits in the spleen which respond to a modified fat and reduced calorie diet
   (e) Is associated with avascular necrosis of bone

4. Lysosomes:
   (a) Are implicated in Zellweger's disease
   (b) Are responsible for acidification of the gastric secretions
   (c) Participate in phagocytosis and killing of ingested microbes
   (d) Cannot be seen in fixed sections of tissues when examined under the electron microscope
   (e) Were discovered by biochemical exploration of fractionated cell contents

5. (a) Fabry's disease is caused by a lysosomal defect manifest predominantly in the endothelial cell
   (b) Fabry's disease is cured by enzyme-replacement therapy
   (c) Gaucher's disease responds to allogeneic bone marrow transplantation.
   (d) Niemann-Pick disease (acid sphingomyelinase deficiency) is characteristically responsible for a frontal lobe syndrome with selective neuronal atrophy in this region of the brain
   (e) Pompe's disease (glycogenosis type II) is characteristically associated with severe hypoglycaemia and hepatic disease

ANSWERS

1a False	2a False	3a True	4a False	5a True
b False	b False	b True	b False	b False
c False	c False	c False	c True	c True
d True	d True	d False	d False	d False
	e True	e True	e True	e False

The Croonian Lecture
Pathophysiology and treatment of malignant tertian malaria

D A Warrell

□ INTRODUCTION

Plasmodium falciparum infection ('malignant tertian malaria') is responsible for enormous human misery and mortality. This has always been a disease of warm climates, and may seem a very distant threat to people living in Britain. However, those contemplating a tropical holiday, for example to popular locations such as coastal Kenya or the Gambia, should be aware of the risk of contracting this potentially fatal infection (Fig. 1).

□ MALIGNANT MALARIA IN ENGLAND

At the time of Dr William Croone, FRS (1633–1684), by whose design these lectures at the Royal College of Physicians were endowed, another type of malaria was rife in England. Judging from the numbers of deaths attributed to this 'marsh fever' or 'marsh ague', it fully deserved to be called 'malignant'. Dobson [1,2] has assessed the death rates and health reputation of more than 600 parishes in Essex, Kent and

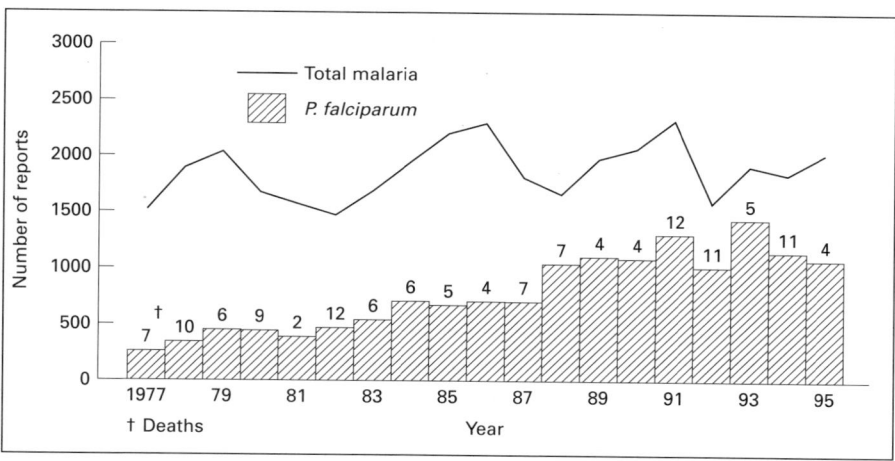

Fig. 1 Reported cases of malaria imported into Britain. Hatched columns represent the proportion of *Plasmodium falciparum* infections. The numbers above each column are the malaria fatalities each year. (Data by courtesy of the PHLS Malaria Reference Laboratory, London School of Hygiene & Tropical Medicine.)

Sussex from 1600 to 1800, comparing those in estuarine or marshland areas with those in the uplands. In about the 1670s, average crude death rates and infant mortality rates (per 1000) were more than 60 and more than 300 respectively in Romney Marsh compared to 20–30 and less than 200 in upland parishes [1]. As late as the early 19th century, life expectancy in north Kent marshes was only 33 years compared to more than 58 years in upland areas. There is persuasive historical evidence that malaria was a major component of the 'marsh fevers' or 'marsh agues' responsible for much of this excess mortality. Clinical descriptions of periodic (tertian and quartan) fever paroxysms, relapses of symptoms several months after the primary attack, progressive anaemia, jaundice and splenomegaly ('ague cake') suggest this diagnosis. Even more convincing was the efficacy of cinchona bark (quinine) although this treatment, as would be expected with *Plasmodium vivax* malaria, did not prevent relapses. These arise from the persistence of latent forms of *P. vivax* (hypnozoites) in the liver. There is convincing epidemiological evidence that many of the marsh fevers were vivax malaria. Their geographical distribution coincided with the habitat of *Anopheles atroparvus* mosquitoes (Fig. 2), the only

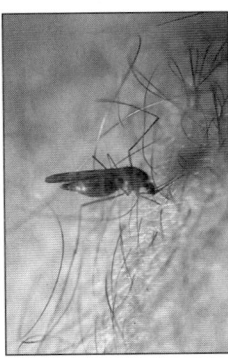

Fig. 2 The major English mosquito vector for *Plasmodium vivax* malaria, *Anopheles atroparvus*. (By courtesy of Professor Chris Curtis, London School of Hygiene & Tropical Medicine.)

potentially effective malaria vector occurring in Britain. The observations that these fevers were non-contagious and seasonal in their incidence and that children and newcomers to the area ('non-immunes') were the most vulnerable also fit well with the epidemiology of malaria [1]. Fortunately, the incidence and severity of marsh fever declined during the 19th century but there were still occasional cases up to 1910, when the diagnosis of *P. vivax* malaria was confirmed parasitologically [3]. Indigenous *A. atroparvus* mosquitoes proved their ability to transmit *P. vivax* during the First World War, when there was an epidemic of more than 500 cases of malaria in the north Kent marshes, introduced by soldiers who had been infected in Greece, Mesopotamia, India and elsewhere [4].

If the marsh fevers of 17th to 19th century England really were caused by *P. vivax*, the apparently high mortality is surprising. Infections by tropical strains of this parasite during the 20th century have proved benign; the rare fatalities result from spontaneous or traumatic rupture of the spleen, severe anaemia, possibly thrombocytopenia and concomitant debilitating illnesses [5]. For example, at the peak of a massive epidemic of *P. vivax* malaria in Sri Lanka in 1969, there were 537 705 cases without a single death [6]. It is possible that the marshlands populations of 17th and 18th century Britain were particularly susceptible to severe or fatal vivax malaria through other acute and chronic infections such as tuberculosis, typhoid, typhus and louse-borne relapsing fever, malnutrition, progressive anaemia and even through the excessive administration of opium to young children [1]. If *P. vivax* had been introduced to Britain relatively recently, there would have been insufficient time for the selection of resistance genes in the population. Erythrocytes of the Duffy negative (a–, b–) blood group (genotype Fy-Fy) resist invasion by *P. vivax*. [7]. This blood group reaches a prevalence of more than 90% in West African countries, where malaria has probably occurred for thousands of years, but does not occur in the indigenous races of northern Europe.

☐ MALIGNANT TERTIAN MALARIA IN THE TROPICS

Plasmodium falciparum, the cause of malignant tertian malaria, causes more deaths than any other single pathogen, except perhaps *Mycobacterium tuberculosis*. More than 40% of the world's population in more than 100 countries is exposed to this infection and there are thought to be more than 250 million symptomatic infections each year with an annual global mortality exceeding 1–2 million [8]. After the failure of the World Health Organization's global malaria eradication campaign (1955–69), which relied on extensive spraying with DDT (chlorophenathone, dicophone) and chloroquine chemoprophylaxis, there has been a re-emphasis on malaria control and improving the treatment of affected patients.

Cerebral malaria: dexamethasone and the 'permeability hypothesis'

Over the past 17 years, work based in the Nuffield Department of Clinical Medicine, University of Oxford, has focused on cerebral malaria, the most familiar clinical manifestation of severe *P. falciparum* infection. In 1979, when the Wellcome– Mahidol University, Oxford Tropical Medicine Research Programme, started up in Thailand, the most challenging aspect of cerebral malaria was a reported case fatality of 0–47% in adult patients [9]. Improving this appalling high mortality surely depended on gaining a better understanding of the underlying mechanism of the condition [10]. At that time, Maegraith's 'permeability hypothesis' was widely accepted as an explanation for the mechanism of cerebral malaria. Results of studies in rhesus monkeys terminally infected with *P. knowlesi* had suggested that a toxic factor released by the parasites increased permeability of the blood-brain barrier resulting in cerebral oedema, coma and death [11]. This concept had encouraged the widespread use of dexamethasone as an ancillary treatment for cerebral malaria, but there had been no clinical trials. A randomized double-blind placebo-controlled trial of dexamethasone in adults with cerebral malaria [12] provided the opportunity to assess the efficacy and safety of this popular treatment and, at the same time, to test the permeability hypothesis, since dexamethasone is the most potent known anti-inflammatory agent acting at the blood-brain and blood-cerebrospinal fluid barriers.

The lack of a generally accepted case definition of cerebral malaria explained the wide variation in reported case fatalities. In Thailand, a pragmatic definition was developed, based on the Glasgow coma scale (Table 1). Pra Pokklao Provincial Hospital in Chantaburi, in eastern Thailand near the Cambodian border, proved to be an excellent site for the study. Immigrants from non-malarious areas of Thailand were attracted by the prospect of gem mining in the jungles of this border region. They commonly contracted severe malaria within a few months of their arrival. Within the space of several months, 100 adult patients conforming to the new definition of cerebral malaria had been recruited to the study. All were started on the standard regimen of quinine by intravenous (i.v.) infusion and were randomized to treatment with dexamethasone (total dose 2 mg/kg over 48 h) or placebo. There was no difference in mortality between the two groups but in the dexamethasone-treated patients coma was prolonged and there was an excess of serious gastrointestinal bleeding and secondary infections (Table 2) [12]. These results were generally confirmed by a second study carried out by Hoffman and his colleagues at Jayapura in Irian Jaya (Table 2) in which a more than five times larger dose of dexamethasone (11.4 mg/kg over 48 h) was given [13]. These data have led to the abandonment of dexamethasone as an ancillary treatment in cerebral malaria. The Chantaburi study yielded other useful observations. The clinical features of cerebral malaria in presumed non-immune Thai adults were documented (Table 3). A number of important clinical phenomena were 'rediscovered' and were later studied in greater detail: hypoglycaemia resulting from quinine-induced hyperinsulinaemia [14],

Table 1 Cerebral malaria in adult patients: case definition [12].

1	Unrousable coma (no localizing response to pain)* persisting for more than 6 h if the patient had experienced a generalized convulsion
2	Asexual forms of *P. falciparum* found in the blood
3	Exclusion of other causes of encephalopathy (eg viral/bacterial/fungal encephalitis)
4	Characteristic cerebral histopathological appearances in fatal cases

*Glasgow coma scale: eye movements <3; best motor response <5; best verbal response <3

Table 2 Dexamethasone in cerebral malaria: randomized, controlled trials.

	Thailand [12]		Irian Jaya [13]	
	Dexamethasone	Placebo	Dexamethasone	Placebo
Patients: dexamethasone or placebo	50	50	19	19
Dose of dexamethasone (mg/kg/48 h)	2	–	11.4	–
Deaths (%)	16	18	21	21
Duration of coma (h; mean ± 1SD)	63±12	47±7	83±49	80±59
Gastrointestinal bleed (%)	8	0	15	0
Infections (%)	38	20	16	?37

Table 3 Cerebral malaria: clinical features in Thai adults. (From Warrell [10] and Warrell et al. [12].)

Coma
Convulsions
Symmetrical upper motor neurone lesion
Abnormal postural responses: extensor/flexor posturing
Dysconjugate gaze
Retinal haemorrhages

retinal haemorrhages [15], hepatic dysfunction [16], malarial anaemia [17] and the dangers of malaria in the last trimester of pregnancy [18]. It is clear from more recent work in the Gambia (by Greenwood, Kwiatkowski and their colleagues), Malawi (by Molyneux, Taylor and their colleagues) and Kenya (by Marsh, Newton and their colleagues) that cerebral malaria in African children is, in many respects, a different disease.

The prolongation of coma by dexamethasone argued against the idea that an inflammatory process and increased cerebral vascular permeability were important pathophysiological processes in cerebral malaria. Other evidence leading to the rejection of the permeability hypothesis was the observation that CSF opening pressures at lumbar puncture were usually normal in adult patients [19], that blood-CSF barrier permeability was unchanged in convalescence as compared to coma [19] and that cerebral oedema was uncommon in cerebral malaria and was usually an agonal phenomenon when assessed during life by computerized tomography (CT) [20] or nuclear magnetic resonance (NMR) scans [21]. An alternative explanation for cerebral malaria, the 'mechanical hypothesis', seemed more attractive.

The mechanical hypothesis

Marchiafava and Bignami had studied patients dying of malignant summer–autumn malarial fevers contracted in the Pontine marshes near Rome towards the end of the 19th century [22]: 'The cerebral capillaries are entirely filled with red blood corpuscles, each one of which contains a parasite with pigment at the centre' (see Plate 3). A century later, Miller and his colleagues observed similar appearances in the small cardiac blood vessels of Aotus monkeys experimentally infected with *P. falciparum* [24,25]. Parasitized erythrocytes appeared to stick to vascular endothelium via electron-dense protuberances (knobs) on their surface. Unfortunately, there was no satisfactory animal model of human cerebral malaria which reproduced both the characteristic clinical features and histopathological appearances [26,27]. However, several of the implications of the mechanical hypothesis could be tested in human patients with cerebral malaria in Thailand (Table 4). An ultrastructural study of postmortem needle necropsy samples of brain showed sequestration of parasitized erythrocytes in the brains of patients dying of cerebral malaria, but not in those dying of non-cerebral malaria. Packing of parasitized erythrocytes was tighter in the brain than in other organs [28]. With the

Table 4 Mechanical hypothesis: implications.

1 Concentration of parasitized erythrocytes in cerebral microvasculature
2 Decreased global cerebral blood flow
3 Cerebral hypoxia with increased lactate production
4 Clinical improvement after reversing cytoadherence/rosetting

help of the late Dr Norman Veall, the Kety–Schmidt method was modified for the measurement of total cerebral blood flow in patients with cerebral malaria in Chantaburi [29]. Cerebral blood flow was low in relation to arterial oxygen content, its principal physiological determinant, but this may have been the result of low arterial pCO_2 [30]. Cerebral oxygen consumption was low during coma and immediately after recovery of consciousness, and cerebral lactate production decreased significantly with recovery from coma suggesting that the unconscious state in cerebral malaria was associated with a switch to cerebral anaerobic glycolysis [29,31].

The molecular basis of cytoadherence

Subsequent laboratory studies have elucidated the molecular basis for cytoadherence, the process that leads to sequestration of erythrocytes containing mature forms of *P. falciparum* in cerebral venules and the microcirculation of other vital organs and tissues [32]. A number of candidate receptors have been identified in human vascular endothelium (Table 5). Some, such as CD36 and thrombospondin, are constitutive (always expressed) in a wide range of vascular beds and bind *in vitro* to all 'wild' isolates of *P. falciparum*. Their expression is not related, qualitatively or quantitatively, to disease severity. Other receptors such as ICAM-1 and E-selectin, are inducible (show increased expression or are only expressed) in the cerebral vessels of patients with cerebral malaria, suggesting that they may have a role in cytoadherence in this disease [33,34]. This induction is mediated by tumour necrosis factor-alpha (TNFα) and other inflammatory mediators [33]. Recently, there has been progress in defining the ligands on the surface of the parasitized erythrocyte that bind to these receptors (Table 6). PfEMP-1 are large (200–350 kDa) proteins concentrated in the electron-dense knobs under the surface of parasitized erythrocytes. During the search for drug-resistant genes in *P. falciparum*, a family of

Table 5 Cytoadherence: candidate endothelial receptors.

Thrombospondin	Adhesive glycoprotein
CD36	Leucocyte differentiation antigen, platelet glycoprotein IV (binds to OKM5)
ICAM-1	Cell adhesion (binds to LFA-1)
VCAM-1	Cell adhesion (binds to VLA-4)
E-selectin	Leucocyte-endothelial adhesion
Chondroitin sulphate A	Glycosaminoglycan

Table 6 Cytoadherence: candidate ligands on the surface of parasitized erythrocytes.

PfEMP-1	(binds to CD36, ICAM-1 ?thrombospondin)
Erythrocyte band 3 anion transporter	(binds to CD36 ? thrombospondin)
Sequestrin	(binds to CD36)

perhaps 150 highly variable ('var') genes were discovered, which constitute about 6% of the whole *P. falciparum* genome. They encode PfEMP-1. Several have now been sequenced, cloned and partially expressed [35–37]. PfEMP-1 binds to CD36, ICAM-1 and possibly thrombospondin. The other two candidate ligands, sequestrin [38] and the erythrocyte band 3 anion transporter [39], also appear to bind to CD36 and/or thrombospondin. Another phenomenon which may contribute to mechanical obstruction is rosetting, the adherence of non-parasitized to parasitized erythrocytes [40]. This phenomenon, so far observed only *in vitro*, is exhibited by parasite strains responsible for severe disease [41].

The toxin/cytokine hypothesis

Over the past 15 years, there has been renewed interest in a malarial toxin. In 1911 Sir Ronald Ross had suggested that a 'toxin' might be released at schizont rupture [42]. This 'toxin', which may be an inositol-free proteolipid (Kwiatkowski D, personal communication), or a complex of malarial surface proteins (MSP-1 and MSP-2) with the erythrocyte membrane's glycosylphosphatidyl-inositol anchor [43], is thought to induce the characteristic fever paroxysms of malaria by stimulating the release of the cytokine TNFα from macrophages. Clark [44] first suggested a role for cytokines in the pathophysiology of malaria and there is now convincing evidence associating high circulating levels of TNFα and other cytokines with the severity, case fatality and incidence of neurological sequelae in African children with cerebral malaria [45,46]. Treatment with an anti-TNF monoclonal antibody produced a dose-related reduction in fever in children with cerebral malaria [47] and a randomized double-blind placebo-controlled trial has been completed in the Gambia (Kwiatkowski D, personal communication). The most convincing evidence of a causative link between TNFα production and cerebral malaria has been provided by genetic studies in the Gambia [48]. Children homozygous for the TNF2 allele in the TNFα promoter region of human chromosome 6 showed a 4.0-fold increased risk of cerebral malaria and a 7.7 increased risk of death or sequelae from cerebral malaria. The TNFα promoter gene joins a growing group of genes responsible for resistance/susceptibility to malaria infection (Table 7). It now seems likely that cytokines and cytoadherence are integrated mechanisms in the pathogenesis of cerebral malaria (Fig. 3). These advances in the understanding of the fundamental mechanisms of pathogenicity in malaria are fascinating in themselves, but also offer the future prospect of new treatments such as synthetic soluble receptor peptides or antibodies that might competitively inhibit cytoadherence, anti-rosetting antibodies, a malarial antitoxin, and malarial vaccines aimed at preventing pathogenic processes rather than infection itself.

Table 7 Malaria resistance genes.

α, β-Globin	Major histocompatibility complex class I & II
Glucose-6-phosphate dehydrogenase	Spectrin
Blood group O	Glycophorin A & B
Erythrocyte band 3	Chemokine receptor (Duffy)
TNFα promoter	

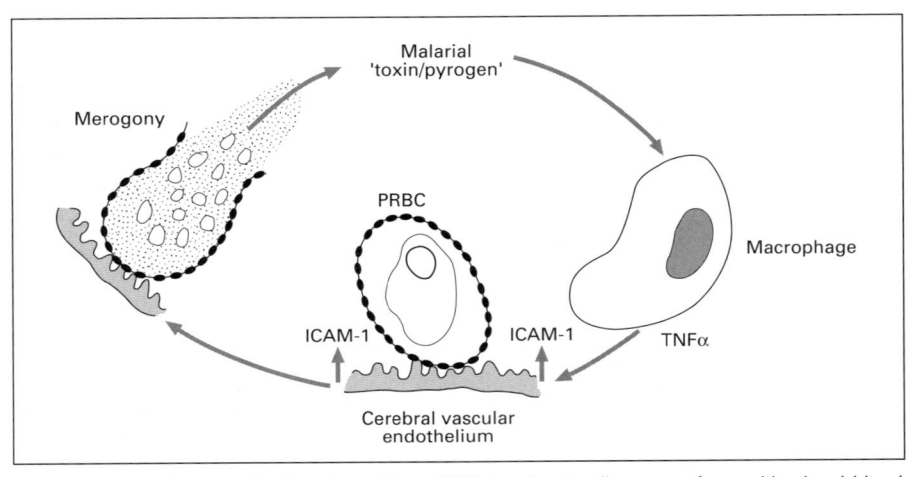

Fig. 3 Possible integrated roles of cytokines (TNFα) and cytoadherence of parasitized red blood corpuscles (PRBC) in the pathogenesis of cerebral malaria.

Chemotherapy of severe falciparum malaria

The chemotherapy of severe falciparum malaria has been greatly complicated over the past 30 years by the emergence of strains of *P. falciparum* resistance to pyrimethamine, chloroquine and other antimalarial drugs [49]. Chloroquine is still the most widely used antimalarial drug, but for the treatment of severe falciparum malaria it has now been largely replaced by quinine. The results of clinical studies by White and his colleagues have led to the development of optimal dosage regimens of quinine and its diastereomer, quinidine, for adults, pregnant women and children [50]. Intravenous treatment must be initiated with a loading dose [50] and patients must be monitored for hypoglycaemia, the most important side effect of the cinchona alkaloids [14]. Unfortunately, there is now evidence of increasing resistance to quinine treatment, especially in Thailand and Vietnam, and increases in dosage have resulted in greater toxicity, especially hypoglycaemia and, in convalescent patients, difficulties with compliance. The group of drugs that are already replacing quinine in some areas are the artemisinin derivatives ('qinghaosu') from the herb *Artemisia annua* which have been traditional treatments for fever in China for more than a thousand years [51]. Results of studies in China, south-east Asia and elsewhere have proclaimed the efficacy and safety of these compounds

[51,52], but there have been worrying reports of fatal neurotoxicity in several species of laboratory animals [53]. Artemisinin derivatives clear *P. falciparum* parasitaemia twice as fast as quinine (Fig. 4) but reduction in mortality and the incidence of neurological sequelae has yet to be demonstrated. Licensing, marketing and use of these drugs in western countries will have to await the results of two large studies that have now been completed: a comparison of artemether and i.v. quinine in children with severe falciparum malaria in Kenya, Malawi, the Gambia and Nigeria and a comparison of artemether and intramuscular quinine in 560 Vietnamese adults with severe falciparum malaria at Cho Quan Hospital, Ho Chi Minh City. Artemisinin derivatives are needed with particular urgency in areas of emerging quinine resistance; for the treatment of pregnant women, in whom the risk of quinine-induced hypoglycaemia is particularly high, and for the treatment of patients with malarial haemoglobinuria attributed to quinine treatment. New compounds containing the active endoperoxide group of artemisinin are now being synthesized [54]. It is to be hoped that improved understanding of pathophysiological mechanisms and the introduction of the new class of antimalarial endoperoxides may at last reduce the high mortality of cerebral malaria (Table 8).

☐ THE DEATH OF DR WILLIAM CROONE, FRS

Dr William Croone died of a fever in London on 12 October 1684 at the early age of 51. It would be very convenient to be able to attribute his death to 'marsh fever' (virulent *P. vivax* malaria) [1,2] which he might have acquired in the 'damp and stinking fens' around Cambridge where he received his Doctorate of Medicine in

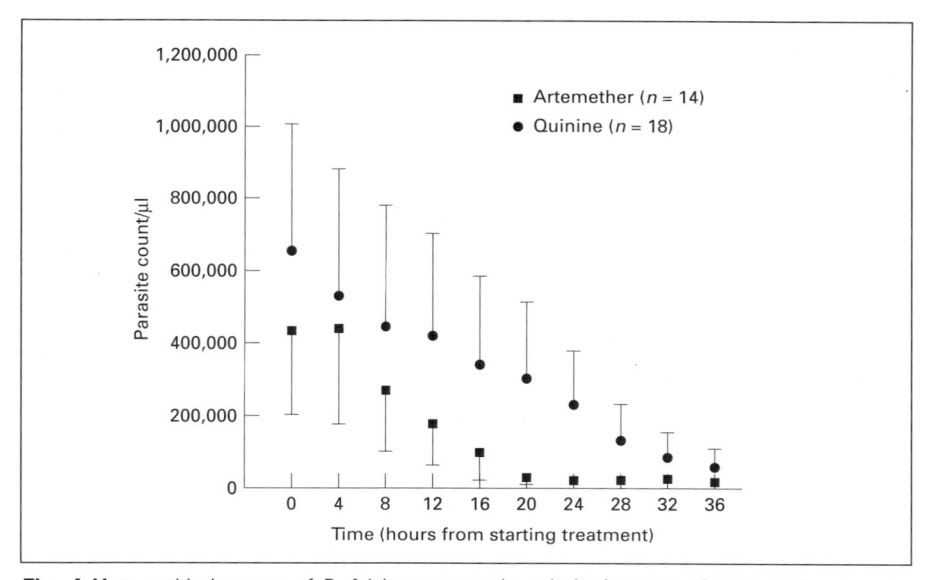

Fig. 4 More rapid clearance of *P. falciparum* parasitaemia by intramuscular artemether than by intravenous quinine in Melanesian adults in Port Moresby, Papua New Guinea. (Unpublished data by courtesy of Seaton RA, Trevett AJ, Lalloo DG, *et al.*) (Geometric mean parasitaemias ± 2 SEM).

Table 8 Case fatality of strictly defined cerebral malaria.

Patients			Fatality		Reference
			n	%	
Children					
Africa		Malawi	131	15.0	Molyneux et al. 1989 [55]
		Gambia	77	24.7	Waller et al. 1995 [56]
		Kenya	185	16.8	Marsh et al. 1995 [57]
		Burkina Faso	368	20.7	Modiano et al. 1995 [58]
Papua New Guinea			68	8.8	Allen SJ et al. 1996 (personal communication)
Adults					
Thailand			100	17.0	Warrell et al. 1982 [12]
Vietnam			280	15.8	Hien TT et al. 1996 (personal communication)
Papua New Guinea			12	41.7	Lalloo et al. 1996 [59]

1663 [60,61]. However, this is probably unlikely. The unhealthy reputation of such lowland and marshy areas would have been well known to someone of Croone's education and he would not willingly have lingered there. In any case, Thomas Sydenham wrote in 1666 that the Jesuit's powder or Peruvian bark (quinine) 'has been famous in London for over five and twenty years' [62]. Had Dr Croone developed symptoms of malaria he would have been treated with quinine, unless his physician, like the occasional doctor in London even today, failed to include malaria in the differential diagnosis of an acute fever in a patient who could have been exposed to that infection.

ACKNOWLEDGEMENTS

This review has drawn on the work of many friends and colleagues in Oxford, Thailand and elsewhere. For their help in the early years of the Wellcome–Mahidol University, Oxford Tropical Medicine Research Programme, I am particularly grateful to Sornchai Looareesuwan, Mary Warrell, Tranakchit Harinasuta, Danai Bunnag, Nick White and Rodney Phillips. Mary Dobson, Dominic Kwiatkowski, Chris Newbold, Anthony Berendt and Gareth Turner have contributed useful discussion of their recent work. I am grateful to David Lalloo, Andrew Trevett, Andrew Seaton and Steve Allen for access to their unpublished data from Papua New Guinea and to Miss Eunice Berry for outstanding administrative and secretarial support. The clinical studies were supported by the Wellcome Trust and the WHO/Rockefeller Foundation Great Neglected Diseases Programme.

REFERENCES

1. Dobson MJ. Malaria in England: a geographical and historical perspective. *Parassitologia* 1993; **36**: 35–60.
2. Dobson MJ. *Contours of Death and Disease in Early Modern England*. Cambridge: Cambridge University Press, 1996.
3. MacArthur W. A brief story of English malaria. *Brit Med Bull* 1951; **8**: 76–9.
4. Bruce-Chwatt LJ, de Zulueta J. *The Rise and Fall of Malaria in Europe: a Historico-Epidemiological Study*. Oxford: Oxford University Press, 1980.
5. Warrell DA, Molyneux ME, Beales PF (eds). Severe and complicated malaria. Second Edition. World Health Organization Malaria Action Programme. *Trans Roy Soc Trop Med Hyg* 1990; **84**: (Suppl) 1–65.
6. Wickramasinghe MB. Malaria and its control in Sri Lanka. *Ceylon Med J* 1981; **26**: 107–15.
7. Miller LH, Mason SJ, Clyde DF, McGinniss MH. The resistance factor to *Plasmodium vivax* in black: the Duffy blood group genotype, Fy-Fy. *New Engl J Med* 1976; **295**: 302–4.
8. World Health Organization. *Practical Chemotherapy of Malaria*. Technical Report Series 805. Geneva: WHO, 1990.
9. Daroff RB, Deller JJ, Kastl AJ, Blocker WW. Cerebral malaria. *J Am Med Assoc* 1967; **202**: 119–22; 679–82.
10. Warrell DA. The impact of clinical investigation on two third world diseases: cerebral malaria and louse-borne relapsing fever. In: Saunders KB (ed). *Advanced Medicine 19*. London: Pitman, 1983: 99–111.
11. Maegraith B, Fletcher A. The pathogenesis of mammalian malaria. *Adv Parasitol* 1972; **10**: 49–75.
12. Warrell DA, Looareesuwan S, Warrell MJ, *et al*. Dexamethasone proves deleterious in cerebral malaria: a double-blind trial in 100 comatose patients. *New Engl J Med* 1982; **306**: 313–9.
13. Hoffman SL, Rustama D, Punjabi NH, *et al*. High-dose dexamethasone in quinine-treated patients with cerebral malaria: a double-blind placebo-controlled trial. *J Infect Dis* 1988; **158**: 325–31.
14. White NJ, Warrell DA, Chanthavanich P, *et al*. Severe hypoglycaemia and hyperinsulinaemia in falciparum malaria. *New Engl J Med* 1983; **309**: 61–6.
15. Looareesuwan S, Warrell DA, White NJ, *et al*. Retinal haemorrhage, a common physical sign of prognostic significance in cerebral malaria. *Am J Trop Med Hyg* 1983; **32**: 911–15.
16. Molyneux ME, Looareesuwan S, Menzies IS, *et al*. Reduced hepatic blood flow and intestinal malabsorption in severe falciparum malaria. *Am J Trop Med Hyg* 1989; **40**: 470–6.
17. Phillips RE, Looareesuwan S, Warrell DA, *et al*. The importance of anaemia in cerebral and uncomplicated falciparum malaria: role of complications, dyserythropoiesis and iron sequestration. *Quart J Med* 1986; **227**: 305–23.
18. Looareesuwan S, Phillips RE, White NJ. Quinine and severe falciparum malaria in late pregnancy. *Lancet* 1985; **ii**: 4–8.
19. Warrell DA, Looareesuwan S, Phillips RE, *et al*. Function of the blood-cerebrospinal fluid barrier in human cerebral malaria: rejection of the permeability hypothesis. *Am J Trop Med Hyg* 1986; **35**: 882–9.
20. Looareesuwan S, Warrell DA, White NJ, *et al*. Do patients with cerebral malaria have cerebral oedema? A computed tomography study. *Lancet* 1983; **i**: 434–7.
21. Looareesuwan S, Wilairatana P, Krishna S, *et al*. Magnetic resonance imaging of the brain in patients with cerebral malaria. *Clin Infect Dis* 1995; **21**: 300–9.
22. Marchiafava E, Bignami A. *On Summer, Autumn Malarial Fevers*. Translated from the 1st Italian edition by JH Thompson. London: The New Sydenham Society, 1894: 112–7.
23. Mannaberg J. *The Malarial Parasites*. London: The New Sydenham Society, 1894.
24. Miller LH. Distribution of mature trophozoites and schizonts of *Plasmodium falciparum* in the organs of *Aotus trivirgatus*, the night monkey. *Am J Trop Med Hyg* 1969; **18**: 860–5.

25. Luse SA, Miller LH. *P. falciparum* malaria ultrastructure of parasitized erythrocytes in cardiac vessels. *Am J Trop Med Hyg* 1971; **20**: 655–60.
26. Warrell DA. Pathophysiology of severe falciparum malaria in man. *Parasitology* 1987; **94 (Suppl)**: S53–S76.
27. Taylor-Robinson AW. Murine models of cerebral malaria: a qualified defence. *Parasitol Today* 1995; **11**: 407–9.
28. MacPherson GG, Warrell MJ, White NJ, et al. Human cerebral malaria: a quantitative ultrastructural analysis of parasitised erythrocyte sequestration. *Am J Pathol* 1985; **119**: 385–401.
29. Warrell DA, White NJ, Veall N, et al. Cerebral anaerobic glycolysis and reduced cerebral oxygen transport in human cerebral malaria. *Lancet* 1988; **ii**: 534–8.
30. Newton CRJC. Intracranial hypertension in Kenyan children with cerebral malaria. Dissertation submitted for Doctorate of Medicine, University of Cape Town, South Africa, 1994: 72.
31. White NJ, Warrell DA, Looareesuwan S, et al. Pathophysiological and prognostic significance of cerebrospinal fluid lactate in cerebral malaria. *Lancet* 1985; **i**: 776–8.
32. Berendt AR, Ferguson DJP, Gardner J, et al. Molecular mechanisms of sequestration in malaria. *Parasitology* 1994; **108**: 519–28.
33. Berendt AR, Simmons DL, Tansey J, et al. Intercellular adhesion molecule-1 is an endothelial cell adhesion receptor for *Plasmodium falciparum*. *Nature* 1989; **341**: 57–9.
34. Turner GDH, Morrison H, Jones M, et al. An immunohistochemical study of the pathology of fatal malaria: evidence for widespread endothelial activation and a potential role for intercellular adhesion molecule-1 in cerebral sequestration. *Am J Pathol* 1994; **145**: 1057–69.
35. Baruch DI, Pasloske BL, Singh HB, et al. Cloning the *P. falciparum* gene encoding PfEMP-1, a malarial variant antigen and adherence receptor on the surface of parasitised human erythrocytes. *Cell* 1995; **82**: 77–87.
36. Su X-Z, Heatwole VM, Wertheimer SP, et al. The large diverse family *var* encodes proteins involved in cytoadherence and antigenic variation of *Plasmodium falciparum*-infected erythrocytes. *Cell* 1995; **82**: 89–100.
37. Smith JD, Chitnis CE, Craig AG, et al. Switches in expression of *Plasmodium falciparum var* genes correlate with changes in antigenic and cytoadherent phenotypes of infected erythrocytes. *Cell* 1995; **82**: 101–10.
38. Ockenhouse CF, Klotz FW, Tandon NN, Jamieson GA. Sequestrin, a CD36 recognition protein on *Plasmodium falciparum* malaria-infected erythrocytes identified by anti-idiotype antibodies. *Proc Nat Acad Sci* 1991; **88**: 3175–9.
39. Sherman IW, Crandall I, Smith H. Membrane proteins involved in the adherence of *Plasmodium falciparum*-infected erythrocytes to the endothelium. *Biol Cell* 1992; **74**: 161–78.
40. Carlson J. Erythrocyte rosetting in *Plasmodium falciparum* malaria – with special reference to the pathogenesis of cerebral malaria. *Scand J Infect Dis* 1993; Suppl **86**: 1–79.
41. Carlson J, Helmby H, Hill AVS, et al. Human cerebral malaria: association with erythrocyte rosetting and lack of anti-rosetting antibodies. *Lancet* 1990; **336**: 1457–60.
42. Kwiatkowski D. The biology of malarial fever. *Bailliere's Clin Infect Dis* 1995; **2**: 371–88.
43. Schofield L, Hackett F. Signal transduction in host cells by a glycosyl-phosphatidylinositol toxin of malaria parasites. *J Exp Med* 1993; **177**: 145–53.
44. Clark IA, Virelizier J-L, Carswell EA, Wood PR. Possible importance of macrophage-derived mediators in acute malaria. *Infect Immun* 1981; **32**: 1058–66.
45. Grau GE, Taylor TE, Molyneux ME, et al. Tumor necrosis factor and disease severity in children with falciparum malaria. *New Engl J Med* 1989; **320**: 1586–91.
46. Kwiatkowski D, Hill AVS, Sambou I, et al. TNF concentration in fatal cerebral, non-fatal cerebral and uncomplicated *Plasmodium falciparum* malaria. *Lancet* 1990; **336**: 1201–4.
47. Kwiatkowski D, Molyneux ME, Stephens S, et al. Anti-TNF therapy inhibits fever in cerebral malaria. *Quart J Med* 1993; **86**: 91–8.

48 McGuire W, Hill AVS, Allsopp CEM, Greenwood BM, Kwiatkowski D. Variation in the TNFα promoter region associated with susceptibility to cerebral malaria. *Nature* 1994; **371**: 508–11.
49 Peters W. *Chemotherapy and Drug Resistance in Malaria.* London: Academic Press, 1987.
50 White NJ. Malaria. In: Cook GC (ed). *Manson's Tropical Diseases,* 20th edition. London: WB Saunders, 1996: 1087–164.
51 Hien TT, White NJ. Quinghaosu. *Lancet* 1993; **341**: 603–8.
52 Wellcome Trust. Artemisinin. Proceedings of a meeting convened by the Wellcome Trust on 25–27 April 1993. *Trans Roy Soc Trop Med Hyg* 1994; **88** Suppl 1: S1/1–65.
53 Brewer TG, Grate SJ, Peggins JO, *et al.* Fatal neurotoxicity of arte-ether and artemether. *Am J Trop Med Hyg* 1994; **51**: 251–9.
54 Meshnick SR, Jefford CW, Posner GH, *et al.* Second-generation antimalarial endoperoxides. *Parasitol Today* 1996; **12**: 79–82.
55 Molyneux ME, Taylor TE, Wirima JJ, Borgstein A. Clinical features and prognostic indicators in paediatric cerebral malaria: a study of 131 comatose Malawian children. *Quart J Med* 1989; **71**: 441–59.
56 Waller D, Krishna S, Crawley J, *et al.* Clinical features and outcome of severe malaria in Gambian children. *Clin Infect Dis* 1995; **21**: 577–87.
57 Marsh K, Forster D, Waruiru C, *et al.* Indicators of life-threatening malaria in African children. *New Engl J Med* 1995; **333**: 1399–404.
58 Modiano D, Sawadogo A, Pagnoni F. *New Engl J Med* 1995; **333**: 1011.
59 Lalloo DG, Trevett AJ, Paul M, *et al.* Severe and complicated falciparum malaria in Melanesian adults in Papua New Guinea. *Am J Trop Med Hygiene* 1996; in press.
60 Payne LM, Wilson LG, Hartley H. William Croone, FRS (1633–1684). *Notes and Records of the Royal Society of London* 1960; **15**: 211–9.
61 Munk W. *The Roll of the Royal College of Physicians of London.* Vol 1, 1518–1700. London: Royal College of Physicians, 1878.
62 Latham RG (ed). *The Works of Sydenham.* London: The Sydenham Society, 1850.

☐ MULTIPLE CHOICE QUESTIONS

1 Human phenotypes associated with genetic resistance to malaria:
   (a) Rhesus negative blood group
   (b) Glucose-6-phosphate-dehydrogenase deficiency
   (c) South east Asian ovalocytosis
   (d) Tropical splenomegaly syndrome
   (e) Diamond–Blackfan anaemia

2 Historical marsh fever in Britain:
   (a) It was caused by *Plasmodium falciparum*
   (b) The vector was probably *Aedes albopictus*
   (c) It was most common in the Scottish Highlands
   (d) The interval between fever paroxysms was 48 or 72 h
   (e) Quinine did not prevent relapses

3 In the chemotherapy of severe falciparum malaria:
   (a) Quinidine is effective treatment
   (b) Artemisinin derivatives clear parasitaemia more quickly than quinine
   (c) Quinine suppresses insulin secretion by the pancreas
   (d) Artemisinin derivatives have proved neurotoxic in experimental animals
   (e) Cinchona alkaloids have been used in China for more than a thousand years

4   Involvement of cytokines in the pathophysiology of severe malaria:
    (a) Release of TNFα is stimulated by erythrocyte invasion
    (b) TNFα is implicated in malarial anaemia
    (c) Treatment with anti-TNF monoclonal antibodies has no effect in malaria
    (d) Schizont rupture is associated with release of lipopolysaccharide endotoxin
    (e) Circulating TNFα levels correlate with prognosis in cerebral malaria

5   Features of human cerebral malaria:
    (a) Cerebral oedema (in a minority of cases)
    (b) Increased expression of ICAM-1 in cerebral vascular endothelium
    (c) Margination of leucocytes and other inflammatory cells in cerebral vasculature
    (d) Cerebral anaerobic glycolysis with increased cerebral lactate production
    (e) Elevated intracranial pressure, judged by CSF opening pressure at lumbar puncture, in most adult patients

ANSWERS

1a False	2a False	3a True	4a False	5a True
b True	b False	b True	b True	b True
c True	c False	c False	c False	c False
d False	d True	d True	d False	d True
e False	e True	e False	e True	e False

The Lord Rayner Lecture*
Social inequalities in cardiovascular disease: their origins and implications

George Davey Smith

☐ INTRODUCTION

The background against which socio-economic differentials in cardiovascular disease risk should be considered is that of large and increasing differentials in all-cause mortality rates in the population. From the years around the 1921 census onwards (with a trial run around the 1911 census), routine statistics on social class mortality differences have been produced, providing the best longitudinal series of such data available internationally. Figure 1 presents mortality rates for middle-aged men from the years around the 1921 census to the years around the 1981 census. Dramatic declines in mortality are seen for social class I and II, while for social class IV and V small and inconsistent decreases in mortality are seen. Increases in both the relative and absolute differentials in mortality between the social class groups have occurred since the early 1950s, a pattern that recent data demonstrate has continued throughout the 1980s [1].

Currently there are large gradients in mortality from all the major cardiovascular diseases according to social class. Figure 2 displays social class differences in ischaemic heart disease, stroke and all-cause mortality for men of working age

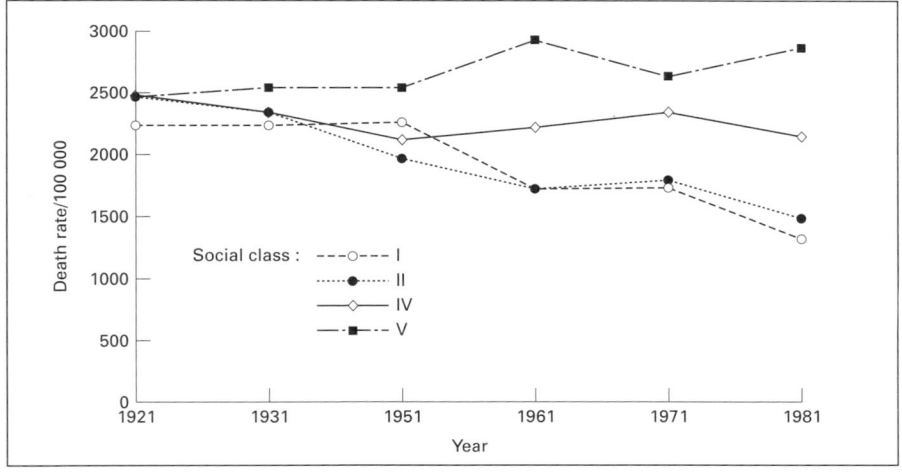

Fig. 1 Death rates per 100 000 men aged 50–64 in England and Wales, 1921–1981.

*This lecture was published in *J R Coll Physicians Lond* 1997; **31**: 414–24.

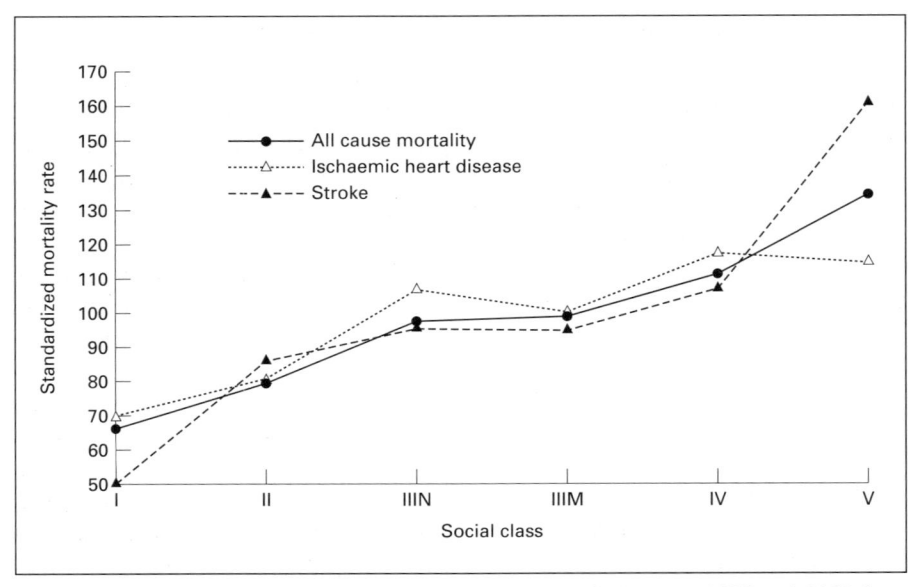

Fig. 2 Social class differences in mortality of men aged 15–64 between 1976 and 1989 from various causes of death. (From Harding [1].)

between 1976 and 1989 [1]. The socio-economic distribution of cardiovascular disease mortality is reflected in morbidity rates. In a survey of nearly 23 000 people aged 35 and over in Somerset and Avon, histories of angina, myocardial infarction and stroke were all more common among individuals living in deprived compared to affluent areas (Table 1) [2].

Table 1 Age standardized prevalence per 100 of self-reported illness by deprivation category. (From Eachus *et al.* [2].)

Condition	1st fifth	2nd fifth	3rd fifth	4th fifth	5th fifth	P value (test for trend)
Males						
Angina	4.4	5.5	5.5	5.5	6.9	<0.001
Myocardial infarction	3.2	3.7	4.0	4.5	4.8	<0.001
Stroke	2.0	1.8	1.3	2.3	2.6	0.03
Females						
Angina	3.8	4.4	4.6	4.4	5.8	<0.002
Myocardial infarction	1.5	1.9	1.7	1.8	2.5	0.03
Stroke	1.6	2.0	2.1	2.2	2.4	0.04

☐ FACTORS CONTRIBUTING TO SOCIO-ECONOMIC DIFFERENTIALS IN HEALTH

Several studies have investigated the contribution of particular health-related behaviours and physiological risk factors to mortality differentials. In the first Whitehall study of London civil servants considerable differences in mortality risk according to two socio-economic measures – employment grade in the civil service and car ownership – were demonstrated. Car ownership was a good indicator of available income in the late 1960s, when this study was established (Fig. 3) [3]. While patterns of smoking behaviour suggested that the lower grade and non-car owning civil servants were more likely to smoke than the higher grade and car owning ones, the pattern of mortality differentials among men who had never smoked was identical to that of the whole cohort (Fig. 4).

The above data are for all-cause mortality, but cardiovascular disease mortality showed very similar associations with employment grade and car ownership as all-cause mortality (Fig. 5). Cholesterol levels were greater among high-grade rather than lower grade civil servants in the late 1960s, when this study was established. Differences in cholesterol levels could not, therefore, account for the higher rates of coronary heart disease among the lower grade employees. This can be taken to suggest that differences in dietary fat intake between grades were not responsible for the coronary heart disease mortality differentials. Indeed, simultaneous consideration of a range of risk factors, including smoking, blood pressure, cholesterol levels and prevalent cardiorespiratory disease, failed to account for the grade differences in cardiovascular and non-cardiovascular mortality [3].

Similar findings have emerged from a study in the west of Scotland, established around the same time as the first Whitehall study [4]. Large differentials in cardio-vascular disease mortality according to both educational attainment and social class existed at a time when blood cholesterol levels were highest in those with the most

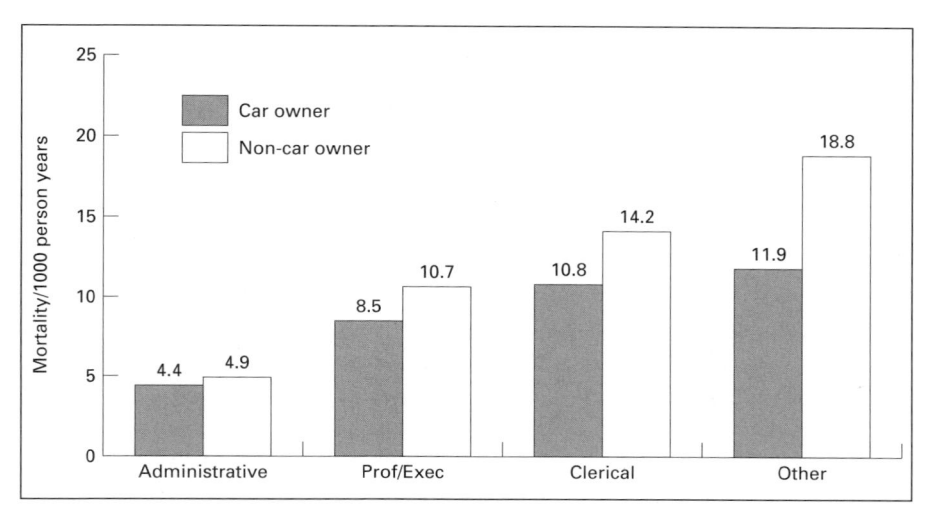

Fig. 3 Mortality by employment grade and car ownership in the Whitehall study. (From Davey Smith et al. [3].)

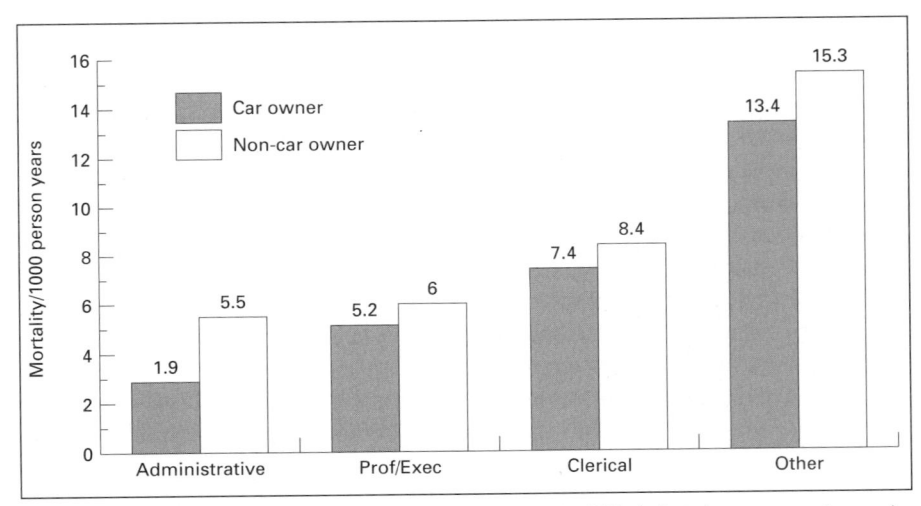

Fig. 4 Mortality by employment grade and car ownership in the Whitehall study: never smokers only. (From Davey Smith et al. [3].)

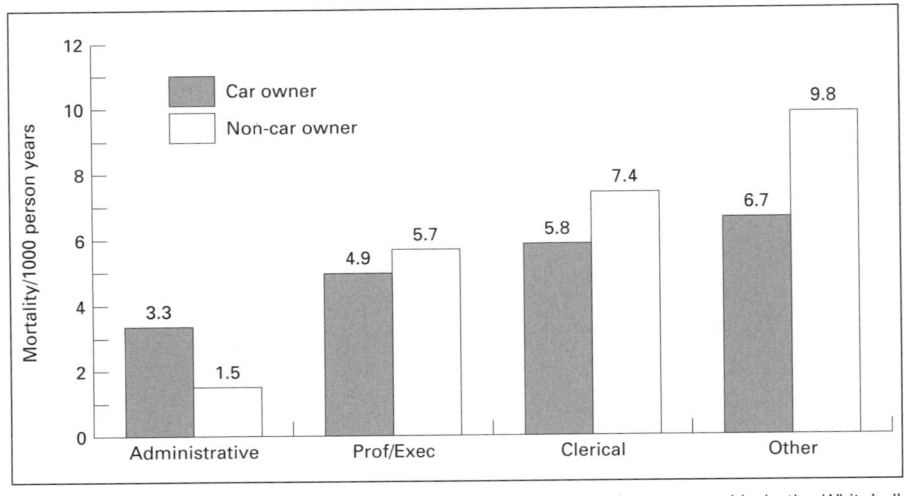

Fig. 5 Cardiovascular disease mortality by employment grade and car ownership in the Whitehall study. (From Davey Smith et al. [3].)

education and in those in the professional and managerial occupations. Adjustments for a wide range of risk factors failed to explain the considerable mortality differentials from cardiovascular disease in this study.

These findings are not limited to British studies. A prospective study of 300 000 men screened for the Multiple Risk Factor Intervention Trial between 1970 and 1973, with 16 years of mortality follow-up, found a strong association between the income level of the area of residence of the men and their risk of mortality from coronary heart disease and stroke [5]. While adjustment for smoking, cholesterol levels, blood pressure and diabetes somewhat attenuated these associations, it did not remove them (Fig. 6).

As a result of the finding that conventional risk factors fail to account adequately for the social distribution of cardiovascular disease, a second Whitehall study was initiated to explore additional psychosocial, behavioural, dietary and metabolic factors that could contribute to the socio-economic differentials in health. The baseline examinations demonstrated that higher grade civil servants, with higher incomes, had lower prevalence of cardiorespiratory disease, among both sexes. Average cholesterol levels were similar in each grade, but concentrations of serum apolipoprotein (AI), the main structural protein of high-density lipoprotein (HDL) cholesterol, showed an association with grade [6] and suggested that characteristic disturbances of lipid metabolism associated with lower occupational status were potentially identifiable.

An opportunistic study that has used data from the Whitehall II civil servants cohort has examined the effect of job insecurity on health status. When the baseline examinations were carried out in the mid-1980s, the civil servants thought they had secure jobs for life. Partly as a response to the initiatives implemented following the reviews of civil service efficiency which Lord Rayner introduced, privatization of some civil service functions was discussed and then implemented. The first civil service department into which these changes were introduced was the Property Services Agency (PSA), for whom, from 1988 on, it became clear that changes were to be made and that jobs were therefore insecure. By 1993, the PSA was fully privatized. The rest of the civil service remained a relatively secure employer, at least until 1990. Thus the health of the group of people undergoing the stress associated with the anticipation, and then the actuality, of their employment being rationalized could be examined. At the time of the repeat examinations in 1990 PSA workers, who had generally better health at the time of the baseline examinations than the rest of the cohort, were reporting more symptoms of ill-health and more health problems in the last years [7]. A relatively acute effect of how people feel about their

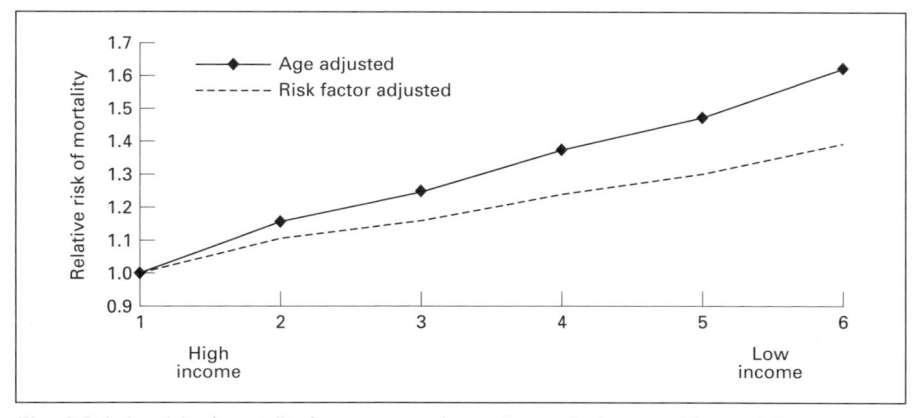

Fig. 6 Relative risk of mortality from coronary heart disease by income: 16 year follow-up of over 300 000 men. (From Davey Smith et al. [5].)

health appears to be caused by anticipation of the loss of secure employment. Two years later, repeat clinical examinations were made, when the PSA employees were actually experiencing rationalization, privatization and loss of secure employment. Cholesterol levels and body mass index (BMI) in men and women had increased in the PSA compared to the other civil service departments. There was an increase in blood pressure for women and a non-significant increase in ischaemia for men and women combined. These effects can be translated into meaningful health differentials, suggesting increased risk of cardiovascular disease among members of the civil service agency first to experience privatization. This study demonstrates how a particular form of social stress could increase cardiovascular disease risk. Further work of high methodological quality on the effects of psychosocial stress on risk of disease is required, since much research in this area is difficult to interpret.

☐ LIFE-COURSE INFLUENCES ON SOCIO-ECONOMIC DIFFERENTIALS IN CARDIOVASCULAR DISEASE RISK

Until recently, the debates regarding inequalities in health generally related to the association between socio-economic circumstances in adulthood and poor health. There has recently been a revival of interest in the effects of poor social circumstances in early life on health in adulthood [8]. The UK Department of Health report *Variations in Health* has recognized the importance of a life-course perspective on inequalities in health. It concludes that it 'is likely that accumulative differential lifetime exposure to health-damaging or health-promoting physical and social environments is the main explanation for observed variations in health and life expectancy'. Few empirical data regarding such cumulative effects exist, however. In a cohort study in the west of Scotland [4,9] in which men have been followed for over 20 years, it was possible to relate mortality experience to the social class of the fathers of the cohort members; to the social class of the first occupation of the men on entering the labour market; and to the social class of their occupation at the time of screening, when aged 35–64. Table 2 shows that cumulative social class, indexed simply by summing the manual and non-manual social class locations of the three stages of the life course, together with other indicators of socio-economic position at the time of screening, are strongly related to mortality risk [4]. When social class at different periods of the life course is related to mortality from specific causes, social class of the fathers of the men and their own social class at the time of screening independently contribute to all-cause and cardiovascular disease mortality. This indicates that there are some long-lasting influences of socio-economic circumstances in childhood on mortality in adulthood.

Socio-economic circumstances in childhood and adulthood have been examined with respect to a variety of cardiovascular disease risk factors in the above-mentioned Scottish cohort [10]. Cigarette smoking was more common among the men in manual than in non-manual occupations, with fathers' social class contributing little to the distribution of smoking behaviour when examined in addition to the social class of the men themselves. This suggests that smoking behaviour is determined mainly by current social environment, rather than by any particular influences of

Table 2 All-cause mortality by cumulative social class, car and deprivation category. Values are age adjusted relative rates. (From Davey Smith et al. [4].)

	Cumulative social class			
	All 3 non-manual	2 non-manual/ 1 manual	2 manual 1 non-manual	All 3 manual
Car	1	1.28 (1.01–1.63)	1.36 (1.08–1.73)	1.57 (1.27–1.95)
No car	1.22 (0.91–1.64)	1.52 (1.19–1.95)	1.76 (1.40–2.21)	2.00 (1.64–2.44)
Deprivation category (1–4) (more deprived)	1	1.25 (1.01–1.56)	1.37 (1.09–1.72)	1.70 (1.39–2.09)
Deprivation category (5–7) (more affluent)	1.06 (0.74–1.52)	1.41 (1.10–1.82)	1.54 (1.25–1.90)	1.74 (1.45–2.09)

childhood environment. Height is associated both with fathers' social class and with own adulthood social class. This could reflect environmental, particularly nutritional, effects from early life, together with the possible contribution of height-related upward social mobility. Body mass index was more strongly associated with fathers' social class than the subjects's own social class, with the reverse being the case for blood pressure and cholesterol levels. Thus, experiences at different stages of the life course appear to make different contributions to particular risk factors for cardiovascular disease. Fibrinogen was not measured in the Scottish cohort, but was included in the Whitehall II study. In this study, fibrinogen levels were associated with indicators both of parental social class and of current socio-economic position [11].

Of particular current research interest are the long-term effects of development during fetal and early infant life on disease risk in adulthood. While many previous exemplars can be found [8] interest was regenerated in early influences on adult cardiovascular disease mortality by the work of Forsdahl [12], who related infant mortality rates earlier this century to present day coronary heart disease mortality rates in Norway. He demonstrated that areas where infant mortality rates had been high in the past, and where, by implication, children had been nutritionally deprived both in early infancy and in childhood, coronary heart disease mortality rates 70 years later were also high. While these data are suggestive of a link, it is precisely those places that had high infant mortality rates at the beginning of this century that remain the most deprived places today. If present day deprivation levels are taken into account in the analysis, there is essentially no residual association between past infant mortality rates and present coronary heart disease mortality rates [13] (Fig. 7). These data do not mean that early life factors have no importance, but do demonstrate that studies are needed with adequate data across the life course of the individuals if the separate effects of early life and later life exposures are to be ascertained.

Since the pioneering work of Forsdahl, a series of ecological and prospective studies have demonstrated that birth weight and weight at 1 year of age are inversely

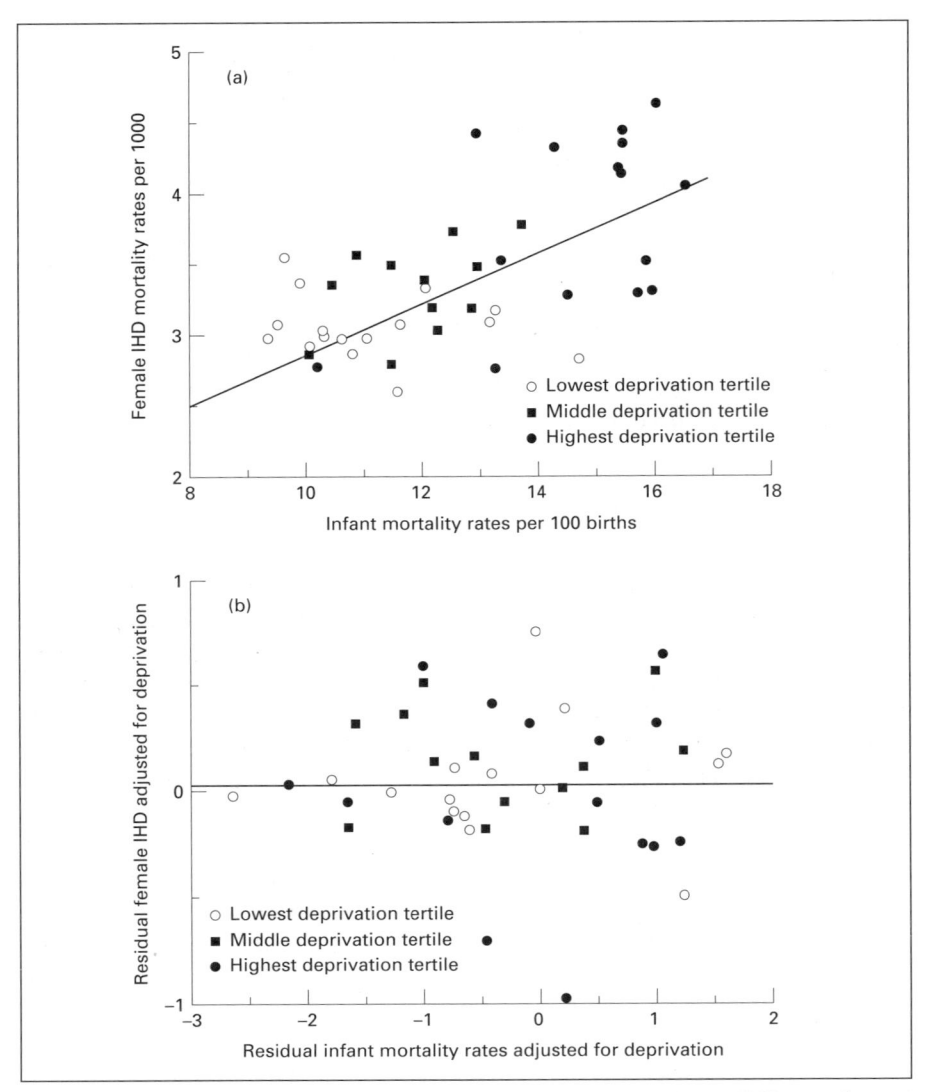

Fig. 7 Infant mortality rates 1895–1908 and female ischaemic heart disease (IHD) mortality age 65–74 in 1969–73 before (a) and after (b) control for measure of adult deprivation. (From Ben-Shlomo and Davey Smith [13].)

related to cardiovascular disease, diabetes and blood pressure in later life [14]. These findings support the proposition that there are important persisting influences on cardiovascular disease risk from early life into adulthood, and encourage the establishment of studies with adequate data across the life course, to take this area of research forward.

In the recent period, little research has been carried out on the effects of childhood nutrition on later disease, although earlier this century it was considered unproblematically obvious that such effects did exist [8]. Preliminary data are now available from a mortality follow-up of the children included in surveys of poverty, nutrition and child health carried out under the auspices of Lord John Boyd Orr in the immediate period before the Second World War. At the time this survey was carried out, it was recognized by one of the investigators, Isabella Leitch, that leg length was a particularly good indicator of childhood socio-economic and nutritional circumstances [15].

In a re-analysis of these data this is clearly the case [16] (Table 3). Age-standardized indicators of total height, leg length and trunk length reveal differential associations with nutritional and socio-economic factors. In particular, it is noticeable that the negative correlations between overcrowding and social class of head of household (scored from 1 for professional groups to 5 for unskilled manual workers) are considerably stronger for leg length than for trunk length, while the positive correlations between weighted *per capita* food expenditure and relative family *per capita* calorie consumption are also stronger for leg length than trunk length. Results for females are similar to those in males.

Leg length in childhood is associated with mortality over the subsequent 60 years (Table 4). These data suggest that there may be important long-term consequences of childhood nutrition on health in later life. They do not, however, paint a one-sided view of rapid growth in childhood. In line with evidence from animal studies and some epidemiological findings, they suggest that cancer risk may be increased by greater calorie intake and growth in early life. Thus reductions in cardiovascular disease mortality in response to socio-economic and nutritional conditions that encourage growth in childhood may, in part, be counterbalanced by increases in cancer mortality.

Studies of birthweight and cardiovascular disease risk factors have suggested that interactions between early life and later life exposures may occur. A study from Uppsala, Sweden, demonstrated that low birthweight babies who became obese adults had elevated blood pressure and high levels of insulin resistance [17]. In the

Table 3 Pearson's correlation coefficients between anthropometry, childhood dietary and socio-economic variables (males). (From Gunnell *et al.* [16].)

Anthropometric, dietary or socio-economic index (n)	'z' score for height	'z' score for leg length	'z' score for trunk length
Birth order (1397)	−0.14*	−0.14*	−0.06*
Number of children (1394)	−0.25*	−0.24*	−0.14*
Weighted per capita food expenditure (1394)	0.31*	0.33*	0.14*
Social class of head of household (1287)	−0.18*	−0.21*	−0.05
Overcrowding (1220)	−0.19*	−0.20*	−0.08*
Relative family per capita calorie consumption (1394)	0.23*	0.26*	−0.08*

* $p < 0.05$.

Table 4 Leg length and mortality: Carnegie survey follow-up. (From Gunnell et al. [16].)

Quintile	Coronary heart disease mortality: fully adjusted relative risk (*95% CI)	Cancer mortality: fully adjusted relative risk (*95% CI)
Males		
1 (shortest)	2.8 (1.1,6.9)	0.4 (0.1,1.1)
2	2.5 (1.0,6.0)	0.4 (0.2,1.1)
3	2.2 (0.9,5.2)	0.6 (0.2,1.5)
4	2.5 (1.1,5.7)	0.8 (0.4,1.8)
5 (tallest)	1.0	1.0
Linear trend test	p = 0.09	p = 0.06
Females		
1 (shortest)	4.2 (0.8,22.2)	1.0 (0.4,2.3)
2	3.5 (0.7,17.8)	1.1 (0.5,2.4)
3	1.9 (0.3,10.6)	1.0 (0.4,2.2)
4	0.9 (0.1,6.6)	0.8 (0.4,2.0)
5 (tallest)		
Linear trend test	p = 0.006	p = 0.77

* Adjusted for age and indices of childhood and adult socio-economic circumstances, calorie consumption and birth order

Caerphilly study, birthweight is inversely related to risk of coronary heart disease in adulthood. This association is robust to adjustment for a wide range of conventional risk factors for cardiovascular disease. The relationship between birthweight and risk of coronary heart disease is, however, restricted to men in the highest body mass index tertile in adulthood (Fig. 8) [18].

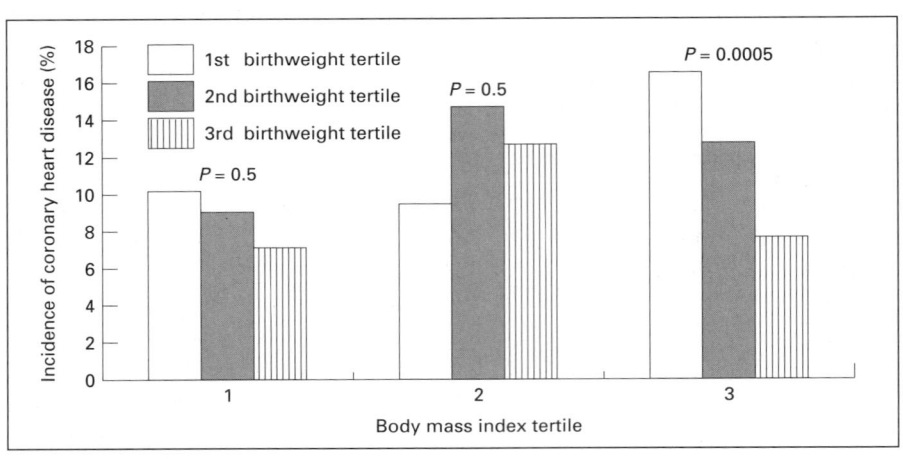

Fig. 8 Coronary heart disease incidence by birthweight and body mass index in the Caerphilly study. (From Frankel et al. [18].)

Recent research has demonstrated important interactions between socially patterned exposures in early life, such as low birthweight and poor growth, and later life exposures, reflected in obesity levels. Studies of how factors accumulate and interact over the life course to generate risk of cardiovascular disease are in their infancy, but offer to advance our understanding of how social phenomena are translated into socio-economic differentials in cardiovascular disease risk.

☐ IMPLICATIONS OF INEQUALITIES IN CARDIOVASCULAR DISEASE RISK

The existence of socio-economic differentials in cardiovascular disease risk provides an important model with which to study the basic causes of cardiovascular disease. Attempts to explain the social patterning of cardiovascular disease should therefore advance our understanding of fundamental issues related to the aetiology and possible prevention of these diseases.

Social inequalities in cardiovascular disease also focus attention on the equitable distribution of health service activities as an important goal. Comparing angiography rates with coronary heart disease mortality rates provides a way of ascertaining whether people are being investigated to the same degree for a given level of need in different areas. In Scotland, people living in areas of high deprivation are less likely to get investigated with angiography than those living in more affluent areas, once coronary heart disease mortality rates, as an index of need, are taken into account [19]. Evidence of an inequitable distribution of cardiovascular investigations in relation to need would be greater if private procedures were taken into account.

Inequities in health service interventions should be investigated and, where possible, remedied. The broader inequity in society is of primary importance in generating inequalities in cardiovascular disease risk, however. These inequalities cannot be simply reduced to behavioural and life-style differences between social groups. Furthermore, even where differences in smoking behaviour, dietary patterns and exercise participation are seen, they should not be considered as simply due to ignorance or fecklessness on the part of people living in materially less-favourable circumstances. In poorer areas, healthy food is less available and is often more expensive than in affluent areas. Similarly, the reason why smoking breaks the rule that households with low incomes cope by decreasing the personal expenditure of adults cannot be reduced to personal failure. Thus, for women caring for children in adverse socio-economic circumstances, smoking may be one of the few activities undertaken solely for themselves and one that provides some respite from the strain of coping with the consequences of material deprivation [20].

Over the recent period when inequalities in health have been widening, many indicators demonstrate increasing social polarization. By 1993, one in three children in the UK lived in households with less than 50% of average UK income after housing costs; in 1979 this was fewer than one in ten. Income inequalities have increased enormously over the same period, with the income after housing costs of the lowest decile group in 1991 being lower than the equivalent income of the lowest decile group in 1979. This growth in income inequality has gone hand-in-hand with growth in socio-economic differentials in mortality, which includes widening inequalities in cardiovascular disease mortality. The only economic argument in support of allowing income inequalities to widen is that the incentive of large increases in income for the already wealthy in some way drives overall economic performance. This doctrine, strongly associated with the Thatcherite agenda of the 1980s, has recently been exploded. Figure 9 plots labour productivity growth between 1979 and 1990 against income inequality in 1980 [21]. It is clear that countries with lower levels of income inequality in 1980 had greater labour productivity growth over the following decade. In 1979 the UK lay at around the average of the countries under consideration for both income inequality and labour productivity growth. Since then inequality has massively increased in the UK and it is now vying with the USA for the unfavourable title of most unequal country. Tackling socio-economic inequalities in cardiovascular disease risk involves addressing the processes leading to increasing social inequalities more generally and making firm decisions about what sort of society we would like to live in.

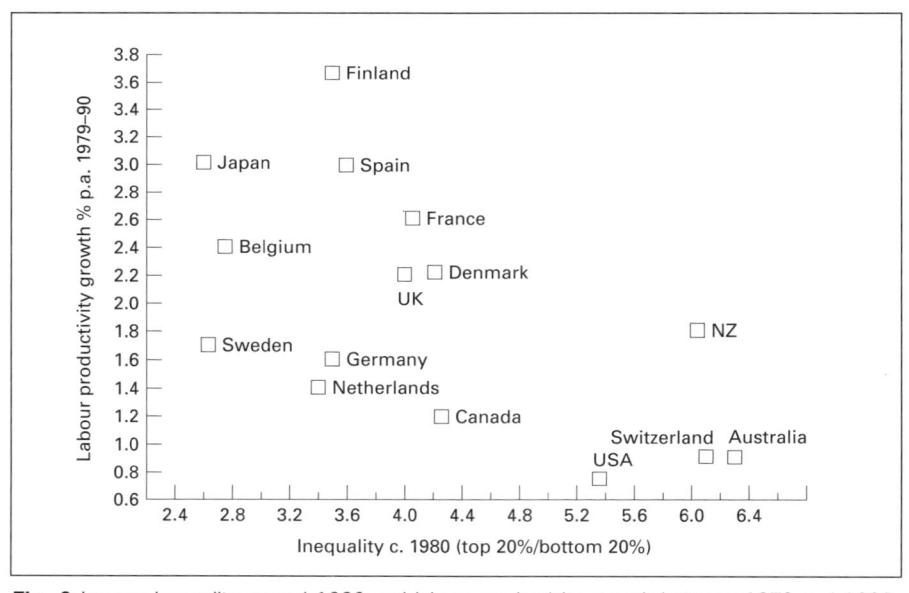

Fig. 9 Income inequality around 1980 and labour productivity growth between 1979 and 1990. (From Glynn and Miliband [21].)

ACKNOWLEDGEMENTS

Analysis of socio-economic differentials in cardiovascular disease mortality in the Scottish cohort was supported by a grant from the NHS Management Executive, Cardiovascular Disease and Stroke Research and Development Initiative. I would like to thank Carole Hart for performing the analyses on the Scottish cohort and Debbie Tope and Anne Rennie for help with preparation of the manuscript.

REFERENCES

1. Harding S. Social class differences in mortality of men: recent evidence from OPCS longitudinal study. *Pop Trends* 1995; **80**: 31–7.
2. Eachus J, Williams M, Chan P, Davey Smith G, Grainge M, Donovan J, Frankel S. Deprivation and cause-specific morbidity: evidence from the Somerset and Avon Survey of Health. *Brit Med J* 1996; **312**: 287–92.
3. Davey Smith G, Shipley MJ, Rose G. The magnitude and causes of socio-economic differentials in mortality: further evidence from the Whitehall study. *J Epidemiol Community Health* 1990; **44**: 260–5.
4. Davey Smith G, Hart C, Blane D, Gillis C, Hawthorne V. Lifetime socioeconomic position and mortality. *Brit Med J* 1997; **314**: 547–52.
5. Davey Smith G, Neaton JD, Wentworth D, Stamler R, Stamler J. Socio-economic differentials in mortality risk among men screened for the Multiple Risk Factor Intervention Trial: Part I – results for 300 685 white men. *Am J Public Health* 1996; **86**: 486–96.
6. Brunner EJ, Marmot MG, White IR, O'Brien JR, Etherington MD, Slavin BM, Kearney EM, Davey Smith G. Gender and employment grade differences in blood cholesterol apolipoproteins and haemostatic factors in the Whitehall II study. *Atherosclerosis* 1993; **102**: 195–207.
7. Ferrie JE, Shipley MJ, Marmot MG, Stansfeld S, Davey Smith G. Health effects of anticipation of job change and non-employment: longitudinal data from the Whitehall II study. *Brit Med J* 1995; **311**: 1264–9.
8. Davey Smith G, Kuh D. Does early nutrition affect later health: views from the 1930s and 1980s. In: Smith D (ed). *The History of Nutrition in Britain in the Twentieth Century: Science, Scientists and Politics*. London: Routledge, 1996: 214–37.
9. Hart C, Davey Smith G, Blane D, Hole D, Gillis C, Hawthorne V. Social mobility, health, and cardiovascular mortality (abstract). *J Epidemiol Community Health* 1995; **49**: 552.
10. Blane D, Hart CL, Davey Smith G, Gillis CR, Hole DJ, Hawthorne VM. The association of cardiovascular disease risk factors with socio-economic position during childhood and during adulthood. *Brit Med J* 1996; **313**: 1434–8.
11. Brunner EJ, Davey Smith G, Marmot M, Canner R, Beksinska M, O'Brien J. Childhood social circumstances and psychosocial and behavioural factors as determinants of plasma fibrinogen. *Lancet* 1996; **347**: 1008–13.
12. Forsdahl A. Are poor living conditions in childhood and adolescence an important risk factor for arteriosclerotic heart disease? *Brit J Prev Soc Med* 1977; **31**: 91–5.
13. Ben-Shlomo Y, Davey Smith G. Deprivation in infancy or in adult life: which is more important for mortality risk? *Lancet* 1991; **337**: 530–4.
14. Barker DJP. Early nutrition and coronary heart disease. In: Davies DP (ed). *Nutrition in Child Health*. London: Royal College of Physicians of London, 1995.
15. Leitch I. Growth and health. *Brit J Nutr* 1951; **5**: 142–51.
16. Gunnell D, Davey Smith G, Frankel S, Nanchahal K, Braddon FEM, Pemberton J, Peters TJ. Childhood leg length and adult mortality – follow up of the Carnegie (Boyd Orr) survey of diet and growth in pre-war Britain. *J Epidemiol Community Health* 1996; **50**: 580–1.
17. Leon J, Koupilova I, Lithell HI, Berglund L, Mohsen R, Vagero D, et al. Failure to realise growth potential in utero and adult obesity in relation to blood pressure in 50 year old Swedish men. *Brit Med J* 1996; **312**: 401–6.
18. Frankel S, Elwood P, Sweetnam P, Yarnell J, Davey Smith G. Birthweight, body mass index in middle age and incident coronary heart disease. *Lancet* 1996; **348**: 1478–80.
19. Findlay IN, Dargie HJ, Dyke T. Coronary angiography in Glasgow: relation to coronary heart disease and social class. *Brit Heart J* 1991; **66A**: 70.
20. Graham H. Women and smoking in the United Kingdom: the implications for health promotion. *Health Promotion* 1988; **3**: 371–82.
21. Glynn A, Miliband D. *Paying for Inequality: The Economic Cost of Social Justice*. London: Rivers Oran Press, 1994.

Helicobacter pylori: clinical implications

G D Bell

☐ INTRODUCTION

Helicobacter pylori (Hp) infects the stomachs of about half the world's population. Evidence suggests that in westernised communities it is acquired in early childhood with the highest incidence occurring in a background of overcrowding and social deprivation.

Until very recently opinion was divided between a faecal-oral and an oro-oral route of transmission. Axon has put forward the novel idea of a gastro-oral mode of transmission. His hypothesis [1] is that the natural route of transmission is by gastric juice, specifically as a result of epidemic vomiting in childhood, the idea being that acute Hp infection is characterized by vomiting of achlorhydric mucus which may serve as a vehicle for transmission.

In the UK, Hp serology testing suggests that the infection rate is about 20% of 20 year olds, with an observed increase of approximately 1% per year in the incidence up to age 60, when it flattens out. This is almost certainly due to a cohort effect and not the fact that 1% of the population is acquiring infection each year. Thus 50 year olds, if they had been tested 30 years ago when they were aged 20, probably had the same prevalence of infection (ie 50%) as they do today.

Most practising physicians wish to be 'brought up to speed' on the most effective form of eradication therapy. With this in mind, I include five tables of some of the latest double-blind, randomized clinical trials presented at the 1995 European Hp meeting in Edinburgh [2]. Finally, I make a few comments of my own based on our extensive experience of eradication therapy and Hp reinfection/late recrudescence rates in Suffolk [3].

☐ PEPTIC ULCER DISEASE AND *HELICOBACTER PYLORI*

Approximately 95% of duodenal ulcer (DU) and 70% of gastric ulcer patients are infected with Hp [4,5]. Acid-lowering drug therapy (ALDT) such as H_2 receptor antagonists (H_2RAs) and proton pump inhibitors (PPIs) in the majority of cases heal the ulcer and relieve symptoms. The 'down side' is the high recurrence rate of ulcers once treatment is withdrawn [4,5]. Continuous maintenance ALDT greatly decreases the incidence of ulcer recurrence but at the expense of considerable long-term cost. Table 1 shows some 1991 data suggesting that 35 million patients world-wide were receiving ALDT at a total cost of over 7.3 billion dollars. One-third of patients on ALDT had ulcer disease but most were taking the drug intermittently to treat ulcer flare-ups rather than continuously to control peptic ulcer disease.

About 10% of men and 4% of women will develop a peptic ulcer at some time in their lives. Once this has occurred, they are liable to have recurrent problems for the next 10–30 years with all the attendant risks of such complications as

Table 1 Use and cost of anti-ulcer drugs – the global market 1991. (From Lehman Brothers Pharmaceutical Research Ltd.)

	Maintenance	Acute	Total	%
Number of patients (millions)				
Reflux	1.25	9.37	10.62	30.3
Peptic ulcer	1.85	11.17	13.02	37.2
Gastritis	1.13	6.80	7.93	22.7
Dyspepsia	0.33	3.10	3.45	9.9
Total	4.56	30.44	35.00	
Market size ($ millions)				
Reflux	750	1405	2155	29.5
Peptic ulcer	1100	1675	2785	38.1
Gastritis	675	1020	1695	23.2
Dyspepsia	200	465	665	9.1
Total	2735	4565	7300	

haemorrhage and perforation. It has been estimated that about 25% of DUs will bleed, though the risk of perforation is much lower. It costs the British taxpayer some 50 million pounds annually to treat the 40 000 hospital admissions in the UK per year with the complications of peptic ulcer disease.

If DU patients undergo Hp eradication, then the incidence of recurrent ulcer formation (and hence its complications) are dramatically reduced [4,5]. Tytgat reviewed 27 studies involving 1881 DU patients and calculated that the annual ulcer relapse was 58% (571/988) in Hp-positive patients compared with 2.6% (23/893) in patients in whom the infection had been successfully eradicated [5]. Penston [4] reviewed the risk of rebleeding in DU patients and found that in three studies the incidence of rebleeding over 9 to 17 months was 27–37% in the infected patients compared with 0% over a similar period in the group rendered free of infection. At least two further studies were published in 1995 confirming this finding [6,7].

The National Institutes of Health (NIH) Consensus meeting on Hp recommended that every Hp-positive ulcer patient be treated with eradication therapy irrespective of whether it was the patient's first presenting episode or a recurrence of a known ulcer (complicated or otherwise) [8]. The evidence for Hp eradication therapy in non-non-steroidal anti-inflammatory drug (non-NSAID) induced gastric ulcers, though at present less strong than for DU, is becoming increasingly persuasive [5].

☐ ECONOMIC SAVINGS FROM *HELICOBACTER PYLORI* ERADICATION IN DUODENAL ULCER PATIENTS

We have shown that in the average peptic ulcer patient who is Hp-positive, at least in Suffolk, it is possible to save about £70 per year per patient by eradicating the organism [9]. However, it is our experience that at least 20% of ulcer patients rendered free from Hp infection will need to continue ALDT mainly because of the presence of gastro-oesophageal reflux/hiatus hernia type problems [9].

In general practice about 0.86% of our Ipswich patients were on acute intermittent or continuous ALDT with about one-third of those in whom either a barium meal or endoscopy had been carried out having a peptic ulcer. Suffolk has a population of 650 000 people and the annual prescription analysis and cost tabulation (PACT) bill for our county for ALDT is about £4 million. We are currently analysing the results of a community-based Hp eradication programme in which all 394 GPs in the 84 general practices in Suffolk were invited to search on their practice computers for patients on ALDT who had proven peptic ulcer disease. Preliminary data suggest an approximately 55% saving in ALDT prescribing following a course of eradication therapy which was successful in just over 90% of cases.

☐ HELICOBACTER PYLORI SCREENING AND ERADICATION THERAPY IN PATIENTS WITH NON-ULCER DYSPEPSIA

Approximately half of non-ulcer dyspepsia (NUD) patients will be Hp-positive. The NIH Consensus on Hp does not recommend the routine use of eradication therapy in NUD patients [8]. In the UK we are eagerly awaiting the outcome of a large Medical Research Council (MRC) sponsored trial which Professor Ken McColl and colleagues are conducting in Glasgow, in which in a prospective double-blind fashion the clinical impact of Hp eradication is being studied in NUD patients.

The risk of a patient developing a DU is 40 times higher in a Hp-positive patient compared with an uninfected individual. If we assume that 95% of DU patients are Hp-positive and the lifetime risk in men of developing a DU is about 10% then one might argue that in infected NUD patients one might be preventing subsequent peptic ulcer development in one-fifth of male patients but in less than one-tenth of females.

Several studies have shown that if one looks at undiagnosed dyspeptic patients under 45 years of age, if the individual has a negative Hp serology test and is not on NSAIDs, then the chances of finding any important pathology at gastroscopy is very small. Some groups now try to confine their endoscopy of the younger dyspeptic patient to those who are Hp-positive and/or on NSAIDs, thereby reducing by up to one-third the number of unnecessary oesophagogastroduodenoscopy (OGDs) in under 45 year olds.

☐ HELICOBACTER PYLORI AND ITS LINK WITH GASTRIC CANCER

The incidence of gastric cancer is falling in the UK but there are still about 10 000 new cases per year and, unlike in Japan, most cases present late and 95% are likely to be dead within 5 years.

Hp has been deemed by the World Health Organization (WHO) to be a class 1 carcinogen. Nested case-control studies have shown that the relative risk of a patient developing gastric cancer is from 2 to 6 times higher in infected individuals.

The lifetime risk of developing gastric cancer is about 1:200 but it can be calculated that in Hp-positive individuals the lifetime risk might be nearer 1:100. The mechanism whereby Hp infection, which is normally acquired in early childhood, might predispose to gastric cancer and gastric ulcer (both conditions associated with gastric atrophy and hypoacidity) in later life is shown in Fig. 1. It

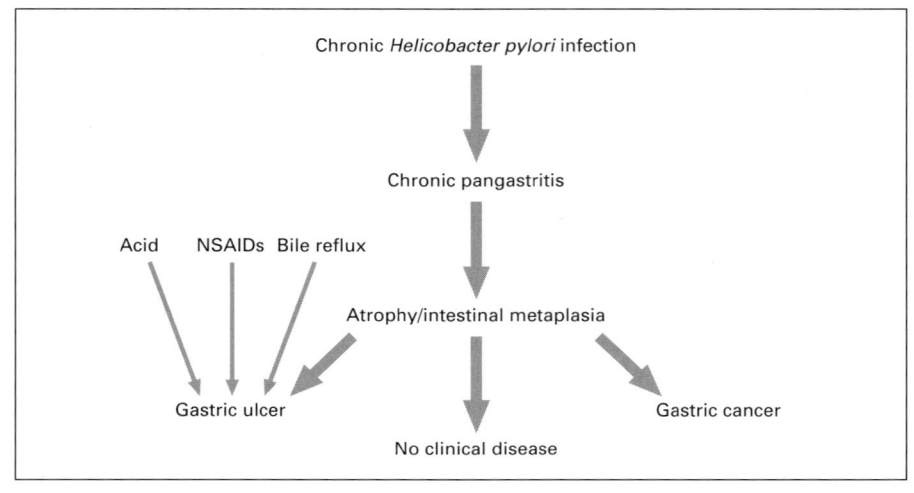

Fig. 1 Possible relationship between *Helicobacter pylori*, gastric ulcer and gastric cancer. (Adapted from Dixon [13].)

must be pointed out that eradicating Hp from the stomach of a 55–65 year old patient with marked gastric atrophy and intestinal metaplasia who may have had his or her infection for over 50 years may not prevent the development of stomach cancer at the age of 70 to 80 years. There are references to studies linking Hp and both gastric cancer as well as the much rarer gastric lymphoma [10].

I am reliably informed by Professor David Foreman, who has done so much of the important early work on the gastric cancer link, that we would need to have a prospective study involving some 30 000 middle-aged men followed up for at least 10 years to know if eradicating Hp from the stomachs of half of them would significantly reduce the chance of developing stomach cancer. I believe that such a study is unlikely to be carried out.

☐ CORONARY HEART DISEASE AND *HELICOBACTER PYLORI* INFECTION

Professor Tim Northfield's group at St George's Hospital were the first to describe the fact that patients attending a cardiac clinic in South London had a significantly higher rate for positive Hp serology than age- and sex-matched controls. Many argued that the association was not causal but merely reflected the fact that both coronary heart disease and Hp infection were commoner in patients coming from an underprivileged background. The St George's group claimed that they had made allowances for such confounding factors and still found a significant increase even after allowing for social class, smoking etc.

If the association between Hp infection and ischaemic heart disease is genuinely causal then what might the possible mechanism be? Fibrinogen acts as an acute-phase protein and in the presence of a persistent chronic infection such as Hp gastritis might be elevated thereby predisposing the patient to an increased risk of developing ischaemic heart disease (IHD). Plasma fibrinogen levels have indeed been shown to be slightly, but statistically significantly, higher in Hp-infected patients than in non-infected cases.

I await with interest to see if other groups can confirm a causal relationship between Hp infection and coronary heart disease. If so then clearly the implications are far reaching.

☐ WHICH *HELICOBACTER PYLORI* ERADICATION THERAPY?

In vitro antibiotic testing has proved disappointing as a predictor of the success or failure of Hp eradication therapy. The most effective single agent is clarithromycin, which when given in a dose of 500 mg three times daily for 2 weeks produces an eradication rate of up to 40% while a similar dose of amoxycillin would be successful in only 20% of cases. Bismuth either in the form of the subcitrate (De-Nol, Yamanouchi) or as ranitidine bismuth citrate (Pylorid, Glaxo) as monotherapy gives eradication figures of less than 10%. Standard bismuth-containing triple therapy (STT) consisting of De-Nol 1 four times daily plus oxytetracycline 500 mg four times daily and metronidazole 400 mg three times daily for 2 weeks will be successful in over 90% of metronidazole-sensitive infections but in under 40% of those with a metronidazole-resistant strain. In Suffolk we find that 20% of Hp isolates are metronidazole-resistant but in inner city areas such as London where there is a large immigrant population the incidence of metronidazole-resistant strains may be as high as 80%.

The great objections to STT are:

- ☐ its high incidence of side effects
- ☐ poor efficacy in metronidazole-resistant infection
- ☐ poor compliance because the patient needs to take a complicated regimen for 2 weeks.

The dual combination of omeprazole 40 mg daily plus amoxycillin 500 mg three times daily for 2 weeks (OA) is much better tolerated but in our hands gave only about a 50% eradication rate. However, by adding 400 mg metronidazole three times daily to OA one can achieve high Hp eradication rates even if the combination is only given for one week [11]. Bazzoli and colleagues have similarly found a 7-day course of omeprazole with clarithromycin 250 mg twice daily and tinadazole 500 mg twice daily effective in over 90% of cases [12].

Tables 2–7 are taken from a short review on six of the latest double-blind studies presented at the Eighth International Workshop on Hp held in July 1995 [2]. It shows that a two-week dual combination of omeprazole and clarithromycin in a dose of 500 mg three times daily is effective in 70–80% of cases (Tables 2 and 3) while the same dose of clarithromycin plus ranitidine bismuth citrate for one month gives

Table 2 Dual therapy of clarithromycin and omeprazole. (From Hunt et al. in reference [2].)

Treatment	Duodenal ulcer healing post-treatment	Hp eradication at 3 months post-treatment	Ulcer recurrence at 6 months post-	
			Hp −ve	Hp +ve
OME + CL	94% (60/63)	72% (41/57)	6% (2/35)	57% (12/21)
OME	88% (62/70)	0% (0/44)	0% (0/1)	74% (42/57)
CL	71% (49/69)	40% (19/48)	12% (2/17)	36% (10/26)

OME + CL = omeprazole (40 mg in the morning) + clarithromycin (500 mg three times daily) for 2 weeks then omeprazole 20 mg daily for further 2 weeks
OME = omeprazole (40 mg in the morning) for 2 weeks then 20 mg daily for further 2 weeks
CL = clarithromycin (500 mg three times daily) for 2 weeks then omeprazole 20 mg daily for further 2 weeks

Table 3 Dual therapy of clarithromycin and omeprazole. (From O'Morain et al. in reference [2].)

Treatment	Duodenal ulcer healing post-treatment	Hp eradication at 4–6 weeks post-treatment	Ulcer recurrence at 6 months post-treatment
OME + CL	99% (151/152)	78% (126/162)	8% (10/125)
OME	97% (156/161)	3% (5/171)	51% (77/150)

OME + CL = omeprazole (40 mg in the morning) + clarithromycin (500 mg three times daily) for 2 weeks then omeprazole 20 mg daily or 40 mg daily for further 2 weeks
OME = omeprazole (40 mg in the morning) for 2 weeks then 20 mg daily or 40 mg daily for further 2 weeks

Table 4 Dual therapy of ranitidine bismuth citrate and clarithromycin. (From Peterson et al. in reference [2].)

Treatment	Hp eradication		6-Month ulcer relapse	
	%	No. of patients	%	95%CI
RBC+CL	82%	14/17*	20%	2.2–37.8
RBC 400 BD	0%	0/20	84%	67.9–100
CL 500 mg TDS	36%	8/22	41%	21.4–60.6
Placebo	0%	0/9	87%	62.9–111

*$p<0.009$ as compared to others
RBC+CL = ranitidine bismuth citrate 400 mg twice daily for 4 weeks plus clarithromycin 500 mg three times daily for 2 weeks
RBC 400 BD = ranitidine bismuth citrate 400 mg twice daily for 4 weeks
CL 500 mg TDS = clarithromycin 500 mg three times daily for 2 weeks

slightly higher but rather variable results (Tables 4 and 5). Table 6 summarizes the trial of Sung et al. and confirms that 2 weeks of OA is better tolerated than bismuth triple therapy but at the price of lower Hp eradication rates. Finally, Table 7 summarizes the results of the MACH1 study (*metronidazole, amoxycillin,*

Table 5 Dual therapy of ranitidine bismuth citrate (GR122311X or GR) and clarithromycin (CL). Intent-to-treat analysis. (From Bardhan et al. in reference [2].)

Results	GR400	GR400 + CL	GR800 + CL
Number of patients with DU	82	75	75
Healing rate at 4 weeks	83%	89%	93%
Relapse rate after 6 months	40%	6%*	9%*
Hp eradication	2%	94%*	84%*
Patients with any adverse event	29%	28%	25%

*$p<0.001$ for comparison of monotherapy with each co-prescription regimen
GR400 = ranitidine bismuth citrate 400 mg twice daily for 4 weeks
GR400 + CL = ranitidine bismuth citrate 400 mg twice daily for 4 weeks plus clarithromycin 250 mg four times daily for first 2 weeks
GR800 + CL = ranitidine bismuth citrate 800 mg twice daily for 4 weeks plus clarithromycin 250 mg four times daily for first 2 weeks

Table 6 Amoxycillin plus omeprazole for 2 weeks (OA2) versus one-week triple therapy (BTM1) for the eradication of Hp and healing of duodenal ulcers. (From Sung et al. in reference [2].)

Results	BTM1	OA2	p
Total number of patients	46	42	–
Patients defaulted follow-up	4	3	–
Patients violated protocol	5	2	–
Ulcer healing at 6 weeks	33/37 (89%)	31/37 (84%)	0.49
Hp eradication	32/37 (86%)	27/37 (73%)	0.15
Side-effects	30/37 (81%)	17/37 (46%)	<0.01

BTM1 = bismuth subcitrate 120 mg, tetracycline 500 mg, metronidazole 400 mg, all four times daily for 7 days
OA2 = omeprazole 20 mg plus amoxycillin 1 g twice daily for 2 weeks

clarithromycin and *Helicobacter pylori*) which is one of the best studies to date on one-week eradication regimens. It can be seen that several combinations of twice daily antibiotics plus omeprazole can achieve eradication rates of over 90%.

☐ *HELICOBACTER PYLORI* REINFECTION OR LATE RECRUDESCENCE?

The 'reinfection' rate in the UK following apparently successful Hp eradication therapy is less than 0.5% per year after the first year but varies during that first year depending on the efficacy of the eradication therapy [3]. This strongly suggests that most 'reinfections' in adults in this country are a late recrudescence of a suppressed infection rather than true reinfection. We feel that ^{13}C- or ^{14}C-urea breath-tests are the best tests to perform post-treatment to confirm successful eradication. Since the eradication therapies now available can obtain eradication rates of about 90% or

Table 7 The MACH1 study: optimal one-week treatment for Hp defined. (From Lind et al. in reference [2].)

Treatment	No. of patients	Eradication	95% CI
OAC500	106/110	96%	93–100
OMC250	105/111	95%	90–99
OMC500	106/118	90%	84–95
OAC250	93/111	84%	77–91
OAM	94/119	79%	72–86
OP	1/115	1%	0–3

Eradication rates and 95% CI according to APT
OAC500 = omeprazole 20 mg plus amoxycillin 1 g and clarithromycin 500 mg twice daily for 7 days
OMC250 = omeprazole 20 mg plus metronidazole 400 mg and clarithromycin 250 mg twice daily for 7 days
OMC500 = omeprazole 20 mg plus metronidazole 400 mg and clarithromycin 500 mg twice daily for 7 days
OAC250 = omeprazole 20 mg plus amoxycillin 1 g and clarithromycin 250 mg twice daily for 7 days
OAM = omeprazole 20 mg plus amoxycillin 1 g and metronidazole 400 mg twice daily for 7 days
OP = omeprazole 20 mg twice daily for 7 days
NB All doses in MACH1 study given twice daily for 7 days. In the case of the OAM regimen it appears important to give the amoxycillin (500 mg) and metronidazole (400 mg) three times daily and not twice daily [11]. Also for OAC the 500 mg dose of clarithromycin seems to be necessary to obtain optimal results if a twice daily dose regimen is adopted.

more it can be argued that it is not necessary to confirm that the infection has been cured in patients with uncomplicated ulcer disease but, as explained above, in patients with a past history of a gastrointestinal bleed it is imperative not to stop maintenance H_2RA therapy until a post-treatment test has confirmed that the anti-*Helicobacter* therapy has worked.

☐ CONCLUSION

At the present time Hp eradication therapy is of proven value only in infected patients with peptic ulcer disease. Screening dyspeptic patients under 45 years of age for infection using a serology test may reduce unnecessary investigations. Treating infected NUD patients is not of proven value. Theoretically Hp eradication may prevent the development of gastric cancer in later life, and may also reduce the risk of coronary heart disease. This, however, is unproven and at the present time there is no indication for widespread screening of asymptomatic middle-aged patients in the UK of whom up to 50% may be infected. Safe and effective one-week eradication therapies are now available which are effective in 90% of cases.

REFERENCES

1. Axon ATR. Review article. Is *Helicobacter pylori* transmitted by the gastro-oral route? *Aliment Pharmacol Ther* 1995; **9**: 585–8.
2. Bell GD. Conference Report. Duodenal ulcer trials reported at the European *Helicobacter pylori* Study Group, Edinburgh 1995. *Aliment Pharmacol Ther* 1996; **10**: 49–54.
3. Bell GD, Powell KU. *Helicobacter pylori*: reinfection after eradication; the Ipswich experience. *Scand J Gastroenterol* 1995; **31**(Suppl 215): 96–104.

4   Penston JG. *Helicobacter pylori* eradication: understandable caution but no excuse for inertia. *Aliment Pharmacol Ther* 1994; **8**: 369–89.
5   Tytgat GNJ. Treatments that impact favourably on the eradication of *Helicobacter pylori* and ulcer recurrence. *Aliment Pharmacol Ther* 1994; **8**: 359–68.
6   Rokkas T, Karameris A, Mavrogeorgis A, Rallis E, Giannikos N. Eradication of *Helicobacter pylori* reduces the possibility of rebleeding in peptic ulcer disease. *Gastrointest Endoscopy* 1995; **41**: 1–4.
7   Jaspersen D, Koerner T, Schorr W, Brennenstuhl M, Raschka C, Hammar C-H. *Helicobacter pylori* eradication reduces the rate of rebleeding in ulcer haemorrhage. *Gastrointest Endoscopy* 1995; **41**: 5–7.
8   NIH Consensus Development Panel on *Helicobacter pylori* in peptic ulcer disease. *J Am Med Assoc* 1994; **272**: 65–9.
9   Powell KU, Bell GD, Bolton GH, Burridge SM, Bowden AF, Rameh B, Hart L, Bradley P, Harrison G, Gant PW, Jones PH, Trowell JE, Brown C. *Helicobacter pylori* eradication in patients with peptic ulcer disease: clinical consequences and financial implications. *Q J Med* 1994; **87**: 283–90.
10 Parsonnet J, Hansen S, Rodriguez L, *et al*. *Helicobacter pylori* infection and gastric lymphoma. *New Engl J Med* 1994; **330**: 1267–71.
11 Bell GD, Powell KU, Burridge SM, Atoyebi W, Bolton GH, Jones PH, Brown C. Rapid eradication of *Helicobacter pylori* infection. *Aliment Pharmacol Ther* 1995; **9**: 41–6.
12 Bazzoli F, Zagari RM, Fossi S, *et al*. Short-term low-dose triple therapy for the eradication of *Helicobacter pylori*. *Eur J Gastroenterol Hepatol* 1994; **6**: 773–7.
13 Dixon M. *Helicobacter pylori* and peptic ulceration: histopathological aspects. *J Gastroenterol Hepatol* 1991; **6**: 125–30.

☐ MULTIPLE CHOICE QUESTIONS

1   *Helicobacter pylori* infection:
    (a) Infects 20% of the world's population
    (b) Usually transmitted sexually
    (c) Usually acquired in childhood
    (d) Present in 95% of gastric ulcer patients
    (e) May be associated with increased incidence of carcinoma of the stomach

2   Duodenal ulcer disease:
    (a) Affects 10% of men at some time in their lives
    (b) Is complicated by haemorrhage in less than 5%
    (c) 90–95% have associated *H. pylori* infection
    (d) If the ulcer has bled once then rebleeding occurs in about a third of untreated cases within 2 years
    (e) *H. pylori* eradication therapy is treatment of choice

3   Non-ulcer dyspepsia:
    (a) *H. pylori* eradication therapy is treatment of choice
    (b) *H. pylori* screening in over 45 year olds may prevent unnecessary investigation
    (c) 50% of cases in UK infected by *H. pylori*
    (d) Particularly common in immigrant populations
    (e) Incidence of *H. pylori* positivity rises with age

4   H. *pylori* treatment:
    (a) Useful in non-NSAID gastric ulcer disease
    (b) Of proven value in prevention of gastric cancer
    (c) Of proven value in duodenal ulcer disease
    (d) Standard two-week triple therapy contraindicated if there is a history of penicillin allergy
    (e) Over 90% *H. pylori* eradication rates possible with a 7-day combination of a proton pump inhibitor and two antibiotics

5   H. *pylori* eradication therapy:
    (a) *In vitro* testing of antibiotics essential
    (b) Clarithromycin monotherapy successful in 20% of patients
    (c) Metronidazole resistance to the infection affects success rate for standard triple therapy
    (d) In UK metronidazole-resistant infections commoner in inner city areas than in rural populations
    (e) Acquired *H. pylori* resistance to amoxycillin is frequent

ANSWERS

1a	False	2a	True	3a	False	4a	True	5a	False
b	False	b	False	b	False	b	False	b	False
c	True	c	True	c	True	c	True	c	True
d	False	d	True	d	False	d	False	d	True
e	True	e	True	e	True	e	True	e	False

Advances in gastrointestinal cancer

A Webb and D Cunningham

☐ INTRODUCTION

Gastrointestinal malignancies present a common and challenging problem for the clinician. Complete surgical resection forms the mainstay of curative treatment for these malignancies. However, long-term survival following curative surgery is still disappointing, with a 5-year survival of approximately 45% in colorectal cancer, 8–15% in oesophago-gastric cancer and less than 5% in pancreatic cancer. A coordinated team effort between surgeons, gastroenterologists and oncologists has resulted in improvements in some of these long-term survival figures. Adjuvant treatment with chemotherapy or chemoradiation following complete surgical resection for colorectal cancer has consistently demonstrated increases in survival up to 15%. However, many patients will present with advanced disease or develop metastatic disease. Recent advances have demonstrated that palliative chemotherapy can provide good quality of life as well as a survival advantage. This article will examine some of the most recent developments and look at future prospects.

5-Fluorouracil (5-FU) is the cytotoxic agent most commonly used in both adjuvant and advanced disease settings. It acts during the S phase of the cell cycle mainly via cytotoxic metabolite fluorodeoxyuridine monophosphate (FdUMP), which binds to thymidylate synthase. Thymidylate synthase is involved in the synthesis of pyrimidine, one of the building blocks for nucleic acids. 5-FU has a short half-life and only 3% of cells are in S phase at any one time, hence most of the advances using this drug are based around methods for prolonging the duration of binding thymidylate synthase.

☐ COLORECTAL CANCER

Colorectal cancer is the second most common cause of cancer death in the western world. However, there are wide geographical variations, with Asia and Africa having a low incidence. There are 26 000 new cases identified each year in the UK.

Staging

The most commonly used classification is a modification of the original Dukes staging. This is based on the depth of tumour invasion and involvement of regional lymph nodes. The invasion of tumour at presentation is closely correlated to overall survival (Table 1). Other pathological features predictive of a poor prognosis are the presence of vascular or neural invasion, or poorly differentiated tumour histology. In the future, molecular markers may be used to identify patients who are at high risk of recurrence. Loss of heterogeneity of the DCC (deleted in colorectal cancer)

Table 1 Modified Astler-Coller modification of Dukes classification and survival in colorectal cancer.

Stage	Pathology	5-year survival (%)
A	Lesion limited to the mucosa	92–86
B_1	Lesion extends into but not through the muscularis propria	82–73
B_2	Lesion through muscularis propria	76–57
B_3	Lesion directly invades other organs/structures	63–51
C_1	As B_1 plus lymph node spread	60–50
C_2	As B_2 plus lymph node spread	55–35
C_3	As B_3 plus lymph node spread	38–29

gene on chromosome 18 and p53 gene short arm of chromosome 17 in the primary tumour correlates with an increased risk of metastases. In addition, loss of the putative anti-metastases gene Nm23 has been demonstrated to have a strong association with the development of liver metastases. Overexpression of p53 and thymidylate synthase also correlates with increased probability of relapse.

Adjuvant therapy

Colon cancer

Adjuvant chemotherapy following complete surgical resection was developed on the basis that micro-metastatic disease could be eradicated in the postoperative period before larger volume disease becomes established. Until the publication of the Intergroup study in 1990, there was no accepted role for adjuvant chemotherapy. However, four large studies have now confirmed survival benefits seen using adjuvant treatment (Fig. 1). The Intergroup study of 929 patients with Dukes C disease randomized between observation, 5-FU plus levamisole for 48 weeks, or

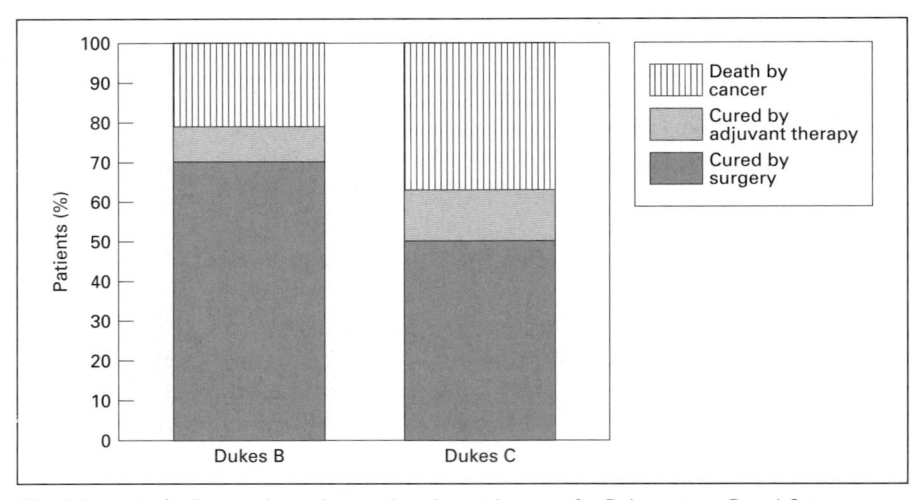

Fig. 1 Impact of adjuvant chemotherapy in colorectal cancer for Dukes status B and C tumours.

levamisole alone was updated in 1995 with a median follow-up of 6.5 years [1]. This demonstrated significant advantage for 5-FU and levamisole, the recurrence rate was reduced by 40% ($p<0.0001$), and the mortality rate by 33% ($p = 0.0007$). The National Surgical Breast and Bowel Project (NSABP) has reported three trials of adjuvant systemic chemotherapy and one of adjuvant chemotherapy delivered via the portal vein. These trials confirmed the survival benefit from chemotherapy and that the benefit is greatest for systemic treatment rather than via the portal vein. These trials also indicate that 5-FU modulated by folinic acid is the most effective regimen. Folinic acid modulates 5-FU by stabilizing the complex formed by FdUMP and thymidylate synthase, and this combination results in higher response rates than 5-FU alone in trials of metastatic disease. Two further large trials have confirmed the efficacy of 6 months therapy with 5-FU/folinic acid in the adjuvant setting. The role of levamisole in this context is still being investigated in a number of randomized trials, but the initial results indicate that levamisole has little or no additive effect. 5-Fluorouracil and folinic acid is a potentially toxic treatment which can cause myelosuppression, stomatitis, diarrhoea, nausea, alopecia, and toxic deaths have been reported. Protracted venous infusion (PVI) of 5-FU administered via a Hickman line using a portable pump has a better toxicity profile as well as having the advantage that more cells are exposed to 5-FU during their S phase. In the advanced disease setting, PVI 5-FU results in improved response rates, less haematological toxicity and no toxic deaths. A randomized study comparing PVI 5-FU with 5-FU/folinic acid in the adjuvant setting is currently underway at the Royal Marsden Hospital, and initial reports confirm the toxicity advantage for PVI 5-FU.

The role for adjuvant chemotherapy in Dukes C tumours has been clearly demonstrated; however, in patients with Dukes B tumour it remains controversial. The Intergroup has recently updated results in 318 patients with Dukes B tumours randomized between treatment for 48 weeks with 5-FU/levamisole or surgery alone. At a median follow-up of 7 years, this study showed a 31% reduction in recurrence rate and a 20% reduction in the cancer-related deaths, but neither reached statistical significance. The NSABP have recently analysed the relative efficacy of adjuvant chemotherapy in 1567 patients with Dukes B compared to 2254 patients with Dukes C tumours and found that the relative reduction of recurrence and mortality was similar in both groups. However, other investigators have not found a significant effect for adjuvant treatment in patients with Dukes B tumour. Most trials have been underpowered and thus unable to detect a significant difference when the number of cancer related events are low. On the basis of current evidence, we recommend adjuvant systemic chemotherapy in most patients with Dukes B_2 tumours. However, the risk:benefit ratio needs to be considered in each individual patient. Features that indicate a high risk of recurrence are vascular or neural invasion, Dukes B_3 tumour or a perforated/obstructing tumour. At the same time, these need to be balanced against the high risk of toxicity in patients with comorbid disease or advanced age (>75 years).

Rectal cancer

The local recurrence of rectal tumours following potentially curative surgery occurs in approximately 10–50% of patients. This difference, compared to colon cancer where the local recurrence rate is low, is due to the rectum lying below the peritoneal reflection. Good surgical technique is of paramount importance in achieving complete tumour resection. Total mesorectal excision is a recently developed technique where the whole tumour field is resected and preliminary reports suggest that the local recurrence rates can be reduced to 4%. Initial studies from NSABP in patients with Dukes B and C rectal cancer comparing surgery alone to adjuvant chemotherapy or adjuvant radiotherapy demonstrated that adjuvant chemotherapy improved overall survival. Adjuvant radiotherapy had no impact on survival but did reduce local regional failures. Subsequent trials compared chemoradiation with radiotherapy alone and, after 7 years of follow-up, chemoradiation reduced the death rate by 29% [2]. Hence, this approach has become standard practice.

A further NSABP trial investigated the role of radiotherapy in rectal tumours by comparing adjuvant chemotherapy with or without radiotherapy. This showed that there was no difference in disease-free or overall survival, but there was a small reduction in the local recurrence rate in the patients who received radiotherapy (11.3% versus 6.7%; $p = 0.045$). This trial raises the question whether radiotherapy is needed in all patients, particularly as surgical techniques improve. Currently, we recommend that all patients who have B_3 or C_3 tumours (invasive of pelvic organs or the pelvic wall) should have adjuvant radiotherapy in conjunction with chemotherapy. However, further improvement with chemoradiation has recently been reported when protracted venous infusion of 5-FU was used instead of bolus 5-FU during the period of pelvic irradiation. This resulted in a 31% reduction in death rate ($p = 0.005$) for patients treated with the PVI 5-FU [3].

Preoperative radiotherapy, with or without chemotherapy, has some potential advantages in that the radiotherapy field is smaller, hence morbidity should be reduced, as well as the possibility of downstaging primary tumours and improving the overall resectability rate. This approach is currently under investigation in randomized trials.

Advanced colorectal cancer

Approximately 25% of patients will have metastatic disease at presentation and ultimately 40–50% of patients die from locally advanced or metastatic disease. A small subgroup of patients who present with solitary/localized liver or lung metastases should be considered for surgical resection since total clearance can result in long-term survival. The patients most likely to benefit from resection of liver metastases are those with three or fewer metastases, Dukes B primary tumour, and at least 12 months between resection of primary tumour and development of metastases.

However, most patients with metastatic disease are unsuitable for surgery and the main object of treatment is improvement or maintenance of quality of life with a secondary aim of increasing survival time. The use of chemotherapy to obtain this goal has been controversial. However, randomized trials comparing chemotherapy to best supportive care have demonstrated a clear, but modest, survival advantage in favour of chemotherapy, with evidence of tumour shrinkage and improvement of symptoms [4–6] (see Table 2). However, these benefits are only achieved in patients

Table 2 Randomized trials of best supportive care versus chemotherapy.

Reference	Number of evaluable patients	Median survival (months)		p value
		Chemotherapy	Best supportive care	
Colorectal cancer				
Scheithauer et al. [4]	36	11	5	<0.006
Allen-Mersh et al. [5]	100	14	7	<0.05
Nordic group [6]	183	14	9	0.02
Gastric cancer				
Pyrhonen et al. [12]	36	12	3	<0.001
Murad et al. [13]	40	10	3	<0.001
Pancreatic cancer				
Mallinson et al. [15]	40	9	2	<0.0001
Leonard et al. [16]	43	8	3.5	<0.002

who have a reasonable performance status, ie able to care for themselves and who are up and about more than 50% of the day.

Folinic acid is the most frequently used 5-FU modulating agent and works by stabilizing the complex form between FdUMP and thymidylate synthase. The meta-analysis of 1381 patients, comparing 5-FU modulated folinic acid with 5-FU alone, demonstrated superior response rates (23% versus 11%) but no survival advantage (11 months for both) [7]. Other modulators of 5-FU, including methotrexate, interferon, α- and n-phosphono-acetyl-l-aspartate, have produced disappointing results in randomized trials. PVI of 5-FU enhances efficacy by increasing the number of cells exposed to 5-FU while in the S phase of the cell cycle as well as resulting in less toxicity. PVI 5-FU can be administered via an indwelling central venous catheter, such as a Hickman line, together with a portable pump allowing patients to be treated continuously while at home. Response rates of 30–35% have been achieved with PVI 5-FU. One randomized trial has demonstrated a higher response rate and less toxicity with the PVI 5-FU when compared to bolus 5-FU [8]. On the basis of data currently available for patients with a suitable performance status, palliative chemotherapy can be offered with either folinic acid modulated 5-FU or PVI 5-FU.

Future developments

There is evidence that cancer cells lose their normal circadian rhythm, hence it is possible to exploit this by giving infusions of 5-FU overnight when the normal cells are less likely to be damaged (chronomodulation). One study has investigated chronomodulated 5-FU administered together with folinic acid and a new drug oxaliplatin when compared with the same drugs given in a flat infusion rate. This resulted in both significantly higher response rates and a survival advantage for patients treated with the chronomodulated drugs [9]. A new specific thymidylate synthase inhibitor (Raltitrexed) has a prolonged intracellular action and hence can be given as an intravenous bolus every 3 weeks. A recent randomized trial demonstrated at least equivalent response and survival when compared to folinic acid modulated 5-FU schedule, but with less toxicity [10]. Two new drugs, irinotecan (CPT-11) and oxaliplatin have shown promising activity in phase II trials in patients who have 5-FU refractory disease. Advances in the understanding of the molecular biology of colorectal cancer may provide openings for therapies such as ADEPT (antibody-directed enzyme pro-drug therapy), gene therapy, tumour vaccines and antisense therapy.

Key points

The key points for colorectal cancer can be summarized as follows:

- Adjuvant chemotherapy in patients with resected Dukes stage C and high-risk stage B saves lives
- High-risk populations should be screened
- Palliative chemotherapy improves symptoms and can prolong life
- 5-Fluorouracil-based regimens are most commonly used but new drugs promise real alternatives

OESOPHAGO-GASTRIC CANCER

Oesophageal cancer accounts for approximately 2% of cancer deaths in the UK annually with an incidence of 6000 cases per year. Gastric cancer is the second most common tumour globally and the fourth most common in the UK with approximately 12 000 new cases per year. Oesophago-gastric cancer is curable by surgery only if detected at an early stage; however, most patients present with locally advanced or metastatic disease and the overall 5-year survival is approximately 10% (Table 3). The geographical incidence of oesophago-gastric cancer varies considerably with the highest incidence being seen in the Far East. A number of risk factors exist, including a range of genetic and environmental factors. *Helicobacter pylori* is the most recent and may provide a target for preventive therapy.

Screening

In Japan, where the incidence of gastric cancer is high, endoscopic screening has increased the proportion of patients presenting with early gastric cancer to approximately 30–40% and, consequently, improvements in overall survival have been seen. The incidence in the USA and Europe is much lower and population screening of asymptomatic patients is not practicable.

Table 3 Staging for gastric cancer and 5-year survival rate in the UK [18].

Stage	Clinical	Pathology	Distribution (%)	5-year survival (%)
I	Radical resection	Muscularis propria −, Serosa −, Nodes −	0.9	72
II	Radical resection	Muscularis propria +, Serosa +/−, Nodes −	5.8	32
III	Radical resection	Muscularis propria +/−, Serosa +/−, Nodes +	13.7	10
IVa	Palliative resection	Residual disease	8.9	<5
IVb	No resection	Biopsy positive only	66.7	<5

Surgery

Surgical resection forms the mainstay of curative management for oesophago-gastric cancer. Extensive lymphadenectomy for gastric cancer is routinely used in Japan, but two randomized trials in Europe investigated the role of limited (R1) versus more extensive (R2) resection. The preliminary results from both studies reported higher operative mortality and morbidity rate in patients undergoing the R2 resection, and survival after 3 years of follow-up suggests that the higher mortality from the R2 resection will at least nullify any survival benefit from the more extensive operation [11].

Adjuvant therapy

A meta-analysis in 1993 of 11 trials in 2096 patients demonstrated no benefit in terms of additional survival for adjuvant chemotherapy. However, this report was later criticized for failing to include two eligible trials, which were found in a more exhaustive search of the literature. When these data were included, the hazard ratio was 0.82 (95% confidence intervals 0.68–0.98) in favour of adjuvant therapy. Newer regimens with higher activity may increase this benefit, but it is likely that the benefit will remain small. Hence, most investigators are now exploring the use of pre-operative (neoadjuvant) chemotherapy, which has the advantage of downstaging large tumours before operation, as well as treating micro-metastases earlier in their natural history. In a recently reported randomized trial in oesophageal cancer, patients treated with preoperative chemoradiation had a 3-year survival of 32% compared to patients who were treated with surgery alone, where the 3-year survival was 6%.

Advanced disease

Several randomized trials have demonstrated both survival and quality of life advantage for patients treated with chemotherapy [12,13] (see Table 2). Oesophago-gastric cancers are certainly chemosensitive and response rates up to 71% have been seen using a regimen called ECF, developed at the Royal Marsden Hospital. This regimen uses PVI 5FU in combination with cisplatin and epirubicin. In a recently reported randomized trial comparing this treatment with the previous best chemotherapy, the ECF regimen demonstrated superior response rates, toxicity, quality of life, cost effectiveness and survival [14] (Table 4). Although this survival

Table 4 ECF versus FAMTX regimens in advanced oesophago-gastric cancer [14].

	ECF	FAMTX	p value
Number of patients	126	130	
Response rate (%)	45	21	0.0002
Median survival (months)	8.9	5.7	0.0009
Median failure free survival (months)	7.4	3.4	0.00006
1 year survival (%)	36	21	

ECF regimen is epirubicin, cisplatin, protracted venous infusion 5-fluorouracil
FAMTX regimen is 5-fluorouracil, adriamycin, methotrexate

advantage is modest (8.9 months versus 5.7 months, $p = 0.0009$), the good toxicity profile allows most patients with reasonable performance status to be considered for palliative chemotherapy. Dysphagia is the most troublesome symptom and the ECF regimen can relieve this in the majority of patients within a few weeks treatment. However, other procedures may also be needed such as endoscopic laser therapy as well as rigid or expandable stents. Radiotherapy is best used only for relatively small locally advanced oesophageal tumours or for the palliation of pain from bone metastases.

Key points

The key points for oesophago-gastric cancer can be summarized as follows:

☐ Second most common cause of cancer death despite reducing incidence

☐ Most patients present with advanced disease

☐ Chemotherapy provides effective palliation and may increase resectability if given preoperatively

☐ The regimen of choice is epirubicin, cisplatin, infusional 5-fluorouracil (ECF)

☐ PANCREATIC CANCER

Pancreatic carcinoma is the fifth most common cause of cancer death in Britain and the prognosis remains very poor with only 3–5% of patients alive at 5 years. The incidence has continued to rise since the 1930s but the reason for this is unknown; the most well established risk factor is cigarette smoking. Adenocarcinomas account for over 80% of pancreatic malignancies but it is imperative that a biopsy sample be obtained because other rarer tumours, such as neuroendocrine tumours and lymphomas, can present in a similar manner and have considerably different natural histories and responsiveness to chemotherapy.

Surgery

Only a small proportion of patients with pancreatic cancer present at an early stage suitable for potentially curative surgery. The standard operative procedure is a pancreatico-duodenectomy which has a high morbidity and mortality. Five-year survival following complete resection is approximately 10–25% depending on patient selection and surgical centre. The value of adjuvant therapy following complete resection is unclear and is currently being evaluated in randomized trials.

Advanced disease

Two randomized trials have demonstrated benefit for chemotherapy compared to best supportive care, with a survival and quality of life advantage for the chemotherapy group [15,16] (see Table 2). These results are controversial and results from confirmation studies are due shortly. Experience from the Royal Marsden Hospital using PVI 5FU and cisplatin demonstrated a 16% response rate with a 7.6 month median survival and 50% of patients deriving symptomatic benefit [17]. In the light of such results, it is important that the oncologist has a frank discussion on an individual patient basis, evaluating the potential risks and benefits. At present, there is no evidence to suggest that combination chemotherapy is any better than 5-FU alone, and for patients with locally advanced disease only the addition of radiotherapy to chemotherapy may be of benefit, although it is not without some added toxicity.

Key points

The key points for pancreatic cancer can be summarized as follows:

☐ Most patients present with advanced disease

☐ Chemotherapy can palliate symptoms but tumour response rates remain low

☐ Combination chemotherapy has no benefit over single agent 5-fluorouracil.

☐ CONCLUSIONS

Cooperation between surgeons, gastroenterologists and oncologists has led to considerable advances in the treatment of gastrointestinal cancer in recent years. In colorectal cancer, improved surgical techniques together with the use of adjuvant chemotherapy with or without radiotherapy has clearly improved long-term survival. Further refinements in the use of 5-FU together with several new drugs provide real options in the palliative treatment of advanced disease. In oesophago-gastric cancer, identification of high-activity regimens such as ECF will hopefully improve survival in the neoadjuvant setting, as well as providing effective palliation in advanced disease. In pancreatic cancer, chemotherapy can provide effective palliation; however, more effective agents are still required.

REFERENCES

1. Moertel CG, Fleming TR, Macdonald JS, et al. Fluorouracil plus levamisole as effective adjuvant therapy after resection of stage III colon carcinoma: a final report. Ann Intern Med 1995; 122: 321–6.
2. Krook JE, Moertel CG, Gunderson LL, et al. Effective surgical adjuvant therapy for high-risk rectal carcinoma. New Engl J Med 1991; 324: 709–15.
3. O'Connell MJ, Martenson JA, Wieand HS, et al. Improving adjuvant therapy for rectal cancer by combining protracted-infusion fluorouracil with radiation therapy after curative surgery. New Engl J Med 1994; 331: 502–7.
4. Scheithauer W, Rosen H, Kornek GV, Sebesta C, Depisch D. Randomised comparison of combination chemotherapy plus supportive care with supportive care alone in patients with metastatic colorectal cancer. Brit Med J 1993; 306: 752–5.
5. Allen-Mersh TG, Earlam S, Fordy C, Abrams K, Houghton J. Quality of life and survival with continuous hepatic-artery floxuridine infusion for colorectal liver metastases. Lancet 1994; 344: 1255–60.
6. Nordic Gastrointestinal Tumour Adjuvant Therapy Group. Expectancy or primary chemotherapy in patients with advanced asymptomatic colorectal cancer: a randomised trial. J Clin Oncol 1992; 10: 904–11.
7. Advanced Colorectal Cancer Meta-Analysis Project. Modulation of fluorouracil by leucovorin in patients with advanced colorectal cancer: evidence in terms of response rate. J Clin Oncol 1992; 10: 896–903.
8. Lokich JJ, Ahlgren JD, Gullo JJ, Philips JA, Fryer JG. A prospective randomized comparison of continuous infusion fluorouracil with a conventional bolus schedule in metastatic colorectal carcinoma: a Mid-Atlantic Oncology Program study. J Clin Oncol 1989; 7: 425–32.
9. Levi FA, Zidani R, Vannetzel JM, et al. Chronomodulated versus fixed infusion rate delivery of ambulatory chemotherapy with oxaliplatin, fluorouracil and folinic acid (leucovorin) in patients with colorectal cancer metastases: a randomized multi-institutional trial. J Natl Cancer Inst 1994; 86: 1608–17.
10. Cunningham D, Zalcberg JR, Rath U, et al. 'Tomudex' (ZD1694): results of a randomised trial in advanced colorectal cancer demonstrate efficacy and reduced mucositis and leucopenia. The 'Tomudex' Colorectal Cancer Study Group. Eur J Cancer 1995; 31A: 1945–54.
11. Cuschieri A, Fayers P, Fielding J, et al. Postoperative morbidity and mortality after D1 and D2 resections for gastric cancer: preliminary results of the MRC randomised controlled surgical trial. Lancet 1996; 347: 995–9.
12. Pyrhonen S, Kuitunen T, Kouri M. A randomised Phase III trial comparing fluorouracil, epidoxorubicin and methotrexate (FEMTX) with best supportive care in non-resectable gastric cancer (Meeting abstract). Ann Oncol 1992; 3(S5): 161.
13. Murad AM, Santiago FF, Petroianu A, Rocha PR, et al. Modified therapy with 5-fluorouracil, doxorubicin and methotrexate in advanced gastric cancer. Cancer 1993; 72: 37–41.
14. Webb A, Cunningham D, Scarffe H, et al. A randomized trial comparing ECF with FAMTX in advanced oesophago-gastric cancer. J Clin Oncol 1996 (in press).
15. Mallinson CN, Rake MO, Cocking JB. Chemotherapy in pancreatic cancer: results of a

controlled, prospective, randomised, multicentre trial. *Brit Med J* 1980; **281**: 1589–91.
16 Palmer KR, Kerr M, Knowles G, Cull A, Carter DC, Leonard RCF. Chemotherapy prolongs survival in inoperable pancreatic carcinoma. *Brit J Surg* 1994; **81**: 882–5.
17 Nicolson M, Webb A, Cunningham D, *et al.* Cisplatin and protracted venous infusion 5-fluorouracil (CF) – good symptom relief with low toxicity in advanced pancreatic carcinoma. *Ann Oncol* 1995; **6**: 801–4.
18 Allum WH, Powell DJ, McConkey CC, Fielding JW. Gastric cancer: a 25-year review. *Brit J Surg* 1989; **76**: 535–40.

☐ MULTIPLE CHOICE QUESTIONS

1 In colorectal cancer, 5-fluorouracil:
   (a) When modulated by folinic acid causes higher response rates but more toxicity than bolus 5-fluorouracil alone
   (b) When given as a continuous infusion causes higher response rates but more toxicity than bolus 5-fluorouracil alone
   (c) Is long-acting with a plasma half-life of 7.4 days
   (d) Works mainly via a cytotoxic metabolite which binds to thymidylate synthase
   (e) Normally results in complete but reversible alopecia

2 Following the complete surgical resection of a Dukes C colon cancer:
   (a) Adjuvant radiotherapy improves overall survival
   (b) Adjuvant chemotherapy improves overall survival
   (c) About 70% of patients are cured without further treatment
   (d) The most common site of recurrence is the lungs
   (e) Only rarely should adjuvant therapy be given

3 Oesophago-gastric cancer:
   (a) Is the second most common cancer worldwide
   (b) Results in overall 5-year survivals of about 25%
   (c) Is not associated with *Helicobacter pylori* exposure
   (d) Is unresponsive to chemotherapy
   (e) Is usually incurable at the time of presentation

4 In pancreatic cancer:
   (a) Chemotherapy rarely palliates symptoms
   (b) Median survival is 12 weeks
   (c) A raised serum CA19-9 is diagnostic
   (d) Biopsy proof of tumour type does not alter management
   (e) Complete surgical resection results in 5-year survival rate of about 50%

5 Features indicating a high risk of recurrence following complete surgical resection of a Dukes B colorectal tumour are:
   (a) Neural or vascular invasion on histology
   (b) Poorly differentiated histology

(c) A normal preoperative serum CEA
(d) A perforating tumour
(e) Overexpression of p53 in the tumour

6   Increased incidence of colorectal cancer is associated with:
(a) Acromegaly
(b) Achrondoplasia
(c) Crohn's disease
(d) Surgical implantation of ureters in to colon
(e) *Trypanosoma cruzi*

ANSWERS

1a True	2a False	3a True	4a False	5a True	6a True
b False	b True	b False	b True	b True	b False
c False	c False	c False	c False	c False	c True
d True	d False	d False	d False	d True	d True
e False	e False	e True	e False	e True	e False

Practical aspects of the brain–gut axis

Q Aziz and D G Thompson

☐ INTRODUCTION

Evidence for the brain's influence on gut function was first provided by William Beaumont, an American surgeon and physiologist, in 1833 [1]. During the course of studies on his patient Alexis St Martin, left with a gastrocutaneous fistula following a gunshot wound, he repeatedly observed alterations in gastric mucosal colour and motor activity in association with variations in St Martin's emotional state.

The role of psychological stress in the aetiology of functional bowel disorders has been the subject of intense study for most of this century, and it is now recognized that more than 70% of patients with irritable bowel syndrome have abnormal scores on psychometric tests [2]. Furthermore, experimental stress whether physical or mental can alter the function of the entire gastrointestinal tract [3]. These studies suggest that the brain exerts a powerful influence on gut function.

☐ THE BRAIN–GUT AXIS: ANATOMICAL CONSIDERATIONS

Gut function is modulated by extrinsic as well as intrinsic neural pathways [4,5]. The myenteric and the submucous plexi provide the intrinsic innervation and are involved in local reflexes, whereas the extrinsic innervation is provided by the splanchnic-'sympathetic' and vagal-sacral 'parasympathetic' nerves. The proximal oesophagus and the external anal sphincter are composed of striated muscle and motor function in these regions is regulated entirely by vagal and sacral nerves respectively. The rest of the gastrointestinal tract is composed of smooth muscle, has its own intrinsic innervation and shows less dependence on extrinsic innervation. Nevertheless, the enteric neural network is subject to descending neural control by the central nervous system (CNS) which helps to co-ordinate motility in different regions of the gut. Sectioning the extrinsic nerves does not paralyse the gut but seriously disrupts its function.

Afferent information from the gastrointestinal tract is carried via both vagal and spinal afferents [4–6]. Cell bodies of vagal afferents lie in the nodose ganglia, while cell bodies of spinal afferents lie in the dorsal root ganglia. The central processes of vagal afferents terminate in the brain stem nucleus of the solitary tract (NTS) from which second-order neurons pass both ipsilaterally and contralaterally to the cingulate as well as the supracingulate cortex, especially the orbitofrontal and the insular cortex. This cortical projection is mediated mainly via the thalamic nuclei; however, some projections also pass via the hypothalamus, tegmentum and the reticular formation. Vagal afferents also constitute the sensory limb of the circuitry involved in vago-vagal reflexes and are connected to the motor limb via projections from the NTS to the vagal efferent neurons in the dorsal motor nucleus (DMN) of the vagus which in turn project to the intrinsic neural ganglia. Second-order neurons of spinal afferents pass either to the CNS predominantly in the spinothalamic tracts which project to the cortex via the ventral and medial nuclear complex of the thalamus or return via the prevertebral ganglia, to the intrinsic neural plexi of the gut to form spinal reflexes. Collaterals from spinal afferents also form short reflex loops with postganglionic sympathetic nerves in the prevertebral ganglion (Fig. 1).

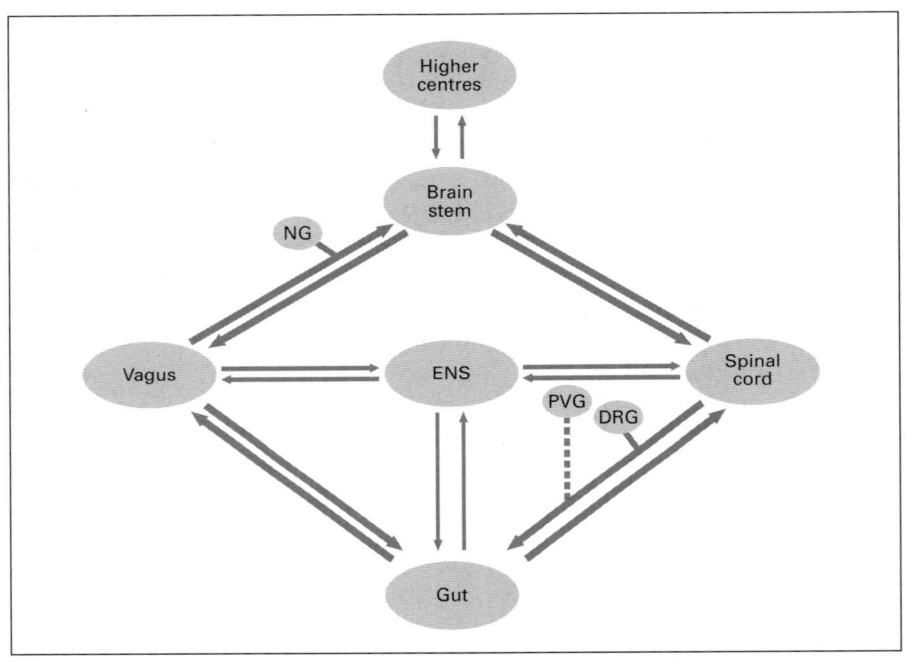

Fig. 1 Schematic representation of the brain–gut neural pathways. Abbreviations: NG, nodose ganglion; DRG, dorsal root ganglia; PVG, prevertebral ganglia; ENS, efferent nervous system. See text for details.

Numerous hormones and neuropeptides have been identified which modulate gut function either by direct action on the gut or indirectly by acting on the brain–gut neural network both centrally and peripherally. Furthermore, evidence for the regulation of the brain–gut axis by the immune system has also been obtained. This 'immune brain–gut axis' regulates gastric secretion and mucosal homoeostasis through the action of various cytokines like interleukin 1. Discussion of the humoral and immune regulation of the brain–gut axis is beyond the scope of this review and the reader is referred to other detailed reviews on the subject [7,8].

Origin of gut sensation

The two afferent pathways conduct different information from the gut viscera [5,6]. Vagal afferents which constitute 70–90% of the vagus nerve conduct vegetative data, for example hunger, satiety and nausea, whereas spinal afferents mediate sensations that inform the brain about potentially noxious events. In contrast to somatic sensation, which is well localized, visceral sensation is vague and poorly localized. This is because visceral afferents are fewer in number than somatic afferents, accounting for only 10% of the total number of spinal afferents despite having a similar surface area to innervate. Owing to convergence of visceral and somatic afferents at the level of the spinal cord, visceral sensation is often referred to somatic structures.

Modulation of gut sensation

Animal studies show that modulation of gut sensation can occur at several sites within the CNS and the peripheral nervous system (PNS) [6,9,10]. The CNS modulates gut sensation via excitatory and inhibitory descending pathways from the cerebral cortex both to the termination of vagal afferents at the level of the brain stem NTS and to the second-order spinal neurons (Fig. 2). Modulation of gut sensation can also occur peripherally, either at the level of the prevertebral ganglia by descending influences from the higher centres [11], or at the level of the primary afferent fibres within the gut wall by local factors such as inflammatory and immune mediators, hormones and neuropeptides which may alter receptor function [12] (Fig. 3). In addition, recent animal studies provide evidence for viscerovisceral reflexes mediated via the brain stem, so that information encoded within vagal afferents can have an inhibitory influence on spinal afferent activity [13].

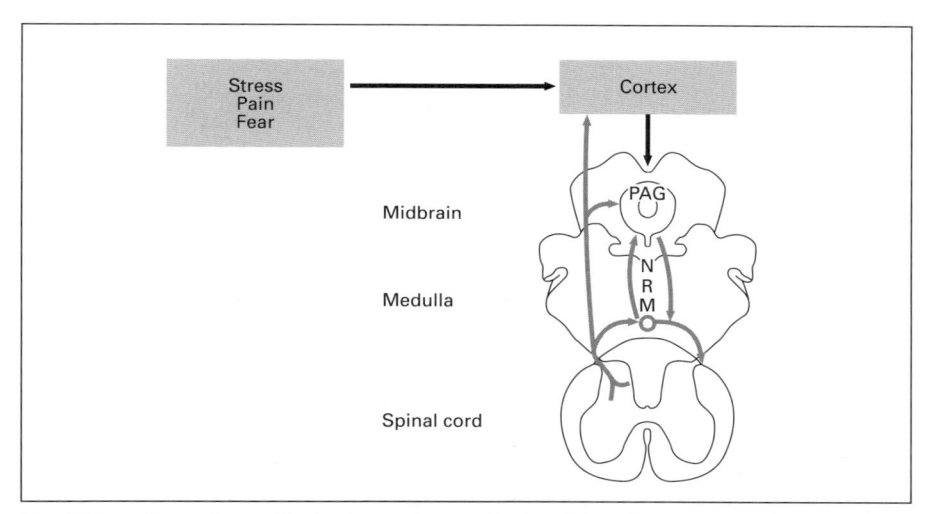

Fig. 2 The pathways involved in the descending modulation of dorsal horn neurons. The corticofugal pathways pass via the periaqueductal grey (PAG) region of the midbrain and the medial and lateral regions of the rostral ventral medulla including the nucleus raphe magnus (NRM) to the dorsal horn of the spinal cord. The primary viscerosomatic spinal afferents ascend in the spinothalamic tract and send collaterals to the NRM and the PAG on their way to the cortex. (Adapted from Besbaum and Fields [11].)

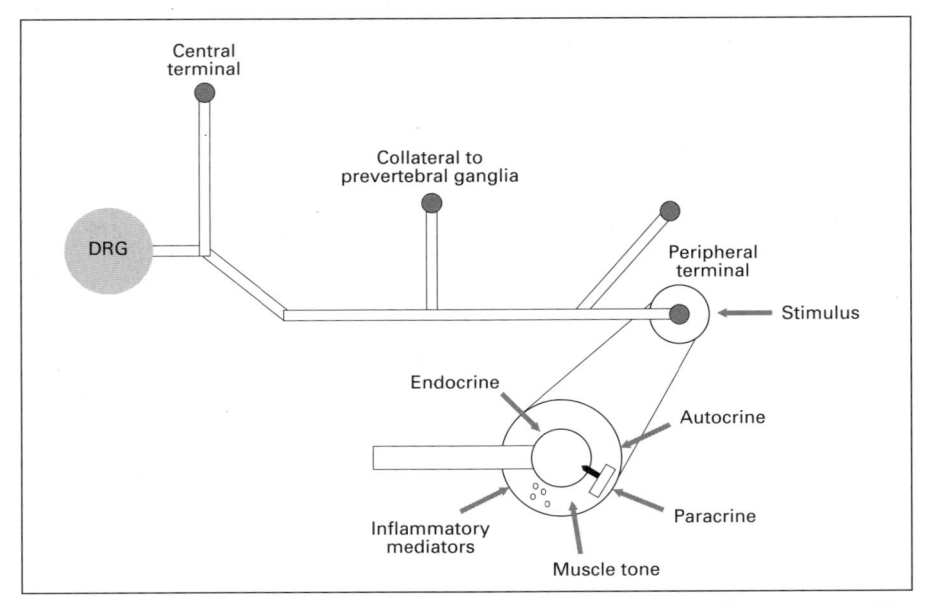

Fig. 3 Schematic representation of the functional anatomy of the spinal afferent neurons. The peripheral terminals with cell bodies in the dorsal root ganglia (DRG) act as mechanoreceptors. The central terminal synapses with second-order neurons in the dorsal horn of the spinal cord. Collaterals also pass to the postganglionic sympathetic neurons in the prevertebral ganglia. The blow-up shows the possible modulating influences on the peripheral terminals. (Adapted from Mayer et al. [12].)

☐ INVESTIGATION OF THE BRAIN–GUT AXIS IN MAN

The neurophysiological characteristics of human visceral afferent pathways and the CNS loci which process sensation are now beginning to be explored in intact subjects using the novel non-invasive neurophysiological techniques of cortical evoked potentials (CEP), magnetoencephalography (MEG), and positron emission tomography (PET). CEP and MEG provide information, respectively, about the electrical and the magnetic fields generated by cortical neurons in response to peripheral stimulation and cortical events occurring from millisecond to millisecond. Because a magnetic field (unlike an electrical field) is not altered as it passes through the skull, the spatial resolution provided by MEG is considerably better than that provided by CEP so that an accurate anatomical location of the sources generating the magnetic field can be obtained by co-registering MEG data on brain magnetic resonance images (MRI). With PET, changes in neuronal activity in the brain can be detected by observing the spatial distribution of intravenously administered positron emitting radioisotopes. PET provides good spatial resolution of cortical and subcortical sources but its temporal resolution is poor so that, despite the precise anatomical localization of neuronal sources, no information is provided about the sequence in which these sources are activated. PET also requires expensive facilities to produce radioisotopes and it involves exposure to radiation so that, while it remains the gold standard for spatial resolution studies, it is not appropriate for repeated or routine use in volunteers and patients [14].

Studies of gut afferent pathways

Despite its major clinical importance, the aetiology of visceral pain syndromes, particularly those of gut origin, remains obscure and the modern techniques described above have only just begun to be used to study visceral sensory physiology. Studies of the processing of gastrointestinal sensation by the brain have been performed using CEPs evoked by distension [15], and by electrical stimulation [16], of the oesophagus and the anorectum [17]. Typical cortical evoked potentials consist of a series of positive and negative potentials (Fig. 4), the spatiotemporal distribution

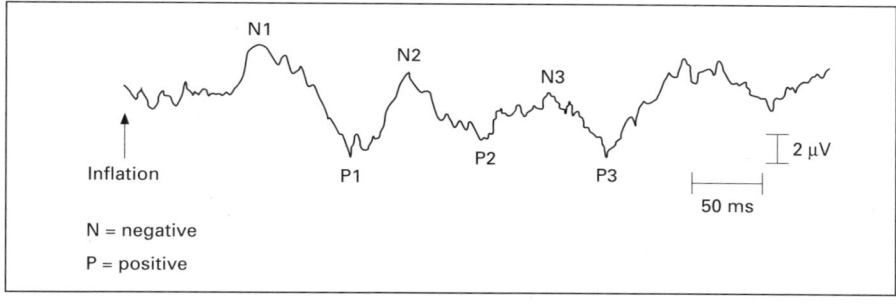

Fig. 4 Typical cortical-evoked response recorded from the vertex following repeated oesophageal balloon distension in a healthy volunteer. The upward and downward deflections represent negative (N) and positive (P) potentials respectively, and are numbered sequentially.

of each potential representing a specific step in the cortical processing of the information. Recent studies of oesophageal evoked cortical potentials suggest that multiple cortical sources process oesophageal sensation. The topographic distribution of these potentials on the scalp suggests that either the primary somatosensory cortex or the insula is the first to receive oesophageal sensory information. Thereafter, secondary processing of this information occurs in the prefrontal and the cingulate cortices (see Plate 4). The potentials representing secondary processing of oesophageal sensation are highly sensitive to changes in sensory perception, suggesting that this technique could be used objectively to assess the subject's response to variable stimulation intensities (Fig. 5). The oesophagus appears to be viscerotopically organized on the cortex, sources for the upper oesophagus being located more anteriorly than those for the lower oesophagus. This indicates that the sensory cortex is also responsible for the discriminative aspects of visceral sensation in a manner similar to that for somatic sensation. Although the potentials can be recorded from both cortical hemispheres, there is evidence of lateralization of these potentials to either the right or the left hemisphere in most subjects. This observation may explain the radiation of oesophageal pain to the left or the right arm and suggests that referral of visceral pain to one or other side of the

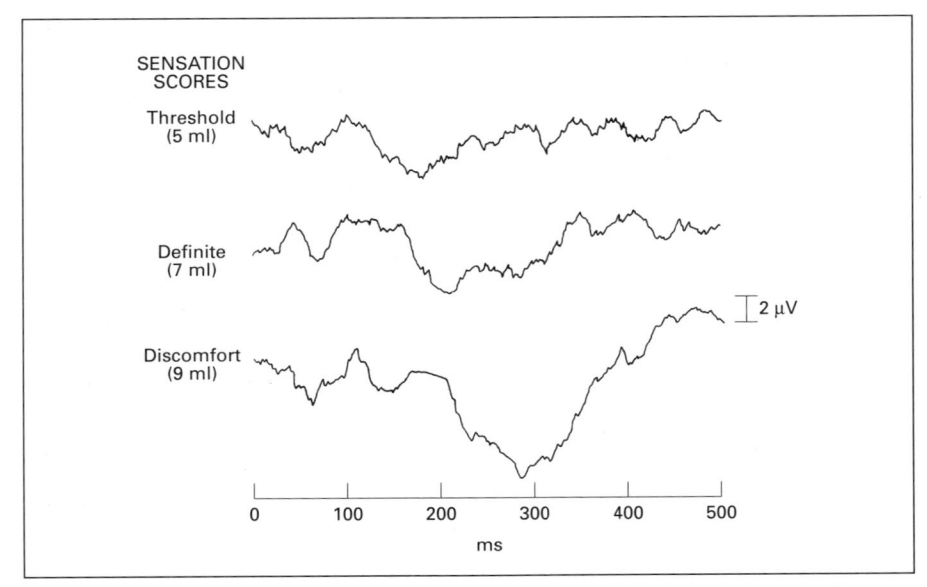

Fig. 5 Cortical-evoked responses recorded from the vertex in a healthy volunteer following oesophageal distension at different volumes. An increase in stimulation intensity produced an increase in amplitude of the late potentials.

body may be related to the hemispheric lateralization of the sensory information for the visceral structure.

Cortical processing of human oesophageal sensation has also been studied using magnetoencephalography [18]. The results show that discrete areas of the primary somatosensory cortex are indeed the first sites to be activated by oesophageal stimulation; thereafter, activation of the insular cortex occurs (see Plate 5).

PET has recently been used to identify the cortical loci that process oesophageal sensation [19]. The results of these studies suggest that, although cortical areas processing both nociceptive and non-nociceptive oesophageal sensation overlap in the primary somatosensory cortex and the insula, nociceptive sensation is processed exclusively in the right anterior insular cortex and the anterior cingulate gyri (see Plate 6).

Studies of gut efferent pathways

Swallowing can be initiated volitionally, suggesting that the cerebral cortex plays an important role in its mediation. A detailed study of the corticofugal pathways to the swallowing tract has, however, not been possible in conscious subjects until the recent development of transcranial magnetic stimulation (TCMS) of the brain.

Magnetic stimulation of human neural tissue is based on the basic principle of electromagnetic induction first described by Michael Faraday in 1831 at the Royal Institution of Great Britain. It states: 'In conducting tissues, a time varying magnetic field induces an electric field and causes current to flow'. Thus the generation of a transient magnetic field over the human cerebral cortex generates an electric field at that site, and produces neural stimulation [20].

TCMS has recently been used to evoke electromyographic (EMG) responses in muscles involved in the oral, pharyngeal and oesophageal phases of swallowing (Fig. 6) [21,22]. The results suggest that these muscles are somatotopically organized on the motor and premotor cortex of each hemisphere, with the oral muscles being located most lateral and the oesophagus most medial. Despite their bilateral cortical representation, the swallowing muscles show evidence of interhemispheric asymmetry which is independent of subject handedness.

Stimulation of the extracranial vagus nerve in the neck using TCMS can also be performed and such stimulation evokes two types of oesophageal EMG responses: a direct response mediated via the vagal motor fibres and an indirect reflex response that may be the result of afferent fibre activation which then excites efferent fibres, via the swallowing centre in the brain stem (Fig. 7). Furthermore, magnetic stimulation of the vagal afferents immediately before cortical stimulation facilitates the cortically evoked oesophageal EMG responses suggesting that sensory feedback plays an important role in the modulation of the swallowing [21].

☐ THE BRAIN–GUT AXIS IN DISEASE

The importance of the extrinsic innervation of the gut in the regulation of gut function is highlighted by the clinical consequences of vagotomy, which increases gastric tone, delays gastric emptying of solids while increasing the emptying of

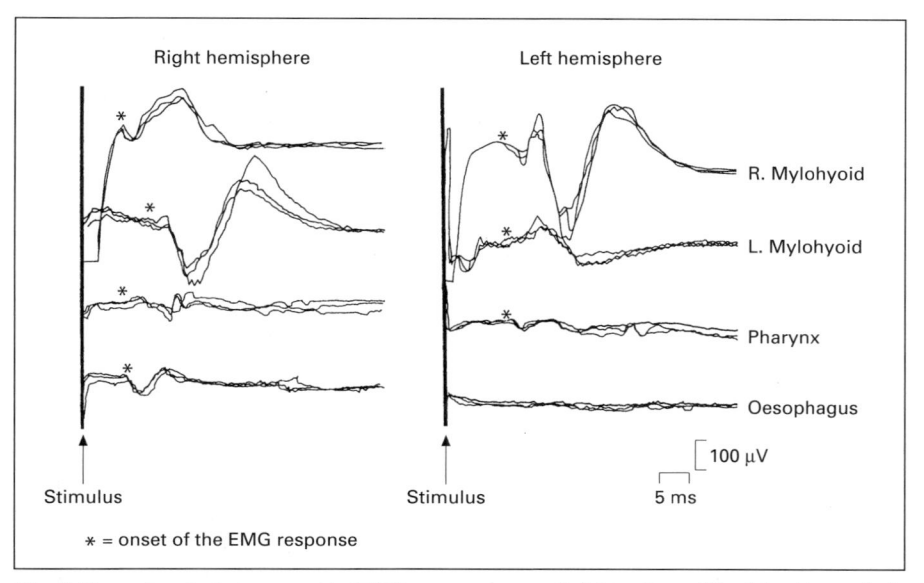

Fig. 6 Shows the electromyographic (EMG) responses recorded from the oral (mylohyoid muscles), pharyngeal and oesophageal muscles following transcranial magnetic stimulation of the right and the left cortical hemispheres in a healthy volunteer. Larger pharyngo-oesophageal EMG responses are evoked following stimulation of the right hemisphere. (Adapted from Hamdy et al. [22].)

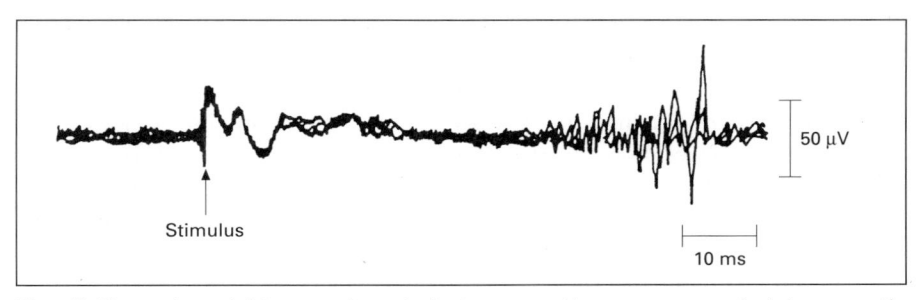

Fig. 7 The early and late oesophageal electromyographic responses evoked by magnetic stimulation of the extracranial vagus nerve in the neck.

liquids, and leads to symptoms such as postprandial pain, bloating and nausea. Furthermore, vagotomized patients demonstrate hypersensitivity to sensory stimuli applied to the stomach. This hypersensitivity may be due to sensitization of mechanoreceptors due to alterations in gastric tone [23].

Abdominal pain is a clinical problem associated with considerable morbidity and is the most common cause of referral to a gastroenterologist [9,10]. Visceral pain from the gastrointestinal tract is associated either with organic diseases, eg inflammation, or with 'functional disorders' without evidence of organic disease, eg non-cardiac chest pain, non-ulcer dyspepsia and irritable bowel syndrome (IBS).

Although clearly defined aetiological factors have not been identified for these functional disorders, it is speculated that an upregulation (innocuous stimulus producing a noxious response) of either primary visceral afferents within the gut wall or neurons within the spinal cord may be occurring due to the effect of local factors, eg inflammatory mediators [9,10]. The loss of the vagal inhibitory influence on spinal afferents has also been implicated in the aetiology of pain in functional bowel disorders [12]. Furthermore, the fact that stress exacerbates functional bowel disorders [2,3,9,10] suggests that abnormal processing of visceral afferent information by the brain is also involved.

Considerable research is being carried out to understand the pathophysiology of visceral pain. However, until recently most data on the subject were available from animal studies. The availability of non-invasive neurophysiological techniques such as CEP, MEG and PET has made it possible to explore the human brain–gut axis in health and disease and useful information is being provided by these early studies.

Comparison of cortical potentials evoked in response to oesophageal balloon distension between healthy subjects and patients with non-cardiac chest pain demonstrates that, despite reduced sensory thresholds, patients have normal CEP amplitudes, suggesting that afferent information arising from the oesophagus is normal and therefore increased perception of oesophageal distension in patients is related to abnormal cortical processing of oesophageal sensation [24]. In contrast, a study of CEPs evoked by rectal distension in patients with chronic constipation and encopresis has implicated a defect in the rectal afferent pathways [25].

In another recent study, PET was used to compare the regional cerebral blood flow patterns between patients with IBS and healthy volunteers during anticipation of rectal pain [26]. The results suggest that IBS patients have a relatively higher level of thalamic blood flow than healthy volunteers, suggesting that dysregulation of central processing of pain information may occur in these patients.

Studies of the cortical control of human swallowing function using TCMS have shown that, although swallowing muscles are represented bilaterally, there is evidence of interhemispheric asymmetry [22]. To determine whether this asymmetric cortical representation of swallowing muscles could be responsible for development of dysphagia following unilateral hemispheric stroke, studies have been performed to test the hypothesis that the hemisphere with a larger representation of swallowing muscles maintains dominant control and therefore damage to this hemisphere will lead to dysphagia, while damage to the non-dominant hemisphere will not affect swallowing function. Patients with and without dysphagia following unilateral hemispheric stroke were studied and swallowing muscle EMGs were recorded following TCMS of both affected and non-affected hemispheres. The results suggest that the magnitude of swallow-muscle representation on the affected hemisphere is poor in both dysphagic and non-dysphagic patients. In contrast, on the unaffected hemisphere, the swallow muscle representation was greater in non-dysphagic patients than in dysphagic patients. This suggests that in non-dysphagic patients the dominant swallowing centre on the unaffected hemisphere is spared, while damage to the dominant cortical swallowing centre located on the affected hemisphere appears to be the basis of dysphagia following unilateral hemispheric stroke [27].

☐ CONCLUSION

The brain–gut axis plays an important role in the modulation of gut function. The availability of non-invasive neurophysiological techniques has now made it possible to study the neurophysiological characteristics of brain–gut neural pathways and to identify the CNS centres that regulate gut function. The use of these techniques in patients with functional bowel disorders and neurogenic dysphagia provides a new insight into the pathophysiology of these diseases. It is hoped that further studies will not only help in the understanding of the aetiology of numerous disorders such as chronic visceral pain where dysfunction of the brain–gut axis is implicated, but will also help in evaluating the outcome of therapeutic interventions aimed at altering the course of disease.

ACKNOWLEDGEMENT

The authors would like to thank Dr S Hamdy for his comments and suggestions, which were very useful in the preparation of the manuscript.

REFERENCES

1 Beaumont W. In: *Experiments and observations on the gastric juice and the physiology of digestion.* Facsimile of the original publication of 1833. New York: Dover Publications, Inc., 1959.

2. Whitehead WE, Bosmajian L, Zonderman AB, Costa PT Jr, Schuster MM. Symptoms of psychological distress associated with irritable bowel syndrome. *Gastroenterology* 1988; **95**: 709–14.
3. Buneo L, Collins S, Junien J-L, eds. In: *Stress and Digestive Motility*. Paris: John Libbey, Eurotext, 1989.
4. Davison JS. Innervation of the gastrointestinal tract. In: Christensen J, Wingate DL, Wright PSG, eds. *A Guide to Gastrointestinal Motility*. Bristol: Wright and Sons, 1983; 1–47.
5. Roman C, Gonella J. Extrinsic control of digestive tract motility. In: Johnson LR, ed. *Physiology of the Gastrointestinal Tract*. New York: Raven, 1987; 507–54.
6. Grundy D, Scratcherd T. Sensory afferents from the gastrointestinal tract. In: Schultz SG, Wood JD, Rauner BB, eds. *Handbook of Physiology*. Vol. 1. Section 6. New York: Oxford University Press, 1989: 593–620.
7. Tache Y. Central control of gastrointestinal transit and motility by brain gut peptides. In: Snape WJ, ed. *Pathogenesis of Functional Bowel Disease*. New York: Plenum Medical Book Company, 1989: 55–78.
8. Uehara A, Kitamori S, Harada K, Takasugi Y. Gastric antisecretory and antiulcer actions of interleukin-1: evidence for the presence of an 'immune-brain-gut axis'. *J Clin Gastroenterol* 1992; **14** (Suppl 1): S149–S155.
9. Mayer EA, Raybould HE. Role of visceral afferent mechanisms in functional bowel disorders. *Gastroenterology* 1990; **99**: 1688–704.
10. Mayer EA, Gebhart GF. Basic and clinical aspects of visceral hyperalgesia. *Gastroenterology* 1994; **107**: 271–93.
11. Besbaum AI, Fields HL. Endogenous pain control systems: brainstem spinal pathways and endorphin circuitry. *Ann Rev Neurosci* 1984; **7**: 309–38.
12. Mayer EA, Raybould H, Koelbel C. Neuropeptides, inflammation and motility. *Dig Dis Sci* 1988; **33** (Suppl): 71S–7S.
13. Randich A, Gebhart GF. Vagal afferent modulation of nociception. *Brain Res Rev* 1992; **17**: 77–99.
14. Crease RP. Biomedicine in the age of imaging. *Science* 1993; **261**: 554–61.
15. Aziz Q, Furlong PL, Barlow J, Hobson A, Alani S, Bancewicz J, Ribbands M, Harding GFA, Thompson DG. Topographic mapping of cortical potentials evoked by distension of the human proximal and distal oesophagus. *Electroenceph Clin Neurophysiol* 1995; **96**: 219–28.
16. Frieling T, Enck P, Wienbeck M. Cerebral responses evoked by electrical stimulation of the esophagus in normal subjects. *Gastroenterology* 1989; **97**: 475–8.
17. Frieling T, Enck P, Wienbeck M. Cerebral responses evoked by electrical stimulation of rectosigmoid in normal subjects. *Dig Dis Sci* 1989; **34**: 202–5.
18. Furlong PL, Aziz Q, Singh K, Holliday I, Barnes I, Harding GFA, Thompson DG. Localization of cortical centres for human esophageal sensation using magnetoencephalography. (Abstr) *Gastroenterology* 1995; A726.
19. Aziz Q, Andersson J, Valind S, Sundin A, Langstrom, Hamdy S, Jones AKP, Thompson DG. Identification of cortical loci processing human oesophageal sensation using positron emission tomography. (Abstr) *Gut* 1996; in press.
20. Jalinous R. Technical and practical aspects of magnetic nerve stimulation. *J Clin Neurophysiol* 1991; **8**(1): 10–25.
21. Aziz Q, Rothwell JC, Barlow J, Thompson DG. Modulation of oesophageal responses to magneto-electric stimulation of the human brain by swallowing and by vagal stimulation. *Gastroenterology* 1995; **109**: 1437–45.
22. Hamdy S, Aziz Q, Rothwell JC, Singh K, Barlow J, Hughes DG, Tallis RC, Thompson DG. The cortical topography of swallowing motor function in man. *Nature Med* 1996; **2**: 1217–24.
23. Stadaas JO. Intragastric pressure/volume relationship before and after proximal gastric vagotomy. *Scand J Gastroenterol* 1975; **10**: 129–34.
24. Smout AJP, DeVore MS, Dalton CB, Castell DO. Cerebral potentials evoked by oesophageal distension in patients with non-cardiac chest pain. *Gut* 1992; **33**: 298–302.

25 Loening-Baucke V, Yamada T. Is the afferent pathway from the rectum impaired in children with chronic constipation and encopresis. *Gastroenterology* 1995; **109**: 397–403.
26 Silverman DHS, Ennes H, Munakata J, Hoh C, Mandelkern M, Phelps M, Mayer EA. Regional cerebral blood flow patterns during experience and anticipation of rectal pain in IBS patients. (Abstr) *Neurogastroenterol Motility* 1995; 7: 135.
27 Hamdy S, Crone R, Aziz Q, Rothwell JC, Tallis RC, Thompson DG. Does dysphagia in unilateral hemispheric stroke depend on cerebral asymmetry of swallowing motor function? (Abstr) *J Physiol* 1996; **491**(P): 118P.

☐ MULTIPLE CHOICE QUESTIONS

1 Neural connections between the brain and the gut:
   (a) Function of the striated muscle of the oesophagus is regulated by the myenteric plexus
   (b) Sectioning of the extrinsic nerves paralyses the smooth muscle regions of the gut
   (c) Cell bodies of vagal afferents lie in the nodose ganglia
   (d) Vagus nerve is predominantly composed of efferent fibres
   (e) Convergence of visceral and somatic afferents occurs at the level of the spinal cord

2 Origin and modulation of gut sensation:
   (a) Vagal afferents transmit information about noxious events
   (b) The central nervous system modulates gut sensation via excitatory and inhibitory descending pathways
   (c) Function of primary afferent fibres within the gut wall may be altered by descending influences from the central nervous system
   (d) Vagal afferents have an excitatory influence on spinal afferents
   (e) Vagal and spinal afferents mediate different gut sensations

3 Investigation of the brain–gut axis in man:
   (a) Cortical evoked potentials represent cortical magnetic fields generated in response to peripheral nerve stimulation
   (b) Magnetoencephalography provides better spatial resolution of cortical sources than cortical evoked potentials
   (c) Positron emission tomography provides information about cortical events occurring from millisecond to millisecond
   (d) Positron emission tomography is not appropriate for repeated studies in healthy volunteers
   (e) Magnetic fields are altered as they pass through the skull

4 Studies of gut afferent and efferent pathways:
   (a) Oesophageal sensation is processed by multiple cortical sources
   (b) The oesophagus is viscerotopically organized on the cerebral cortex
   (c) Nociceptive oesophageal sensation is processed exclusively in the primary somatosensory cortex

(d) Swallowing muscles are symmetrically represented on each cortical hemisphere
(e) Sensory feedback plays an important role in the modulation of swallowing

5 Brain–gut axis in disease:
(a) Dysphagia only occurs following bilateral cortical damage
(b) In functional gut disorders abdominal pain occurs in the absence of organic disease
(c) Loss of spinal inhibitory influence on vagal afferents is responsible for pain in functional bowel disorders
(d) In patients with irritable bowel syndrome processing of painful sensation by the central nervous system may be abnormal
(e) Dysphagia following unilateral hemispheric stroke may occur due to damage to the dominant cortical swallowing centre

ANSWERS

1a False	2a False	3a False	4a True	5a False
b False	b True	b True	b True	b True
c True	c False	c False	c False	c False
d False	d False	d True	d False	d True
e True	e True	e False	e True	e True

Management of acute liver failure

J G O'Grady

☐ INTRODUCTION

There are at least 500 hospitalizations to specialist centres in the UK annually for acute liver failure. The combination of advances in the medical and surgical treatment has brought more hope and determination to the management of this emergency. Early recognition and referral of appropriate patients maximizes their chances of getting the full benefit of the available treatment options which now offer survival rates of between 40% and 90%, depending on aetiology and category.

☐ TERMINOLOGY

Acute liver failure is a heterogeneous condition with the underlying aetiology and the rate of progression of the disease, in particular, influencing the manifestation of the syndrome. New terminology has been proposed to render the clinical syndromes more meaningful with respect to the assessment of prognosis and management [1]. The core term is acute liver failure (ALF) and this is prefixed by hyper- or sub- to describe the two cohorts at either end of the temporal spectrum (Table 1).

Hyperacute liver failure (HALF)

Paradoxically this group has the highest likelihood of recovery with medical management irrespective of the underlying prognosis. This is despite the rapid deterioration, the high incidence of cerebral oedema and the severe prolongation of prothrombin time (PT).

Table 1 Characteristics of subgroups of patients with acute liver failure.

	Hyperacute liver failure	Acute liver failure	Subacute liver failure
Encephalopathy	Yes	Yes	Yes
Duration of jaundice	0–7 days	8–28 days	29–84 days
Cerebral oedema	Common (69%)	Common (56%)	Unusual (14%)
PT – mean peak	64 s	72 s	46 s
Survival rates 1973–85[*]	36%	7%	14%

[*] For all cases with grade 3–4 encephalopathy admitted to the liver unit during that period and before the application of liver transplantation to patients with ALF

Acute liver failure (ALF)

This group best fits the classic image of this condition with high mortality, high incidence of cerebral oedema and marked prolongation of PT.

Subacute liver failure (SALF)

This is also characterized by high mortality despite a very low incidence of cerebral oedema. The much less dramatic prolongation of PT, together with the slow and often erratic deterioration, may mask the severity of the condition leading to delay in referral to a specialist unit.

☐ AETIOLOGY AND DIAGNOSIS

The aetiology of ALF varies geographically as illustrated by the breakdown of underlying causes in the UK, France and the USA (Table 2). Paracetamol remains a disproportionately high contributor in the UK and there is little evidence to suggest a decrease in its incidence. Viral hepatitis, however, is the most common aetiology worldwide, with hepatitis A (HAV) and hepatitis B with or without hepatitis D accounting for the vast majority of cases of definable aetiology. Asymptomatic chronic carriers of the hepatitis B virus (HBV) are at risk of ALF through super-infection with the hepatitis D virus (HDV) or as a consequence of a spontaneous increase in viral replication manifest by a sharp rise in circulating HBV deoxyribonucleic acid (DNA) levels. The role of hepatitis E (HEV) is mainly confined to endemic areas such as the Indian subcontinent, although occasional cases are seen in the UK. Hepatitis C (HCV) is a very rare cause of ALF and the early indications are that hepatitis G is unlikely to account for many of the cases of ALF so far attributed to non-A,non-B hepatitis. This group remains the single most common cause of ALF worldwide and is currently being referred to as having seronegative hepatitis, non-A-E hepatitis or ALF of indeterminate aetiology.

Table 2 Geographical variations in the main aetiologies of acute liver failure.

Aetiology	Acute liver failure (%) in		
	UK	France	USA
Paracetamol overdose	54.1	2	16
Viral	36.5	70	65
hepatitis A	4.9	4	7
hepatitis B ± D	9.0	45	18
seronegative hepatitis*	16.5	18	39
other viral causes	0.6	3	0.6
drug reactions	6.9	14.5	10
Miscellaneous	3.9	12	9

*Also called cryptogenic and of indeterminate aetiology

Ecstasy (methylenedioxymethamphetamine) is a synthetic amphetamine used recreationally and its ingestion is being recognized as an important emerging cause of ALF. It has been documented to cause all the syndromes of ALF ranging from hyperacute liver failure with the added clinical feature of hyperpyrexia to subacute liver failure. Wilson's disease may present as ALF, typically during the second decade of life, and in the majority of cases is characterized by a Coomb's negative haemolytic anaemia and demonstrable Kayser–Fleischer rings. Other less common causes of ALF are listed in Table 3. The incidence, diagnosis and epidemiology of the main aetiologies of ALF are given in Table 4.

☐ MANAGEMENT STRATEGIES

The current management of ALF is a combination of the treatment of multivisceral failure together with the use of liver transplantation in those with a particularly poor prognosis. As mentioned above, early recognition and prompt referral of cases to specialist centres is important. Guidelines for the referral of paracetamol-induced ALF are given in Table 5. SALF now represents the group where delayed referral most frequently affects the management options, as many of these patients have developed sepsis, malnutrition or other (relative) contraindications to liver transplantation by the time they present to specialist centres. Guidelines for referral of aetiologies other than paracetamol are given in Table 6.

Different criteria have been identified for use in specialist centres to identify the cohort most in need of liver transplantation (Table 7) [2]. These are now widely used, are simple and fast, and have recently been described as the best available [3]. However, they are not perfect and are liable to modification with improvement in survival rates with both medical management and liver transplantation. In the original analysis the discriminatory power of a metabolic acidosis with an arterial pH <7.30 on the second or subsequent day after a paracetamol overdose was very

Table 3 Causes of acute liver failure.

Viral
Hepatitis A, hepatitis B ± D, hepatitis E, seronegative presumed viral hepatitis.
Rare viral causes include hepatitis C, herpes simplex, human herpes virus 6, varicella, cytomegalovirus and Epstein-Barr virus.

Drug and chemical
Paracetamol, halothane, 'ecstasy', carbon tetrachloride, *Amanita phalloides* (mushroom poisoning) and idiosyncratic reactions to a range of drugs including non-steroidal anti-inflammatory drugs (NSAIDs), benoxyprofen, gold, sulphonamides, tetracycline, ketoconazole, monoamine oxidase inhibitors (MAOIs), tricyclic antidepressants, flutamide, allopurinol, sodium valproate, carbamazepine, phenytoin, disulphiram, methyldopa, amiodarone, propylthiouracil, 2,3-dideoxyinosine (ddI).

Other causes
Wilson's disease, pregnancy related syndromes (fatty liver of pregnancy, toxaemia related, HELLP syndrome), vascular insults including Budd-Chiari syndrome, autoimmune disease (often only positive for anti-KLM autoantibodies), malignancy (especially lymphoma and breast), sepsis and hyperthermia.

Table 4 Incidence, diagnosis and epidemiological features of main aetiologies of acute liver failure.

Aetiology	Incidence (%)	Diagnosis	Epidemiology
Hepatitis A	0.14–0.35	Immunoglobulin (IgM) HAV	Increasing incidence, especially in older people
			Vaccine available for those at risk
Hepatitis B	1–4	Acute – IgM anticore Recurrence – HBV DNA	Vaccine available for those at risk
Hepatitis E	?	Research tool	Water-borne infection in endemic areas
			Risk greatest in pregnancy, especially last trimester
Seronegative hepatitis	2.3–4.7	Diagnosis of exclusion	Sporadic, female predominance
Paracetamol	—	History of ingestion Blood levels may be useful	Enzyme induction by alcohol or drugs increases risk
Halothane hepatitis	—	More than one exposure	Incidence dramatically reduced
Other idiosyncratic drug reactions	Variable	History of exposure	Sporadic and largely unpredictable
			Increase in cases due to anti-TB therapy
Ecstasy	Unknown	History, toxicology	Increasing, especially 16–25 year olds

Table 5 Guidelines for referral of patients to specialist centres following paracetamol overdose.

Day 2	Day 3	Day 4
Arterial pH <7.30	Encephalopathy	Encephalopathy
International ratio (INR) >3.0 or PT >50 s	Arterial pH <7.30	INR >6 or PT >100 s
Hypoglycaemia	INR >4.5 or PT >75 s	Progressive rise in PT irrespective of value
Oliguria	Oliguria	Oliguria
Creatinine >200 µmol/l	Creatinine >200 µmol/l	Creatinine >250 µmol/l
Severe thrombocytopenia		

Table 6 Guidelines for referral of patients to specialist centres for other aetiologies. The presence of *any* feature should prompt referral.

Hyperacute	Acute	Subacute
Encephalopathy	Encephalopathy	Encephalopathy
PT >30 s	PT >30 s	PT >20 s
Renal failure	Renal failure	Renal failure
		Serum sodium <130 µmol/l
		Shrinking liver volume

Table 7 Selection criteria for liver transplantation.

Paracetamol	Other aetiologies
Arterial pH <7.30*	PT >100 s or INR >6.7
or *all three* of following:	or *any* three of following:
PT >100 s	Unfavourable aetiology (seronegative hepatitis,
Creatinine >300 μmol/l	halothane hepatitis or drug reaction)
Grade 3–4 encephalopathy	Jaundice >7 days before encephalopathy
	Age <10 or >40 years
	PT >50 s or INR >4.0
	Serum bilirubin >300 μmol/l

NB All patients with Wilson's disease developing encephalopathy should be considered for transplantation
* Threshold reduced to pH <7.25 in some centres (see text)

strong. Changes in subsequent medical practices, especially the more liberal use of N-acetylcysteine and more aggressive early rehydration, appear to have improved the survival rate in these patients and consequently the discriminatory threshold has been reduced to pH <7.25 in some centres. This practice awaits validation. Survival rates for the first 10 years of liver transplantation for ALF were in the 50–65% range in most centres and consequently it was only considered for patients who otherwise had a less than 20% chance of recovery. As will be discussed later, the survival rates after transplantation are belatedly showing the improvement previously documented for the overall transplant population. As a result, if survival rates of 80–90% are consistently attainable for transplantation in ALF, it may be considered reasonable to extend transplantation to patients with a 20–40% chance of recovery with medical management. It is possible that biotechnological developments may also impact on the construction of management strategies in the future.

☐ GENERAL MEASURES

A considerable number of general management measures have been tested in ALF and are reviewed elsewhere (Table 8), but those that have been subjected to controlled trials have produced disappointing results [4]. An exception was the use of N-acetylcysteine in paracetamol-induced ALF, despite not being started until 36–80 h after ingestion of the drug [5]. The patients receiving N-acetylcysteine had significantly lower incidences of cerebral oedema and haemodynamic instability, and a higher survival rate than the control group. These findings, together with the observations of the beneficial effects that N-acetylcysteine had on oxygen debt, have led to an extended role for this drug in paracetamol-induced ALF. The possible value of N-acetylcysteine in ALF of other aetiologies has not been adequately tested. Extracorporeal circuits incorporating hepatocytes of pig, tumour cell lines and normal human hepatocytes are under development, but will need to be assessed by carefully constructed controlled studies.

Table 8 General management measures in acute liver failure.

Measure	Controlled trials	Comment
Corticosteroids	Yes	Old study, no benefit seen
Interferon	No	No benefit seen in larger study
Insulin and glucagon	Yes	No survival benefit
Prostaglandin E_1	Yes	No survival benefit
N-Acetylcysteine	Yes	Beneficial in paracetamol cases
Bowel decontamination	Yes	Inconclusive results
Charcoal haemoperfusion	Yes	No survival benefit, re-emerging as component of some extracorporeal circuits incorporating hepatocytes
Resin haemoperfusion	No	Preliminary studies only, inconclusive
Extracorporeal circuits	No	In development, studies awaited

☐ SPECIFIC COMPLICATIONS

ALF has the potential to result in complex multiorgan failure requiring specialist intensive care [4,6]. The main complications and the salient points of their management are outlined in Table 9. Cerebral oedema, sepsis and haemodynamic instability are the most important complications and account for the majority of deaths in these patients. Cerebral oedema is seen mainly in HALF and ALF and is best managed using multimodality monitoring of intracranial pressure, cerebral blood and perfusion pressures, electroencephalograms (EEG) and brain oxygen utilization. The threat from cerebral oedema persists during and for the first 24 hours after liver transplantation and failure of brain recovery has been documented after otherwise successful transplants. Mannitol remains the first-line therapy, while barbiturates, low tidal volume hyperventilation and hepatectomy may be transiently helpful in very unstable situations. The maximization of the cerebral perfusion pressure and oxygen delivery to the brain are also critical in the more advanced stages of this complication.

Sepsis is a common cause of disqualification from eligibility for transplantation as well as a major cause of death. The diagnosis of both bacterial and fungal infections may be very difficult, and low indices of suspicion coupled with aggressive intervention with antimicrobial agents are necessary. Sepsis is also a factor driving the profound haemodynamic instability frequently encountered in these patients. High and escalating inotrope requirements may also constitute a contraindication to transplantation. Vasopressor agents should be combined with microcirculatory protection with N-acetylcysteine or prostacycline to prevent a deleterious effect on oxygen delivery and consumption.

☐ LIVER TRANSPLANTATION

Orthotopic liver transplantation has revolutionized the management of ALF by offering a lifeline to those cases that have a poor prognosis despite all the advances

Table 9 Specific complications of acute liver failure.

Complication	Incidence	Comments and treatment
Cerebral oedema	HALF 69%	Intensive monitoring required in HALF and ALF
	ALF 56%	Minimize auditory and tactile stimuli
	SALF 14%	Treat as per text
Renal failure	Paracetamol 75%	Continuous haemofiltration systems preferred
	Other aetiologies 30%	Early intervention advised
Sepsis	Bacterial 85%	Early and aggressive treatment
	Fungal 30%	
Hypotension	Very common	Aggressive monitoring and treat as per text
Hypoglycaemia	Very common	Hourly blood glucose estimations
Respiratory failure	Common	Multifactorial in causation
		Early ventilatory support, inhalation of NO in severe cases
Coagulopathy	Universal	Treat significant bleeding only (unless decision with respect to transplantation has already been made)
		Pay special attention to platelet count
		Prophylactic gastric mucosal protection
Pancreatitis	Paracetamol 15%	High index of suspicion required
	Rest – less common	May contraindicate transplantation if severe
Malnutrition	Increases with duration of illness	Parenteral feeding generally tolerated
Electrolytes	Very common	Sodium, potassium, phosphate, magnesium especially important
Acid–base abnormalities	Common	Metabolic alkalosis dominates apart from most severe paracetamol cases

in supportive care. As mentioned above, until recently survival rates after transplantation ranged from 50% to 65% in most centres, but the latest reports cite survival rates in excess of 85% [7]. Studies that have addressed the applicability of liver transplantation to ALF have consistently shown that about half of all cases (excluding paracetamol-induced cases) that are admitted are transplanted. The remainder are, to varying degrees, patients not considered to need transplants, patients dying while awaiting transplantation and patients considered to have contraindications to transplantation at the time of presentation. The equivalent figure for paracetamol-induced cases in the UK is much lower due to the rapidly progressive disease and the need to consider socio-psychiatric as well as medical criteria.

Heterotopic and orthotopic auxiliary liver transplantation have been used and this approach is especially attractive for cases that have the capacity to regain normal liver function after recovery from ALF. This allows immunosuppression to be withdrawn after the native liver has recovered, sparing the patient the need for lifelong immunosuppressive therapy. The precise indications for this approach are not yet clear as some of the immediate advantages of liver transplantation result from the removal of the necrotic liver rather than the implantation of functioning tissue. Therefore data are required to define the critical mass of native necrotic liver tolerated, and functional transplanted liver required, at the main evolutionary stages of the disease.

REFERENCES

1. O'Grady JG, Schalm SW, Williams R. Acute liver failure: redefining the syndromes. *Lancet* 1993; **342**: 273–5.
2. O'Grady JG, Alexander GJM, Hayllar KM, Williams R. Early indicators of prognosis in fulminant hepatic failure. *Gastroenterology* 1989; **97**: 439–45.
3. Lake JR, Sussman NL. Determining prognosis in patients with fulminant hepatic failure: when you absolutely have to know the answer. (Editorial) *Hepatology* 1995; **21**: 879–82.
4. O'Grady JG, Portmann BC, Williams R. Fulminant hepatic failure. In: Schiff E, Schiff L, eds. *Diseases of the Liver*. Philadelphia: JB Lippincott Co, 1993: 1077–90.
5. Harrison PM, Keays R, Bray GP, Alexander GJM, Williams R. Late *N*-acetylcysteine administration improves outcome for patients developing paracetamol-induced fulminant hepatic failure. *Lancet* 1990; **i**: 1572–3.
6. Lee WM. Medical progress. Acute liver failure. *New Engl J Med* 1993; **329**: 1862–72.
7. Ascher NL, Lake JR, Emond JC, Roberts JP. Liver transplantation for fulminant hepatic failure. *Arch Surg* 1993; **128**: 677–82.

☐ MULTIPLE CHOICE QUESTIONS

1. Acute liver failure:
   (a) Is diagnosed on the basis of a prolonged prothrombin time
   (b) Is due to hepatitis B when HBsAg is positive in serum
   (c) Is rarely due to hepatitis C
   (d) May be due to 'ecstasy'
   (e) Is increasingly caused by hepatitis A

2. Isolated bad prognostic indicators in acute liver failure include:
   (a) Age under 10 years
   (b) Pregnancy related aetiologies
   (c) Rapid onset of encephalopathy
   (d) Prothrombin time >100 s in paracetamol cases
   (e) Prothrombin time >100 s in non-paracetamol cases

3. The following are of proven benefit in the management of acute liver failure:
   (a) Corticosteroids
   (b) Mannitol
   (c) *N*-Acetylcysteine
   (d) Interferon
   (e) Prostaglandin E_1

4. Liver transplantation for acute liver failure:
   (a) Is used in about half the non-paracetamol cases

(b) Carries survival rates under 50%
   (c) May use auxiliary grafts orthotopically
   (d) May be preceded by hepatectomy by up to 20 h
   (e) May be followed by failure of neurological recovery

5 The complications of acute liver failure include:
   (a) Renal failure in 75% of paracetamol cases
   (b) Pancreatitis in 15% of viral cases
   (c) Metabolic alkalosis
   (d) Oxygen debt
   (e) Hypercalcaemia

ANSWERS

1a False	2a True	3a False	4a True	5a True
b False	b False	b True	b False	b False
c True	c False	c True	c True	c True
d True	d False	d False	d True	d True
e True	e True	e False	e True	e False

Management of chronic viral hepatitis

M Ahmed and E Elias

☐ INTRODUCTION

Viral hepatitis is an infection of the liver by one or more of the hepatitis viruses resulting in inflammation. There are seven lettered hepatitis viruses: A, B, C, D, E, F (as yet uncharacterized) and G (Table 1). Hepatitis A and E can cause acute hepatitis but do not result in chronic liver disease. However, hepatitis B, C, G and D (in the presence of hepatitis B virus) may result in chronicity.

☐ HEPATITIS B

Hepatitis B virus (HBV) is a DNA virus belonging to the hepadnavirus family (Fig. 1). Chronic HBV infection is a serious health problem globally, with an estimated 300 million HB surface antigen (HBsAg) positive individuals accounting for approximately 5% of the world's population. Some 80% of these chronic carriers are of Oriental origin. In adult-acquired infection, chronicity results in approximately 10% of cases, while perinatal infection results in chronicity in 90%

Table 1 Characteristics of the hepatitis viruses.

Virus	Nucleic acid	Family	Size	Transmission	Clinical course
Hepatitis A (HAV)	Ribonucleic acid (RNA)	Picornavirus	~27 nm	Faeco-oral, enteric, water-borne	Acute, never chronic
Hepatitis B (HBV)	Deoxyribonucleic acid (DNA)	Hepadnavirus	42 nm	Parenteral especially blood transfusion and needle injection, sexual, mother to child	Acute and chronic. Carrier state exists. Increased risk of hepatoma
Hepatitis C (HCV)	RNA	Flavivirus, Pestivirus	55 nm	Parenteral especially blood transfusion and needle injection, many covert infections	Acute and chronic. Increased risk of hepatoma
Hepatitis D (HDV)	RNA	Plant viroid, virusoids or plant satellite RNA (?)	36 nm (some 40 nm)	As for HBV	Acute and chronic. Associated with chronic HBV infection
Hepatitis E (HEV)	RNA	Calcivirus	32–34 nm	As for HAV	Acute, never chronic, high mortality in pregnancy
Hepatitis G (HGV)	RNA	Flavivirus	?	?As for HCV	Acute and chronic. Long-term effect not known

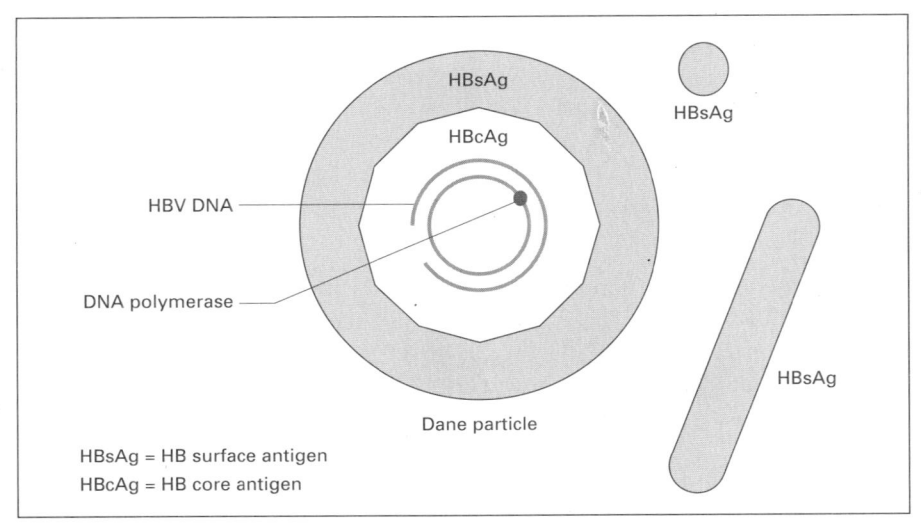

Fig. 1 Hepatitis B virus.

of cases. The natural history of liver disease caused by persistent HBV infection can be variable and is summarized for adult-acquired infection in Fig. 2.

Chronic HBV infection

Chronic HBV infection may be divided into three phases (Fig. 3). These phases can be summarized as follows.

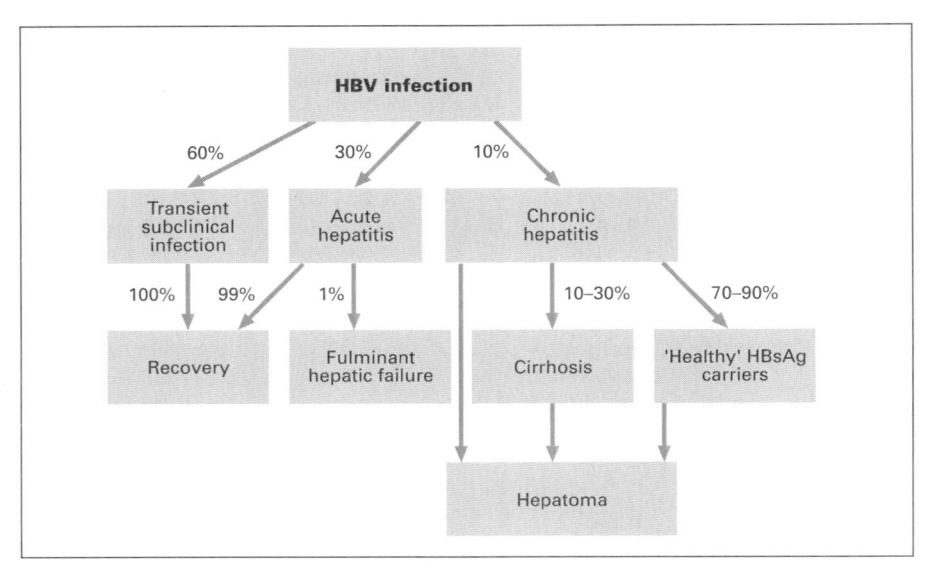

Fig. 2 Outcome of HBV infection acquired in adulthood.

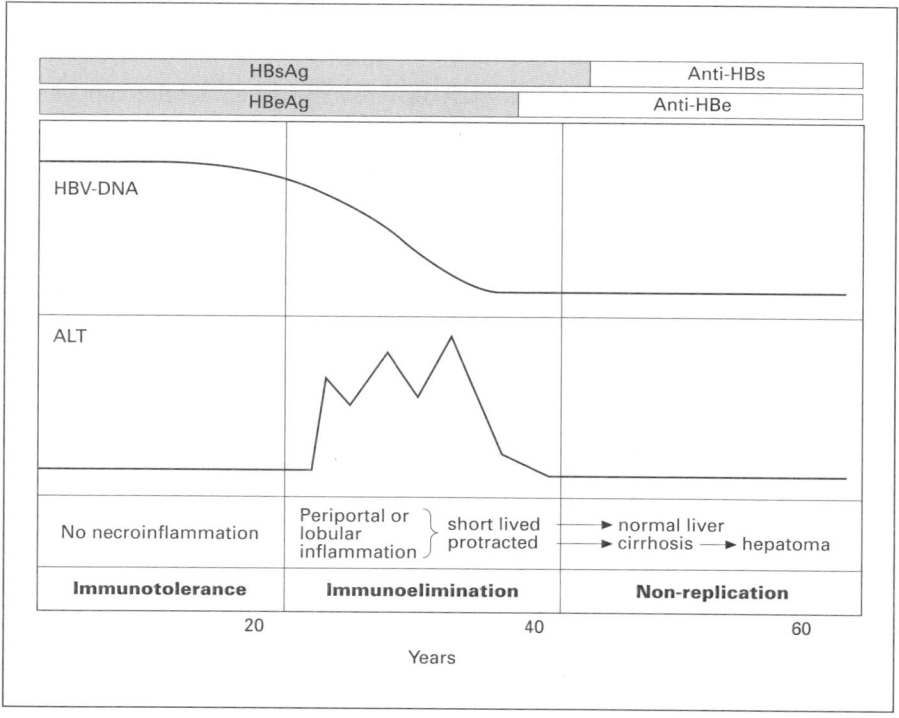

Fig. 3 Natural history of HBV (wild type).

1. *Viral replication associated with immunotolerance:*
   - Virus is replicating
   - Host is immunotolerant
   - High titres of HBsAg, anti-HBc, HBV DNA and HBeAg
   - Normal serum ALT (aminotransferase) levels
   - No necroinflammation in liver.

2. *Viral replication associated with immunoelimination (seroconversion):*
   - Virus is fluctuating or constant level of viraemia
   - Host shows immunoelimination
   - Persistence of HBsAg, HBV DNA and HBeAg or anti-HBe; raised immunoglobulin (IgM) anti-HBc
   - Raised serum ALT levels
   - Necroinflammatory activity in liver.

3. *Viral non-replication (latent infection):*
- ☐ Virus is non-replicating
- ☐ HBsAg is present (1–2% will lose HBsAg ever year and develop anti-HBs); HBeAg and HBV DNA negative
- ☐ Normal serum ALT levels
- ☐ Variable liver histology ranging from normal to cirrhosis.

Treatment of chronic hepatitis B virus

Aims of treatment

The primary aims of treating chronic HBV are to suppress HBV replication, to reduce infectivity and to induce remission of associated liver disease. The secondary aims of treatment are to eradicate HBV (rendering the host HBsAg negative), to prevent development of cirrhosis and hepatoma and to improve survival.

When to treat chronic HBV

Antiviral therapy for HBV is indicated for patients with chronic infection who have active viral replication within the liver. Such patients are HBsAg positive, HBeAg positive (unless pre-core mutant virus is present) and HBV DNA positive by hybridization assay.

Interferon for chronic HBV

Table 2 lists the agents evaluated in humans for the treatment of chronic HBV infection. At present, interferon-alpha is the only licensed treatment in USA and UK. Interferons (IFN) are a family of naturally occurring proteins produced by certain cells in response to stimuli such as foreign nucleic acids, foreign cells, bacteria and viral antigens. The three main types of IFN are designated alpha, beta and gamma. They have a wide range of effects, including direct antiviral and antitumour responses as well as modulation and enhancement of the cell-mediated immune system.

IFN-alpha is the most widely used agent for the treatment of chronic HBV infection. About 30% of patients treated with IFN-alpha clear HBeAg and HBV DNA from serum and 3–24% also clear HBsAg. Two recently published meta-analyses confirmed that IFN-alpha treatment was better than no therapy, with loss of markers of viral replication (HBeAg and HBV DNA) occurring 20% more often in treated patients and loss of HBsAg occurring 6% more often in treated patients [1,2]. Successful antiviral response is usually accompanied by biochemical and histological evidence of improvement of liver disease. Generally, successful treatment requires at least 3 months of IFN-alpha at a dose of 5–10 MU administered three times a week (Fig. 4).

Interferon treatment for HBV – prognostic indicators

Factors that predict the likelihood of response to IFN-alpha are listed in Table 3. Favourable factors include low levels of viral DNA, high serum ALT levels and active

Table 2 Agents evaluated in humans for the treatment of chronic HBV infection.

Interferon
- ☐ alpha
- ☐ beta
- ☐ gamma

Antiviral agents
- ☐ Acyclovir
- ☐ Foscarnet
- ☐ Azidothymidine (zidovudine)
- ☐ Adenine arabinoside (Ara A and Ara-AMP)
- ☐ Fialuridine (FIAU)
- ☐ Dideoxyinosine
- ☐ Ribavirin
- ☐ Lamivudine

Immunomodulation
- ☐ Prednisolone
- ☐ Levamizole
- ☐ Interleukin-2 (IL-2)
- ☐ Granular macrophage colony-stimulating factor (GM-CSF)

Combination
- ☐ IFN-alpha + prednisolone
- ☐ IFN-alpha + Ara AMP
- ☐ IFN-alpha + levamisole
- ☐ IFN-alpha + IL-2
- ☐ IFN-alpha + acyclovir
- ☐ More than one type of IFN

Others
- ☐ Phyllanthrus amarus

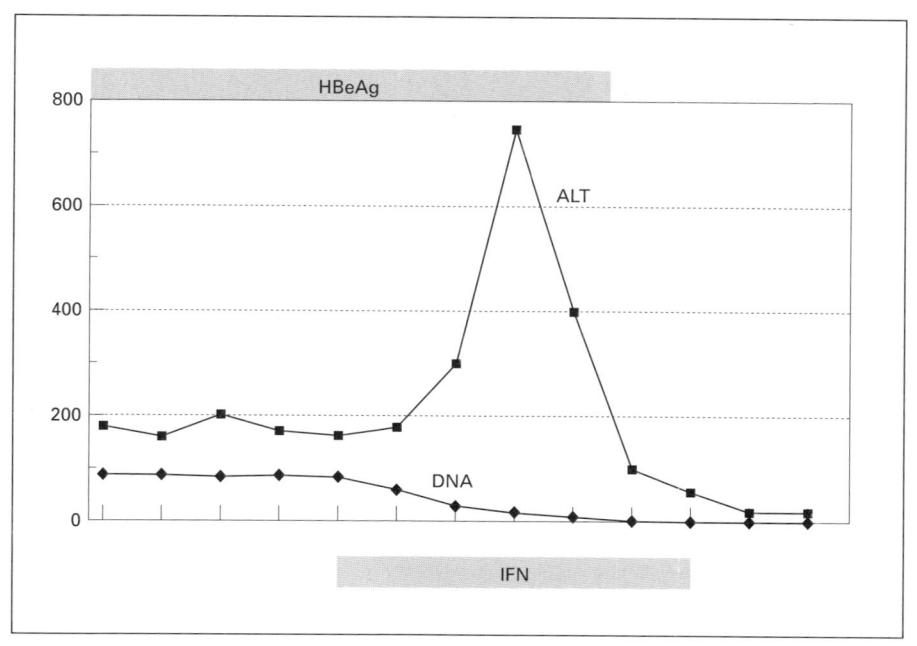

Fig. 4 Successful treatment of chronic HBV infection with IFN-alpha 6 MU three times a week for 6 months. Note the ALT 'flare' prior to the clearance of HBeAg.

Table 3 Factors associated with response to IFN-alpha in chronic HBV.

Favourable	Unfavourable
Caucasian	Asian
Female	Male
Recent onset	Long-standing
Icteric	Anicteric
Active liver histology	Inactive liver histology
High transaminase	Low transaminase
Low HBV DNA	High HBV DNA
Heterosexual	Homosexual
anti-HIV negative	anti-HIV positive
anti-HDV negative	anti-HDV positive

liver histology. These factors reflect a strong host immune response attempting to lyse infected hepatocytes.

Steroid pretreatment

Retrospective analysis of studies performed in the 1970s suggested that withdrawal of corticosteroids frequently resulted in an acute flare in transaminase levels which was thought to represent 'immunological rebound'. Several randomized control studies have compared the response rates of IFN alone to that of prednisolone pretreatment followed by IFN. No single randomized control trial shows a statistically significant difference between the two treatments. However, a recent meta-analysis suggests that, in patients with low or normal pretreatment ALT levels, sequential prednisolone-IFN treatment may be useful [3]. Patients with normal pretreatment ALT levels generally have high serum levels of HBV DNA (Fig. 5).

Non-responders

About 60% of treated patients do not respond to a 4 month course of IFN. In most studies, a second course of therapy has been shown to be unhelpful. The EUROHEP study group is currently looking into the effect of an additional 4 month treatment in the non-responder group. An alternative approach to the management of patients who have failed to respond is prednisolone pretreatment followed by IFN. Another approach would be to re-treat patients during a phase when they appear to be better candidates for therapy, for example when they have high ALT levels and low HBV DNA levels (Fig. 6).

Delayed reactivation of HBV

In the first year following IFN-alpha treatment, reactivation of HBV replication has been reported in 5–50% of patients. Delayed reactivation after the first year (mostly

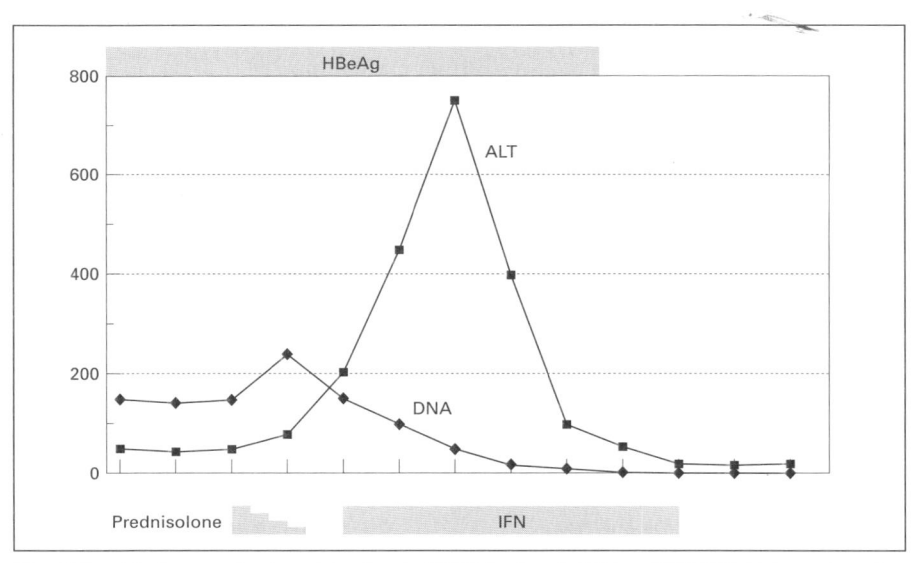

Fig. 5 Prednisolone pretreatment in chronic HBV infection if ALT low/HBV DNA high, eg tapering course of prednisolone over 6 weeks starting at 60 mg per day followed by 2 treatment-free weeks prior to 6 months of IFN therapy.

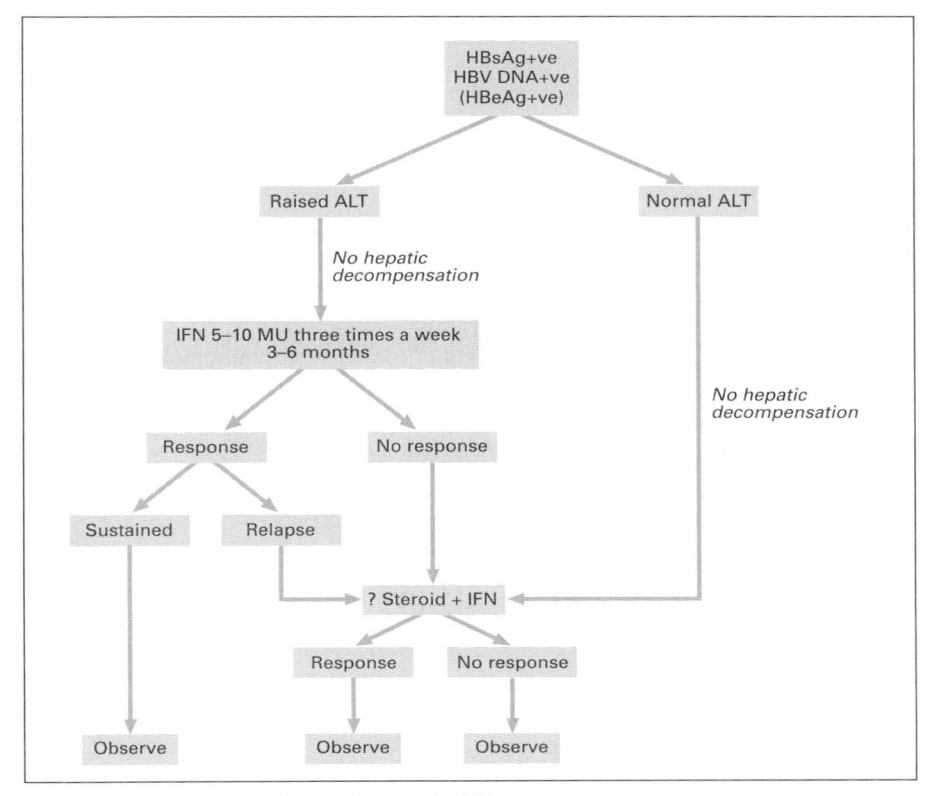

Fig. 6 Suggested strategy for treating chronic HBV.

during the second year) has been reported in 10–20% of initial responders. The management of these patients requires further evaluation.

Liver transplant for HBV related end-stage liver failure

Cirrhosis, hepatoma and end-stage liver failure (ESLF) are important sequelae of chronic HBV infection. Liver transplantation is the only effective therapy for ESLF (Fig. 7). Viral recurrence following transplantation is common, particularly in

```
                    End-stage liver failure
                         due to HBV
                    ┌──────────┴──────────┐
        Low levels of HBV          High levels of HBV replication
     replication pre-transplant        pre-transplant
      (HBeAg–ve, HBV DNA–ve)        (HBeAg+ve, HBV DNA+ve)
                │                             │
     Transplant with long-term HBIg    ? Transplant with alternative
              prophylaxis              prophylaxis, eg lamivudine
```

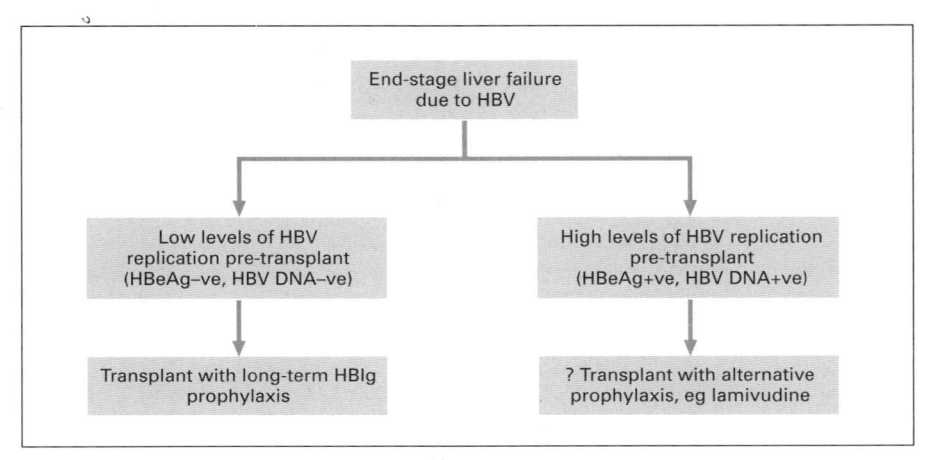

Fig. 7 Suggested strategy for management of end-stage liver failure due to HBV.

patients with markers of active viral replication (HBeAg and HBV DNA), prior to transplantation [4]. Aggressive viral recurrence may occur in the presence of immunosuppression, resulting in early cirrhosis and subacute liver failure due to fibrosing cholestatic hepatitis. Consequently graft and patient survival are poor compared to liver transplantation for other conditions.

Long-term immunoprophylaxis with polyclonal HBV immunoglobulin (HBIg) has been shown to be useful in preventing HBV recurrence in patients with low levels of viral replication (HBeAg negative/HBV DNA negative by hybridization assay) prior to transplant. In patients with high levels of viral replication (HBeAg positive/HBV DNA positive), alternative strategies using novel antiviral agents such as lamivudine or famcyclovir are currently being evaluated.

☐ **HEPATITIS D**

Chronic HDV tends to be a severe form of hepatitis related to a dual infection with HDV and HBV. HDV was originally described in Italy and seems to be most common in southern European countries. Patients with chronic HDV are more likely to develop cirrhosis (which occurs in 60–70% of cases) and liver failure than patients with chronic HBV alone.

Preliminary reports suggested that a 3–4 month course of IFN-alpha resulted in suppression of HDV replication and improvement in liver disease in some patients. However, in almost all cases discontinuation of therapy was followed by relapse. Farci et al. [5] found that, even after 12 months of IFN-alpha (9 MU three times a week), the majority had recurrence of hepatitis. The relapse was often delayed, sometimes occurring over a year after completion of treatment.

☐ HEPATITIS C

Hepatitis C (HCV) is an enveloped positive-stranded RNA virus related to the flaviviridae family (Fig. 8). In 1989, Choo et al. [6] isolated and cloned HCV from

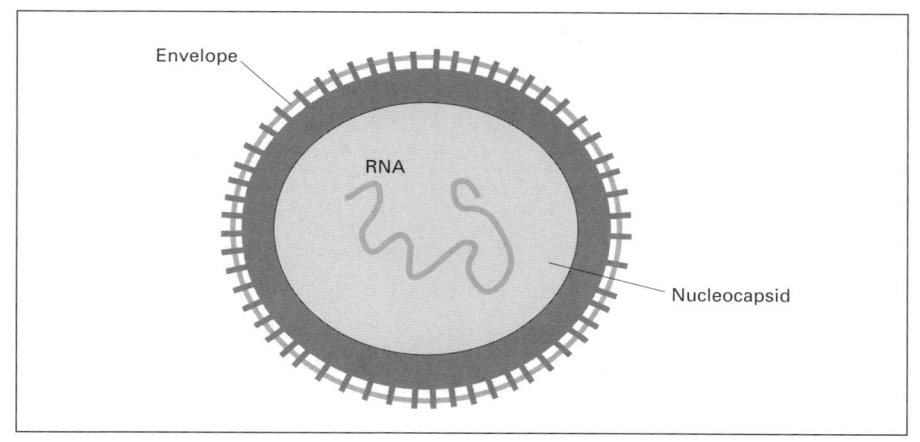

Fig. 8 Hepatitis C virus.

highly infectious chimpanzee plasma using a recombinant immunoscreening approach. Since then it has been shown that HCV accounts for the majority of cases of post-transfusion non-A non-B hepatitis (NANB).

The HCV RNA strand is approximately 10 000 nucleotides in length with a single, long, open reading frame. There are at least six major genotypes, which differ substantially in their nucleotide sequence and geographical distribution. Within each major genotype there may be a number of subtypes. HCV, like other RNA viruses, has a high rate of mutation. Infecting viruses may develop minor genetic variations and circulate as 'quasispecies' in patients.

The prevalence of HCV infection varies between countries and anti-HCV positivity is seen in 0.01–1.5% of blood donors worldwide. Infection by HCV is usually acquired parenterally, for example following transfusion of infected blood or blood products or in abusers of intravenous drugs. However, covert exposure also accounts for a large number of cases. Vertical and sexual transmission of HCV seem to be uncommon.

The natural history of HCV is incompletely understood (Fig. 9). Following acute infection, chronicity develops in at least 60% of patients. Chronic HCV is slowly progressive but at least 20% of infected patients may develop cirrhosis after 10 or 20

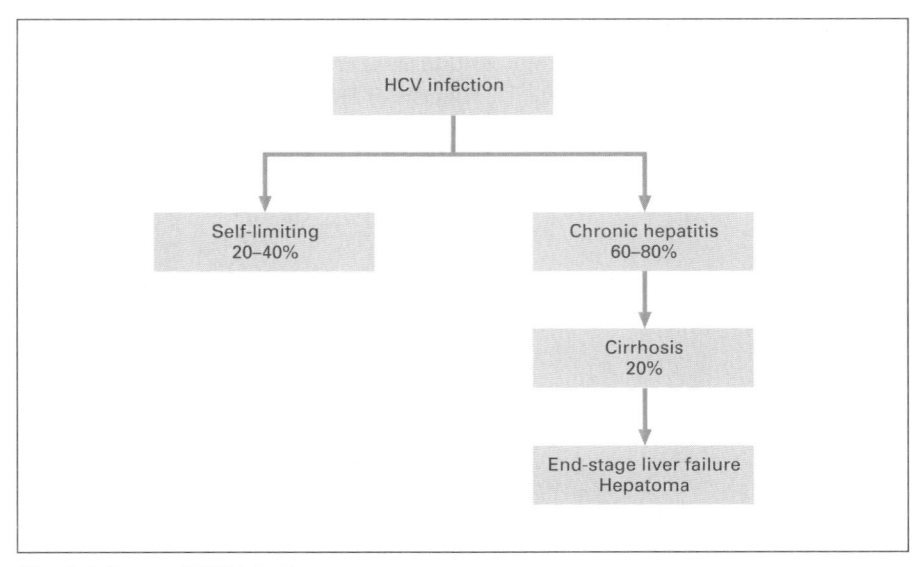

```
                    HCV infection
                   /            \
          Self-limiting      Chronic hepatitis
            20–40%              60–80%
                                   |
                                Cirrhosis
                                  20%
                                   |
                          End-stage liver failure
                                Hepatoma
```

Fig. 9 Outcome of HCV infection.

years. Cirrhotic patients may develop end-stage liver failure and are at an increased risk of developing hepatoma.

The treatment of patients with HCV depends on the stage of their disease. Most HCV-infected patients seen by clinicians have chronic asymptomatic disease. Patients with HCV-related cirrhosis and end-stage liver failure requiring liver transplantation are an increasingly important group.

Treatment of chronic HCV infection

Aims of treatment

The aims of treatment are to reduce disease progression, to eradicate HCV, to prevent development of cirrhosis and hepatoma and to improve survival.

Assessment of response

Generally, serial serum alanine aminotransferase (ALT) levels and changes in liver histology are used to monitor response to treatment. *Complete response* is said to occur if ALT levels are normal at the end of the treatment period, while *sustained response* is said to occur if ALT levels remain within normal limits in the follow-up period after cessation of treatment.

Objective assessment of histological changes is achieved using a scoring system such as the one proposed by Knodell *et al.* [7] or a modification as used on our unit (Table 4). The polymerase chain reaction (PCR) may be used to monitor HCV RNA in the serum and liver tissue. HCV quantitation may also be achieved using signal amplification with branched-chain DNA (bDNA).

Table 4 Assessment of liver biopsy using a histological activity index (HAI).

Inflammation

(i) Portal activity	(ii) Periportal activity	(iii) Lobular activity
0 none/minimal	0 none	0 none
1 mild	1 mild	1 spotty inflammation/necrosis
2 moderate	2 moderate	2 zonal necrosis
3 severe	3 severe	3 bridging necrosis

Fibrosis
0 none
1 mild expansion
2 early septa and spurs
3 established septa
4 cirrhosis

HAI = sum of the scores in the four categories; 0 is best, 13 is worst

Interferon for chronic HCV

At present IFN-alpha-2b is the only licensed treatment of chronic HCV in the USA and UK. IFN was first used for the treatment of NANB hepatitis in 1986 at the National Institutes of Health [8]. This was a small uncontrolled study where 10 patients with NANB hepatitis were treated with varying doses of IFN-alpha for up to 12 months. The promising results from this pilot study led to a series of large-scale randomized controlled trials (reviewed by Ahmed and Elias [9]). These studies showed that in about 50% of IFN-treated patients serum ALT levels return to normal during treatment and this biochemical response is associated with a decrease in histological activity. However, the relapse rate following cessation of treatment was high and only about 20% of treated patients had a sustained biochemical response.

Tine *et al.* [10] performed a meta-analysis of 17 randomized clinical trials where recombinant or lymphoblastoid interferon was used to treat NANB hepatitis. These trials enrolled a total of 916 patients from Europe, North America and Australia. Despite the variability in the IFN treatment schedules used, the meta-analysis showed that there was homogeneity in the direction of treatment effect favouring IFN-treated patients.

Dose and duration of interferon

In the early studies, relatively small doses of IFN were used for the treatment of chronic HCV compared to chronic HBV infection. The dose and duration of IFN used in these studies tended to vary widely. At present, a 'typical' regimen would be 3 MU three times a week for 6 to 12 months. However, the search for the optimum dose and duration continues. Some studies have suggested that treatment for 12 months may be superior to 6 months treatment. Trials looking at treatment for 18 months have also been performed, though numbers are small.

Interferon treatment for HCV – prognostic indicators

As with HBV, it is possible to predict those patients who are more likely to respond to treatment using several prognostic indicators. These indicators may be divided into patient and viral factors (Table 5). Favourable prognostic indicators of response

Table 5 Factors associated with response to γ-IFN in chronic HCV.

	Favourable	Unfavourable
Patient factors	Young age	Old age
	Non-cirrhotic	Cirrhotic
	Mild inflammation	Severe inflammation
	Heavy alcohol intake	
Viral factors	Short duration of illness	Prolonged illness
	Genotype 2 and 3	Genotype 1
	Low viral load	High viral load
	Low viral diversity (quasispecies)	High diversity
	No co-infection with HIV	Co-infection with HIV

to interferon include young age, short duration of illness and mild inflammation on liver biopsy. The presence of cirrhosis is a poor prognostic indicator. Viral factors predictive of poor response include high pretreatment levels of viraemia, genotype 1 (particularly type 1b), a high level of viral diversity (quasispecies) and possibly coinfection with HIV. Heavy alcohol usage in patients with HCV may accelerate hepatocellular damage, potentiate development of hepatoma, reduce survival and reduce the response rate to IFN.

When to treat chronic HCV

Most patients with HCV seen by the clinician are asymptomatic or minimally symptomatic. It is difficult to recommend an optimum selection protocol when deciding which patients require treatment (Fig. 10). Patients with decompensated cirrhosis, severe cytopaenia, psychosis or associated autoimmune disease generally should not be treated because of the potential for adverse effects. In HCV patients positive on confirmatory (RIBA) testing who do not have contraindications, our current policy is to base the decision to treat primarily on the appearance of the initial liver biopsy. The liver biopsy is assessed using a histological activity index (HAI, range 0–13, see Table 4).

Patients with a HAI of 6 or more but without advanced cirrhosis are offered treatment with IFN-alpha-2b at a dose of 3 MU three times a week for 12 months. Patients are seen in the clinic weekly for two weeks, then fortnightly for four weeks and then monthly. Haematological profile and ALT are performed at each visit and thyroid function tests performed every two months. Treatment is discontinued if there is no biochemical response by three months.

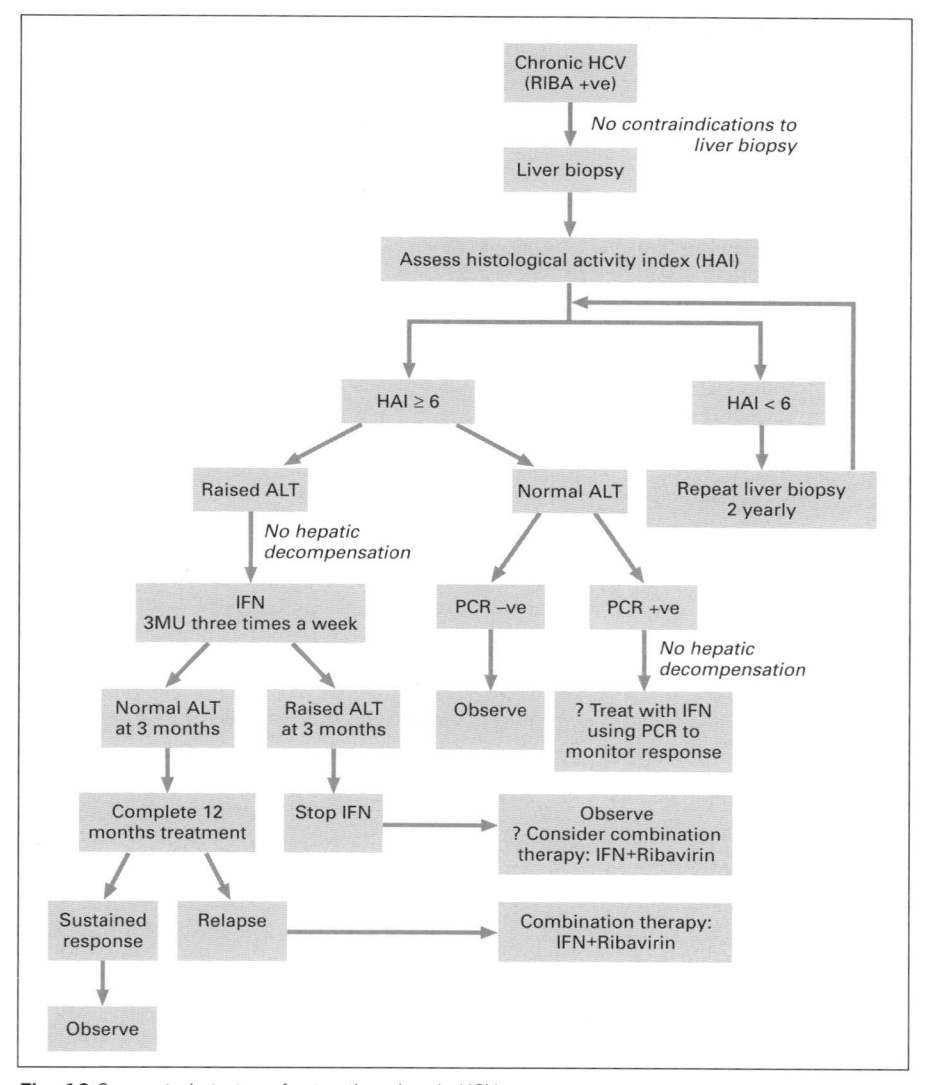

Fig. 10 Suggested strategy for treating chronic HCV.

Patients with an initial HAI of less than 6 are not treated with IFN but are followed up in clinic on a 6 monthly basis and are re-biopsied every two years to monitor histological progression. If the follow-up biopsy shows a HAI of 6 or more, then treatment is offered. All patients with heavy alcohol usage (>21 units a week for men or >14 units a week for women) are advised to reduce alcohol intake to no more than half these limits.

Relapses and non-responders

Approximately 50% of patients with chronic HCV treated with IFN show no biochemical response. Of the 50% who show a complete response, more than half subsequently relapse. Possible management strategies in relapsers include longer duration of treatment, repeated courses of IFN, long-term low-dose therapy or alternative treatment. The optimum management of non-responders and relapsers is under evaluation.

Alternative treatment

A number of alternatives or adjuncts to IFN have been proposed for the treatment of chronic HCV (Table 6). Ribavirin is the most promising of these adjuncts. Ribavirin is an orally administered guanosine analogue with a broad spectrum of antiviral activity against both DNA and RNA viruses including those of the flavivirus family. Its main side effect is dose-related reversible haemolysis, which is generally mild.

Recent data indicate that ribavirin and IFN may act synergistically in chronic HCV. For example, Brillanti *et al.* [11] treated previously IFN-unresponsive patients with a combination of interferon-alpha and ribavirin for 6 months. Nine months after treatment, sustained normalization of ALT levels associated with sustained loss of serum HCV RNA was observed in 40% (4/10) compared with none of the patients treated with IFN-alpha alone. At present large randomized controlled studies are in progress comparing combination therapy with IFN alone.

Liver transplant for HCV related end-stage liver failure

ESLF due to chronic HCV is an important indication for liver transplantation. Viral recurrence following transplantation is common. HCV RNA can be detected in 85–90% of patients, sometimes as early as the first week post-transplant. In one study, the actuarial rate of recurrent hepatitis at 4 years after orthotopic liver transplantation (OLT) was 72% [12]. The severity of the recurrent hepatitis varies widely. Usually, HCV infection in transplanted patients produces a mild disease state. Many patients with graft re-infection will remain asymptomatic with good graft function at least in the short term, even with immunosuppressive therapy.

Table 6 Treatments evaluated in humans for chronic HCV.

Interferon: alpha, beta and gamma
Ribavirin
Thymosin
Azidothymidine (zidovudine)
Ursodeoxycholic acid
N-Acetylcysteine
Quinalones
Non-steroidal anti-inflammatory drugs
Prednisolone
Venesection

However, progression to symptomatic chronic hepatitis and cirrhosis within a few years of OLT have been reported. Rapidly progressive recurrent disease requiring re-transplantation has also been reported. Genotype 1b is associated with more severe graft injury [13].

In contrast to HBV re-infection, currently there are no methods to prevent HCV graft re-infection. Experience with treatment of recurrent HCV with IFN-alpha is limited. In a study from San Francisco, treatment of recurrent HCV with IFN resulted in biochemical response in 28% (5/18) with a reduction in HCV RNA levels during treatment, but the HCV RNA levels subsequently returned to pretreatment levels [14]. Prophylactic use of IFN before the onset of hepatitis does not seem to prevent the appearance of HCV RNA or halt progression of histological activity. Concern about the use of IFN relates to upregulation of expression of HLA class I and II antigens which may increase the risk of graft rejection. Indeed, cases of acute vanishing bile-duct syndrome after IFN treatment therapy for recurrent HCV infection have been reported.

As an alternative, ribavirin monotherapy has been used in a small study from King's College, London. Serum ALT levels normalized in 4/7 patients but all remained HCV PCR positive. A preliminary report by Bizollon *et al.* [15] suggests that combination therapy using IFN and ribavirin may be beneficial in preventing the progression of HCV related graft disease.

☐ HEPATITIS G

Hepatitis G virus is a novel positive-stranded RNA virus which is related to the flaviviridae family [16]. The HGV genome codes for a polypeptide comprising 2900 amino acids and has 26% homology to the HCV genome. HGV is thought to be identical to the newly described GBV-C virus.

HGV is transmitted parenterally and 60% of infected patients have chronic elevation of ALT levels. HGV can be detected by RT-PCR and currently there are no antibody tests. The long-term consequences of chronic HGV infection are uncertain and at present there are no guidelines for treatment.

☐ SUMMARY

HBV and HCV are the commonest causes of chronic viral hepatitis. In both cases, IFN-alpha is currently the only licensed treatment.

For chronic HBV, IFN treatment is recommended for patients with evidence of active viral replication. Response is likely in about one-third of cases. Good prognostic indicators include low viral DNA levels, raised ALT levels and an active histology. In patients with normal ALT levels the likelihood of response may be improved with steroid pretreatment.

For chronic HCV, IFN treatment is recommended for patients with significant changes in their liver histology. Sustained biochemical response is likely in about 20% of cases. The role of combination therapy using IFN and ribavirin is currently being evaluated.

REFERENCES

1. Tine F, Liberati A, Craxi A, Almasio P, Pagliaro L. Interferon treatment in patients with chronic hepatitis B: a meta-analysis of published literature. *J Hepatol* 1993; **18**: 154–62.
2. Wong DKH, Cheung AM, O'Rourke K, Naylor CD, Detsky AS, Heathcote J. Effect of alpha-interferon treatment in patients with hepatitis B e antigen-positive chronic hepatitis B: a meta-analysis. *Ann Intern Med* 1993; **119**: 312–23.
3. Cohard M, Poynard T, Mathurin P, Zarski JP. Prednisolone-interferon combination in the treatment of chronic hepatitis B: direct and indirect meta-analysis. *Hepatology* 1994; **20**: 1390–8.
4. Samuel D, Muller R, Alexander G, *et al*. Liver transplantation in European patients with the hepatitis-B surface-antigen. *New Engl J Med* 1993; **329**: 1842–7.
5. Farci P, Mandas A, Coiana A, *et al*. Treatment of chronic hepatitis D with interferon-alfa-2a. *New Engl J Med* 1994; **330**: 88–94.
6. Choo Q-L, Kuo G, Weiner AJ, Overby LR, Bradley DW, Houghton M. Isolation of a cDNA clone derived from a blood-borne non-A,non-B viral hepatitis genome. *Science* 1989; **244**: 359–62.
7. Knodell KG, Ishak KG, Black WC, *et al*. Formulation and application of a numeric scoring system for assessing histological activity in asymptomatic chronic hepatitis. *Hepatology* 1981; **1**: 1431–5.
8. Hoofnagle JH, Mullen KD, Jones DB, *et al*. Treatment of chronic non-A,non-B hepatitis with recombinant human alpha-interferon. *New Engl J Med* 1986; **315**: 1575–8.
9. Ahmed M, Elias E. Hepatitis C virus infection – who to treat? In: Farthing MJG, ed. *Clinical Challenges in Gastroenterology*. London: Martin Dunitz, 1996: 188–209.
10. Tine F, Magrin S, Craxi A, Pagliaro L. Interferon for non-A,non-B chronic hepatitis. *J Hepatol* 1991; **13**: 192–9.
11. Brillanti S, Garson J, Foli M, *et al*. A pilot study of combination therapy with ribavirin plus interferon-alfa for interferon-alfa resistant chronic hepatitis C. *Gastroenterology* 1994; **107**: 812–7.
12. Feray C, Gigou M, Samuel D, *et al*. The course of hepatitis C virus infection after liver transplantation. *Hepatology* 1994; **20**: 1137–43.
13. Gane EJ, Portmann BC, Naoumov NV, *et al*. Long-term outcome of hepatitis C infection after liver transplantation. *New Engl J Med* 1996; **334**: 815–20.
14. Wright TL, Combs C, Kim M, *et al*. Interferon-alpha therapy for hepatitis C virus infection after liver transplantation. *Hepatology* 1994; **20**: 773–9.
15. Bizollon T, Ducerf C, Trepo C. New approaches to the treatment of hepatitis C virus infection after liver transplantation using ribavirin. *J Hepatol* 1995; **23**: 22–5.
16. Linnen J, Wages J, Zhangkeck ZY, *et al*. Molecular cloning and disease association of hepatitis G virus – a transfusion-transmissible agent. *Science* 1996; **271**: 505–8.

☐ MULTIPLE CHOICE QUESTIONS

1. In chronic HBV, the following are favourable prognostic indicators for response to IFN therapy:
   (a) High pretreatment ALT level
   (b) High pretreatment HBV DNA level
   (c) Inactive cirrhosis prior to treatment
   (d) Female sex
   (e) HDV superinfection

2. Hepatitis C virus:
   (a) Is a RNA virus

(b) Results in chronic liver disease in 30% of cases
   (c) Has a genome that is 50% homologous to that of HGV
   (d) Accounts for most cases of post-transfusion NANB hepatitis
   (e) Has a high vertical transmission rate

3 In chronic HCV, the following are favourable prognostic indicators for response to IFN therapy:
   (a) HCV genotype 1b
   (b) HCV genotype 2
   (c) Low quasispecies diversity
   (d) High pretreatment levels of viraemia
   (e) Cirrhosis

4 Following liver transplantation for HBV:
   (a) Viral recurrence is common in patients who were HBV DNA positive prior to transplantation
   (b) Short-term HBIg immunoprophylaxis usually prevents viral recurrence in patients who were HBV DNA positive pre-transplant
   (c) Viral recurrence may result in fibrosing cholestatic hepatitis
   (d) Cirrhosis may develop within 2 years of transplantation
   (e) Long-term HBIg immunoprophylaxis is useful in preventing recurrence in patients who were HBV DNA negative pre-transplant

5 Interferon-alpha treatment:
   (a) For 6 months in chronic HCV results in sustained biochemical response in 50% of patients
   (b) For 6 months in chronic HCV results in complete biochemical response in 25% of patients
   (c) In combination with oral ribavirin may improve response rates in chronic HCV
   (d) For 6 months in chronic HBV results in loss of HBeAg in approximately one-third of patients
   (e) For chronic HDV results in sustained clearance of HDV in the majority of patients

ANSWERS

1a True	2a True	3a False	4a True	5a False
b False	b False	b True	b False	b False
c False	c False	c True	c True	c True
d True	d True	d False	d True	d True
e False	e False	e False	e True	e False

Diagnosis and management of Cushing's syndrome

J A H Wass

☐ INTRODUCTION

Cushing's syndrome is due to chronic glucocorticoid excess and may result from a variety of causes (Table 1). Cushing's disease refers to the pituitary secretion of excess adrenocorticotrophic hormone (ACTH) and this causes bilateral adrenocortical hyperplasia with the excessive production of cortisol, adrenal androgens and other steroids that cause the clinical and biological effects of the disease.

From the epidemiological point of view, in adults Cushing's disease is the most frequent cause of the syndrome (65%). There is a female preponderance of 3 to 1 and it most commonly presents between the ages of 25 and 45. Prevalence figures vary but one estimate suggests that there are three new cases per million per year [1]. In children the distribution of causes is different, with adrenal adenomas being more common than Cushing's disease (30% of the total).

☐ DIAGNOSIS OF CUSHING'S SYNDROME

There are two steps in the diagnosis of the hypercortisolaemic state (Table 2). First it should clearly be established that Cushing's syndrome is present. Second, the

Table 1 Causes of Cushing's syndrome.

ACTH-dependent	ACTH-independent
Pituitary ACTH oversecretion:	Adrenal adenoma (14% of total)
Cushing's disease (65% of total)	Adrenal carcinoma (11% of total)
Tumours producing CRH (corticotrophin-releasing hormone)	Bilateral adrenocortical nodular hyperplasia (0.2%)
Hypothalamic	**Iatrogenic**
Ectopic	Exogenous glucocorticoids
Non-pituitary ACTH oversecretion:	Exogenous ACTH
Ectopic ACTH secretion (9% of total)	

Table 2 Steps in diagnosis of Cushing's syndrome.

Establish Cushing's syndrome	Differential diagnosis
Dexamethasone suppression	ACTH levels
Midnight cortisol levels	High-dose dexamethasone
Insulin tolerance test	CRH test
Urinary cortisol levels	

cause needs to be shown; this has important prognostic and therapeutic implications.

The establishment of the existence of Cushing's syndrome can be extraordinarily difficult and the correct diagnosis of the cause is one of the most challenging aspects of clinical endocrinology. Numerous pitfalls await the unwary or inexperienced. Some tests do not give clear differentiation and abnormalities in them may have a number of different causes. Drugs may interfere with tests and patients with severe Cushing's syndrome can be extremely ill both physically and psychologically. Lastly, hypercortisolaemic states may exist in cyclical form and this applies to Cushing's disease, ectopic ACTH secretion and adrenal adenoma. Diagnostic certainty is imperative before recommending further investigation and treatment.

Establishing the hypercortisolaemic state

In Cushing's syndrome the normal circadian rhythm of cortisol is absent and midnight cortisol levels above 50 nmol/l provide a sensitive index of cortisol hypersecretion. These must be carried out after 48 h in hospital and intercurrent illness of any sort may elevate the midnight value above normal.

Urinary cortisol metabolites measured as 24 h urinary cortisol excretion also provide a useful marker of excessive cortisol secretion, but this measurement is not as sensitive as the suppression tests (below) and mild cortisol excess may be associated with a normal 24 h urinary cortisol (Table 3).

Table 3 Diagnosis of Cushing's syndrome.

	Sensitivity	Cortisol criterion
Low-dose dexamethasone (2 mg/day, 48 h)	98%	<50 nmol/l
Midnight cortisol (asleep) after 48 h in hospital	100%	<50 nmol/l
Urinary free cortisol	95%	elevated

Suppression tests

The classic low-dose dexamethasone suppression test as described by Liddle [2] remains the preferred reference test in the diagnosis of Cushing's syndrome. It is performed by the administration of 0.5 mg of dexamethasone every 6 h for eight doses starting at 09:00. Cortisol is measured at 0, 24 and 48 h and should be undetectable by 48 h. Less than 5% of patients with Cushing's syndrome show normal suppression. Conditions that may be associated with abnormal suppression after dexamethasone treatment include heart failure, intercurrent illness, due for example to malignant disease, severe depression and alcoholism.

The overnight 1 mg dexamethasone suppression test [3] (Table 4) has also been used quite widely. Dexamethasone (1 mg) is administered at midnight and blood cortisol measured the next morning at 09:00. Cortisol should not be detectable at

Table 4 Overnight dexamethasone suppression test.

Dexamethasone 1 mg at 2300–2400 h	
Plasma cortisol measured at 0800–0900 h	
Positive (no suppression): 13% obese 23% hospital inpatients	False-positive: on oestrogen enzyme-inducing drug

this time and it is important that the morning sample is not delayed. The test itself suffers from lack of specificity and has been found to be positive (ie lacking normal suppression) in as many as 13% of obese subjects and in 23% of hospitalized or chronically ill patients [4]. Therefore it may be useful to exclude Cushing's syndrome with this test, but a significant proportion of patients will need to go on and have a full 2 mg dexamethasone suppression test carried out if normal suppression is lacking with the overnight test.

☐ ESTABLISHING THE CAUSE OF CUSHING'S SYNDROME

The measurement of ACTH clearly differentiates adrenal from other causes of ACTH-dependent Cushing's syndrome. ACTH was one of the first radioimmunoassays to be developed and used clinically in man. Its measurement is complicated by the fact that ACTH is rapidly destroyed in blood and therefore special care is needed to obtain valid measurements. Because of its rapid degradation, blood samples should be spun and frozen within 15 minutes of collection.

Undetectable ACTH values clearly indicate an adrenocortical tumour, either an adenoma or a carcinoma, as the cause of Cushing's syndrome. However, ACTH values do not clearly differentiate between the various ACTH-dependent causes of Cushing's syndrome and there is a very clear overlap between those values found in ectopic ACTH syndrome and pituitary-dependent disease.

Further tests are imperative in the differentiation of these two conditions. These tests include the potassium, the high-dose dexamethasone test and the CRH test.

The plasma potassium is helpful in the diagnosis of ectopic ACTH secretion and in almost all patients with this condition who are not taking diuretics it is less than 3.2 mmol/l (Table 5).

High-dose dexamethasone suppression test

This was first described by Liddle [2]. A 2 mg dose of dexamethasone is given orally

Table 5 Cushing's syndrome – differential diagnosis.

	Ectopic (%)	Pituitary-dependent (%)
Hypokalaemia	100	10
High-dose dexamethasone – suppression (8 mg/day, 48 h)	10	80
CRH test (rise in ACTH >50%)	<1	>95

every 6 h for 48 h, beginning at 09:00. Urinary cortisol is measured on 24 h for 48 h and plasma cortisol at 0, 24 and 48 h. Urinary cortisol and plasma cortisol should fall by 50% and this occurs in 80% of patients with Cushing's disease. Unfortunately, responsiveness to high-dose dexamethasone suppression is also seen in 20% of patients with ectopic ACTH secretion, so this test does not provide definitive differentiation between the two conditions.

Metyrapone test

In this test, 750 mg of metyrapone is given every 4 h for six doses. Urinary steroids are measured the day before, the day of and the day after metyrapone administration. This test differentiates even less well than high-dose dexamethasone suppression tests and is not routinely used in most endocrine units.

Corticotrophin-releasing hormone test

Corticotrophin-releasing hormone (CRH) was isolated and characterized in 1981 by Vale *et al.* [5]. CRH is the hypothalamic peptide that stimulates pituitary ACTH release and this has led to the CRH test in which 100 µg of CRH is administered intravenously and responses of ACTH and cortisol are followed over 120 minutes. In pituitary-dependent Cushing's syndrome, CRH causes a rise of ACTH of more than 50% in 95% of patients. In patients with ectopic ACTH secretion, no rise in ACTH is seen. Only rare exceptions occur.

Adrenal imaging

In patients with undetectable ACTH values, adrenal imaging is clearly indicated. No adrenocortical tumour causing Cushing's syndrome will not be picked up by abdominal computerized tomography (CT) scan. Adrenocortical carcinomas are larger and will also be picked up with ease.

Pituitary imaging

The majority of pituitary tumours causing Cushing's disease are small. Only 50% will be picked up by CT but T1 weighted magnetic resonance imaging (MRI) typically shows a hypointense signal which increases after gadolinium enhancement and is seen in around 70% of patients. This is therefore the technique of choice.

Diagnostic pitfalls

The diagnosis of Cushing's syndrome may be difficult in a number of ways. Some drugs, particularly oestradiol, for example in the pill and during pregnancy, raise cortisol-binding globulin levels. This means that cortisol levels are elevated and in these circumstances dexamethasone suppression may be abnormal. Urinary levels of free cortisol are normal in these circumstances.

Drugs such a phenytoin and rifampicin, by their action as liver-enzyme inducers, accelerate dexamethasone metabolism and this again may result in false-positive dexamethasone suppression tests.

Intercurrent illness of any sort, including cardiac failure, chronic renal failure and malignant disease, all interfere with the normal circadian rhythm of ACTH and cortisol and result in cortisol levels that are detectable at midnight.

Lastly, a number of conditions cause hypercortisolaemia without Cushing's syndrome but nevertheless diagnostic confusion can occur. Thus, in depression, anorexia nervosa and alcoholism, circadian rhythms of ACTH and cortisol are abnormal.

☐ INVESTIGATIVE STRATEGY

If the tests described point clearly to either an adrenal or pituitary adenoma then this can be treated. If the results of the tests are equivocal, that is one or other but not both of the high-dose dexamethasone suppression test or CRH test points to pituitary-driven disease or perhaps there is not a clear abnormality on the pituitary MRI scan, petrosal sinus sampling may be carried out as this technique has the power to differentiate pituitary-driven disease from ectopic ACTH secretion.

Catheters are introduced bilaterally through the femoral vein into the inferior petrosal sinuses. In pituitary-dependent disease there is an ACTH gradient between the central catheter sample and the periphery that is usually greater than 2. However, in patients with ectopic ACTH secretion the gradient is less than 2 and usually less than 1.7. The administration of CRH increases the differentiation between pituitary and ectopic ACTH secretion by increasing the central to peripheral ratio of ACTH. If the results of the tests point to ectopic ACTH secretion, this may derive from several sources including foregut carcinoids in the bronchus, pancreas etc, phaeochromocytoma and medullary carcinoma of the thyroid. Delineation of the cause of ectopic ACTH secretion requires careful imaging of the chest and abdomen.

☐ TREATMENT OF CUSHING'S DISEASE

Surgery

The primary treatment of Cushing's disease is surgical. The tumours are small and surgery offers a rapid response. There is evidence that the experience of the surgeon is important, but despite apparently adequate surgery relapse of Cushing's disease occurs. Recently a better assessment of the postoperative outcome has enabled various postoperative cortisol levels to predict the likelihood of subsequent relapse. Thus ideally after operation the cortisol level should be undetectable and in these circumstances late recurrence of Cushing's disease is rare (9% at 5 years). If a postoperative cortisol is low/normal (as opposed to undetectable) the recurrence rate rises. Undetectable cortisol levels are achieved after surgery in experienced hands in 42% (Table 6).

Complications occur and these include hypopituitarism (10%), cerebrospinal fluid (CSF) leak and meningitis (Table 7). If the initial operation is not successful

Table 6 Results of pituitary surgery for Cushing's disease. (Data from Endocrinology Department, St Bartholomew's Hospital.)

First operation		Second operation	
Cortisol undetectable	42%	Cortisol undetectable	50%
<300 nmol/l	65%		

Table 7 Complications after pituitary surgery for Cushing's disease.

Mortality	1.9%	Bleeding	1.3%
Meningitis	2.8%	Diabetes insipidus	3.0%
Cerebrospinal fluid leak	4.6%	Pulmonary embolism	0.6%

with selective surgery, more radical surgery will result in the cure of a further 50% of patients.

Complication rates of second attempts at surgery are higher, but hypopituitarism is preferable to prolonged glucocorticoid excess, which may be difficult to control and which has both a mortality and a morbidity.

Conventional radiotherapy

Conventional radiotherapy can be effective in 50% of patients [6], but response to radiotherapy is slow and it may take months or years for the full effect to develop. Hypopituitarism develops in a proportion of patients but serious complications such as optic nerve damage and late malignancy are rare though they have been reported in some series.

Gamma knife stereotactic radiosurgery is a technique that is gaining popularity in America and Stockholm. It is a technique capable of high precision which delivers radiation doses that are fixed to areas ranging from a few centimetres to a few millimetres without side effects. Treatment can be completed within 30 minutes and success rates in Cushing's disease of 76% are reported [7]. Currently the technique is not widely available and more experience is needed.

Medical treatment

Medical treatments include metyrapone, ketoconazole and op-DDD (Table 8). Metyrapone [8] acts as an 11β-hydroxylase inhibitor thus blocking the last step in adrenal steroid biosynthesis. This drug can be a useful adjunct in the treatment of Cushing's disease or indeed in the treatment of any patient with Cushing's syndrome. In the majority, using doses of between 750 and 3000 mg per day, cortisol levels can be reduced to an average of between 200 and 300 mmol/l. In this way the drug may be used acutely to try to improve a patient who at presentation is seriously ill or after unsuccessful surgery while awaiting the full effect of pituitary radiation. Ketoconazole is an imidazole derivative which interferes with cortisol synthesis at

Table 8 Medical treatment of Cushing's disease.

Drug	Action	Side effect
Metyrapone	11β-Hydroxylase inhibitor	Hirsutism
op-DDD	Adrenolytic	G.i. 30%
		Neurological
Ketoconazole	20–22 Desmolase + 11β-hydroxylase	Toxic hepatitis

two levels, namely 20 to 22 desmolase and 11β-hydroxylase. It has a beneficial effect in doses between 300 and 1200 mg per day. It may rarely cause severe hepatic failure, and liver biochemistry should therefore carefully be monitored especially in the early stages of treatment. op-DDD is an adrenolytic drug which is highly lipophilic. It is usually used in doses of 3 g per day and it produces selective necrosis of the adrenal cortex. It is not widely available in the UK.

☐ CONCLUSION

The investigation of a patient with Cushing's syndrome remains one of the most intriguing clinical challenges that an endocrinologist can face. Recent advances in our understanding of the physiology of ACTH release, the isolation of CRH, the improvement in imaging techniques and the clear delineation of different outcomes of surgery have enabled the majority of patients with Cushing's disease to be treated successfully.

REFERENCES

1. Etxabe J, Vazquez JA. Morbidity and mortality in Cushing's disease: an epidemiological approach. *Clin Endocrinol* 1994; **40**: 479–84.
2. Liddle GW. Tests of pituitary–adrenal suppressibility in the diagnosis of Cushing's syndrome. *J Clin Endocrinol Metab* 1960; **20**: 1539–60.
3. Nugent CA, Nichols T, Tyler FH. Diagnosis of Cushing's syndrome – single dose dexamethasone suppression tests. *Arch Intern Med* 1965; **116**: 172–6.
4. Crapo L. Cushing's syndrome – a review of diagnostic tests. *Metabolism* 1979; **28**: 955–77.
5. Vale W, Spiess J, Rivier CJ. Characterisation of the 41-residue ovine hypothalamic peptides that stimulate secretion of corticotrophin and beta endorphin. *Science* 1981; **213**: 1394–7.
6. Howlett TA, Plowman PN, Wass JAH, Rees LH, Jones AE, Besser GM. Megavoltage pituitary irradiation in the management of Cushing's disease and Nelson's syndrome: long term follow-up. *Clin Endocrinol* 1989; **31**: 309–23.
7. Degerblad M, Rahn T, Bergstrand G, Thoren M. Long-term results of stereotactic radiosurgery to the pituitary gland in Cushing's disease. *Acta Endocrinol* 1986; **112**: 310–4.
8. Jeffcoate WJ, Rees LH, Thomlin S, Jones AE, Edwards CRW, Besser GM. Metyrapone in the long-term management of Cushing's disease. *Brit Med J* 1977; **2**: 215–7.

☐ MULTIPLE CHOICE QUESTIONS

1. Tests to establish a diagnosis of Cushing's syndrome:
   (a) CRH test

(b) Urinary cortisol levels
  (c) ACTH levels
  (d) Midnight cortisol levels
  (e) High-dose dexamethasone suppression test

2   Tests to establish the cause of Cushing's syndrome:
    (a) ACTH levels
    (b) Insulin tolerance test
    (c) High-dose dexamethasone test
    (d) CRH test
    (e) Metyrapone

3   In relation to pituitary surgery:
    (a) The postoperative cortisol level affects recurrence rate
    (b) Preoperative MRI shows an adenoma in 95% of cases
    (c) Postoperative hypopituitarism occurs in more than 20% because the tumour is small and often cannot be found
    (d) Second operations cure up to 50% if the first operation is not successful

4   Tests for excluding a diagnosis of Cushing's syndrome:
    (a) Dexamethasone suppression test
    (b) Urinary free cortisol
    (c) Midnight cortisol after 48 h in hospital
    (d) Pyrogen test
    (e) Synacthen test

ANSWERS

1a	False	2a	True	3a	True	4a	True
b	True	b	False	b	False	b	True
c	False	c	True	c	False	c	True
d	True	d	True	d	True	d	False
e	False	e	False			e	False

The management of thyroid lumps

J A Franklyn

☐ INTRODUCTION

Enlargement of the thyroid is common. The Whickham survey, carried out in the north-east of England, revealed that small goitres (those palpable but not visible) are present in 8.6% of the population, while obvious goitres (palpable and visible) are present in 6.9%, goitres being four times more common in females than in males [1]. The presence of nodular thyroid disease may be even more common than such epidemiological studies suggest, as postmortem studies have shown that up to 50% of the population have either single or multiple nodules in the thyroid, many of which are very small. Studies using high-resolution ultrasound scans have similarly revealed discrete nodules in up to 50% of people over 50 years old.

In contrast to the marked prevalence of thyroid nodules outlined above, thyroid cancer is rare, accounting for less than 0.5% of all new malignancies in England and Wales and less than 0.5% of all cancer deaths. Thyroid cancer is reported to have been found in between 6% and 14% of single thyroid nodules selected for surgery on clinical grounds [2], while cancer risk is even lower in multinodular goitre. The picture is, however, complicated by postmortem studies that describe the presence of occult cancer in up to 5% of thyroid glands normal to palpation. Most occult cancers are small, being only several millimetres in diameter, and the substantial prevalence of occult cancer in those who have died from unrelated disease suggests that this is an entity without clinical significance. The overwhelming challenge to the clinician is therefore to identify the small number of patients presenting with significant neoplastic disease of the thyroid from the majority without, thus sparing up to 90% of patients unnecessary surgery.

☐ HISTORY, LABORATORY TESTS AND EXAMINATION OF THYROID NODULES

The history of a patient may increase the likelihood of that patient having a malignant lesion, although for the vast majority of subjects presenting with one or more thyroid nodules the history is not helpful in determining the nature of the underlying disease. Prior exposure to radiation is a risk factor for both benign and malignant nodular thyroid disease, and patients with such a history should be evaluated with care. There are conflicting reports regarding the effect of age on cancer risk, but thyroid nodules are uncommon in childhood and their presence should be viewed with suspicion. Likewise, there may be an increased risk of cancer in nodules developing over the age of 65 years, and undifferentiated thyroid cancer generally occurs in this age group. Gender is an important determinant of neoplasia risk, since thyroid cancer is relatively more common in thyroid nodules present in males than in females. A family history of thyroid cancer, especially medullary cancer, may be especially pertinent and should lead to a suspicion of multiple endocrine neoplasia syndrome type II or familial medullary thyroid cancer.

A history of symptoms such as dysphagia, dyspnoea or hoarseness may suggest local invasion from a malignant lesion, although such symptoms also occur with benign thyroid enlargement, especially in association with large multinodular goitres. A malignancy rate of 71% has been reported in a group classified 'high risk' on the basis of symptoms suggesting a compressive lesion, as well as signs such as firmness, fixation to adjacent structures, vocal cord paralysis and cervical lymphadenopathy [3], although fewer than 5% of patients presenting with nodular thyroid disease have such symptoms or signs. While it is recognized that thyroid cancer is less common in multinodular goitre than in clinically solitary thyroid nodules, review of our own consecutive series of 461 patients presenting to a specialist thyroid clinic with thyroid enlargement revealed a significant prevalence of neoplasia in those with multinodular or diffuse thyroid enlargement as well as in those with solitary nodules, indicating that further investigation of those with multinodular and diffuse goitre, at least among a population referred to hospital, is justified [4].

Laboratory tests

No laboratory test specifically distinguishes benign from malignant thyroid enlargement. Circulating concentrations of thyroid hormones and thyroid-stimulating hormone (thyrotrophin; TSH) should, however, be measured to exclude hyper- or hypo-thyroidism, which themselves warrant specific treatment, and which, if present, markedly reduce the likelihood of any thyroid enlargement reflecting thyroid neoplasia. Serum concentrations of thyroglobulin are raised in patients with goitre, but values are similar in those with benign and malignant nodules. Measurement of serum thyroglobulin therefore has no value in the initial assessment of the patient presenting with nodular thyroid disease, although its role in the long-term follow-up of patients treated for differentiated thyroid cancer is clear. Serum calcitonin is the tumour marker for medullary thyroid cancer and, although this diagnosis accounts for less than 10% of thyroid malignancies, it has recently been suggested that routine measurement of serum calcitonin has a role in the assessment of patients presenting with nodular thyroid disease. While measurement of serum calcitonin in patients with a family history of medullary thyroid cancer is clearly indicated, further studies are needed to determine whether the prevalence of the disease and the relevance of early diagnosis justify routine measurement of circulating calcitonin [5].

Assessment of thyroid size

In addition to evaluating the nature of nodular thyroid enlargement as discussed below, management is also determined in part by the size of the thyroid lesion and in particular by the presence or absence of tracheal compression. Plain X-ray examination of the trachea may reveal deviation or compression of the airway, although comparison of the specificity and sensitivity of plain radiology with findings from computer-assisted tomography (CT) scanning of the trachea has revealed that plain X-ray findings are often misleading. Assessment of a respiratory flow volume loop is regarded as the best method for evaluating upper airways obstruction (Fig. 1), and we have recently performed a prospective study of this

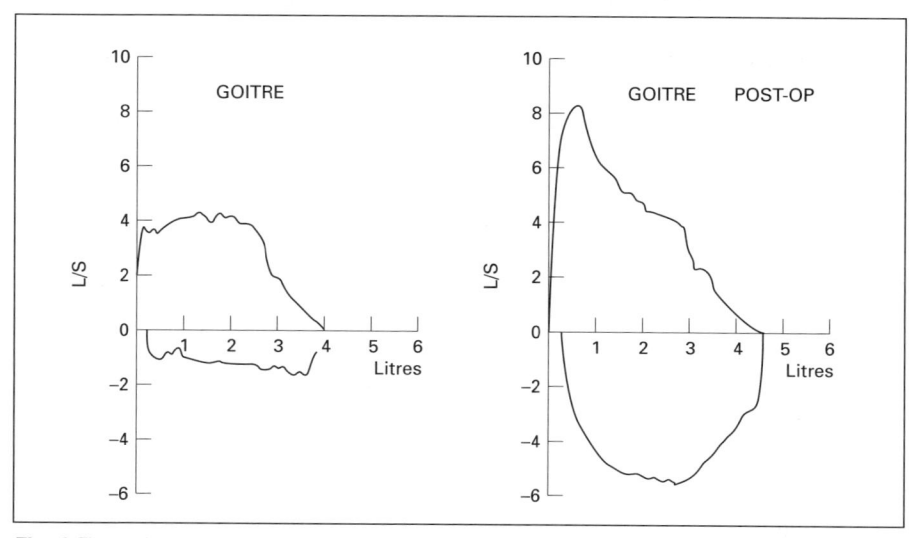

Fig. 1 Flow volume loops of a female patient aged 37 with upper airways obstruction, before partial thyroidectomy for goitre and after surgery.

method for assessment of the airway. We found that inspection of flow volume loops revealed upper airways obstruction in up to one-third of patients presenting with nodular thyroid disease. Symptoms such as choking or breathlessness were poor predictors of this functional upper airways obstruction [6]. It is not yet clear whether flow volume loop evidence of tracheal obstruction in the asymptomatic patient warrants surgical treatment.

Radionuclide imaging

Technetium-99m (^{99m}Tc) pertechnetate is the radionuclide most frequently used in thyroid imaging (Fig. 2). Although the majority of thyroid malignancies do not concentrate radioisotopes (and thus appear 'cold'), less than 20% of 'cold' nodules are due to cancerous lesions, the remaining 80% being due to colloid nodules, haemorrhage, cysts or inflammatory lesions such as Hashimoto's thyroiditis. Radionuclide imaging may also reveal multifocal abnormalities in patients thought clinically to have solitary nodules, mixed areas of hyper- and hypo-function being characteristic of multinodular goitres and less commonly Hashimoto's thyroiditis. Although the incidence of cancer is lower in multinodular goitres than in solitary nodules, the presence of 'cold' areas on such scans leads to concern regarding the underlying pathology, since the presence of a multinodular goitre does not prevent the development of thyroid malignancy as a second abnormality.

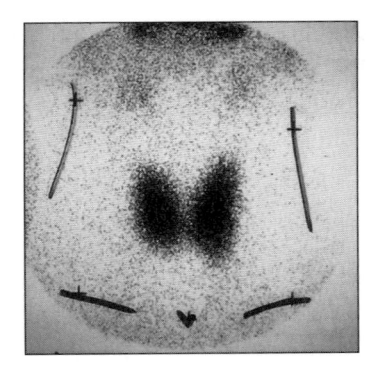

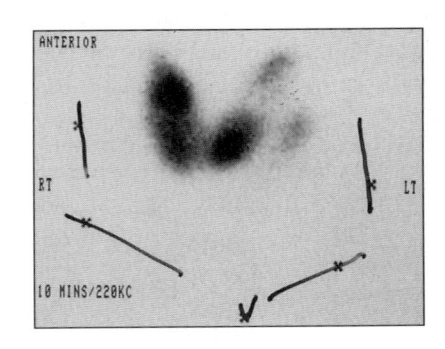

Fig. 2 Radioisotope scans of a thyroid indicating a normal pattern of uptake of isotope (a) and patchy uptake of technetium-99m with an apparent 'cold' area in the left upper lobe (b), raising the suspicion of malignancy. This defect disappeared after aspiration of cyst fluid.

In view of these limitations of radionuclide scanning it is not surprising that this approach does not specifically distinguish benign from malignant lesions. This is illustrated by Ashcraft and Van Herle's review of 22 series [7], in which more than 5000 patients underwent surgery, irrespective of the functional status of the nodule defined by isotope scanning. Of these, 84% were 'cold', 10.5% 'warm' and 5.5% 'hot' lesions. Malignancy was present in 16% of the 'cold', 9% of the 'warm' and 4% of the 'hot' nodules. Thus malignant nodules are more likely to be 'cold' than 'hot', but most 'cold' lesions are benign and the presence of a 'warm' or 'hot' nodule does not exclude malignancy. There are therefore no specific features to indicate the benign or malignant nature of a thyroid nodule, and this poor specificity has led many centres to abandon radionuclide scintigraphy in the routine investigation of those presenting with nodular thyroid disease.

Ultrasound scanning

High-resolution ultrasonography can detect thyroid lesions as small as 1 mm in diameter, and the technique is therefore better in detecting nodules than either physical examination or radionuclide imaging. A high prevalence of nodular thyroid disease of up to 50% is revealed by such high-resolution scanning as mentioned above. In addition, in as many as 40% of those patients thought clinically to have a solitary nodule, multiple nodules in the thyroid are revealed by ultrasonography (Fig. 3). Since data on the incidence of malignancy in nodular thyroid disease are related to clinically palpable goitres, it is unclear whether such multiple nodules detected ultrasonography are associated with a similar or a lower risk of malignancy than those nodules obvious only on clinical examination.

Ultrasonography is of value in distinguishing solid from cystic lesions of the thyroid. Ultrasound scanning has been reported to classify nodules as solid, mixed cystic and solid or cystic with greater than 90% accuracy. It has become clear, however, that no sonographic criteria can define benign or malignant disease with high specificity. In Ashcraft and Van Herle's review [8], more than 1000 patients with

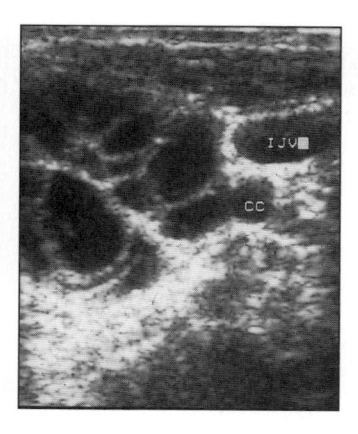

Fig. 3 Ultrasound scan of the thyroid indicating the presence of multiple cysts. IJV = internal jugular vein, CC = common carotid artery.

thyroid nodules underwent conventional ultrasonography before proceeding to surgery. Some 80% were classified preoperatively as solid or mixed solid cystic lesions and 20% were cystic. At surgery, 17% of all the lesions were malignant. Although solid or mixed cystic lesions harboured most of the malignancies, 6% of tumours occurred in those lesions originally thought to be cystic, probably reflecting the observation that some carcinomas undergo cystic degeneration.

The poor specificity of ultrasonography in indicating the underlying pathology, together with the difficulties that arise if impalpable nodules are revealed by ultrasound scanning, means that such scanning is often not considered helpful in patients presenting with nodular thyroid disease. This has led to its routine use being questioned.

Thyroid hormone suppression

Attempts have been made to distinguish benign from malignant nodules by seeking a change in nodule size in response to thyroxine, perhaps related to dependency on TSH for growth. The incidence of malignant disease in patients who demonstrate an apparent response to thyroid hormone suppression is not known, but it is well established that some carcinomas may respond to suppression by decreasing in size. Conversely, a lack of response to a trial of thyroid hormone suppression is not specific for malignancy, the incidence of cancer in non-responders being only between 12% and 40%.

Fine needle aspiration cytology

Fine needle aspiration has emerged as a valuable tool in the diagnosis and management of nodular thyroid disease. In contrast to the techniques already described, which provide at best an indirect evaluation of the nature of the disease, fine needle aspiration provides a means of obtaining thyroid tissue for direct cytological examination without the need for surgery. The technique requires practice, in order to reduce sampling error and to obtain a high frequency of satisfactory smears, and most importantly the skills of an expert cytopathologist (Fig. 4).

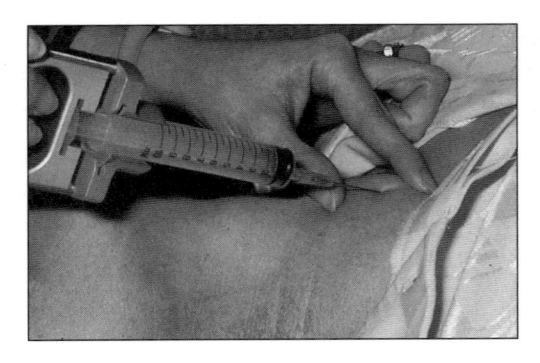

Fig. 4 Technique for fine needle aspiration of the thyroid. The syringe may be hand-held or placed in a carrier as illustrated.

The procedure can be performed in an outpatient department, is well tolerated by the patient, and can be repeated. The cytopathologist can report that an adequate smear contains normal cells only, cells from benign non-tumorous conditions such as lymphocytic thyroiditis, or suspicious (indeterminate) or obviously malignant cells (see Plates 7 and 8). The report that is indeterminate or suspicious of malignant change should be regarded as an indication to proceed to surgical exploration – in the same way as a report of unequivocal malignancy indicating papillary, follicular or medullary carcinoma.

Prolonged evaluation of the technique, especially in Sweden where it has been applied for more than 25 years, has demonstrated that in the hands of a skilled cytopathologist excellent diagnostic accuracy (up to 90%) can be achieved. A false positive report of malignant change is extremely rare but the rate of false negatives (ie tissue thought to be benign at cytology but found to show malignant change at surgery) is 5–10% in most series [9]. This is due in part to difficulty in distinguishing benign adenomas from malignant follicular neoplasms; surgical excision of all such lesions is therefore required (see Plate 9). An analysis from Cusick et al. [10] suggested, however, that the technique may be less reliable than is widely accepted. Analysis of their original data revealed an overall accuracy of 92% but audit of a further prospective evaluation showed an accuracy of only 69% [10]. Conflicting data in reported studies may relate to the clinical nature of the swellings included (multinodular, isolated or dominant), frequency of operation and methods used to calculate accuracy.

Since 1984 we have routinely carried out fine needle aspiration in all euthyroid patients presenting with thyroid enlargement. We have examined outcome in 629 consecutive patients followed for a minimum of 12 months after first aspirate. Patients were classified as having benign or suspicious/malignant cytological features after their first aspirate (see Plate 10). The former group (83% of the total) was managed conservatively, apart from those requiring surgery because of thyroid size or patient preference, and the latter group (17%) proceeded to histological examination. In total, 76% of patients were observed and 24% underwent partial or subtotal thyroidectomy. Of 529 patients with benign cytological findings, clinical follow-up of all patients and surgery in a minority suggested that 'true negative' cytology was present in 520. There were nine 'false negative' reports related to sampling error – three cases of papillary carcinoma, two follicular carcinomas and four follicular adenomas. Seventeen 'malignant' cytological reports correctly identified thyroid malignancy and there was one false positive report; 82 'suspicious' reports prompting surgery identified 39 'true positive' cases of thyroid neoplasia (including cancers and follicular adenomas); 43 of this group had benign colloid goitre. These results indicate a diagnostic accuracy of the cytological findings of up to 92%.

A diagnosis of thyroid cyst was made in 14% of our series of patients presenting with solitary nodules on clinical examination. These patients were investigated only by fine needle aspiration, but had they proceeded to radionuclide scanning such lesions would have appeared 'cold'. Approximately 50% of such patients were cured by simple aspiration of cyst fluid, so avoiding thyroid surgery. Thus, in addition to its diagnostic role, aspiration of thyroid nodules may be of therapeutic importance.

☐ NON-SURGICAL TREATMENT OF NODULAR THYROID DISEASE

Injection of simple cysts with tetracycline as a sclerosant has been shown to be of value for recurrent cysts. More recently, ethanol sclerotherapy, with or without ultrasound guidance, has been advocated. The reports suggest a marked reduction in the size of cystic lesions on follow-up, with minimal adverse effects.

Thyroxine (T_4) therapy in doses that suppress serum TSH to below the normal range has been studied extensively in terms of its short-term and long-term effect on goitre or nodule size. The results of such studies have been conflicting and most show little or no benefit from suppressive therapy (reviewed in [11]), either in patients with solitary thyroid nodules or in those with multinodular goitre. Nonetheless, T_4 therapy continues to be widely used in the hope of inducing a reduction in thyroid size. A trial of T_4-suppressive therapy, perhaps for up to one year, has been judged to be appropriate [11] to determine if a clinically relevant shrinkage in thyroid size results. However, caution needs to be exercised, especially in postmenopausal females in whom it is possible that T_4 therapy is associated with a loss of bone mineral density and hence increased risk of osteoporotic fracture.

A further option in non-surgical treatment that has recently received attention is radioiodine therapy. Radioiodine treatment of multinodular goitre has been reported to induce reduction in goitre size without any short-term increase in size leading to compressive symptoms. Radioiodine treatment has thus been judged to be clinically efficacious and safe, although the long-term risk of inducing hypothyroidism remains unclear.

☐ STRATEGY FOR INVESTIGATION

The appropriate diagnostic evaluation of the patient presenting with nodular thyroid disease remains controversial, despite the frequency of the problem. Several alternative strategies have been proposed, ranging from immediate surgery of all lesions to selective surgery after one or more of a series of investigations including radionuclide imaging, ultrasound scanning, a trial of thyroid hormone suppression and fine needle or large needle biopsy. Molitch et al. [2] used decision analysis to examine the value of these different strategies. They balanced possible long-term benefits of increased life expectancy after surgery against the risk of operative complications, and the value of imperfect diagnostic techniques that alter surgical selection. In view of the good prognosis for most patients with differentiated thyroid cancer, it is not surprising that only small differences can be demonstrated between the predicted value of each strategy for investigation and management. At age 20, aspiration cytology provides a benefit of 0.05% of life expectancy over thyroid hormone suppression, which in turn outweighs immediate surgery by 0.16%.

Considerations other than life expectancy therefore need to be taken into account. Fine needle aspiration cytology, as a sole investigation, followed by selective surgery, is emerging as an appropriate scheme for patient management. This scheme has resulted in a reduction in the number of radionuclide and ultrasound scans and the number of operations performed in many clinics. In our own series, surgery was performed to remove neoplastic tissue in 40% of cases, compared with a predicted rate of 9.6% if all solitary nodules have been removed. Several groups have reported a minimum 25% reduction in frequency of operation for single thyroid swellings and an increase from 31% to 50% in the proportion of operations for neoplastic disease after routine use of aspiration cytology [12]. This approach not only spares many patients with benign disease unnecessary surgery but leads to substantial financial savings.

In centres where large numbers of patients with solitary nodules are seen and where expert cytological skills are available, fine needle aspiration cytology is to be recommended for routine use in the diagnostic evaluation of such patients. In these circumstances we would recommend that patients with malignant or suspicious cytological findings, or where clinical suspicion is high, be referred for selective surgery. Definition of an optimum management strategy does depend, however, on the long-term follow-up of patients with negative results by such centres.

ACKNOWLEDGEMENTS

I am grateful to Professor MC Sheppard, Mr JC Watkinson and Mrs J Daykin for their support in the thyroid clinic and collection of our data. I also gratefully acknowledge Dr Jennifer Young, Senior Lecturer in Pathology, for her expert interpretation of cytological findings.

REFERENCES

1. Tunbridge WMG, Evered DC, Hall R, et al. The spectrum of thyroid disease in a community: the Whickham survey. *Clin Endocrinol* 1977; 7: 481–93.
2. Molitch ME, Beck JR, Dreisman M, et al. The cold thyroid nodule: an analysis of diagnostic and therapeutic options. *Endocr Reviews* 1985; 5: 185–99.
3. Hamming JF, Goslings BM, van Steenis GJ, et al. The value of fine needle aspiration biopsy in patients with nodular thyroid disease in patients divided into groups on suspicion of malignant neoplasms on clinical grounds. *Arch Intern Med* 1990; **150**: 113–6.
4. Franklyn JA, Daykin J, Young J, Oates GD, Sheppard MC. Fine needle aspiration cytology in diffuse or multinodular goitre compared with solitary thyroid nodules. *Brit Med J* 1993; **307**: 240.

5   Sheppard MC. Should serum calcitonin be measured routinely in all patients with nodular thyroid disease? *Clin Endocrinol* 1995; **42**: 451–2.
6   Gittoes NJL, Miller MR, Daykin J, Sheppard MC, Franklyn JA. Upper airways obstruction in patients presenting with thyroid enlargement. *Brit Med J* 1996; **312**: 484.
7   Ashcraft MW, Van Herle AJ. Management of thyroid nodules. II. Scanning techniques, thyroid suppressive therapy and fine needle aspiration. *Head Neck Surg* 1981; **3**: 297–322.
8   Ashcraft MW, Van Herle AJ. Management of thyroid nodules. I. History and physical examination, blood tests, X-ray tests and ultrasonography. *Head Neck Surg* 1981; **3**: 216–30.
9   Mazzaferri EL. Management of a solitary thyroid nodule. *New Engl J Med* 1993; **328**: 553–9.
10 Cusick EL, MacIntosh CA, Krukowski ZH, Williams VMM, Ewen SWB, Matheson NA. Management of isolated thyroid swellings: a prospective six year study of fine needle aspiration cytology in diagnosis. *Brit Med J* 1990; **301**: 318–21.
11 Cooper DS. Thyroxine suppression therapy for benign nodular disease. *J Clin Endocrinol Metab* 1995; **80**: 331–4.
12 Gharib H. Current evaluation of thyroid nodules. *Trends Endocrinol Metab* 1994; 5:365–9.

☐ MULTIPLE CHOICE QUESTIONS

1   Risk factors for the development of thyroid cancer are:
    (a) External irradiation
    (b) Radioiodine treatment for hyperthyroidism
    (c) Pregnancy
    (d) Family history of phaeochromocytoma
    (e) Carbimazole treatment

2   Tumour markers for differentiated thyroid cancer include:
    (a) Thyroxine binding globulin
    (b) Thyroglobulin
    (c) Calcitonin
    (d) Parathyroid hormone
    (e) Tri-iodothyronine

3   Cold lesions on radionuclide scanning are consistent with a diagnosis of:
    (a) Thyroid cyst
    (b) Hashimoto's thyroiditis
    (c) Toxic nodular goitre
    (d) Thyroid cancer
    (e) Colloid nodule

4   Fine needle aspiration cytology:
    (a) Can differentiate follicular adenomas from carcinomas
    (b) Provides a diagnostic accuracy of around 50%
    (c) Is a risk factor for local invasion of thyroid cancer
    (d) Is performed with a Trucut needle
    (e) Can cure simple thyroid cysts

ANSWERS

1a True	2a False	3a True	4a False
b False	b True	b True	b False
c False	c True	c True	c False
d True	d False	d True	d False
e False	e False	e True	e True

Molecular genetics of multiple endocrine neoplasia type 1

R V Thakker

☐ INTRODUCTION

Multiple endocrine neoplasia type 1 (MEN1), which has also been referred to as Wermer's syndrome, is characterized by the combined occurrence of tumours of the parathyroid glands, pancreatic islet cells and anterior pituitary gland. In addition to these tumours, which constitute the major components of MEN1, adrenal cortical, carcinoid and lipomatous tumours have also been described [1,2]. These MEN1 tumours may either be inherited in an autosomal dominant manner or they may occur sporadically, ie without a family history. However, this distinction between sporadic and familial cases may sometimes be difficult; in some sporadic cases the family history may be absent because the parent with the disease may have died before developing symptoms. In addition, the combinations of the affected glands and their pathologic features, eg hyperplasia or single or multiple adenomas of the parathyroid glands, have been reported to differ in members of the same family [2,3]. The manifestations of MEN1 that are related to the sites of the tumours and to their products of secretion are summarized in Table 1.

☐ MOLECULAR GENETICS OF NEOPLASIA

The development of tumours may be associated with mutations or inappropriate expression of specific normal cellular genes, which are referred to as oncogenes [4]. Two types of oncogene, referred to as dominant and recessive oncogenes, have been described. An activation of dominant oncogenes leads to transformation of the cells containing them, and the genetic changes that cause this activation have recently been elucidated. For example, chromosomal translocations affecting such dominant oncogenes are associated with the occurrence of chronic myeloid leukaemia and Burkitt's lymphoma. In these conditions, the mutations that lead to activation of the oncogene are dominant at the cellular level, and therefore only one copy of the mutated gene is required for the phenotypic effect. Such dominantly acting oncogenes may be assayed in cell culture by first transferring them into recipient cells and then scoring the numbers of transformed colonies; this is referred to as the transfection assay. However, in some inherited neoplasms which may also arise sporadically, such as retinoblastoma, tumour development is associated with two recessive mutations that inactivate oncogenes; these are referred to as recessive oncogenes.

In the inherited tumours, the first of the two recessive mutations is inherited via the germ cell line and is present in all the cells. This recessive mutation is not expressed until a second mutation, within a somatic cell, causes loss of the normal

Table 1. Characteristic tumours and associated biochemical abnormalities of MEN1.

MEN1 tumours	Biochemical features
Parathyroids	Hypercalcaemia and ↑ PTH
Pancreatic islets	
Gastrinoma	↑ Gastrin and ↑ basal gastric acid output
Insulinoma	Hypoglycaemia and ↑ insulin
Glucagonoma	Glucose intolerance and ↑ glucagon
Vipoma	↑ VIP and WDHA
PPoma	↑ PP
Pituitary (anterior)	
Prolactinoma	Hyperprolactinaemia
GH-secreting	↑ GH
ACTH-secreting	Hypercortisolaemia and ↑ ACTH
Non-functioning	Nil or ↑ α subunit
Associated tumours	
Adrenal cortical	Hypercortisolaemia or primary hyperaldosteronism
Carcinoid	↑ 5-HIAA
Lipoma	Nil

Abbreviations: ↑, increased; PTH, parathyroid hormone; VIP, vasoactive intestinal peptide; WDHA, watery diarrhoea, hypokalaemia and achlorhydria; PP, pancreatic polypeptide; GH, growth hormone; ACTH, adrenocorticotrophin; 5-HIAA, 5-hydroxyindoleacetic acid

dominant allele (Fig. 1). The mutations causing the inherited and sporadic tumours are similar, but the cell types in which they occur are different. In the inherited tumours, the first mutation occurs in the germ cell, whereas in the sporadic tumours both mutations occur in the somatic cell. Thus, the risk of tumour development in an individual who has not inherited the first germ-line mutation is much smaller, as both mutational events must coincide in the same somatic cell. In addition, the apparent paradox that the inherited cancer syndromes are due to recessive mutations but are dominantly inherited at the level of the family is explained because, in individuals who have inherited the first recessive mutation, a loss of a single remaining wild-type allele is almost certain to occur in at least one of the large number of cells in the target tissue. This cell will be detected because it forms a tumour, and almost all individuals who have inherited the germ-line mutation will express the disease, even though they inherited a single copy of the recessive gene. This model involving two (or more) mutations in the development of tumours is known as the 'two hit' hypothesis [4]. The normal function of these recessive oncogenes appears to be in regulating cell growth and differentiation, and these genes have also been referred to as anti-oncogenes or tumour suppressor genes. An important feature that has facilitated the investigation of the genetic abnormalities associated with tumour development is that the loss of the remaining allele, which occurs in the somatic cell and gives rise to the tumour, often involves a large-scale loss of chromosomal material (see Fig. 1). This represents a much larger target than the inherited mutation, which

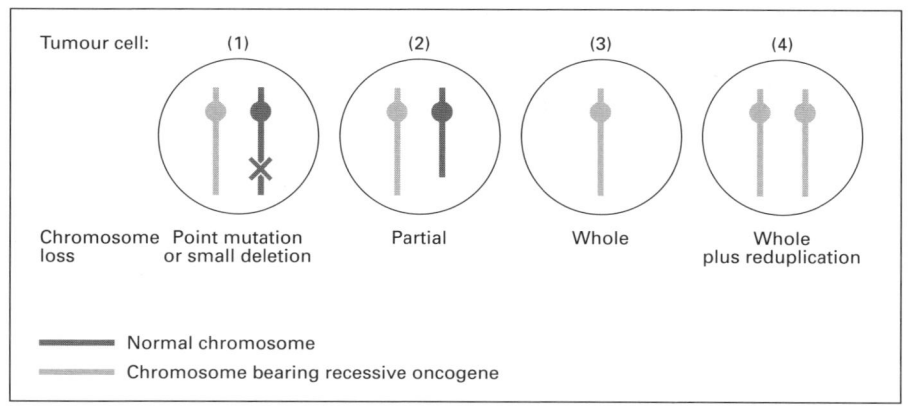

Fig. 1 Chromosomal mechanisms involved in the 'second hit' of Knudson's hypothesis. A pair of chromosomes, one normal and the other bearing the recessive oncogene, are schematically represented in each of four tumour cells (1–4). Four main forms of the 'second hit' involving the normal chromosome, ie the normal dominant allele, are shown. In tumour cell (1), there has been a point mutation or a small deletion, whereas in tumour cells (2) and (3), partial and complete losses of the normal chromosomes have occurred respectively. A complete loss of a chromosome, resulting in autosomal monosomy, may be disadvantageous to cell growth, and reduplication of the chromosome bearing the recessive oncogene may occur, as shown in tumour cell (4). These 'second hits' involving the normal dominant allele would lead to an unmasking of the recessive oncogenic mutation and thereby result in tumour development. (From Thakker [5] with permission.)

may be a small deletion or point mutation, in the search for the genetic loci involved in the development of different inherited tumours.

☐ INVESTIGATION OF GENETIC ABNORMALITIES IN TUMOUR DEVELOPMENT

The investigation of the genetic abnormalities involved in tumour development and the search for these inherited cancer genes has become possible as a result of advances in molecular biology that have provided cloned human DNA sequences to detect these mutations (Fig. 2). These cloned DNA probes identify restriction fragment length polymorphisms (RFLPs), which are the result of variations in the primary DNA sequence of individuals and may be due to either single base changes, deletions, additions or translocations. These changes in DNA sequence occur frequently, approximately once every 250 base pairs (bp) in the non-coding regions, do not usually affect gene function and are often at a distance away from the disease gene. These polymorphisms may, however, lead to the presence or absence of a cleavage site for a restriction enzyme, which cleaves DNA in a sequence-specific manner. The information obtained from these cloned DNA probes may sometimes be limited as many of them are often not highly polymorphic. To gain maximal genetic information, highly polymorphic genetic markers are required and the polymerase chain reaction (PCR) is used to detect directly DNA sequence polymorphisms that are length variations in microsatellite tandem repeats, eg $(CA)_n$, where $n = 10$ to 60. In addition to tandem repeats in the sequence CA, microsatellite tandem repeats consisting of $(AT)_n$, $(GA)_n$, $(ATT)_n$, $(ATTT)_n$ and the hexanucleotide

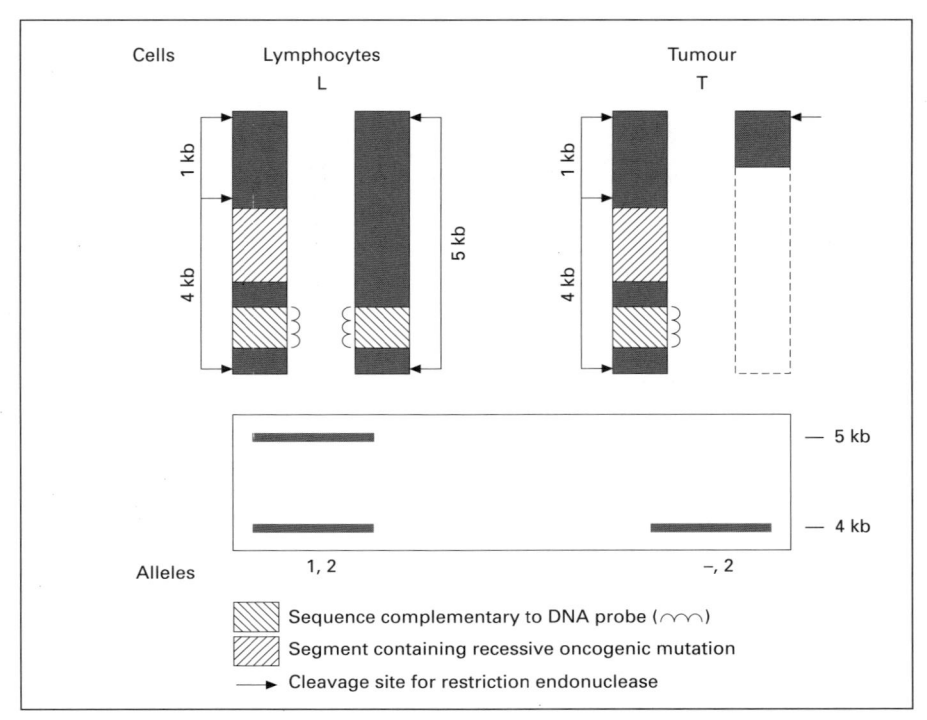

Fig. 2 Schematic representation of the use of restriction fragment length polymorphisms (RFLPs) to investigate the chromosomal mechanisms involved in the 'second hit'. This example is a partial loss of the normal chromosome in the tumour, ie tumour cell (2) in Fig. 1. RFLPs obtained from the leucocyte (L) and tumour (T) DNA of a patient are compared to detect deletions in the tumour tissue. The leucocytes are heterozygous (alleles 1,2) and one of the chromosome pairs in the leucocytes contains the segment incorporating the recessive oncogenic mutation, whereas the other chromosome contains the normal dominant allele. In the example illustrated, there has been a partial loss of the normal chromosome in the tumour, ie tumour cell (2) in Fig. 1, and this is detected by a loss of one of the RFLPs, which have been designated alleles. This abnormality in the tumour cells has been referred to as loss of heterozygosity, loss of alleles, or allelic deletions. (From Thakker [5] with permission.)

$[T(Pu)T(Pu)T(Pu)]_n$ have also been reported. These tandem repeats, which are highly polymorphic and are inherited in a Mendelian manner, are estimated to occur once in every 50 to 100 kilobase pairs (kbp). Thus, these microsatellite polymorphisms and the PCR represent valuable techniques in obtaining a detailed genetic map around a disease locus, for example MEN1. In this approach, oligonucleotide primers are synthesized on either side of the repeat, and PCR is used to amplify the repeat sequence (Fig. 3). The smaller and the larger fragment length polymorphisms in these repetitive sequences are detected by separation on either a polyacrylamide sequencing gel or an agarose gel respectively. These DNA sequence polymorphisms, due to either RFLPs or variations in the tandem repeat of microsatellites, were used in two complementary approaches to identify the genetic abnormalities involved in the development of tumours in MEN1. In one approach, RFLPs and microsatellite polymorphisms obtained from a patient's leucocyte DNA

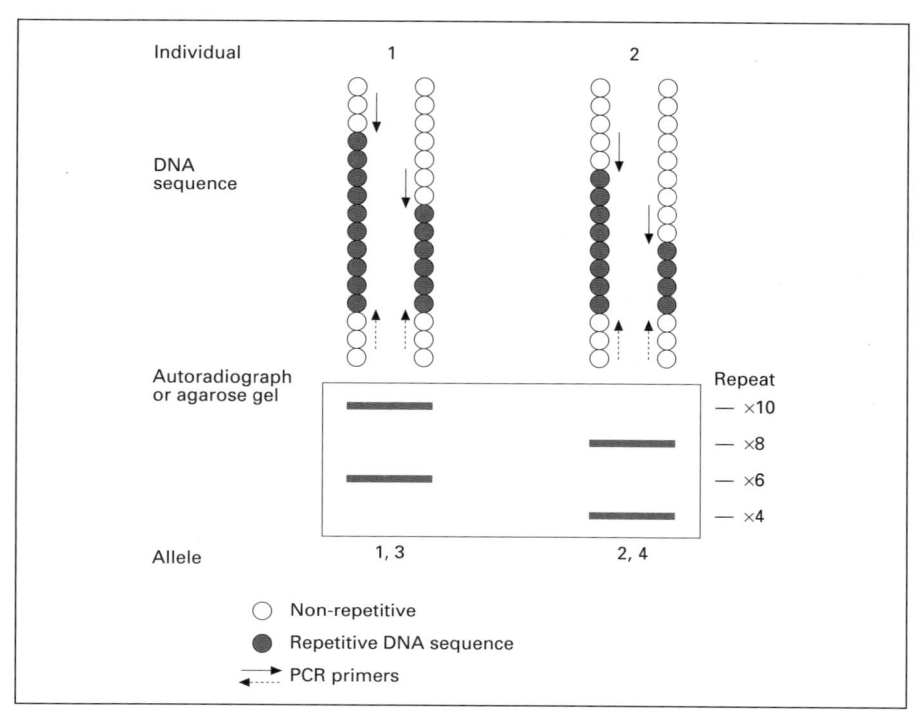

Fig. 3 Schematic representation of polymorphisms in microsatellite tandem repetitive DNA sequences, which may consist, for example, of the dinucleotide CA, or the trinucleotide ATT, or the tetranucleotide ATTT, or the hexanucleotide TATATG. Oligonucleotide primers corresponding to the non-repetitive sequences on either side of the repetitive DNA sequence are synthesized and the polymerase chain reaction (PCR) is used to amplify the repeat in genomic DNA obtained from different individuals. The resulting PCR products are separated either by polyacrylamide gel or agarose gel electrophoresis, and the polymorphisms are revealed by autoradiography or by viewing of an ethidium bromide-stained agarose gel under ultraviolet light. Thus, of the pair of chromosomes from individual (1), one has ten repeats and the other has six repeats, whereas of the pair of chromosomes from individual (2) one has eight repeats and the other has four repeats. Following PCR amplification and separation by gel electrophoresis, these variations in the length of the repeats will be revealed by the differences in the size of the bands, which have been designated alleles; for example, the larger band consisting of ten repeats is designated allele 1, and those consisting of eight, six and four repeats are designated alleles 2, 3 and 4 respectively. These microsatellite tandem repetitive sequences, which are highly polymorphic, show Mendelian inheritance (see Fig. 5) and can be used as genetic markers in MEN1 families. (From Thakker [5] with permission.)

were compared to those obtained from tumour DNA, and differences were sought. In the second approach, these polymorphisms were used as genetic markers in linkage studies of affected families to localize the gene causing MEN1.

☐ TUMOUR DELETION MAPPING STUDIES IN MEN1

A two-stage genetic mutational model has been proposed for the development of tumours in MEN1, and this is analogous to that reported for retinoblastoma. A comparison of the alleles obtained from leucocyte DNA and tumour DNA using either RFLPs or microsatellite polymorphisms can facilitate the detection of the chromosomal abnormalities associated with the 'second hit' in tumour DNA (Fig. 2). A restriction enzyme is used to cleave leucocyte and tumour DNA, and the resulting DNA fragments are separated according to size by agarose gel electrophoresis and transferred by Southern blotting to a nylon membrane, which is hybridized with a single-stranded radiolabelled DNA probe. The labelled DNA probe will anneal to any fragments that have a complementary sequence, and these restricted fragments of varying lengths (RFLPs) are revealed by autoradiography. The exact number and size of RFLPs will vary in relation to the number of recognition sites for the restriction enzyme (see Fig. 2). In this example, the two chromosomes from the leucocytes differ in the number of restriction enzyme cleavage sites; one chromosome has three cleavage sites and the other has two cleavage sites. Following digestion and hybridization, two fragments will be revealed at autoradiography. The chromosome bearing the recessive oncogenic mutation has three cleavage sites, and although two fragments, of 4 kilobases (kb) and 1 kb, will result from the enzymic cleavage, only the 4 kb fragment will be visualized at autoradiography as it contains the complementary sequence to the radiolabelled DNA probe. However, the normal chromosome, ie the one not containing the recessive oncogenic mutation, has a loss of one restriction enzyme cleavage site due to a change in the DNA sequence, and following digestion only restriction fragments of 5 kb in size will result. A single 5 kb RFLP is observed at autoradiography. Alleles can be designated to these RFLPs; for example, the larger 5 kb RFLP is designated allele 1 and the smaller 4 kb RFLP is designated allele 2. Thus, the leucocytes in this example are heterozygous (alleles 1, 2) and the chromosome bearing the recessive oncogenic mutation has allele 2, while the normal chromosome with the dominant allele has allele 1. A partial loss of the normal chromosome, ie the 'second hit' (see Fig. 1), associated with the development of the tumour would be detected by the loss of the 5 kb RFLP (allele 1). Thus, the tumour cells would be hemizygous (allele –, 2) (see Fig. 2) or they may be homozygous (allele 2, 2) if a reduplication of the chromosome bearing the recessive oncogenic mutation had occurred (see Fig. 1). This type of analysis, involving paired leucocyte and tumour DNA, which has been referred to as the detection of a loss of alleles, or allelic deletions, or a loss of heterozygosity in tumours, has been used in localizing the tumour suppressor gene causing MEN1. Microsatellite polymorphisms can also be used in a similar way to detect loss of heterozygosity in tumour DNA (Fig. 4). A loss of alleles involving the whole of chromosome 11 is observed in the parathyroid tumour of a patient with familial MEN1. This loss of alleles in the tumour results from the loss of chromosomal regions containing the marker loci; the complete absence of alleles suggests that this abnormality has occurred within all the tumour cells studied and indicates a monoclonal origin of the tumour. In addition, combined pedigree and tumour studies have demonstrated that such tumour-related allelic deletions of chromosome 11 occur on the chromosome inherited from the normal parent and not the one from the affected parent [3,7]. Thus, the second mutation involves the normal dominant allele and these studies provided additional evidence for the proposed two-stage recessive mutation model for the development of tumours in MEN1.

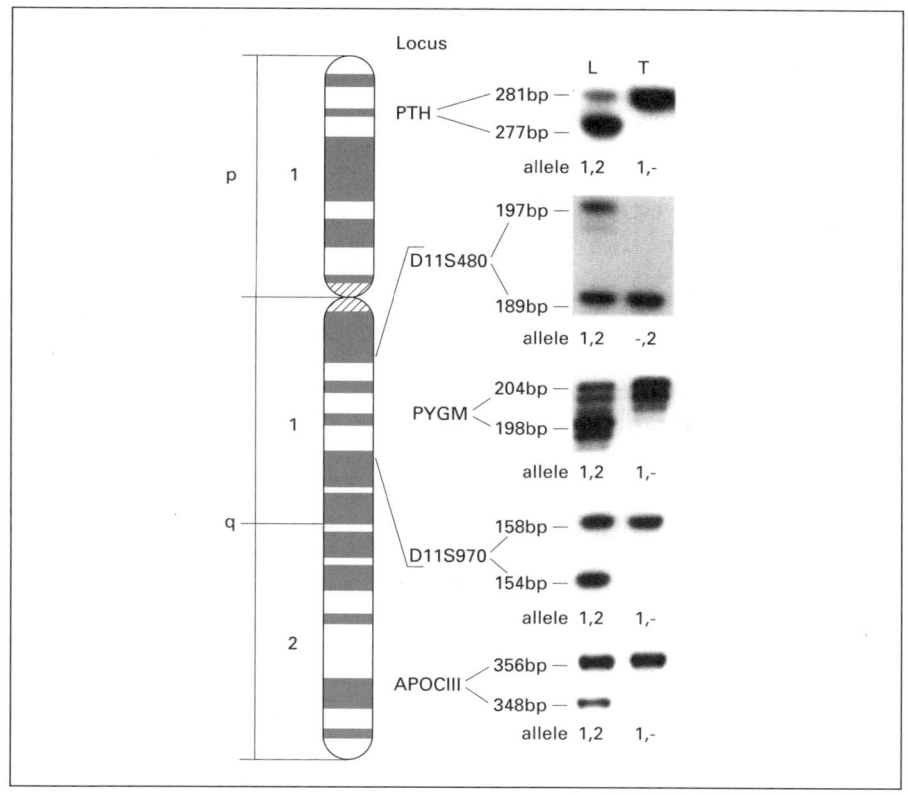

Fig. 4 Loss of alleles on chromosome 11 in a parathyroid tumour from a patient with familial MEN1. The microsatellite polymorphisms obtained from the patient's leucocyte (L) and parathyroid tumour (T) DNA at the PTH, D11S480, PYGM, D11S970 and APOCIII loci are shown. These microsatellite polymorphisms have been identified using specific primers or sequence tagged sites (STSs) for each of the loci that have been localized to chromosome 11, and are shown juxtaposed to their region of origin on the short (p) and long (q) arms of chromosome 11. The microsatellite polymorphisms are assigned alleles (see Fig. 3). For example, D11S480 yielded a 197bp product (allele 1) and a 189bp product (allele 2) following PCR amplification of leucocyte DNA, but the tumour cells have lost the 197bp product (allele 1) and are hemizygous (alleles –,2). Similar losses of alleles are detected using the other DNA markers, and an extensive loss of alleles involving the whole of chromosome 11 is observed in the parathyroid tumour of this patient with MEN1. In addition, the complete absence of bands suggests that this abnormality has occurred within all the tumour cells studied, and indicates a monoclonal origin for this MEN1 parathyroid tumour. (From Pang & Thakker [6] with permission.)

Studies of MEN1 and non-MEN1 parathyroid tumours, insulinomas and anterior pituitary tumours have revealed that allelic deletions on chromosome 11 are also involved in the monoclonal development of these tumours. A detailed examination of such tumours has revealed allele loss within tumours involving smaller regions of chromosome 11, and these studies have mapped the MEN1 locus to the region within chromosome band 11q13 [1]. These results indicate that the MEN1 gene is telomeric to the PYGM locus, which encodes human muscle glycogen phosphorylase, and centromeric to the locus D11S146. In addition, these studies have demonstrated that allelic deletions of chromosome 11 are involved in the development of sporadic non-MEN1 parathyroid tumours, gastrinomas, prolactinomas and somatotrophinomas, and thus the region 11q13 appears to be involved in the development of non-MEN1 and MEN1 endocrine tumours [1].

☐ FAMILY LINKAGE STUDIES IN MEN1

To localize the gene causing MEN1, family linkage studies were used as a parallel and complementary approach to the deletion mapping studies. This investigation of the tumour suppressor gene involved in the MEN1 syndrome was facilitated by the use of RFLPs and microsatellite polymorphisms as genetic markers in studies of affected families. These polymorphisms are inherited in a Mendelian manner and their inheritance can be followed together with a disease in an affected family. The consistent inheritance of a polymorphic allele with the disease indicates that the two genetic loci are close together, ie linked. Genes that are far apart do not consistently co-segregate but show recombination because of the crossing-over during meiosis. By studying recombination events in family studies, the distance between two genes and the probability that they are linked can be ascertained [4]. The distance between two genes is expressed as the recombination fraction (θ), which is equal to the number of recombinants divided by the total number of offspring resulting from informative meioses within a family. The value of the recombination fraction θ can range from 0 to 0.5. A value of zero indicates that the genes are very closely linked, while a value of 0.5 indicates that the genes are far apart and not linked. The probability that the two loci are linked at these distances is expressed as a 'LOD score', which is $\log_{10}$ of the odds ratio favouring linkage. The odds ratio favouring linkage is defined as the likelihood that two loci are linked at a specified recombination (θ) versus the likelihood that the two loci are not linked. A LOD score of +3, which indicates a probability in favour of linkage of 1000 to 1, establishes linkage between two loci, and a LOD score of –2, indicating a probability against linkage of 100 to 1, is taken to exclude linkage between two loci. LOD scores are usually evaluated over a range of recombination fractions (θ), thereby enabling the genetic distance and the maximum (or peak) probability favouring linkage between two loci to be ascertained. This is illustrated in Fig. 5 for family 16/91, which suffers from MEN1.

In family 16/91 (Fig. 5) the disease and INT2 loci are co-segregating in nine out of the ten children, but in one individual (III.6), assuming a 100% penetrance (see below) in early childhood, recombination is observed. Thus, MEN1 and INT2 are co-segregating in 9/10 of the meioses and not segregating in 1/10 meioses, and the likelihood that the two loci are linked at $\theta = 0.10$ is $(9/10)^9 \times (1/10)^1$. If the disease and the INT2 loci were not linked, then the disease would be associated with allele 1 in one-half ($1/2$) of the children and with allele 2 in the remaining half ($1/2$) of the children, and the likelihood that the two loci are not linked is $(1/2)^{10}$. Thus, the odds ratio in favour of linkage between the MEN1 and INT2 loci at $\theta = 0.10$, in this family, is therefore $(9/10)^9 \times (1/10)^1 \div (1/2)^{10} = 39.67:1$, and the LOD score is 1.60 (ie $\log_{10}$ 39.67). Additional studies from other families have also demonstrated positive LOD

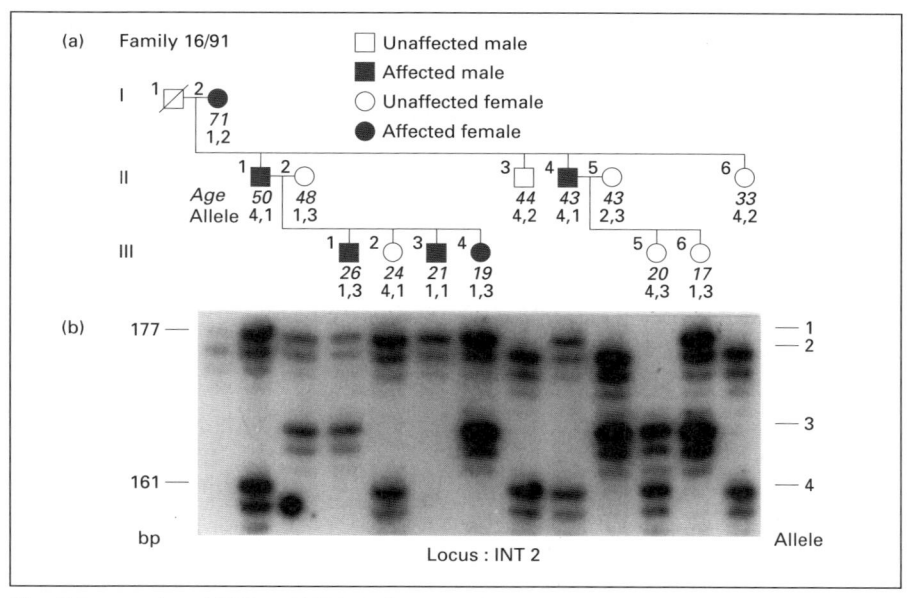

Fig. 5 Segregation of INT2 and MEN1 in family 16/91. Genomic DNA from the family members (a) was used with $\gamma^{32}P$ adenosine triphosphate (ATP) for PCR amplification of the polymorphic repetitive element $(TG)_n$ at this locus. The PCR amplification products were detected by autoradiography on a polyacrylamide gel (b). PCR products were detected from the DNA of each individual; these ranged in size from 161 to 177 base pairs (bp). Alleles were designated for each PCR product and are indicated on the right. For example, individuals II.1 and II.4 reveal two pairs of bands on autoradiography. The upper pair of bands is designated allele 1 and the lower pair of bands is designated allele 4; and these two individuals are therefore heterozygous (alleles 1, 4). A pair of bands for each allele is frequently observed in the PCR detection of microsatellite repeats. The upper band in the pair is the 'true' allele and the lower band in the pair is its associated 'shadow' which results from slipped-strand mispairing during the PCR. The segregation of these bands and their respective alleles together with the disease can be studied in the family members whose alleles and ages are shown. In some individuals, the inheritance of paternal and maternal alleles can be ascertained; the paternal allele is shown on the left. The MEN1 phenotypes in this family were determined by biochemical screening and the age-related penetrance values derived from Fig. 6 were used in linkage analysis, as described in the text. Individual II.1 is affected and heterozygous (alleles 4, 1) and an examination of his affected children (III.1, III.3 and III.4) and his mother (I.2) and sibling (II.4) reveals inheritance of allele 1 with the disease. The unaffected individuals II.3, II.6, III.2 and III.5 have not inherited this allele 1. However, the daughter (III.6) of individual II.4 has inherited allele 1, but remains unaffected at the age of 17 years; this may either be a representation of age-related penetrance, or a recombination between the disease and INT2 loci. (From Thakker [8] with permission.)

scores between MEN1 and the INT2 locus. LOD scores from individual families can be summated, and the peak LOD score between MEN1 and the INT2 locus has exceeded +3 (Table 2), thereby establishing linkage between MEN1 and INT2 loci.

This segregation analysis relies on an accurate assignment of the MEN1 phenotype (ie affected or unaffected) and this depends on the methods used to detect MEN1 and the age of the individual (Fig. 6). The age-related onset, which helps in the estimation of the penetrance of MEN1 and is detailed below in screening studies, was used in the phenotypic assessment of individuals in MEN1 families, and linkage

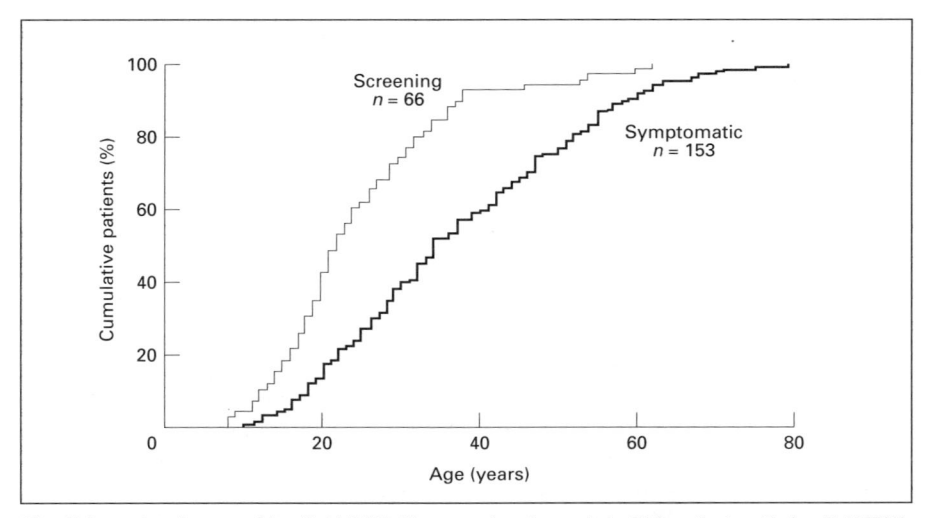

Fig. 6 Age-related onset of familial MEN1. The ages for diagnosis in 219 patients with familial MEN1 were found to range from 8 to 79 years. The patients were subdivided, depending on the method used to detect MEN1, into two groups. The symptomatic group consisted of 153 patients and the age-related onset for MEN1 in these members at 20, 35 and 50 years of age was 18%, 52% and 78% respectively. In another 66 asymptomatic patients, MEN1 had been detected by biochemical screening and the respective age-related onset for MEN1 in these members increased to 43%, 85% and 94%. Thus biochemical screening detected an earlier onset of MEN1 in all age groups. (From Trump et al. [2] with permission.)

was established (ie LOD score > +3) between MEN1 and the 11q13 loci, PYGM and INT2 [3,7]. Recombinants between INT2 and MEN1 have been observed, and this indicates that the oncogene INT2 is not the MEN1 gene itself. No recombinants between MEN1 and PYGM have been observed in affected individuals from two large studies of six and 27 [9] families with MEN1. The genetic map of this region (11q13) has been defined with polymorphic markers to be 11pter-D11S288-D11S149-11cen-PGA-PYGM-D11S97-D11S146-INT2-11qter, and linkage between MEN1 and six of these markers has been established (Table 2). In addition, the MEN1 gene has been located to a region telomeric to PGA and centromeric to D11S97 and in the vicinity of PYGM. The region containing the MEN1 gene has

Table 2. LOD scores for linkage of chromosome 11 markers and MEN1. (From Thakker et al. [9] with permission.)

Locus	Peak LOD score	Recombination fraction (θ)
D11S149	6.29	0.032
PGA	7.78	0.023
PYGM	13.71	0.047
D11S97	13.76	0.076
D11S146	8.27	0.000
INT2	7.04	0.059

been identified to be approximately 2 to 3 centiMorgans (cM) in size. The genetic markers defining this small region around the MEN1 locus are proving useful in further studies of cloning the gene and in identifying individuals within a family who are at risk of developing the disorder.

☐ FAMILY SCREENING IN MEN1

The detection by biochemical screening for the development of MEN1 tumours in asymptomatic members of families with MEN1 is of great importance, as earlier diagnosis and treatment of these tumours reduces morbidity and mortality. The attempts to screen for the development of MEN1 tumours in the asymptomatic relatives of an affected individual have depended largely on measuring the serum concentrations of calcium, gastrointestinal hormones and prolactin [1,2].

Screening in MEN1 is difficult because the clinical and biochemical manifestations in members of any one family are not uniformly similar and because the age-related penetrance (ie the proportion of gene carriers manifesting symptoms or signs of the disease by a given age) has not been established. The proportion of affected individuals who have been detected at a certain age by clinical symptoms or biochemical screening in different series has ranged from 11% to 47% at 20 years of age, 52–94% at 35 years and 85–100% at 50 years; biochemical screening, which detects asymptomatic patients, increased the proportion of affected individuals at all ages [1,2]. Thus, the likelihood of wrongly attributing an 'unaffected' status to an individual with no manifestations of the disease at the age of 35 years may be as high as 1 in 2 or approaching 1 in 20 and depends on whether clinical symptoms alone or biochemical screening methods are used to detect the disease. Further biochemical screening and systematic family studies have been undertaken to improve this situation. Results from a recent study [2] in which 220 patients with familial MEN1 were investigated are shown in Fig. 6. This reveals that the age-related onset for MEN1 detected by clinical manifestations (symptomatic group), at 20, 35 and 50 years of age is 18%, 52% and 78% respectively. The respective age-related onset for MEN1 detected by biochemical screening is markedly improved to 43%, 85% and 94%. However, the identification of individuals at risk in an affected family can still be difficult and the recent availability of DNA markers for MEN1 has helped to reduce these problems.

The use of DNA markers, which may enable carriers of the mutant MEN1 gene to be detected within a family, may help to identify those individuals who need to undergo repeated screening tests for the development of tumours. This is illustrated in Fig. 5 for a family suffering from MEN1. The alleles of each individual at the INT2 locus, which reveals a <6% recombination rate with MEN1 (Table 2) are shown. Individual I.2 is an affected female who is heterozygous (allele 1, 2) and is the mother of four children; her affected children, II.1 and II.4, indicate segregation of allele 1 and the disease. Her other children, II.3 and II.6, who are 44 and 33 years old respectively, are biochemically normal and this indicates that they have a low probability ($\leq$ 15% respectively) of being gene carriers. In addition, the results of genetic marker analysis reveal that II.3 and II.6 have inherited allele 2, which is not associated with the disease in this family, and this indicates a low probability (< 6%) for these being gene carriers. The use of a closer flanking marker, for example PYGM, would help to reduce this probability to <1%. The two daughters (III.5 and III.6) of the affected male II.4 who is heterozygous (alleles 4,1) are in a younger age group (17 to 20 years) and have not developed the disease. The finding of normal serum biochemistry in these individuals still indicates a residual 57% risk of their being gene carriers. However, individual III.5 has inherited allele 4 from her affected father II.4, and this indicates a low probability (< 6%) of her being a gene carrier. In contrast, individual III.6 has inherited allele 1 from her affected father and is at high risk of developing the disease, as the probability of being a gene carrier exceeds 94%. The use of a closer flanking marker such as PYGM (Table 2) would help to confirm and increase this probability to 99.5%. This individual should undergo regular biochemical screening. Thus, the application of DNA markers has helped to determine the carrier risk status of many individuals, and this has substantially altered the screening strategy [2,8] and clinical management of these patients.

The advantages of DNA analysis are that it requires a single blood sample and does not need to be repeated, unlike the biochemical screening tests [4]. This is because the analysis is independent of the age of the individual and provides an objective result. The limitations of DNA analysis are that blood samples needed for the analysis must be available from two or more affected family members to conclude which allele of the marker is inherited with the MEN1 gene. In addition, DNA analysis may be subject to a small but significant error rate because of recombination between the marker and the gene. This error rate can be minimized by the use of flanking DNA markers. The ultimate cloning of the gene itself will help to identify mutations directly and thereby remove this limited uncertainty. At present, an integrated programme of both DNA screening, to identify gene carriers, and biochemical screening, to detect the development of tumours, is recommended. Thus, a DNA test identifying an individual as a mutant gene carrier is likely to lead not to immediate medical or surgical treatment but to earlier and more frequent biochemical screening, whereas a DNA result that leaves an individual with a residual carrier risk of less than 1% will lead to a decision for either infrequent or no screening.

☐ CONCLUSIONS

At present it is suggested that individuals at high risk of developing MEN1 should be screened once a year. Screening should start in early childhood, as the disease has developed in some individuals by the age of 8 years, and should continue for life as some individuals have not developed the disease until over 80 years old [2]. Screening history and physical examination should be directed towards eliciting the symptoms and signs of hypercalcaemia, nephrolithiasis, peptic ulcer disease, neuroglycopenia, hypopituitarism, galactorrhoea and amenorrhoea in women, acromegaly, Cushing's disease, visual field loss and the presence of subcutaneous lipomata [1,2]. Biochemical screening should include serum calcium and prolactin estimations in all individuals, and measurement of gastrointestinal hormones and more specific endocrine function tests should be reserved for individuals who have symptoms or signs suggestive of a clinical syndrome. Thus, the recent advances in molecular biology that have enabled the localization of the gene causing MEN1 have helped in the clinical management of patients and their families with this disorder.

ACKNOWLEDGEMENTS

I am grateful to: the Medical Research Council (MRC) for support; to the clinical and scientific colleagues who have provided valuable resources for these studies; to Ms Carol Wooding, Dr Joanna Pang and Dr Mark Pook for help in preparation of some of the Figures; and to Ms Marilyn Cohda for typing the manuscript.

REFERENCES

1. Thakker RV. Multiple endocrine neoplasia type 1 (MEN1). In: DeGroot LJ, Besser GK, Burger HG, Jameson JL, Loriaux DL, Marshall JC, Odell WD, Potts JT, Rubinstein AH, eds. *Endocrinology* (3rd edn). Philadelphia; WB Saunders, 1994: 2815–31.
2. Trump D, Farren B, Wooding C, Pang JT, *et al.* Clinical studies of multiple endocrine neoplasia type 1 (MEN1). *Q J Med* 1996; **89**: 653–69.
3. Thakker RV, Bouloux P, Wooding C, Chotai K, Broad PM, Spurr NK, Besser GM, O'Riordan JLH. Association of parathyroid tumors in multiple endocrine neoplasia type 1 with loss of alleles on chromosome 11. *New Engl J Med* 1989; **321**: 218–24.
4. Thakker RV, Ponder BAJ. Multiple endocrine neoplasia. In: Sheppard MC, ed. *Clinical Endocrinology and Metabolism.* Vol. 2, No. 4. Molecular biology and endocrinology. London: Baillière Tindall, 1988: 1031–67.
5. Thakker RV. The molecular genetics of the multiple endocrine neoplasia syndromes. *Clin Endocrinol* 1993; **38**: 1–14.
6. Pang JT, Thakker RV. Multiple endocrine neoplasia type 1. *Eur J Cancer* 1994; **30A**: 1961–8.
7. Larsson C, Skogseid B, Oberg K, Nakamura Y, Nordenskjold MC. Multiple endocrine neoplasia type 1 gene maps to chromosome 11 and is lost in insulinoma. *Nature* 1988; **332**: 85–7.
8. Thakker RV. Molecular mechanisms of tumor formation in hereditary and sporadic tumors of the MEN1 type: the impact of genetic screening in the management of MEN1. In: Gagel RF, ed. *Endocrinology and Metabolism Clinics of North America.* Philadelphia: WB Saunders, 1994: 117–35.
9. Thakker RV, Wooding C, Pang J, Farren B. MEN1 Collaborative Group. Linkage analysis of 7 polymorphic markers at chromosome 11p11.2-11q13 in 27 multiple endocrine neoplasia type 1 families. *Ann Hum Genet* 1993; **57**: 17–25.

☐ MULTIPLE CHOICE QUESTIONS

1 Multiple endocrine neoplasia type 1 (MEN1):
 (a) An autosomal recessive disorder
 (b) Characterized by parathyroid, pancreatic islet cell and posterior pituitary tumours
 (c) Frequently has involvement of thyroid C-cells, producing calcitonin
 (d) Due to a gene located on chromosome 11
 (e) Likely to involve a tumour suppressor (recessive) oncogene

2 Tumours frequently observed in patients with MEN1:
   (a) Insulinomas
   (b) Prolactinomas
   (c) Phaeochromocytomas
   (d) Neuromas
   (e) Gastrinomas

3 The following are useful genetic markers:
   (a) Microsatellite polymorphisms
   (b) Plasmid sequence polymorphisms
   (c) Restriction fragment length polymorphisms
   (d) The histocompatibility (HLA) loci
   (e) The ABO blood groups

4 Regarding genetic linkage studies:
   (a) The recombination fraction (θ) indicates the distance between two genes
   (b) A LOD score of <+3 establishes linkage between two loci
   (c) A recombination fraction (θ) of 0.01 indicates that the two loci are close together
   (d) A LOD score of <−2 excludes linkage between two loci
   (e) To establish linkage with a disease locus, the disease must occur at a high frequency in the population

5 Regarding multiple endocrine neoplasia type 1 (MEN1):
   (a) Gastrinomas are associated with peptic ulcers
   (b) Watery diarrhoea, hypokalaemia and achlorhydria (WDHA) occur in association with PPomas
   (c) Glucagonomas are associated with hypoglycaemia
   (d) Insulinomas are associated with glucose intolerance
   (e) Carcinoid tumours are associated with raised 5-hydroxyindoleacetic acid (5-HIAA)

ANSWERS

1a False	2a True	3a True	4a True	5a True
b False	b True	b False	b False	b False
c False	c False	c True	c True	c False
d True	d False	d True	d True	d False
e True	e True	e True	e False	e True

Reappraisal of insulin therapy

E A M Gale

☐ INTRODUCTION

Insulin therapy is one of the great triumphs of 20th century medicine. It converted a miserable wasting illness with an average life expectancy of around 18 months into a state of full activity and well-being. These benefits are still apparent 75 years later, but it is frustratingly evident that insulin replacement therapy does not offer freedom from disabling late complications. Why should this be? At onset, insulin-dependent diabetes mellitus (IDDM) is a condition of straightforward insulin deficiency, and its complex metabolic derangements could all, in theory, be reversed by adequate physiological insulin replacement. Further, there is now incontrovertible evidence that microvascular complications can be prevented by improved glycaemic control. All this suggests that ineffective treatment is the main reason why late complications are so prevalent in the diabetic population. This review will describe some of the inbuilt limitations of current insulin therapy, and will consider ways in which they may partly be overcome.

☐ PHYSIOLOGY OF INSULIN SECRETION

Near normal control of blood glucose is most likely to be achieved by therapeutic imitation of physiological insulin secretion, but several features of the natural system are currently almost impossible to reproduce. In the first place, physiological insulin secretion is under feedback control, mediated by glucose-sensing systems within the β-cell, and this feedback loop maintains very effective regulation of circulating glucose despite the metabolic demands of active life. Second, the pancreas secretes insulin into the portal circulation, and a large but variable proportion, usually quoted at around 50%, is cleared on the first pass through the liver. Portal insulin levels are therefore much higher than systemic levels. A third consideration is that basal insulin secretion achieves relatively constant peripheral insulin levels in healthy individuals during the night and between meals, whereas food ingestion produces a rapid burst of secretion achieving peak levels 5–10 times above baseline. These bursts are closely tailored to metabolic requirements, and the short half-life of insulin (3–5 minutes) means that insulin levels are rapidly restored towards baseline following each burst of secretion.

    Current insulin replacement therapy cannot match this control system [1]. In the first place, insulin has to be administered in advance of metabolic requirements. The amount taken with each injection is not regulated by any feedback mechanism, but is instead based on an informed guess as to the number of units needed to balance anticipated food intake and energy expenditure over the next few hours. Injected insulin then enters subcutaneous tissue whence it diffuses into the systemic circulation. In consequence, patients on insulin are routinely exposed to slightly higher systemic levels of insulin, and considerably lower portal levels, than are healthy individuals. Further, absorption from subcutaneous tissue is slow and erratic, and results in late and sustained peaks of insulin, which are poorly matched to meal-time requirements. These characteristics will be explored in more detail in the following sections, but they help to explain the old dictum that insulin is administered *in the wrong place, at the wrong time*, and *in the wrong amount*.

☐ THE INSULIN INJECTION

Early insulin preparations were relatively crude pancreatic extracts which often produced painful red lumps in the skin when patients started insulin treatment. These ceased to appear after a while, presumably as immune tolerance was acquired. Progressive improvements in the purity of insulin eradicated this phenomenon, although disfiguring cavities in subcutaneous fat known as lipoatrophy remained common until the introduction of highly purified insulins in the 1970s. Fatty lumps under the skin due to repeated injection into the same spot (lipohypertrophy) are still an occasional problem, and regular inspection of the injection site remains an important part of the routine of diabetes management.

Although insulin is designed for injection into subcutaneous fat, unintended intramuscular injection is common. This is because insulin needles are 11–13 mm in length, sufficient to traverse subcutaneous fat layers on the thighs and abdomen of many non-obese people, particularly men and children. Intermittent intramuscular injection is therefore frequent in such individuals and increases the variability of insulin absorption [2]. Further variation is introduced by differences in the rate of absorption from the three major sites, so that insulin is absorbed more rapidly from the abdomen than from the arm, and more rapidly from the arm than from the thigh [1]. Attention to details of technique and injection site will often suggest simple and practical ways of sorting out clinical problems and of achieving more reproducible control. Even so, insulin absorption remains highly variable, and the intra-individual coefficient of variation for T_{50} of absorption is more than 25% even when injections are performed at the same site and with carefully standardized technique [3].

Insulin injected under the skin will have no metabolic effect until it has been absorbed, has entered the circulation, and has reached the cell receptors with which it will interact. This process is shown diagrammatically in Fig. 1. If an intermediate acting preparation is used, the first step will be separation of insulin from the crystal structure of the depot preparation. Its natural configuration is in hexamers formed around a zinc core, and these must dissociate into dimers and monomers before insulin can enter the blood stream in any quantity. This process of *insulin absorption* causes substantial delay before peak insulin action is obtained [4]. Soluble insulin preparations take 1–2 hours to reach their peak effect, after which hyperinsulinaemia persists for longer than desired, increasing the risk of hypoglycaemia. Better matching of food and insulin can be achieved by asking patients to inject 20–40 minutes before eating. This does, however, represent a considerable

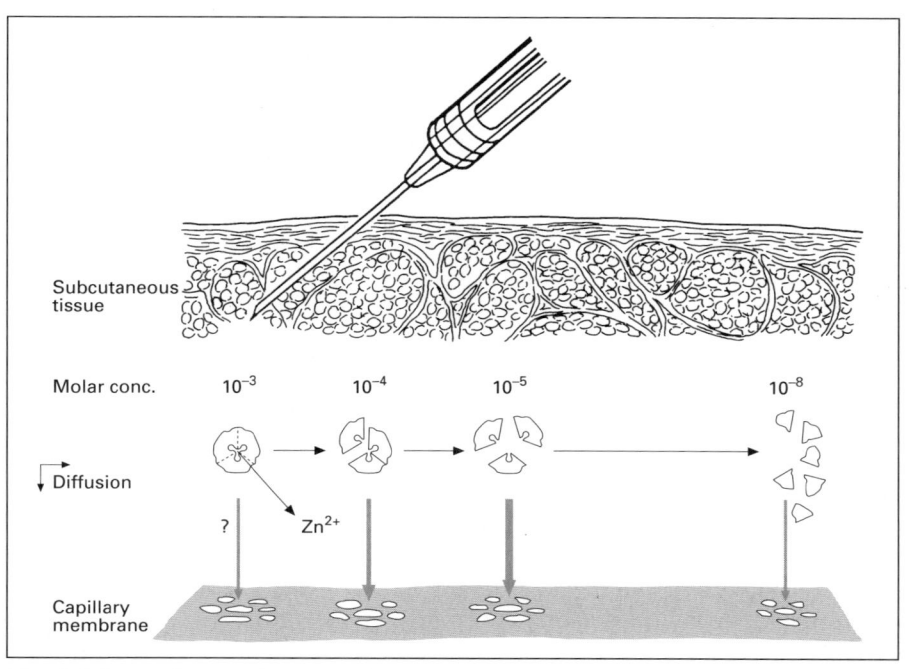

Fig. 1 Scheme of events following subcutaneous injection of insulin. Hexameric insulin diffuses down a concentration gradient. A 50–100-fold dilution is required for dissociation into the dimeric form, and a further 1000-fold dilution is required for dissociation into the monomeric form. (From Brange et al. [4] with permission.)

imposition, and the advice is often more honoured in the breach than in the observance.

☐ PHARMACOLOGY OF INSULIN

The quest for non-immunogenic insulin prompted the move from bovine insulin, which differs from human in three amino acid residues, to pork insulin, which differs by only one. The subsequent introduction of biosynthetic human insulin, although a major technical achievement, produced little clinical advantage over highly purified pork insulin. Insulin is provided either in soluble form, or formulated with zinc or protamine to retard its absorption into the circulation. Soluble insulin is ideally given with each meal to mimic physiological meal-time insulin secretion, and its limitations in this role have already been noted. The main limitation of intermediate insulin preparations, which are used to cover basal insulin requirements, is that injected insulin inevitably peaks and declines, whereas endogenous insulin secretion is relatively constant. In consequence, patients taking intermediate insulins for overnight control characteristically show a dip in glucose around 03:00 (3 am), sometimes resulting in hypoglycaemia, followed by a rapid rise as the insulin effect wears off. Fluctuating fasting blood glucose levels and intermittent nocturnal hypoglycaemia are common clinical consequences.

INSULIN REGIMENS

Traditional once or twice daily insulin therapy remains the mainstay for most patients around the world. Since few obtain acceptable glycaemic control on one injection a day, this is best reserved for those with adverse circumstances or a limited life expectancy. Twice daily injection is best given using free or fixed mixtures of soluble and intermediate insulin, with rather more of the insulin in the longer-acting form. Offered the choice, the majority of younger patients opt for multiple daily injections and take soluble insulin before each meal (usually with a pen device) and intermediate insulin to cover the overnight period. Multiple injections may be preferred more for the flexible lifestyle they allow than because of a serious quest to obtain better glycaemic control. For this reason the term *intensified insulin therapy* should be reserved for motivated patients with appropriate education and support, who are using multiple insulin injections, regular blood tests and modifications of diet and lifestyle to achieve near-normoglycaemia. The patterns of insulin delivery achieved by twice daily insulin and by a multiple injection regimen are shown in Fig. 2.

AIMS OF INSULIN THERAPY

The central aim of insulin therapy is to achieve the best possible approximation to normoglycaemia, at the least possible cost in terms of hypoglycaemia and

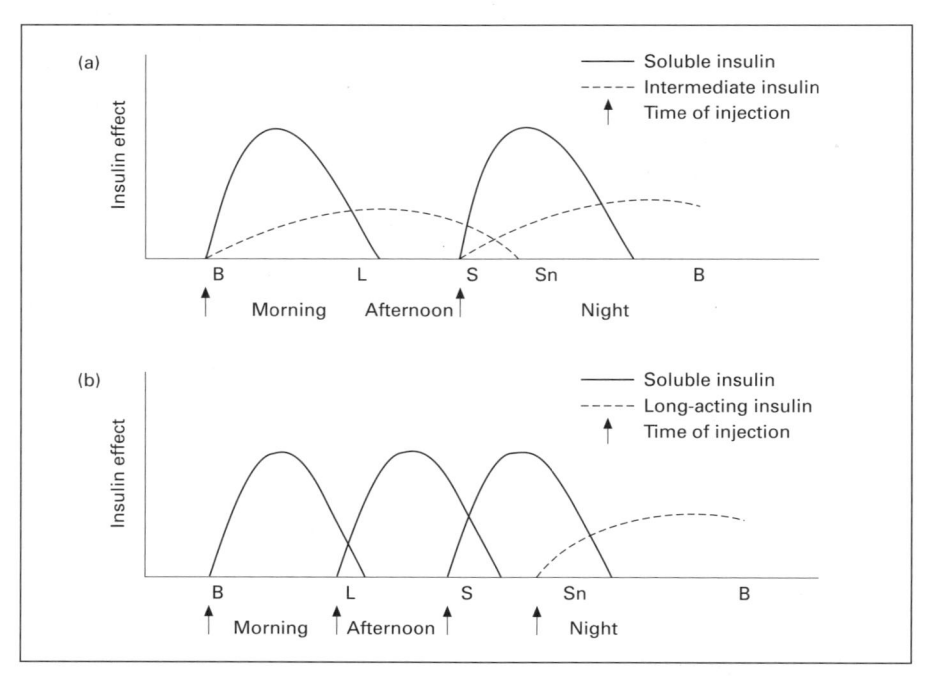

Fig. 2 Insulin regimens. (a) Twice daily soluble and intermediate insulin. (b) Three times daily soluble insulin with long-acting insulin given before supper. B = breakfast; L = lunch; S = supper; Sn = snack (bedtime). (From Tattersall RB, Gale EAM. *Diabetes: Clinical Management*. Edinburgh: Churchill Livingstone, 1990, with permission.)

constraints on lifestyle. These conflicting aims indicate, correctly, that insulin treatment is a compromise between benefits, many of which are long-term, and disadvantages that are usually more immediate. Patients are most likely to accept short term risk and inconvenience when the longer term advantages of so doing are clear, and when they have trust and confidence in the person advising them. The quest for good glycaemic control thus needs to be guided by consideration of the balance of advantage to the patient. In pregnancy, for example, the need for short term control is so urgent that it may have to be paid for by more frequent hypoglycaemia. Conversely, control may reasonably be less rigorous in the elderly or others with limited life expectancy, in those with multiple disease processes, very adverse social circumstances, or subject to frequent and disabling hypoglycaemia. It would be inappropriate to insist on a single standard of control for all patients on insulin, but this does not absolve the clinician of the duty to aim for the best possible level of glucose control within the appropriate context.

☐ IMPORTANCE OF GLYCAEMIC CONTROL

There is now overwhelming evidence that careful control of diabetes can prevent, or at least delay, its small vessel complications. This conclusion was reached by the Diabetes Control and Complications Trial (DCCT), a gargantuan study that compared conventional with intensified insulin therapy [5]. A total of 1441 patients were recruited, aged from 13 to 39 years. They were divided into two cohorts, a primary prevention cohort of 726 patients with a 1–5 year history of diabetes and no detectable complications, and a secondary prevention cohort of 715 with mild (background) retinopathy without overt proteinuria. Patients in each cohort were randomized to conventional therapy, meaning one or two daily injections together with urine or blood testing, or to intensified therapy. The intensified treatment regimen was extremely demanding. Patients had three or more injections per day (less usual in the USA than in Europe) or insulin pump treatment. They measured their blood glucose four times every day, adjusted their treatment frequently to meet very strict blood glucose targets, were seen every month and were contacted by telephone between visits to check that all was well.

Control was substantially better in the intensified treatment group. Glycated haemoglobin (HbA1c) levels of around 7% were maintained over 6 years (normal range up to 6.1%), as against levels of around 9% in the conventionally treated group. After 6.5 years, the effects of improved control were so manifest (Fig. 3) that the trial was brought to an end (Table 1).

The risk of macrovascular disease was also reduced although not to a significant extent, partly because this was a relatively young group of patients and few major cardiovascular events occurred.

The results of this trial are unequivocal. Strict control of blood glucose levels prevents or delays the onset of microvascular complications. There were other important implications.

1 *There is no 'safe level' of blood glucose.* The risk of complications falls progressively in parallel with mean blood glucose, but there is no zone of

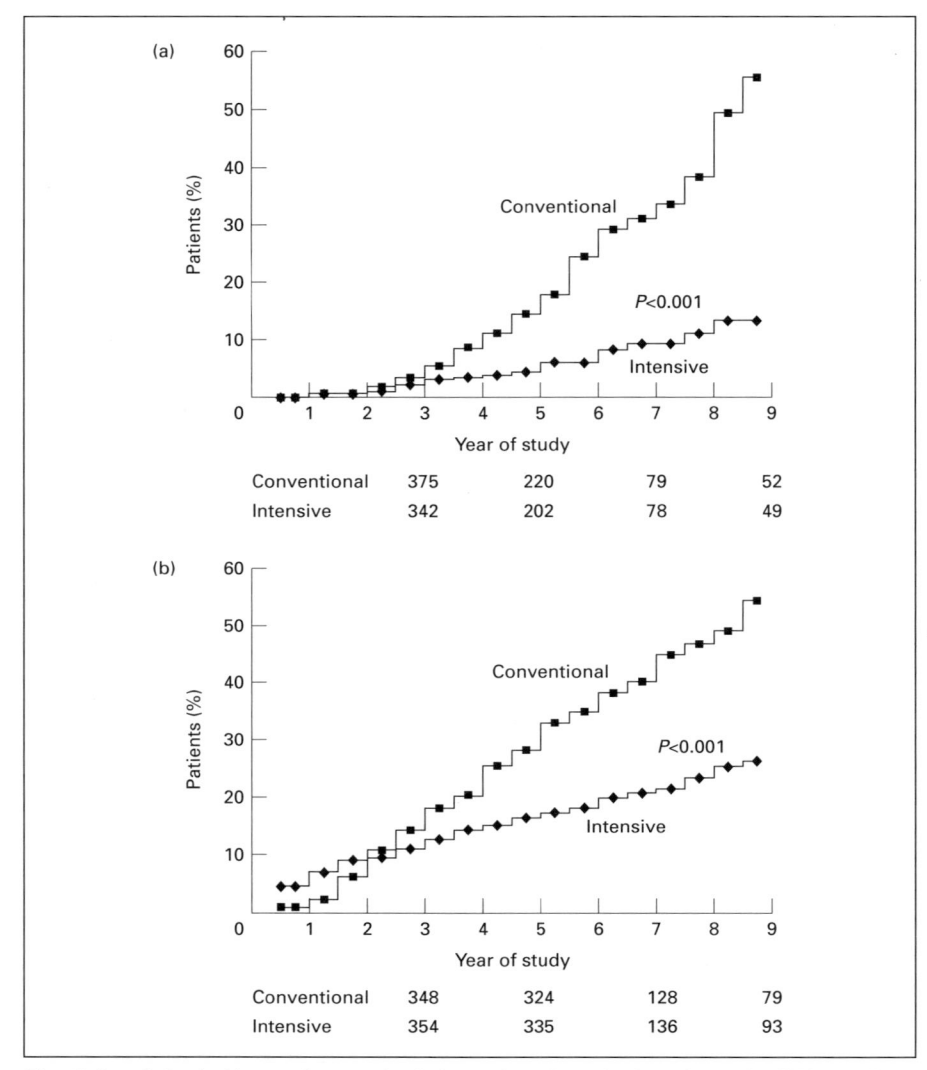

Fig. 3 Cumulative incidence of a sustained change in retinopathy in patients with IDDM receiving intensive or conventional therapy. (a) Primary prevention cohort receiving intensive therapy showed a 76% reduction in the adjusted mean risk of onset of retinopathy during the study compared with conventional therapy ($p < 0.001$). (b) Secondary intervention cohort receiving intensive therapy showed a 54% reduction in the adjusted mean risk of retinopathy progression compared with conventional therapy ($p < 0.001$). The numbers of patients in each therapy group evaluated at 3, 5, 7 and 9 years are shown below the figure. (From Diabètes Control and Complications Trial Research Group [5], with permission.)

safety other than normoglycaemia – itself an impracticable target with current methods of control.

2   *The better the blood glucose, the greater the risk of hypoglycaemia.* Patients on intensified treatment were initially three times as likely to experience severe

Table 1. The results of DCCT [5].

In the primary prevention cohort:
  development of retinopathy was reduced by 76%
  development of microalbuminuria was reduced by 34%
  development of clinical neuropathy was reduced by 69%
In the secondary prevention cohort:
  progression of retinopathy was reduced by 54%
  progression to albuminuria was reduced by 43%
  progression to clinical neuropathy was reduced by 57%

hypoglycaemia as those on conventional treatment; hypoglycaemia emerged as the main obstacle to improved control.

3   *Success is not just a matter of technique.* Although the media quickly caught on to the idea that multiple injections were the key to improved control, the reality was more complex. Good control was achieved because the patients were highly motivated, highly educated and relentlessly encouraged during the trial.

4   *Good control is very demanding, and very expensive.* Patients for the trial were self selected, and backed by large and active clinical teams. The costs of providing equivalent care to all patients with IDDM would be astronomical.

Some questions were left unanswered. Is very strict control appropriate for patients with non-insulin-dependent diabetes mellitus (NIDDM)? Small vessel complications are the main cause of excess mortality in the young, but atherosclerosis is the main cause of death in older patients. Earlier studies found little or no evidence that large vessel disease was influenced by good glycaemic control, and the DCCT produced no conclusive evidence that aggressive insulin therapy is beneficial. Equally, many of these patients are also at risk from other cardiovascular risk factors, such as hypertension and hyperlipidaemia. At present it seems wiser to aim for all-round reduction of coronary risk rather than to focus exclusively on the blood glucose level.

There are some very positive lessons to be drawn from the trial, but techniques for achieving safe normoglycaemia are lacking. Enthusiasm must be tempered with common sense if we are to avoid psychological consequences such as guilt or a sense of failure when very demanding targets are not achieved, or well-meaning advice leads to demoralizing episodes of hypoglycaemia.

☐ HYPOGLYCAEMIA

Hypoglycaemia is the major, most common, and most feared complication of insulin therapy. It has been estimated that an average patient may expect some 2000–4000 episodes of symptomatic hypoglycaemia in the course of 40 years of treatment, and that at least 10% will expect severe hypoglycaemia with coma in the course of a given year. The DCCT confirmed earlier studies in showing a powerful inverse relationship with glycaemic control; the better the HbA1c, the greater the risk of severe hypoglycaemia (Fig. 4). One reason for this is that repeated exposure to low blood glucose levels can itself lead to impairment of counter-regulatory responses and warning symptoms of hypoglycaemia. It has been demonstrated that these responses and symptoms are not irrevocably lost, but are instead triggered at progressively lower blood glucose levels. The patient may by then be so incapacitated

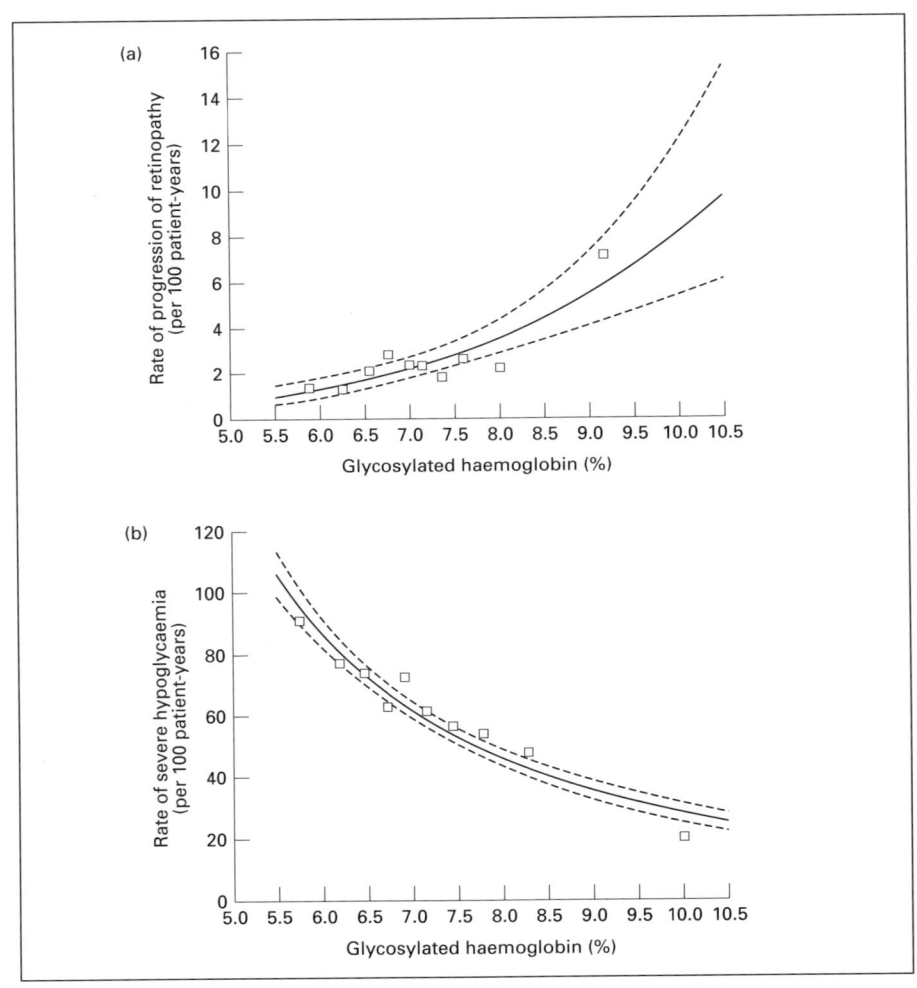

Fig. 4 Risk of sustained progression of retinopathy (a) and rate of severe hypoglycaemia (b) in patients receiving intensive therapy, according to their mean glycosylated haemoglobin values during the trial. (a) Glycosylated haemoglobin values were the mean of values obtained every 6 months. (b) Mean monthly values. □, crude rates within deciles of mean glycosylated haemoglobin values during the trial; each square corresponds to more than 400 patient-years. ——, regression lines estimated as a function of the log of the mean glycosylated haemoglobin value in (a) and the log of the glycosylated haemoglobin value in (b). – – –, 95% confidence intervals. (From Diabetes Control and Complications Trial Research Group [5].)

by neuroglycopenia as to be unable to recognise his condition and to respond effectively. It is, however, encouraging to note that symptoms may be restored if the patient's control is relaxed [6].

Although the acute morbidity and mortality of severe hypoglycaemia are remarkably low compared with other causes of coma, there are worrying indications that recurrent severe hypoglycaemia can lead to progressive cognitive impairment [7]. From the more practical point of view, it is worth emphasizing that the ability to recognize hypoglycaemia, and perhaps also the ability to sustain low blood glucose levels without mishap, is very unevenly distributed within the diabetic population. Some patients achieve near-normoglycaemia much more safely than others. These considerations make it clear that the balance of advantage between improved glycaemic control and disability due to hypoglycaemia can only be determined empirically, which is why clinical skill and judgement form such a large component of effective insulin therapy.

☐ WHAT ARE THE INGREDIENTS OF GOOD CONTROL?

Somewhat inevitably, attention has focussed on the technology of improved glycaemic control rather than on its psychology. This is a pity, since there is powerful evidence that the human factor is of great importance. For example, one classic study compared the effect of home blood glucose monitoring with that of urine testing alone in patients receiving an equal amount of clinical attention, and found that both groups showed equal improvement in glycaemic control [8]. The conclusion from this is not that blood glucose testing is unnecessary; it has established itself as a mainstay of good diabetes management. Instead, the study demonstrates that increased attention and interest improves patient motivation, and that this alone can produce a marked improvement in control – an example of the Hawthorne effect. A survey of the diabetes literature suggests that most reports of techniques for improving control have failed to correct adequately for the Hawthorne effect, and that many of the remainder serve only to emphasize its importance. We may conclude that patient motivation is essential to good control of diabetes, and is most likely to be achieved in patients who feel confident and at ease with their therapy rather than feeling that they themselves are the victims of its demands.

☐ INSULIN ANALOGUES

Genetic engineering opened the way for the development of modified insulin molecules manufactured specifically for pharmacological use. The main benefits we might expect from such new insulins are improved pharmacokinetics, with greater day-to-day reproducibility of effect, more physiological time-action characteristics, or both [9]. We have seen that absorption of soluble insulin is delayed because time is needed for it to dissociate from the hexameric to the monomeric form following injection. The clinical consequences are an overshoot of blood glucose after food and the risk of hypoglycaemia before the next meal is due. Several attempts have been made to produce an insulin with a reduced ability to form monomers, and one known as LysPro (Humalog®) has recently been marketed [10]. This has the useful property of forming hexamers in concentrated solution in the insulin vial, which improves its stability under conditions of storage, but dissociates into monomers much more rapidly than soluble insulin in dilute solution, or after subcutaneous injection.

The modification was based on comparison with the human insulin-like growth factor (IGF) molecule, which is closely related in structure to insulin, yet self-aggregates much less readily. This property is linked to reversal of proline and lysine, which occupy positions 28 and 29 respectively on the C-terminal end of the B-chain of the insulin molecule. LysPro differs from human insulin only in reversal of these two amino acids; the remainder of the molecule is unchanged. This modification is so slight that there is no detectable effect on the metabolic action of the altered insulin, which behaves just like human insulin when injected intravenously.

Potential clinical benefits of the new formulation include better matching of peak insulin action to food absorption following meals, better glycaemic control in the immediate postprandial period, and less risk of hypoglycaemia before the next meal is due. An important practical advantage is that the injection can be given shortly before meals, whereas a 20–30 minute gap is recommended for soluble insulin.

Extensive premarketing studies, mostly based on open comparisons with soluble insulin, suggest that LysPro insulin is safe, and have revealed no major disadvantage compared with soluble insulin. Postprandial glucose levels are 1–2 mmol/l lower than with soluble insulin, but no study has shown any reduction in HbA1c. A double-blind comparison of the two preparations showed that *preprandial* glucose levels were significantly higher on LysPro. This effect, presumably due to the shorter action of the new insulin, probably explains the lack of improvement in overall control. Some of the preregistration studies have also shown a reduction in the frequency of minor hypoglycaemic episodes, which might be related to the increase in preprandial blood glucose, but no difference in severe episodes has been demonstrated. Patient convenience is therefore the main current advantage of LysPro, although it has the potential to improve glucose control when combined with better basal insulin replacement therapy. Formulation of LysPro as a mixture with a variant of neutral protamine Hagedorn (NPH) insulin has been achieved, and premarketing studies are under way. These combinations may be able to combine the advantage of rapid onset of action while maintaining better control of preprandial glucose levels.

☐ FUTURE DEVELOPMENTS

In the longer term, the future holds out the prospect of alternative solutions to the problems of insulin injection therapy. Potential solutions include pancreatic islet transplantation, genetically engineered β-cells and prevention of IDDM itself. In the interim, which is likely to be many years, progress will depend on improvements in standard insulin injection therapy. Implantable glucose sensors or hypoglycaemia alarms would be of great value, but reliable models are unlikely to reach the market within the next few years. At present, a patient-centred approach to insulin therapy that emphasizes the importance of education and motivation offers the key to improved glycaemic control.

REFERENCES

1. Zinman B. The physiologic replacement of insulin: an elusive goal. *New Engl J Med* 1989; **321**: 363–70.
2. Thow J, Home P. Insulin injection technique. *Brit Med J* 1990; **301**: 3–4.
3. Galloway JA, Spradlin CT, Nelson RL, Wentworth SM, Davison JA, Warner JL. Factors affecting the absorption, serum insulin concentration and blood glucose responses after injections of regular insulin and various insulin mixtures. *Diabetes Care* 1981; **4**: 366–76.
4. Brange J, Owens DR, Kang S, Volund A. Monomeric insulins and their experimental and clinical implications. *Diabetes Care* 1990; **13**: 923–54.
5. Diabetes Control and Complications Trial Research Group. The effect of intensive treatment of diabetes on the development and progression of long-term complications in insulin-dependent diabetes mellitus. *New Engl J Med* 1993; **329**: 977–86.
6. Cranston I, Lomas J, Maran A, Macdonald IA, Amiel SA. Restoration of hypoglycaemia unawareness in patients with long duration insulin-dependent diabetes. *Lancet* 1994; **344**: 283–7.
7. Langan SJ, Deary IJ, Hepburn DA, Frier BM. Cumulative cognitive impairment following recurrent severe hypoglycaemia in adult patients with insulin-treated diabetes. *Diabetologia* 1991; **34**: 337–44.
8. Worth R, Home PD, Johnston DG, Anderson J, Ashworth L, Burrin JM, Appleton D, Binder C, Alberti KGMM. Intensive attention improves glycaemic control in insulin-dependent diabetes without further advantage from home blood glucose monitoring: results of a controlled trial. *Brit Med J* 1982; **285**: 1233–40.
9. Galloway JA. New directions in drug development: mixtures, analogues, and modeling. *Diabetes Care* 1993; **16** Suppl 3: 16–23.
10. Howey DC, Bowsher RR, Brunelle RL, Woodworth JR. [Lys(B28), Pro(B29)] – human insulin: a rapidly absorbed analogue of human insulin. *Diabetes* 1994; **43**: 396–402.

☐ MULTIPLE CHOICE QUESTIONS

1. Following subcutaneous insulin injection:
   (a) Circulating insulin peaks more rapidly if the injection is given into the arm rather than into the abdomen
   (b) Inadvertent intramuscular injection is very uncommon
   (c) Control of postprandial glucose levels will be improved if the injection is given at least 20 minutes before eating
   (d) Insulin diffuses into the circulation in the hexameric form
   (e) Lipoatrophy is still an occasional complication

2. Insulin-induced hypoglycaemia:
   (a) There is no evidence that recurrent hypoglycaemia may result in permanent cognitive impairment
   (b) Loss of hypoglycaemic warning symptoms can sometimes be reversed

(c) Nocturnal hypoglycaemia is most common around midnight
(d) Hypoglycaemia is more common after injection into the abdomen
(e) Recurrent hypoglycaemia may induce loss of hypoglycaemic warning symptoms

3   The DCCT study:
(a) Showed that insulin pump therapy is more effective than multiple injections
(b) Showed that proteinuria can be reversed by good glycaemic control
(c) Showed that near-normoglycaemia could be achieved without increasing the frequency of severe hypoglycaemia
(d) Showed that intensified insulin therapy only reduced the rate of progression to retinopathy, renal disease and neuropathy when there was no evidence that these were already present in an early form
(e) Showed that intensified insulin therapy reduced the risk of myocardial infarction in NIDDM

ANSWERS

1a	False	2a	False	3a	False
b	False	b	True	b	False
c	True	c	False	c	False
d	False	d	False	d	False
e	False	e	True	e	False

Management of non-insulin-dependent diabetes mellitus

R C Turner

☐ SPECTRE OF DIABETIC COMPLICATIONS

Non-insulin-dependent (Type 2) diabetes mellitus (NIDDM) is often regarded as being a 'mild' form of diabetes by patients and their physicians. This term is a misnomer that arose because: (i) it can often be managed by diet or tablet therapy, rather than by insulin; (ii) patients are then usually symptom-free and appear to be fit and well, even though glucose levels continue to be raised; (iii) when urine glucose is measured it is often absent, and even when glycosuria is present it is often ignored since the patient is apparently well.

The major problem is that patients with NIDDM are likely to develop morbidity and premature mortality from macrovascular and microvascular complications. Patients with NIDDM have a threefold increased risk of all atheroma-related cardiovascular diseases [1] and when diabetes presents in patients in their 40s or 50s there is a twofold increase in total mortality compared with the general population [2]. Patients with NIDDM develop the same ophthalmic, renal and peripheral neuropathy complications as patients with IDDM, leading to blindness, renal failure and amputations.

NIDDM and IDDM require expensive health-care resources [3]. They are the most common cause of blindness in middle age, and lead to more than 50% of all non-accidental amputations and more than 50% of cases of end-stage renal failure. Angina, intermittent claudication and minor strokes increasingly lead to angiography, angioplasty or bypass operations, so the direct hospital costs of diabetes increase.

☐ PATHOPHYSIOLOGY OF DIABETES

NIDDM arises from a combination (Fig. 1) of impaired insulin sensitivity at the liver, muscle and adipose tissue, sometimes termed 'insulin resistance', and impaired β-cell secretion.

Insulin resistance is a major predisposing feature that is particularly prevalent in ethnic groups with a high incidence of diabetes, eg Asian Indians, AmeroIndians (eg Pima Indians) and Hispanics (Mexican Americans). While insulin resistance may in part be due to specific genetic determinants, the major factors are obesity, central adiposity (since intra-abdominal fat particularly releases free fatty acids affecting hepatic and peripheral glucose metabolism) and impaired physical activity. Insulin resistance is apparent by the time impaired glucose tolerance is present. It does not get markedly worse as diabetes develops, which is predominantly due to an additional, progressive decrease in insulin secretion [4].

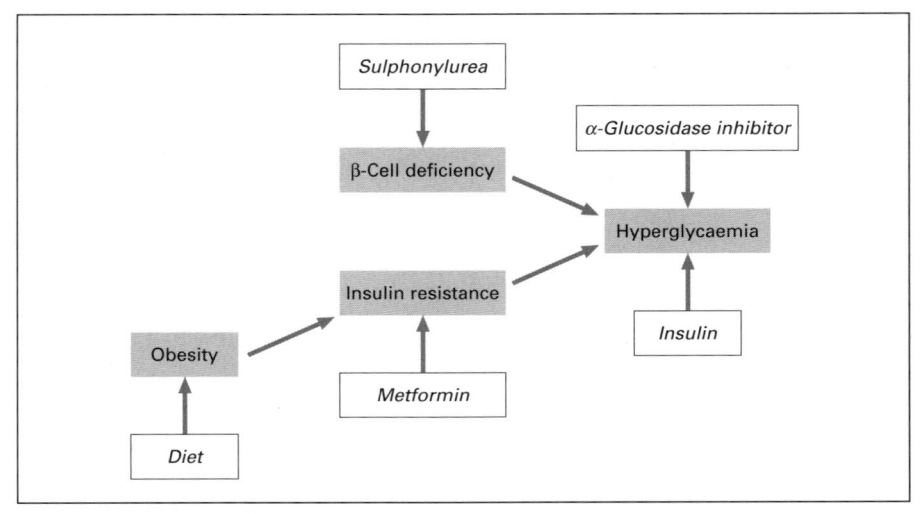

Fig. 1 The pathophysiology of the hyperglycaemia of NIDDM, together with the sites of action of different therapies.

☐ NATURE OF THE GLYCAEMIC ABNORMALITY

The 24 h glucose concentrations that occur in diet-treated patients are shown in Fig. 2. Two separate abnormalities occur: first, a raised baseline glucose concentration that is characteristic for each person for a given state of nutrition, and second, abnormally large postprandial glucose excursions that occur from the raised baseline in each individual (Fig. 2).

☐ CLINICAL MANAGEMENT OF DIABETES

Monitoring diabetes control by fasting glucose concentrations in general practice

Since the two glucose abnormalities, raised fasting concentrations and increased postprandial excursions occur *parri passu*, the fasting plasma glucose provides a simple, relevant index of glucose control in diet-treated patients. Since sulphonylurea and metformin primarily reduce the fasting glucose concentrations (Fig. 3), the fasting plasma glucose is also a relevant index of control for all patients treated by diet or an oral hypoglycaemic agent [6].

In general practice, monitoring diabetes control is feasible by having monthly morning clinics, which fasting patients can attend, with a nurse to measure a finger-prick blood glucose on a meter. As discussed below, the degree to which the fasting blood glucose should be lowered is uncertain, but a conservative aim may be <8 mmol/l. When this is achieved, 3–4 monthly check measurements are needed.

Haemoglobin A1c provides an overall index of glucose control. It is an essential index of control in insulin-treated Type 2 diabetic patients. In Type 1 diabetic patients a conservative aim is for <8%. It is not known whether this or <7% would be appropriate for patients with NIDDM.

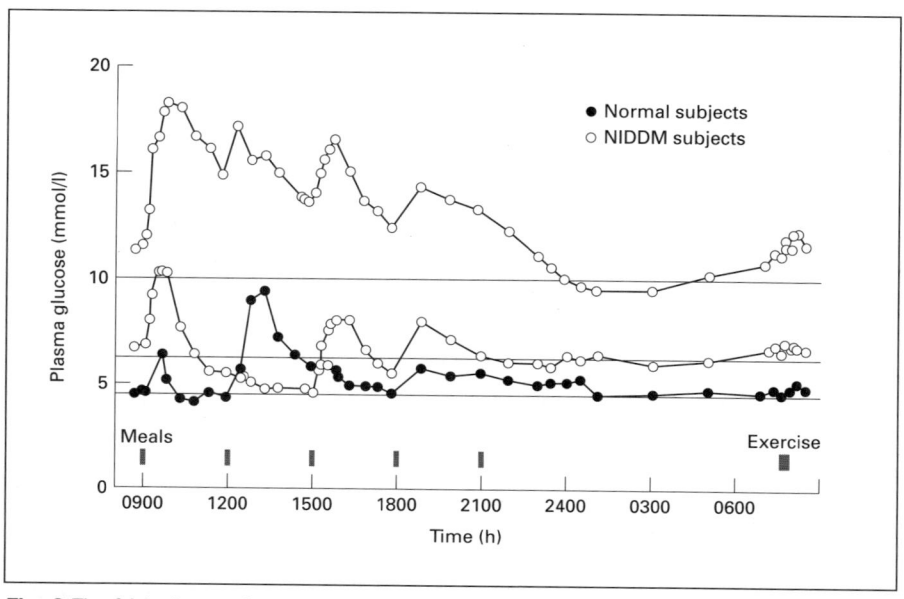

Fig. 2 The 24 h plasma glucose concentration in non-diabetic subjects and two groups of NIDDM subjects treated by diet alone. All the diabetic subjects had a stable, raised overnight glucose concentration, on which were superimposed exaggerated postprandial glucose excursions. (From Holman and Turner [5] with permission.)

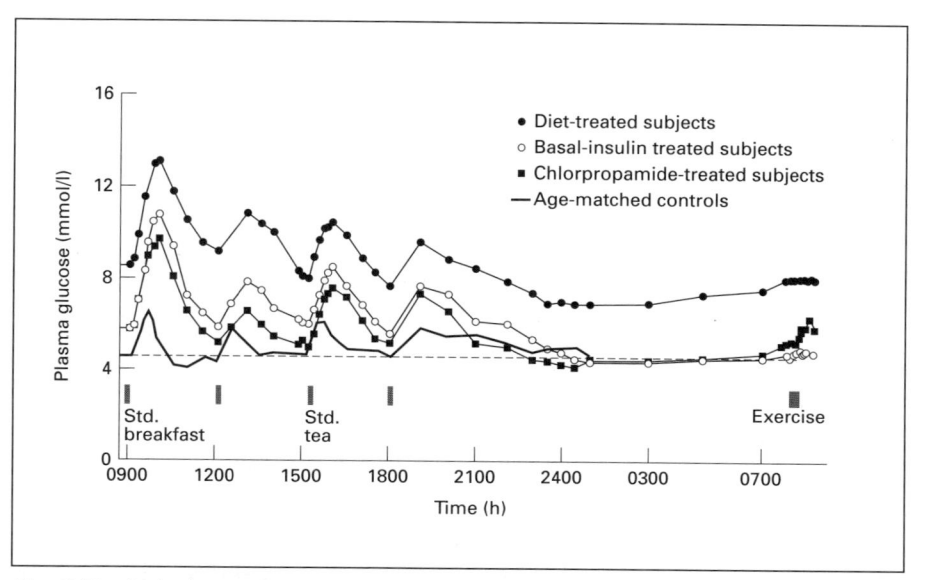

Fig. 3 The 24 h plasma glucose concentrations in diet-treated diabetic subjects who were also treated with the sulphonylurea, chlorpropamide or a basal insulin supplement from once daily ultralente insulin, both of which reduced only the raised basal glucose concentration. (From Holman and Turner [7] with permission.)

Glucose control and its effect on diabetes complications

Microvascular disease

The Diabetes Complications and Control Trial in Type 1 diabetic patients confirmed hyperglycaemia as being the major risk factor for microvascular disease. The study randomized 1441 Type 1 diabetic patients, mean age 27 years, either to intensive control with home blood-glucose monitoring, with an insulin pump or multiple insulin injections, or to conventional therapy with twice daily insulin, attaining a mean haemoglobin A1c of 7.1% and 9.0% respectively over 9 years [8]. The group with intensive therapy had a marked reduction in progression of retinopathy, nephropathy and neuropathy. A study in non-obese Japanese diabetic subjects with NIDDM gave similar results.

The mechanisms by which hyperglycaemia can lead to tissue damage have been described [9,10] (Table 1) and maintaining near-normal glucose concentrations is accepted to be a major factor in preventing microvascular disease.

Control of glucose by diet therapy and healthy living advice

Since obesity and diabetes usually have arisen secondary to overnutrition and a sedentary lifestyle, and correction of these can markedly improve glucose control, they are the first line of therapy. In practice it is difficult to obtain more than 5 kg weight loss, and even then only 15% of patients attain a near-normal glucose level, <6 mmol/l. In two-thirds of these patients, the glucose level subsequently increases. Thus healthy living advice is usually insufficient on its own.

Table 1 Mechanisms by which hyperglycaemia can induce diabetic tissue damage.

1	**Glycosylation of proteins by direct, non-enzymic coupling of glucose with amine groups** This leads to production of active metabolites, eg 3-deoxyglucosone, and formation of insoluble advanced glycosylation end products (AGE) on proteins that can: ☐ *Cause cross-linking of proteins*, eg collagen ☐ *Induce impaired protein function*, eg glycosylated low-density lipoprotein (LDL) cholesterol is less avid for hepatic receptors; antithrombin III becomes inactive when glycosylated ☐ *Increase susceptibility to oxidation*, eg glycosylated LDL cholesterol when oxidized is more likely to be taken up by macrophages to form foam cells in arterial wall. ☐ *Induce removal of AGE on tissues by macrophages*. Although normally protective, this can be pathogenic when large number of AGE are present, as macrophages can release cytokines, eg tumour necrosis factor (TNF) or interleukins, leading to tissue damage
2	**Protein kinase C activation** ☐ Hyperglycaemia-induced activation of protein kinase C β-isoform can lead to increased vascular perfusion and increased vascular permeability
3	**Increased glucose flux through sorbitol pathway** ☐ Hyperglycaemia induces increased intracellular sorbitol concentrations that can lead to compensatory decreased myoinositol concentrations, which are part of the intracellular phosphatase-signalling mechanisms ☐ Increased flux alters the redox state and this can affect synthetic pathways

Effect of oral hypoglycaemic therapy and insulin therapy for hyperglycaemia on macrovascular disease

There are no clinical data to show that improving glucose control will retard development of the atheroma-related complications of diabetes. Indeed, the only available evidence from the Universities Group Diabetes Program, reported in 1971, raised the possibility that sulphonylurea and biguanide therapies may actually increase the incidence of myocardial infarction rather than being protective [11]. Sulphonylureas block ATP-sensitive channels in the heart as well as the pancreas. When ischaemia occurs, the decrease in ATP concentrations opens channels, and the potassium release allows local vasodilatation. It is plausible that sulphonylurea therapy will prevent this and thus aggravate ischaemic damage.

High insulin concentrations *in vitro* induce lipid synthesis and growth of arterial fibroblasts. It has been suggested that long-term insulin therapy may thus predispose to development of atheroma.

Epidemiological studies suggest that any increase in blood glucose concentrations above normal may be pathogenic and that it makes little difference if the fasting glucose level is 6 or 16 mmol/l. Thus it is possible the degree of reduction in glycaemia that is feasible with available therapy is insufficient to be clinically beneficial in relation to cardiac disease. Thus potential, harmful effects of therapy on the heart might outweigh any beneficial effect of reducing glycaemia on heart disease [12].

Efficacy of therapies in relation to progressive hyperglycaemia

While at first sight treatment is available to counter each of the pathophysiological processes leading to diabetes (Fig. 1), in practice there are major problems.

Each of the therapies is moderately weak. Thus in diabetic patients with fasting plasma glucose level of about 8–10 mmol/l, sulphonylurea and metformin therapy only reduce the fasting plasma glucose on average by 1.8 mmol/l and haemoglobin A1c by 0.8%. Acarbose therapy provides a similar reduction in haemoglobin A1c, although side-effects of diarrhoea and flatulence can prevent it being used.

Side-effects of sulphonylurea and insulin treatment, ie hypoglycaemic episodes and weight gain, can limit their clinical efficacy. In theory, insulin doses could be increased to produce normoglycaemia, but in practice patients' and physicians' perception of the risk of hypoglycaemia and weight gain are limiting.

Progressive impairment of the insulin secretory capacity leads to a marked increase in glycaemia that is difficult to prevent (Fig. 4).

Since metformin does not cause the weight gain and hypoglycaemic reactions induced by sulphonylurea, it is often preferred as first-line therapy, particularly in obese subjects [4]. Therapy with sulphonylurea, metformin or insulin improves the haemoglobin A1c, but by 4 years the effect has been nullified by the deteriorating β-cell function and the haemoglobin A1c has often increased to the previous level. Thus each therapy temporarily 'holds the disease' at a similar level of control for 4 years rather than providing a marked, long-term improvement in glucose control (Fig. 4).

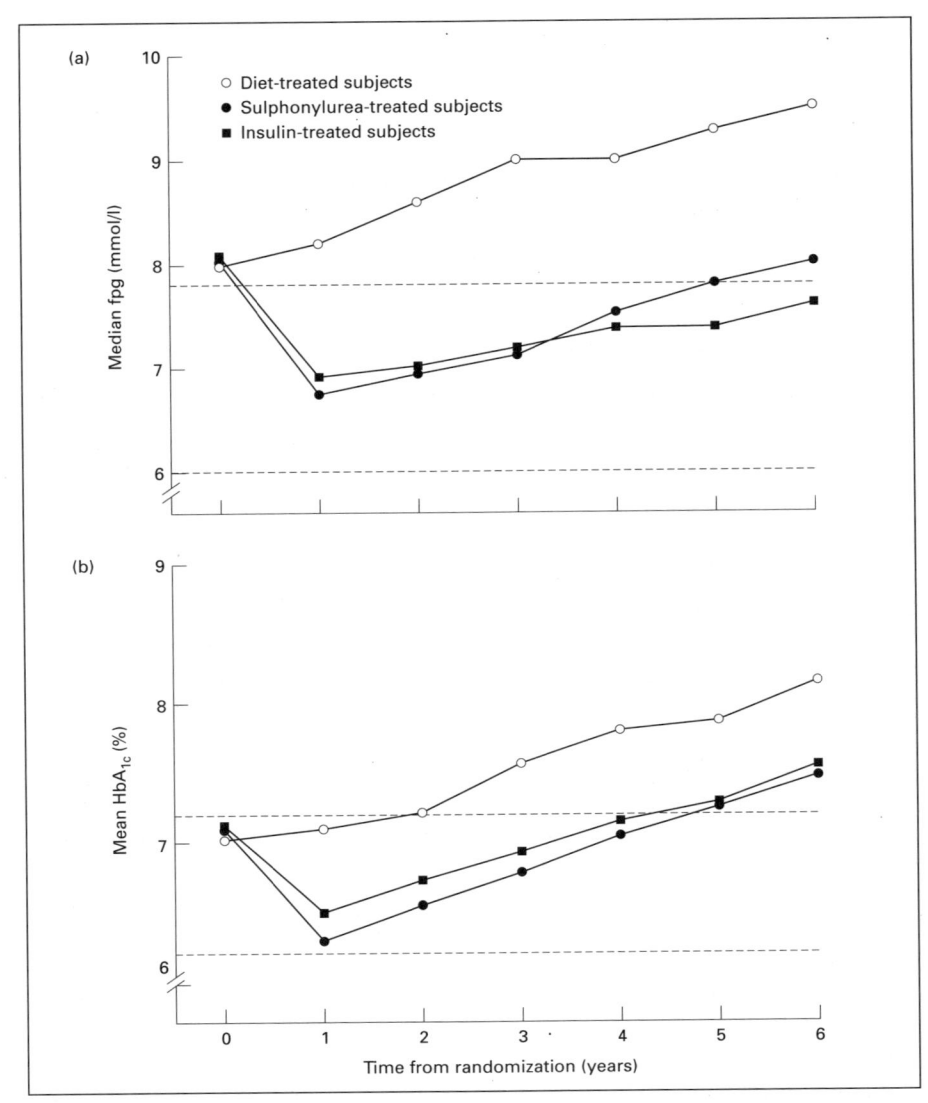

Fig. 4 Data from the UK Prospective Diabetes Study in patients who after 3 months diet were asymptomatic but had raised fasting plasma glucose levels of 6–15 mmol/l and who were allocated to diet, sulphonylurea or insulin treatment. Both therapies initially decreased the fasting plasma glucose (fpg) (a) and haemoglobin A1c (HbA1c) (b), but subsequently the glucose control progressively deteriorated [4]. (With permission of *Diabetes*.)

Need for constant review of requirement for additional therapies/polypharmacy

Since each individual therapy is only modestly and temporarily effective, if improved glucose control is to be maintained it is usually necessary, in a structured manner, to add additional therapies to maintain a certain level of control [12]. These can be summarized as follows:

- ☐ Diet only
- ☐ Metformin *or* sulphonylurea
- ☐ Metformin *and* sulphonylurea
- ☐ Metformin, sulphonylurea and basal insulin (from bedtime isophane or ultralente insulin)
- ☐ Basal and prandial insulin therapy:

    either twice daily soluble/isophane

    or thrice daily soluble/isophane or ultralente

When the α-glucosidase inhibitor, acarbose, should be added is uncertain. It reduces postprandial glycaemia, whereas all the other therapies reduce primarily the fasting plasma glucose. Thus it can be added as an adjunct at any stage of the above regimen.

What level of glucose control is required?

This is the big, unanswered question, given that therapies are potentially dangerous and it is not known whether the major complication, cardiovascular disease, will benefit from improved glucose control. The UK Prospective Diabetes Study is a long-term, randomized controlled trial of the clinical benefit of improved control in preventing clinical complications. It will report in 1998 and until then there are few reliable guidelines. The simplest assumption is that improved glucose control will prevent microvascular disease, in which case epidemiological data suggest that it may be advisable to aim for fasting blood glucose <8 mmol/l, which is reported to be an approximate threshold for microvascular disease. Indeed, a fasting plasma glucose >7.8 mmol/l was chosen as a criterion for diabetes as above that level retinopathy and albuminuria occurred. Figure 5 illustrates two possible approaches. Figure 5(a) shows the common approach to therapy of NIDDM, in which each therapy is only added when the fasting glucose level becomes above 12 mmol/l, which is when sufficient glycosuria occurs to induce symptoms. The inevitable effect is that the glucose concentrations are constantly raised, and are in the region that development of both microvascular and macrovascular disease would be expected.

Figure 5(b) shows the approach that would be needed if one were to aim for a fasting glucose level of below 8mmol/l. Polypharmacy would often be required, with transfer to insulin therapy at a much earlier stage than is usually practised.

Physicians have treated patients with NIDDM for 50 years with oral hypoglycaemic agents, not knowing whether they are safe and not knowing for which level of glucose control they should aim. It is hoped that in 1998 UKPDS will provide data on which a rational choice of therapies can be made.

Risk factors for cardiovascular disease

Cardiovascular disease in patients with NIDDM results from raised low-density lipoprotein (LDL) cholesterol, low high-density lipoprotein (HDL) cholesterol,

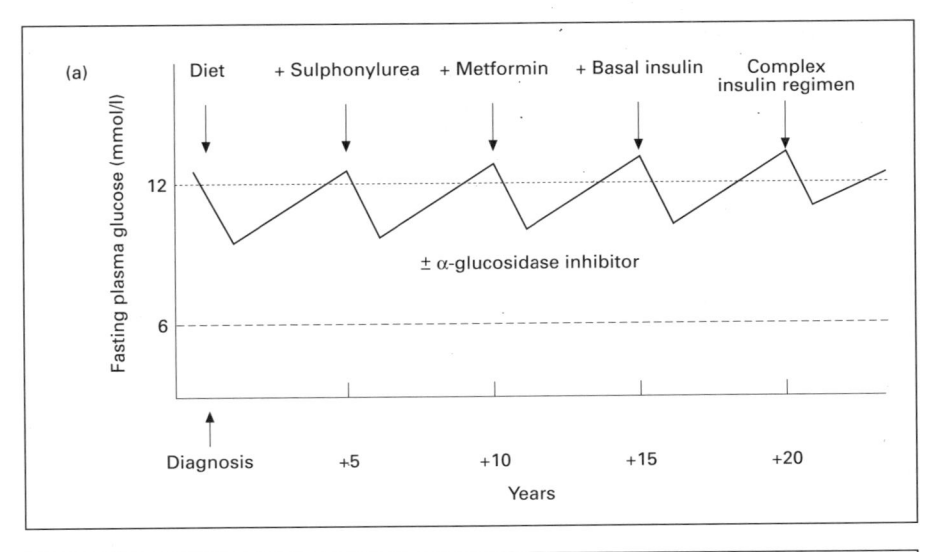

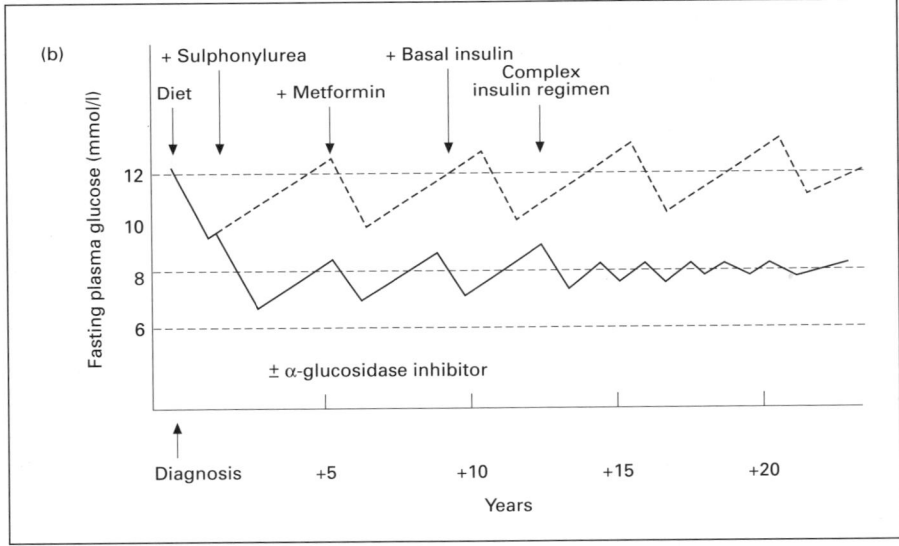

Fig. 5 Illustrative diagram (a) of a common method of treating Type 2 diabetic subjects, when therapies are only introduced when symptoms of thirst develop, arising from glucosuria when the fasting plasma glucose concentration is in the order of 12 mmol/l. The response to therapies and the increase of fasting plasma glucose levels are taken from UKPDS data (see Fig. 4). Diagram (b) illustrates the likely outcome if therapies were added to maintain fasting plasma glucose <8 mmol/l. Polypharmacy would be required at an earlier stage, with insulin therapy being required considerably earlier than is usual.

hypertension and smoking as well as from hyperglycaemia *per se*. Thus attention to preventing smoking, and appropriate treatment of hypertension and of dyslipidaemia is required. In view of the high incidence of vascular problems, 75 mg of aspirin a day may be advisable, but the appropriate clinical trials have not been done.

Prevention of blindness and amputations

These major complications are largely preventable by annual assessment to detect the development of treatable conditions. Ophthalmic examination should include retina ophthalmoscopy for new vessels and visual acuity assessment to detect early maculopathy, both of which can respond to laser therapy.

Foot examination should be undertaken so that ischaemic feet or neuropathic feet can receive appropriate foot care, eg good fitting shoes, and regular podiatry including nail care and therapy of hyperkeratoses. This will help to prevent development of ulcers and amputations.

The future

In theory, appropriate care of hyperglycaemia, hypertension, raised cholesterol levels, smoking prevention, low-dose aspirin therapy and eye and foot screening should manage to prevent the complications of diabetes. The major problems are that better organization of healthcare is needed, with clinical trials to show that the pharmaceutical agents are actually safe and effective. In 1998 both the UKPDS, assessing the benefit of improved glucose control, and the Hypertension in Diabetes Study, assessing the benefit of improved hypertension control, will be published. If these studies show benefit from improved therapy, they will help to encourage more prophylactic therapy to maintain patients' health.

☐ CONCLUSIONS

In patients with NIDDM, diabetes therapy is often directed primarily at preventing symptoms from glycosuria or tiredness. In theory, tighter glucose control may be preferred to prevent the long-term microvascular and macrovascular complications of diabetes. It is known that improved glucose control will delay progression of microvascular disease, but there is no evidence that it will prevent the macrovascular disease which is the major cause of the morbidity and mortality of the disease. Indeed, it is possible that sulphonylurea, biguanide and insulin therapy each might induce cardiac pathology. Diabetes can be monitored in routine clinical practice by fasting blood glucose concentrations and it is possible that therapy should aim for <8 mmol/l to decrease the progress of microvascular disease. However, NIDDM is characterized by progressive increase in glycaemia, and to achieve this aim it would often be necessary to use all available oral hypoglycaemic agents, with insulin often being required. In addition, a high incidence of hypoglycaemic reactions limits the degree to which near-normal glucose concentrations can be obtained. The UK Prospective Diabetes Study is a long-term randomized control trial of different therapies. In 1998 it will report whether the improved glucose control that can in practice be achieved will maintain health of diabetic patients and whether any particular therapies have any specific advantages or disadvantages.

REFERENCES

1   Garcia MJ, McNamara PM, Gordon T, Kannell WB. Morbidity and mortality in diabetics in the Framingham population: sixteen year follow-up. *Diabetes* 1974; **23**: 105–11.

2   Panzram G. Mortality and survival in Type 2 (non-insulin-dependent) diabetes mellitus. *Diabetologia* 1987; **30**: 123–31.
3   Laing W, Williams DR. *Diabetes, a Model for Health Care Management*. London: Office of Health Economics, 1989.
4   UKPDS Group. UK Prospective Diabetes Study 16. Overview of six years' therapy of type 2 diabetes – a progressive disease. *Diabetes* 1995; **44**: 1249–58.
5   Holman RR, Turner RC. The basal plasma glucose: a simple, relevant index of maturity-onset diabetes. *Clin Endocrinol* 1980; **14**: 279–86.
6   Holman RR, Turner RC. A practical guide to basal and prandial insulin therapy. *Diabetic Med* 1985; **2**: 45–53.
7   Holman RR, Turner RC. Basal normoglycaemia attained with chlorpropamide in mild diabetes. *Metabolism* 1978; **27**: 539–47.
8   DCCT Research Group. The effect of intensive treatment of diabetes on the development and progression of long-term complications of insulin-dependent diabetes mellitus. *New Engl J Med* 1993; **329**: 977–86.
9   Brownlee M. Glycation and diabetic complications. *Diabetes* 1994; **43**: 836–41.
10 Porte D, Schwartz MW. Diabetes complications: why is glucose potentially toxic? *Science* 1996; **272**: 699–700.
11 Genuth S. Exogenous insulin administration and cardiovascular risk in non-insulin-dependent and insulin-dependent diabetes mellitus. *Ann Intern Med* 1996; **124**: 104–9.
12 Stout RW. Insulin and atherosclerosis. In: Stout RW, ed. *Diabetes and Atherosclerosis*. Dordrecht: Kluwer Academic Publishers, 1992: 165–201.

☐ MULTIPLE CHOICE QUESTIONS

1   The Diabetes Complications and Control Trial in Type 1 diabetic subjects showed that improved blood glucose control:
    (a) Delayed progress of microvascular disease
    (b) Delayed progress of macrovascular disease
    (c) Increased weight
    (d) Increased incidence of hypoglycaemia

2   Non-insulin-dependent diabetes:
    (a) Is characterized solely by high glucose levels after meals
    (b) Has raised fasting plasma glucose levels that are a useful indicator of severity
    (c) May induce complications due to glycosylation of tissues
    (d) Has a high incidence of complications because of the effect of hyperglycaemia alone
    (e) Should involve attention to hypertension, raised cholesterol and smoking

3   Treatment of non-insulin-dependent diabetes:
    (a) Can be with metformin, sulphonylureas, α-glucosidase inhibitors or insulin
    (b) If haemoglobin A1c is reduced to <7% the incidence of macrovascular and microvascular complications will be reduced
    Should include annual assessment:
    (c) By ophthalmoscopy for new vessels
    (d) Of visual acuity for maculopathy
    (e) Of feet for ischaemia and neuropathy

ANSWERS

1a True	2a False	3a True
b False	b True	b False
c True	c True	c True
d True	d False	d True
	e True	e True

Brain, fat and the fulfilling of prophecies

G Williams

☐ INTRODUCTION

Body weight and fat mass in humans span a relatively wide spectrum, which in westernized societies is becoming progressively skewed towards overweight. Obesity is common, dangerous to health and an important drain on health-care resources, yet tends to be neglected by the medical profession. It has an unexciting image, for several reasons. It is commonly perceived as an essentially cosmetic problem which falls short of being a 'real' disease, and the frustrating failure of most attempts to induce weight loss can make it easier to ignore than treat. The poor understanding of its causes has also made obesity scientifically unappealing.

However, the fortunes of obesity research have improved dramatically during the last few years, and the rapid unravelling of the secrets of energy homoeostasis has renewed hopes of developing rational and effective anti-obesity drugs. The new insights into the neurobiology and endocrinology of obesity will occupy most of this chapter, but the medical and social problems of obesity first deserve brief mention.

☐ IMPACT OF OBESITY

Obesity is a major curse of the 'westernized' lifestyle, with its overplentiful high-energy food and reduced levels of physical activity. In the UK, the prevalence of significant obesity has doubled during the last decade, and 15–20% of British adults are now sufficiently overweight to potentially shorten their life expectancy [1]. The threat of obesity has become so obvious that even the government has recognized the need to reduce the population's weight, in the current *Health of the Nation* report.

Several recent studies have re-emphasized the strong relationships between obesity and diseases such as non-insulin-dependent diabetes (NIDDM), hypertension and atheroma, and ultimately with premature death. Any lingering misconceptions about the health hazards of obesity should be dispelled by the very large follow-up study of American nurses [2]. This showed that, after removing the confounding effects of smoking, the risk of premature death increases progressively as the body-mass index (BMI) rises; worryingly, mortality begins to increase above a BMI of only 19 m/kg^2, considerably lower than the recommended limits for the general population (see Fig. 1).

Obesity is already an expensive disease in affluent countries, both through its well-known medical sequelae and through less obvious effects such as poor mobility and time lost off work; the damage to the quality of life of obese people must also be vast, but so far has eluded financial analysis. The true costs to society are difficult

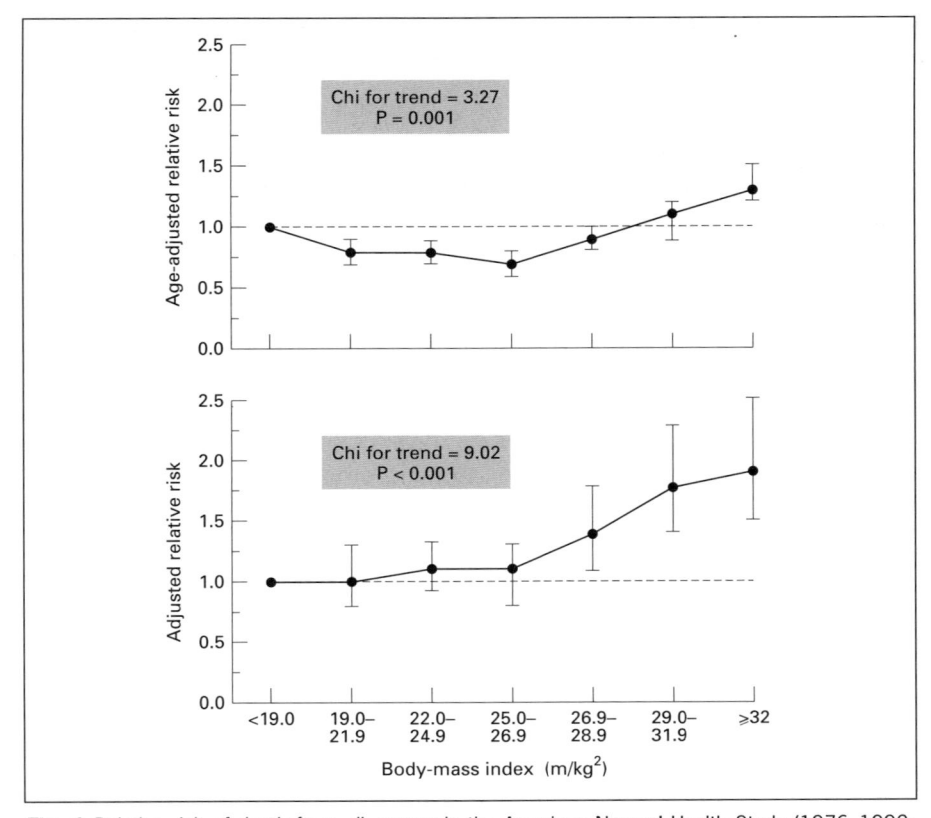

Fig. 1 Relative risk of death from all causes in the American Nurses' Health Study (1976–1992; n = 115 195). (a) All subjects, with relative risks adjusted for age, showing 'J-shaped' relationship with increasing BMI. (b) Lifelong non-smokers only, showing progressive rise in mortality as BMI increases. Data are mean ±95% confidence intervals. (Reproduced from Manson et al. [2], with permission.)

to calculate. In 1986, the health-care costs attributed to obesity in the USA were estimated at US$ 56 billion, about 8% of that country's total health budget [3]; the current bill could be twice as high. The invasion of westernization into developing countries ('Coca-colonization') is already being followed by dramatic increases in obesity and NIDDM, which the Third World can ill afford.

☐ BRAIN AND FAT: FUNDAMENTALS OF ENERGY HOMOEOSTASIS

Under stable conditions, body weight and fat mass of mammals are maintained with incredible precision, to within 0.5%. Moreover, weight and fat content are restored accurately to their respective 'set-points' after temporary disturbances in energy balance, through impeccably co-ordinated adaptive responses that involve both sides of the energy-balance equation. During food deprivation, energy expenditure falls progressively to limit the consumption of the body's fat stores, while the animal becomes hungry and channels its activity into seeking food. When food is found, the animal overeats initially; hyperphagia and reduced energy expenditure persist but diminish gradually until the energy deficit has been corrected and fat mass restored to its set-point.

The ability to regulate the body's energy stores so precisely must involve a homoeostatic loop, with signals that indicate fat mass (presumably carried in the bloodstream) acting on the central nervous system (CNS) to produce appropriate changes in energy balance (Fig. 2). In a classic negative-feedback loop, these signals

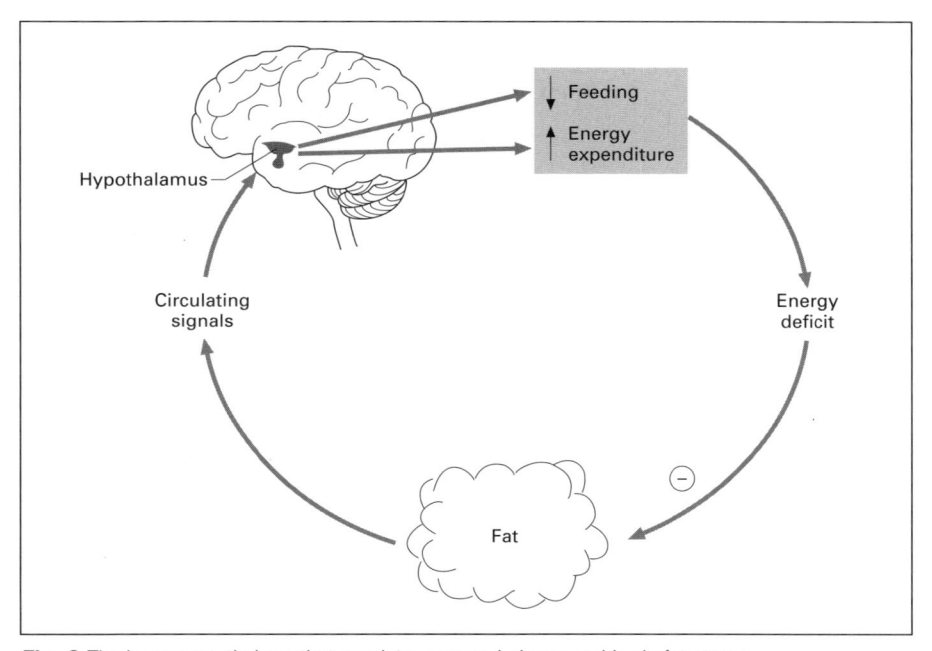

Fig. 2 The homoeostatic loop that regulates energy balance and body fat stores.

would be predicted to inhibit food intake and/or stimulate energy expenditure. Much work has pointed to the hypothalamus as the command centre for this loop, but the key links in the chain, namely the circulating fat-derived signal and the neurones that perceive it, remained a mystery until recently.

In theory, obesity would result if this loop were interrupted at various points. In particular, the signal from fat might not be generated or reach the hypothalamus, or the hypothalamus might fail to perceive it. As discussed below, both these mechanisms have now been demonstrated in genetically obese rodents, but their relevance to human obesity is uncertain.

☐ FAT MICE: FROM BASIC PHYSIOLOGY TO MOLECULAR GENETICS

Basic research in energy balance owes much to various mutant mice and rats, which display morbid (indeed, virtually spherical) obesity, with severe insulin resistance and glucose intolerance or overt NIDDM (see Table 1). Particularly generous in this regard have been the *ob/ob* and *db/db* mice, which are phenotypically similar but have different genetic lesions; the *ob* and *db* loci have been known for some years to lie on chromosomes 6 and 4 respectively, but the gene products and the nature of the mutations were unknown. Obesity develops early in both mutants, and is accompanied by worsening insulin resistance and a compensatory increase in insulin secretion; ultimately, hyperinsulinaemia is no longer able to overcome insulin resistance, when blood glucose levels rise into the diabetic range.

Table 1 Examples of genetically obese rodents.

Model	Nature of mutation	Chromo-some	Obesity	Insulin resistance	Hyper-glycaemia
ob/ob mouse	Leptin (premature termination or complete deletion)	6	+++	+++	+++
db/db mouse	Leptin receptor (OB-Rb; intracellular portion truncated)	4	+++	+++	+++
fa/fa rat	Leptin receptor (point mutation in extracellular portion)	5	+++	+++	±

Hyperglycaemia: +++ = overtly diabetic; ± = moderate glucose intolerance

The energetic basis of obesity in these mutants has been much investigated. Both are pushed into positive energy balance by the combination of hyperphagia and reduced energy expenditure. The reduction in energy expenditure is more important, as obesity still develops (albeit less dramatically) in *ob/ob* or *db/db* mice that are only allowed to eat the same amount as their lean counterparts. In rodents, a major thermogenic tissue is the specialized form of fat known as brown adipose tissue (BAT), in which noradrenaline released from its dense sympathetic innervation acts through β_3-adrenoceptors to stimulate lipolysis and the oxidation of free fatty acids. The expression of 'uncoupling protein', unique to BAT, is also stimulated. Uncoupling protein short-circuits proton flow across the mitochondrial membrane, effectively uncoupling oxidative phosphorylation and generating heat instead of adenosine triphosphate (ATP). In *ob/ob* and *db/db* mice, the defect in energy expenditure is due to underactivity of the sympathetic innervation, rather than defects in BAT itself. Another abnormality that occurs very early in these syndromes is hypersecretion of insulin, resulting in part from overactivity of the parasympathetic (vagal) nerve supply to the pancreatic B cells, which promotes fat deposition [4].

Overall, these abnormalities can be explained by a hypothalamic 'autonomic imbalance', in which the parasympathetic system dominates the sympathetic [4]. Numerous abnormalities in hypothalamic neurotransmitters have been identified in genetically obese rodents, and there has been much speculation about which of these might mediate obesity. The identification of the *ob* and *db* gene products is helping to resolve these issues, and will provide important information about the normal function of one of the most complex parts of the brain.

☐ LEPTIN

The search for the *ob* gene finally ended with the publication in late 1994, by Friedman's group in New York, of a paper that has opened an entire new chapter in endocrinology [5]. The *ob* gene was located by positional cloning, sequenced and its product expressed. *ob* messenger ribonucleic acid (mRNA) was found only in white adipose tissue, making it a prime candidate for the elusive circulating signal of fat mass. The gene was predicted to encode an 18 kDa protein with a cleavage point that would liberate a 16 kDa portion that could be secreted from cells. The common strain of *ob/ob* mouse was found to have a nonsense mutation (Arg → stop) about two-thirds of the way along the coding sequence, which yields a truncated protein, presumably biologically inactive. A variant *ob/ob* strain had a mutation in the regulatory region upstream of the coding sequence that resulted in the complete absence of *ob* mRNA (Fig. 3).

Friedman christened the *ob* gene product 'leptin' (from the Greek for thin), and

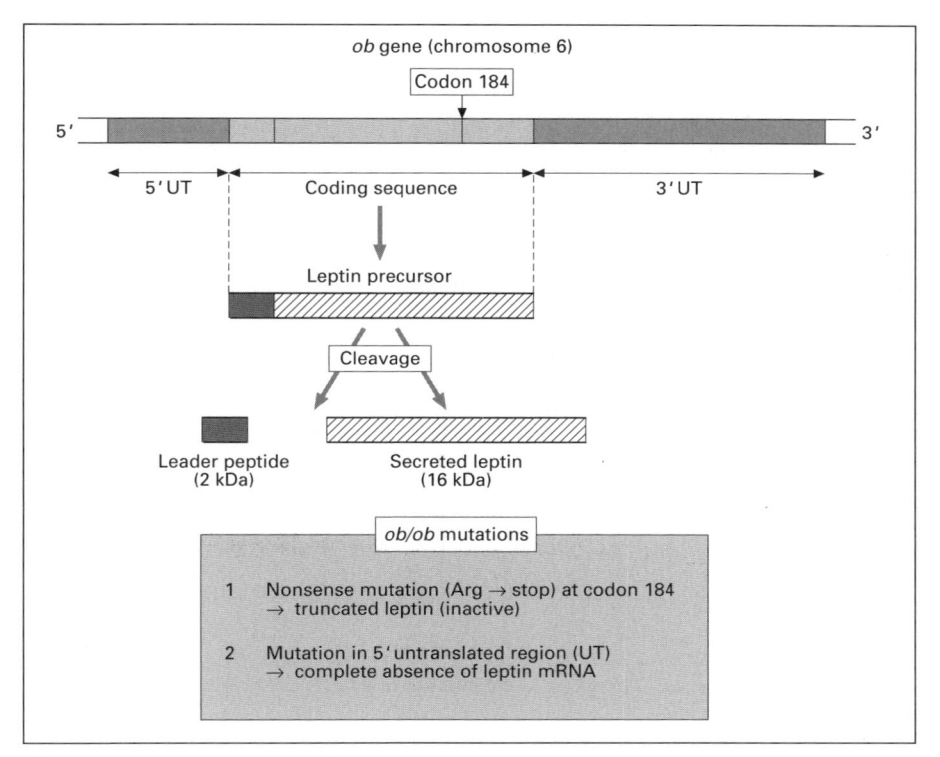

Fig. 3 The leptin gene and sites of mutations in different strains of *ob/ob* mouse.

postulated that it acted as an anti-obesity factor that regulated body fat mass, and that absence of leptin would lead to obesity. This conclusion was the final confirmation of an ingenious series of cross-circulation ('parabiosis') studies, carried out some 30 years previously by Coleman, who deduced that obesity in the *ob/ob* mouse was due to failure of production of a factor that inhibited feeding and caused weight loss.

The properties of leptin have been very rapidly characterized and have largely fulfilled its predicted role. It is present in the circulation of rodents and man, at levels that generally parallel fat mass, although there is considerable individual variation. When injected systemically into normal rodents and *ob/ob* mice, leptin reduces food intake and, if given repeatedly for several days, causes loss of fat and body weight [6] (Fig. 4). The same effects are seen when much smaller dosages are injected into the

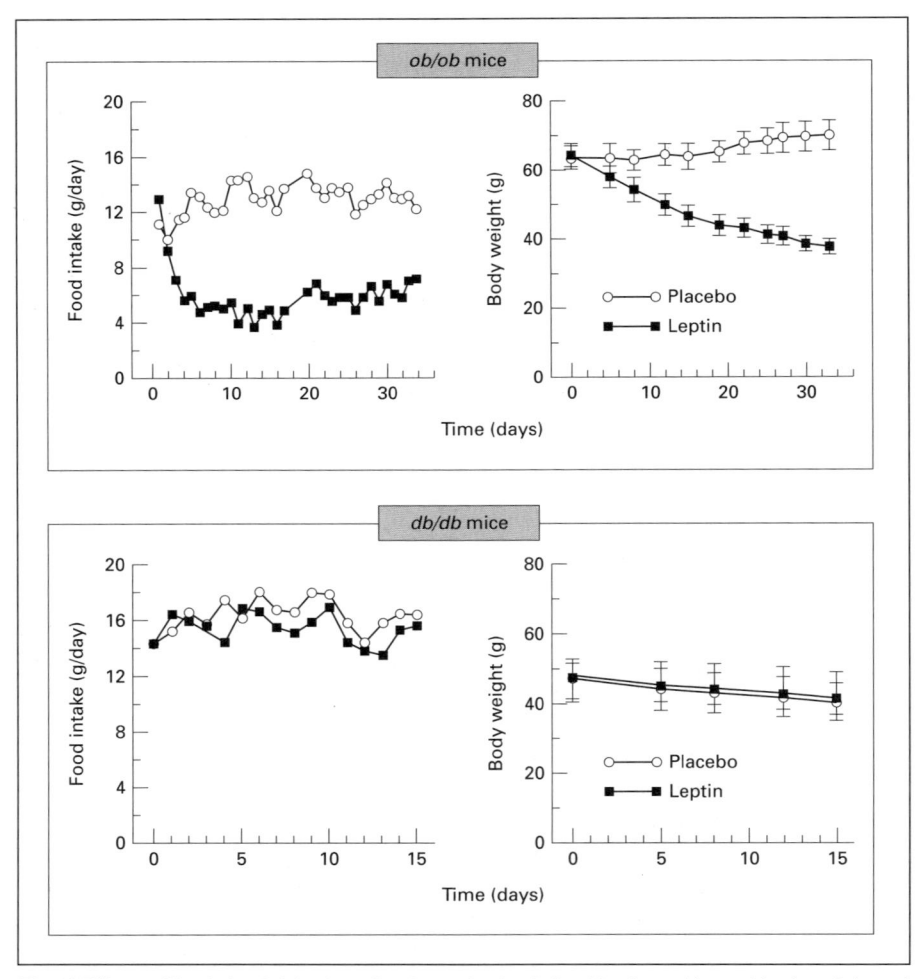

Fig. 4 Effects of leptin in *ob/ob* mice, showing reduction in food intake and loss of body weight and fat content (a). In *db/db* mice, leptin has no effect (b). (From Halaas *et al.* [6], with permission.)

cerebral ventricles, pointing to the CNS as its likely target. Consistent with the contributions of both hyperphagia and reduced thermogenesis in the *ob/ob* syndrome, leptin was found to stimulate energy expenditure as well as inhibit feeding. Expression of uncoupling protein in BAT increases acutely after leptin administration, apparently as a result of increased activity of the sympathetic outflow [7]. As would be predicted, leptin can therefore redress the 'autonomic imbalance' that underlies obesity in the *ob/ob* mouse. Leptin replacement can also correct other neuroendocrine and behavioural abnormalities in the *ob/ob* mouse, including subfertility and reduced physical activity.

☐ LEPTIN RECEPTORS

Coleman's parabiosis experiments had predicted that the *db/db* mouse was insensitive to the anti-obesity factor that was missing in the *ob/ob* mouse, and this was confirmed by demonstrating that leptin was inactive in the *db/db* mouse, even at high dosages [6] (see Fig. 4). These observations prompted a search for the leptin receptor in the CNS, and for evidence that this was the seat of the *db* mutation. Of additional interest was the fatty *fa/fa* Zucker rat, also renowned for its obesity, which can be explained by the same autonomic imbalance as in the *ob/ob* and *db/db* mice; moreover, the *fa* gene had been localized to the region of rat chromosome 5 that is analogous to the *db* locus on mouse chromosome 4.

A leptin receptor (OB-R), isolated by expression cloning, was first reported by Tartaglia *et al.* [8], just over 12 months after Friedman's paper. This receptor was expressed at high levels in the choroid plexus, lungs and kidney, with relatively little in the hypothalamus. The OB-R gene lay tantalizingly close to *db*, but was intact in *db/db* mice. The mystery was subsequently solved by the demonstration that the leptin receptor gene mRNA transcript was processed differently in various tissues, yielding several splice variants of varying length (designated OB-Ra, OB-Rb, etc) (Fig. 5). The full-length product is a single-chain peptide, structurally resembling certain interleukin receptors, which spans the cell membrane. The variant described by Tartaglia and co-workers [8] has only a short intracellular tail which lacks the two domains (boxes) that are thought to initiate intracellular signalling when the receptor is activated by leptin binding to the extracellular portion. An extended form (OB-Rb), which includes both signalling boxes, is expressed in the hypothalamus; this form is affected by the *db* mutation that truncates the protein and removes the second signalling box [9]. The leptin insensitivity of the *db/db* mouse is therefore due to failure of signal transduction by the leptin receptor. By contrast, the *fa* mutation in the extracellular portion of the receptor (Gln → Pro at position 269) may interfere with its ability to bind leptin [10].

The properties and functions of the various leptin receptor isoforms are not yet clear. The short form (OB-Ra) may be involved in transporting leptin from blood into cerebrospinal fluid (CSF) in the choroid plexus and perhaps in clearing the peptide in the lungs and kidney. An even shorter form (OB-Re) comprises only the extracellular portion and may function as a circulating leptin-binding protein, analogous to the growth hormone-binding protein that is now known to be the

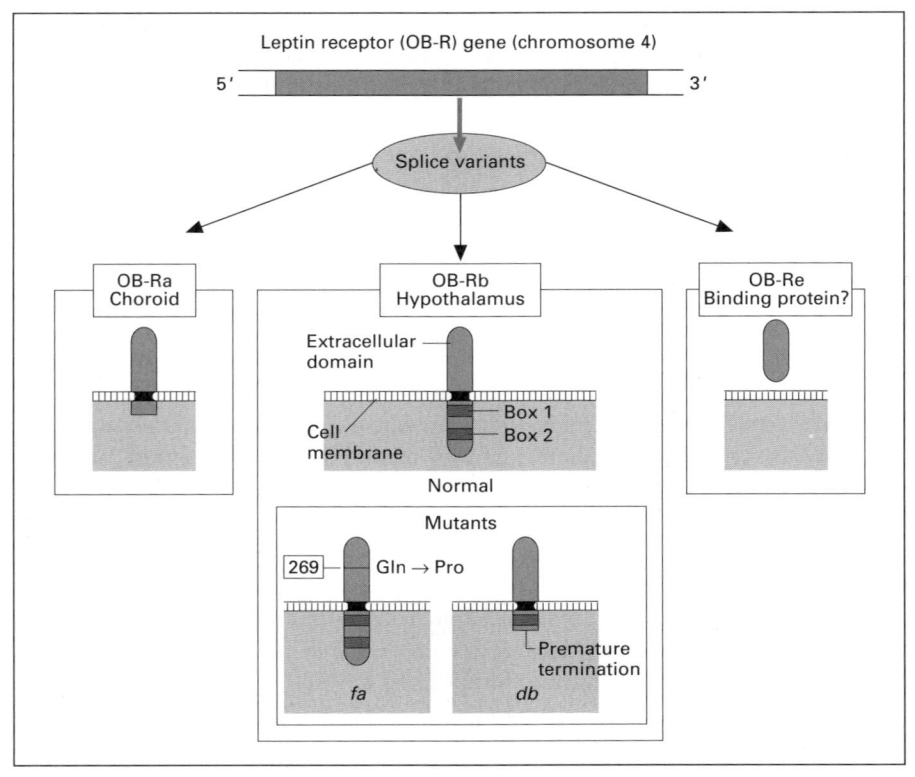

Fig 5 The leptin receptor (OB-R), showing some of the splice variants that are expressed in different tissues and the *fa* and *db* mutations.

extracellular part of the growth hormone receptor. The hypothalamic form (OB-Rb) may mediate leptin's hypophagic and thermogenic actions. Interestingly, radio-labelled leptin injected into the bloodstream has been shown to enter the mediobasal hypothalamus and arcuate nucleus, where the blood-brain barrier is specially modified to allow the passage of large molecules [11].

Leptin in context

Leptin convincingly fills the role of a fat-derived signal that acts on the CNS to regulate fat mass, and is obviously important in keeping rodents slim. However, several other circulating factors have been proposed to control energy homoeostasis, and the place of leptin in the overall hierarchy of such signals is not known. Of particular importance is insulin which, like leptin, circulates at levels proportional to fat mass and (perhaps unexpectedly) can enter the CSF and mediobasal hypothalamus, where specific insulin receptors are expressed. Furthermore, insulin injected into the hypothalamus causes hypophagia, increased thermogenesis and weight loss, effects now known to be shared by leptin. These observations prompted Porte and colleagues to suggest, over a decade ago, that insulin acted physiologically as a satiety factor and regulator of energy balance and body fat content [12]. The advent of leptin does not invalidate this proposal, and highlights the need to determine how these various signals might interact in the periphery and in the CNS.

☐ HYPOTHALAMIC NEUROTRANSMITTERS AND ENERGY HOMOEOSTASIS

A crucial focus of interest is the neural pathways in the hypothalamus and other brain regions which sense and respond to signals such as leptin and insulin. The hypothalamus is notorious for its anatomical complexity and its wide variety of neurotransmitters and neuropeptides, many of which are thought to influence energy balance; some of these are shown in Table 2 [13]. Those that inhibit feeding include serotonin (5-hydroxytryptamine; 5-HT) and the peptides cholecystokinin (CCK), corticotrophin-releasing factor (CRF) and bombesin. Serotonin is the basis of the appetite-suppressing effects of dexfenfluramine, which enhances serotonin's action by stimulating its release and by blocking its re-uptake presynaptically. CCK is a gut-derived satiety factor, which apparently acts on neural pathways converging on the hypothalamus that, interestingly, also release CCK. CRF, as well as releasing corticotrophin (ACTH), also causes profound hypophagia and increased BAT activity and thermogenesis, when injected into the central hypothalamus. Bombesin, the mammalian analogue of a peptide first isolated from frog skin, acts on the hypothalamus and medulla to inhibit feeding.

Relatively few hypothalamic peptides and neurotransmitters stimulate feeding. Noradrenaline injected into the central hypothalamus causes hyperphagia and can induce obesity, while a role for dopamine is inferred from the fatal anorexia that develops in transgenic mice whose dopaminergic neurones have been 'knocked out'. Galanin induces transient overeating but neither sustained hyperphagia nor obesity. Melanin-concentrating hormone (MCH) is a recently described feeding stimulant which is overexpressed in the hypothalamus of the *ob/ob* mouse.

The most convincing appetite stimulant, and probably the front runner among putative regulators of energy balance, is neuropeptide Y (NPY) [14]. This 36 amino acid peptide, structurally related to pancreatic polypeptide, is one of the most abundant peptides in the mammalian brain. A population of NPY neurones in the arcuate nucleus (ARC) at the base of the third ventricle in the mediobasal hypothalamus appears to play a pivotal role in energy homoeostasis. These neurones

Table 2 Examples of neurotransmitters and neuropeptides which may act in the hypothalamus to influence food intake and energy balance.

Inhibitors of feeding	Stimulators of feeding
Serotonin (5-HT)	Noradrenaline
Cholecystokinin (CCK)	Dopamine
Corticotrophin-releasing factor (CRF)	Neuropeptide Y
Bombesin	Galanin
Many others.....	Melanin-concentrating hormone (MCH)

project to the paraventricular and dorsomedial nuclei (PVN, DMH), areas that are crucial in the hypothalamic control of energy balance. The PVN is particularly densely innervated with NPY-containing terminals, and 'push-pull' sampling of extracellular fluid using a stereotactic cannula confirms that it is a site of active NPY release (Figs 6 and 7).

NPY stands out against the many other candidate regulators of energy balance, for several reasons. Firstly, it exerts extremely powerful, specific and co-ordinated effects on energy balance, which lead to fat accumulation. When injected into the PVN or DMH, it is the most powerful appetite stimulant known; it also inhibits the sympathetic stimulation of BAT and reduces energy expenditure. Furthermore, it stimulates insulin secretion, presumably through increased vagal outflow to the

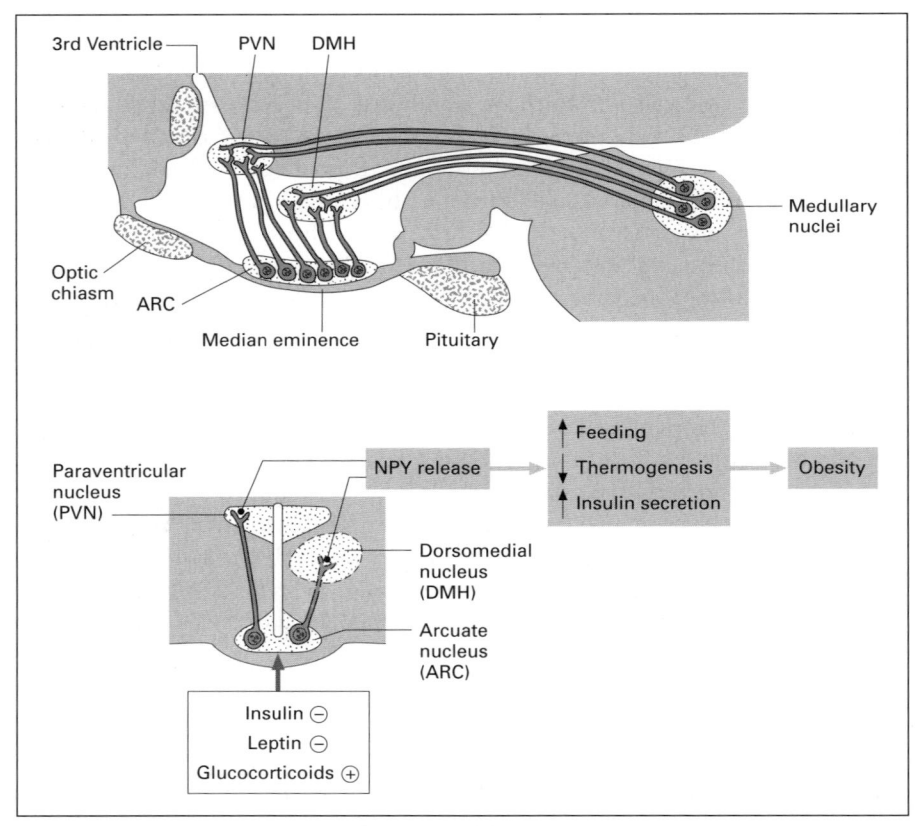

Fig. 6 Anatomy of NPY neurones in the hypothalamus. The paraventricular (PVN) and dorsomedial nuclei (DMH) receive NPY-containing fibres that originate mainly from cell bodies in the ARC. These are thought to play a crucial role in sensing energy deficits and in responding by increasing NPY release in the PVN and DMH, which acts through Y5 'feeding' receptors to stimulate feeding; other effects of NPY in the PVN include reduced sympathetic stimulation of BAT and decreased thermogenesis, and enhanced insulin secretion. Factors suggested to modulate the ARC NPY neurones include circulating leptin and insulin (inhibitory) and glucocorticoids (stimulatory). NPY neurones in the medulla also project to the PVN and DMH; their involvement in energy homoeostasis is uncertain.

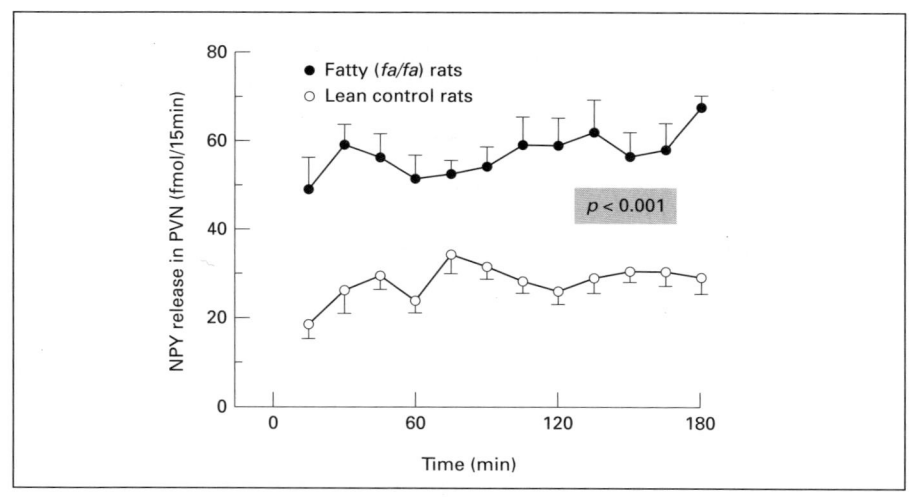

Fig. 7 NPY release in the PVN of fatty (*fa/fa*) Zucker rats is increased compared with lean controls. NPY secretion was measured *in vivo* using continuous 'push-pull' sampling of the extracellular fluid in the PVN, collected using a stereotactically-implanted cannula. (From Dryden et al. [15], with permission.)

islets. After only a few days of repeated or continuous administration, NPY causes obesity and insulin resistance, a property unique among the hypothalamic peptides studied so far. Indeed, NPY administration causes a concerted autonomic imbalance, favouring the parasympathetic system, which mimics that in the *ob/ob* mouse.

There is convincing evidence that the ARC NPY neurones function physiologically to defend body weight. These neurones become overactive under conditions of energy deficit such as starvation and insulin-deficient diabetes; NPY mRNA levels in the ARC, NPY concentrations in the ARC, PVN and DMH, and NPY release in the PVN are all increased. This overactivity would be predicted to cause hunger, hyperphagia and reduced thermogenesis. These are precisely the compensatory changes that occur in these conditions, and that tend to restore energy balance. The function of the ARC NPY neurones may therefore be to sense and correct energy deficits; in effect, an anti-starvation mechanism that could complete the homoeostatic circuit shown in Fig. 1 (compare Fig. 8).

NPY gains further credibility because of convincing evidence that genetic obesity in the *ob/ob* and *db/db* mice and the *fa/fa* Zucker rat may be due, at least in part, to overactivity of the ARC-PVN projection. The *fa/fa* rat shows increased hypothalamic NPY mRNA levels together with enhanced NPY secretion in the PVN (Fig. 7). In the *ob/ob* and *db/db* mice, regional NPY levels and NPY secretion *in vivo* have not yet been reported, but NPY mRNA levels in the ARC are known to be raised.

There is no doubt that many neuronal systems and neurotransmitters participate in controlling food intake and energy expenditure, processes that are so fundamental to survival that they perhaps could not be entrusted to a single system. Indeed, the

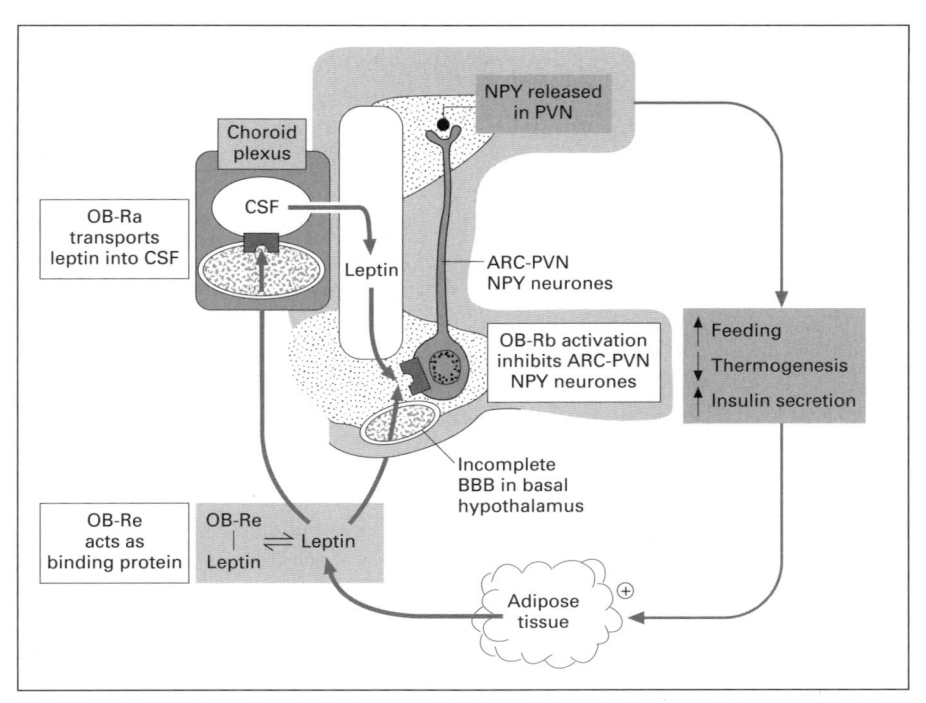

Fig. 8 Leptin-NPY interactions in the homoeostatic loop that controls energy balance and body fat mass. The NPY neurones in the ARC are probably regulated by other factors, including insulin (inhibitions) and glucocorticoids (stimulatory). Leptin can also act through other neural pathways, as it can still inhibit feeding in the NPY knockout mouse [16].

recently reported NPY knockout mouse shows remarkably normal food intake [16], suggesting that other neuronal systems are able to assume command in this model. However, in adult rodents at least, the available evidence strongly suggests a central role for NPY, and indicates that failure to restrain the activity of the ARC neurones leads to obesity. This raises important questions about the factors that normally control the NPY neurones, and whose abnormal action leads to obesity.

☐ REGULATION AND DYSREGULATION OF ARC NPY NEURONES

The ARC receives neural inputs and is accessible to various circulating factors, by virtue of its specially modified blood-brain barrier. It is apparent that the central metabolic actions of NPY (hyperphagia, reduced thermogenesis, fat accumulation) directly oppose those of leptin, and that absence of leptin in the genetically obese rodents results in increased activity of the arcuate NPY neurones. These findings raised the possibility that leptin enters the ARC, which it has now been shown to do [11], and inhibits the NPY neurones. There is some evidence for this, in that leptin administered systemically can lower the raised NPY mRNA in *ob/ob* mice, and when given intracerebroventricularly (ICV) to normal rats decreases both NPY mRNA levels and NPY concentrations in the ARC, PVN and DMH [7,17]. Interestingly, if leptin is injected ICV before NPY it attenuates the latter's hyperphagic action, pointing to a separate, postsynaptic inhibitory effect. The ARC contains mRNA for the long form of the leptin receptor, and recent studies using *in situ* hybridization indicate that this is expressed by the NPY neurones themselves. According to this scheme, obesity in the genetically obese rodents would be due to disinhibition of the NPY neurones, resulting from lack or blockade of the leptin signal (Fig. 8).

Insulin, whose central metabolic actions resemble those of leptin, may also inhibit the NPY neurones, as the ARC contains insulin receptors, and some studies suggest that insulin injected ICV can inhibit NPY expression in the ARC [12,14]. Interestingly, the *fa/fa* Zucker rat is resistant to the hypophagic effect of ICV insulin, and also fails to show the suppression of NPY mRNA levels that is seen in lean animals. The *fa/fa* Zucker might therefore be resistant to insulin at hypothalamic level, as well as in its peripheral tissues [12]. These observations are yet to be reconciled with the fact that the *fa* mutation affects the leptin receptor.

☐ LESSONS FOR HUMAN OBESITY AND ITS TREATMENT

These advances have begun to illuminate the difficult questions of what causes human obesity, and how to treat it. In man, as in rodents, leptin is expressed by fat and secreted into the circulation, where its concentration generally increases as BMI rises (Fig. 9). It can be detected in the CSF, which implies a transport mechanism of some sort, and the extended leptin receptor has recently been demonstrated in the human hypothalamus.

Despite its importance in rodents, leptin is of uncertain significance in humans.

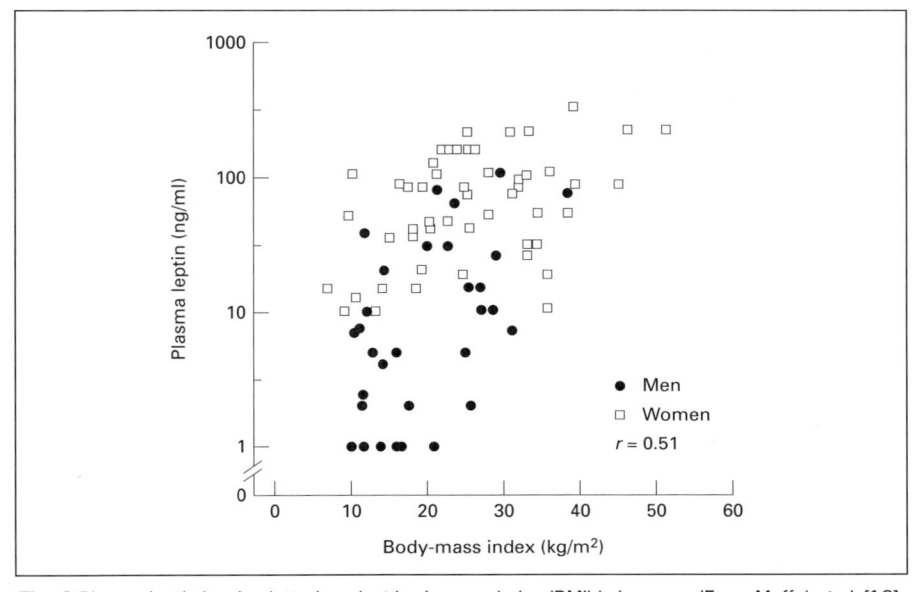

Fig. 9 Plasma leptin levels plotted against body-mass index (BMI) in humans. (From Maffei *et al.* [18], with permission.)

It is now accepted that the common type of human obesity is not due to leptin mutations [19], and the hypothalamic receptor also appears to be intact [20]. Some recent work may suggest more subtle involvement of leptin. Some cases of severe obesity show genetic linkage with the *ob* gene, hinting at abnormalities in the regulatory region upstream of the leptin coding sequence and perhaps at a defect in the control of leptin production [21]; the wide individual variation in plasma leptin levels could, theoretically, conceal some people whose leptin levels are higher than in lean subjects but low in proportion to their fat mass (see Fig. 9). Furthermore, some obese subjects show CSF leptin levels that are disproportionately low in relation to their plasma levels, which might point to impairment of transport from the bloodstream into CSF [22]. In both these cases, attenuation of the leptin signal might cause the CNS to underestimate body fat stores, thus effectively raising the set-point and favouring fat accumulation.

There remain many gaps in our knowledge about NPY and its role in man. NPY neurones are found in the human hypothalamus, but basic information about their connections, regulation and activity in states of altered energy balance is almost totally lacking.

☐ NEW DRUGS FOR OBESITY: PROMISING AVENUE OR BLIND ALLEY?

Novel approaches to treat human obesity could include amplifying the leptin signal, or reducing or blocking NPY action within the hypothalamus (Fig. 10). In theory, leptin could be given therapeutically (possibly by nasal spray to circumvent the need for injections), or its release from fat could be stimulated by specific secretagogues

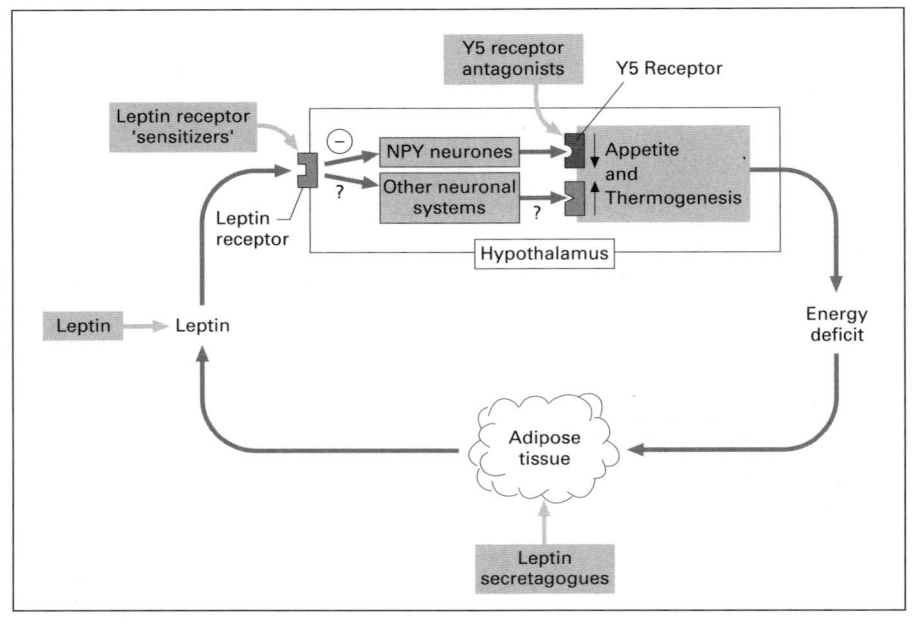

Fig. 10 Possible targets for novel anti-obesity drugs.

(as yet hypothetical). Alternatively, the putative leptin-binding protein could be manipulated to increase the circulating concentrations of free biologically active leptin. These approaches are currently being explored extremely enthusiastically by several major pharmaceutical companies. However, the possibility that leptin transport into the CNS is defective in at least some obese subjects must raise some doubts about whether raising circulating leptin levels will be effective.

A more rewarding strategy may involve targets within the hypothalamus, notably the leptin receptor and the ARC NPY neurones. Rapidly increasing knowledge about the leptin receptor and its signal transduction mechanisms may lead to drugs that sensitize the receptor, in the same way that the thiazolidinedione compounds (now being evaluated in the treatment of NIDDM) enhance insulin action. Modulation of NPY release or action is another option, and the recent identification and cloning of a specific NPY receptor subtype (Y5) that mediates the peptide's hyperphagic effects in rats is a major step forward [23]. Prototype Y5 antagonists have already been shown to inhibit feeding, apparently with reasonably high specificity. However, Y5 receptors are present in brain areas outside the hypothalamus, possibly pointing to other actions (and therefore side-effects), and the status of the Y5 receptor in man at the time of writing is still unknown.

☐ CONCLUSIONS

The pace of discovery in this field has accelerated greatly during the last couple of years and has already produced several outstanding papers that are destined to become citation classics. It is very likely that these advances will lead to new strategies to treat human obesity.

REFERENCES

1 West R. *Obesity*. Paper No. 112. London: Office of Health Economics, 1994.
2 Manson JE, Willett WC, Stampfer MJ, Colditz GA, et al. Body weight and mortality among women. *New Engl J Med* 1995; 333: 677–85.
3 Colditz G. Economic costs of obesity. *Am J Clin Nutr* 1992; 55: 5035–75.
4 Jeanrenaud B. Central nervous system and peripheral abnormalities: clues to the understanding of obesity and NIDDM. *Diabetologia* 1994; 37 (Suppl. 2): S170–8.
5 Zhang V, Proenca R, Maffei M, Barone M, et al. Positional cloning of the mouse *obese* gene and its human homologue. *Nature* 1994; 372: 425–32.
6 Halaas JL, Gajiwala KS, Maffei M, Cohen SL, et al. Weight-reducing effects of the plasma protein encoded by the *obese* gene. *Science* 1995; 269: 543–6.
7 Wang Q, Bing C, Al-Barazanji K, Mossakowaska DE, et al. Interactions between leptin and hypothalamic neuropeptide Y neurons in the control of food intake and energy homeostasis in the rat. *Diabetes* 1997 (in press).
8 Tartaglia LA, Dembski M, Wang X, Deng N, et al. Identification and cloning of a leptin receptor, OB-R. *Cell* 1995; 83: 1263–71.
9 Chen H, Charlat O, Tartaglia LA, Woolf EA, et al. Evidence that the *diabetes* gene encodes the leptin receptor – identification of a mutation in the leptin receptor gene in *db/db* mice. *Cell* 1996; 84: 491–5.
10 Phillips MS, Liu Q, Hammond HA, Dugan V, et al. Leptin receptor missense mutation in the *fatty* Zucker rat. *Nature Genetics* 1996; 13: 18–9.

11 Banks WA, Kastin AJ, Huang WT, Jaspan JB, Maness LM. Leptin enters the brain by a saturable system independent of insulin. *Peptides* 1996; **17**: 305–11.
12 Schwartz MW, Figlewicz DP, Baskin DG, Woods SC, Porte D. Insulin in the brain: a hormonal regulator of energy balance. *Endocr Rev* 1992; **13**: 387–413.
13 Williams G, Wilding JPH. The central nervous system and diabetes mellitus. In: Pickup JC, Williams G, eds. *Textbook of Diabetes*, 2nd edition. Oxford: Blackwell Science, 1996: ch. 65.
14 Frankish HM, Dryden S, Hopkins D, Wang Q, Williams G. Neuropeptide Y, the hypothalamus and diabetes: insights into the central control of metabolism. *Peptides* 1995; **16**: 757–71.
15 Dryden S, Pickavance L, Frankish HM, Williams G. Increased neuropeptide Y secretion in the hypothalamic paraventricular nucleus of obese *(fa/fa)* rats. *Brain Res* 1995; **690**: 185–8.
16 Erickson JC, Clegg KE, Palmiter RD. Sensitivity to leptin and susceptibility to seizures of mice lacking neuropeptide Y. *Nature* 1996; **381**: 415–8.
17 Stephens TW, Basinski M, Bristow PK. The role of neuropeptide Y in the antiobesity actions of the obese gene product. *Nature* 1995; **377**: 530–2.
18 Maffei M, Halaas J, Ravussein E, *et al*. Leptin levels in humans and rodents: measurement of plasma leptin and *ob* mRNA in obese and weight-reduced subjects. *Nature Med* 1995; **1**: 1155–61.
19 Considine RV, Considine EL, Williams CJ, Nyce MR, *et al*. Mutation screening and identification of a sequence variation in the human *ob* coding region. *Biochem Biophys Res Commun* 1996; **220**: 735–9.
20 Considine RV, Considine EL, Williams CJ, Hyde TM, Caro JF. The hypothalamic leptin receptor in humans: identification of incidental sequence polymorphisms and absence of *db/db* mouse and *fa/fa* rat mutations. *Diabetes* 1996; **45**: 992–4.
21 Reed DR, Ding Y, Xu WZ, Cather C, *et al*. Extreme obesity may be linked to markers flanking the human OB gene. *Diabetes* 1996; **45**: 691–4.
22 Schwartz MW, Peskind E, Raskind M, Boyko EJ, Porte D. Cerebrospinal fluid leptin levels: relationship to plasma levels and to adiposity in humans. *Nature Med* 1996; **2**: 587–93.
23 Gerald C, Walker MW, Criscione L, *et al.*. A receptor subtype involved in neuropeptide Y-induced food intake. *Nature* 1996; **382**: 168–71.

Delivering optimal care to patients with asthma

Martyn R Partridge

☐ INTRODUCTION

Medical students are taught to regard asthma as a condition characterized by 'generalized narrowing of the airways which varies over short periods of time either spontaneously or as a result of treatment'. This definition is based on the original Ciba Symposium definition and has stood the test of time in terms of its value in diagnosis of the condition. However, the definition does not include many of the key features of our current understanding of asthma and these need to be understood if we are to appreciate the need for change in the way in which we approach patients. The physiological definition also excludes mention of the symptoms of asthma which are cough, breathlessness, chest tightness and wheezing, with the key feature being that these are often worse at night or after exercise. The definition also excludes description of the state of airway hyper-responsiveness which, although not specific to asthma, is a cardinal feature of the condition.

☐ WHAT IS ASTHMA?

In the mid-1980s Finnish workers rediscovered the inflammatory basis of asthma. They, and subsequently others, have shown that significant structural and cellular changes of inflammation may be present in the airways of people with asthma, even when they are well and free from symptoms [1]. More recent work has suggested that if this inflammatory process is not controlled it may lead to remodelling of the airways with the condition becoming less responsive to treatment with time. The enlargement of our understanding of asthma from a diagnostic physiologically based definition to a wider description of asthma that encompasses both symptoms and the concept of airway hyper-responsiveness and inflammation has meant that a greater proportion of people with asthma than before are regarded as having a long-term condition. Asthma can no longer be regarded as a series of acute episodes of bronchospasm, and the new understanding means a greater proportion of patients than before taking regular anti-inflammatory treatment to prevent asthma and to prevent long-term lung damage. Even if we have appreciated this changed understanding, our patients' knowledge may be inadequate. A recent survey revealed that at the time of diagnosis a third of adults did not realize that the diagnosis of asthma might involve them in taking long-term treatment (Table 1).

One challenge facing us all therefore is to help patients benefit maximally from the drugs available. The need is for us all to stand back and think clearly about our current understanding of asthma and the challenges facing us, but we also need to

Table 1 National Asthma Campaign 1993 poll. A random sample of 2500 people in the UK National Asthma Campaign membership data base were sent a questionnaire and 1631 patients responded. They were asked how they felt at the time of diagnosis.

Bewildered	15%
Angry	9%
Extremely worried	29%
Frightened	20%
Did not realize would need regular treatment	28%

recognize the challenge which faces us for the future. That challenge is to find out why so many more people have asthma now than 10 to 20 years ago. The increase in prevalence of the condition is a real phenomenon and not just a question of diagnostic transfer. Throughout the world we have evidence of an increasing prevalence of asthma, especially in children, in whom the latest UK figures suggest a prevalence of 13.7%.

☐ PREVALENCE OF ASTHMA

Why is the prevalence of asthma increasing?

The tendency to atopy is inherited (probably on more than one gene) and the population will not have changed its genetic constitution over the past 20-year period, so it must be something in the environment that is activating the inherited tendency in more people now than it did 10 to 20 years ago.

Studies in rural China and in rural parts of the African subcontinent suggest that the prevalence of the condition is much lower than in more developed countries. It is important that premature conclusions are not drawn concerning the factors responsible for this increased prevalence. Scientific evaluation involves large-scale population studies to determine factors that may correlate with the increased prevalence, but this needs to be coupled with the realization that an association may not, of course, be causal. Once possible associations are identified, there needs to be an evaluation of the likelihood of there being a genuine connection (based on a scientific evaluation of likelihood), but the importance of such a correlation can only be assessed by further immunological and epidemiological research, followed by intervention studies. These studies are extremely difficult to perform and it is most unlikely that only one single factor is responsible for the increasing prevalence.

☐ FACTORS INVOLVED IN THE INCREASING PREVALENCE OF ASTHMA

Likely candidates responsible for increasing prevalence are environmental factors to which the fetus, newborn or young child are exposed. These include maternal smoking, which has been shown to be associated with increased prevalence of wheezing illnesses in the young, and in adults there is a proven association between exposure to certain occupational sensitizers and the development of asthma. Both of these factors represent a potential area for the primary prevention of the condition. Most of the other factors remain speculative, but they include the possibility that changes in our home environment over the past 10 or 20 years have led to the increased prevalence of asthma. Changes include less ventilation in homes because fireplaces and chimneys have been blocked off, insulation is better, and double-glazing eliminates draughts. Such changes may have an adverse effect on humidity so that house dust mites introduced into this environment are more likely to multiply. It is possible, but not proven, that we expose young children today to larger concentrations of this particular allergen than we did some years ago. This will be enhanced not only by the changes in humidity but by the increased use of fitted carpets and soft furnishings. Diminution in ventilation in our homes may also result in concentration of other allergens and indoor pollutants such as passive smoking and oxides of nitrogen released by the use of gas cookers.

Our diet has also changed over the past 10 to 20 years and it has been suggested that a reduction in intake of fresh vegetables and fresh, especially oily, fish may have altered antioxidant levels in such a way that we are more predisposed to the development of asthma. Atmospheric pollution has attracted the attention of the media as a possible explanation for increased asthma, but less than 5% of our time is spent out of doors, and the recent COMEAP report (Committee on the Medical Effects of Atmospheric Pollution) has reviewed this subject and concluded that it is unlikely that traffic pollution is a significant factor in the increasing prevalence of the condition, although it may of course make established disease worse. In this context it is important to recall that New Zealand, which suffers little pollution, has one of the highest prevalences of asthma. Also a higher prevalence has been reported in the Isle of Skye compared with some urban areas of Scotland. An adverse synergistic effect of traffic pollution and some other environmental factor has not been excluded.

The final factor currently attracting attention is the potential effect of viral infections in early life. While we recognize that such infections are a common trigger of asthma in those who already have the condition, it has been postulated that viral infections in early life may in some way be beneficial and that this effect may be mediated by an early protective activation of the immune system. Such a hypothesis could explain the higher rate of the condition among first-born who are less likely to be exposed to viral infections brought into the home by siblings in the early days or weeks of life.

☐ PREVENTION AND TREATMENT OF ASTHMA

The challenge for the future and the challenge for now

The challenge for the future is the challenge of primary prevention, ie preventing asthma from developing in the first place. It is possible that in 5, 10 or 15 years time we may be able to sit down with a potential mother-to-be, who may be at risk of having an atopic infant by virtue of personal or family history of atopic disease, and advise the mother to stop smoking, to take a certain form of diet and to modify her home so that we can reduce the risk of her having an atopic baby who may go on to develop asthma. However, at present we cannot give such advice, and so the challenge for now is the challenge of preventing attacks of asthma in those who already have the condition. It is the challenge of preventing hospitalization from asthma, and preventing the risk of undertreated asthma giving rise to permanent lung damage, or death. Such prevention is likely to involve drug therapy, but we should not become so prescription-orientated that we ignore the potential, in some patients at least, of environmental manipulation.

The problem, of course, is that despite excellent therapies being available there is still considerable suffering. We know that three-quarters of all adult admissions to hospital could probably have been avoided by better community care, and that 25% of patients in primary care may be over-reliant on bronchodilators. We also know that sufferers are more likely to be readmitted to hospital with acute asthma if the first admission was not under a specialist, or if the reasons for the first attack were not properly investigated and treatment and management changed as a result. So we need to look carefully at the possible reasons why the available effective treatments may not be reaching patients.

Why is good treatment not reaching the patient?

Optimal asthma care involves there being well educated health professionals working in a well organized way within an adequately funded system, and delivering treatment in a way that ensures the patient takes it. However, all too often there are delays in diagnosis. This used to be most problematical in the young, but it is likely now that delays occur equally often among elderly patients when there is often a failure to differentiate asthma from chronic obstructive pulmonary disease (COPD) or other diseases. Until the correct diagnosis is made, the correct treatment is unlikely to be given.

The availability of effective treatments will similarly not benefit patients if the wrong type of treatment is used or if doses are too low. This is likely to occur when patients or doctors underestimate severity, so that there is an over-reliance on bronchodilators or an underuse of anti-inflammatory agents. We also need to recognize that in some countries good asthma care may appear to be too expensive for either the individual or the state. Even in this country for the 20% of those with asthma who do not get free prescriptions the prescription charge may act as a deterrent to compliance and this may be a particular problem with the current trend towards multiple drug regimens.

Most of these are issues for health professionals and for health professional education, and in this country we have some excellent guidelines on the management of asthma which have now been revised three times since they were first produced six years ago [2–5]. These guidelines were produced by a rigorous evaluative process involving the writing of extensive review papers which were peer reviewed, adapted and published, and as a result of this extensive process of review of the literature a detailed consensus was achieved as to how asthma should be managed in patients of all ages and under a variety of circumstances.

Routine management of asthma

The aim of the routine management of asthma is to gain control of the condition. This is achieved by the prompt administration of anti-inflammatory therapy, given in adequate dosage, to all who require the use of bronchodilators on more than a very infrequent basis (Fig. 1). Once control is achieved, as shown by optimal lung function, minimal need for bronchodilators and resolution of symptoms, the treatment is reduced to the minimum that maintains that state. Guidelines containing this advice, and advice on the management of acute attacks in both adults and children, in hospital and in primary care, have been summarized in a number of charts [5]. These have been widely disseminated among health care professionals. We may ask the question as to whether such guidelines work. Published evaluations of guidelines suggest that there can be improvements in both the process of care and the outcome of care after implementation of guidelines [6]. Those most likely to be associated with a successful outcome are those about whom there is active education of health professionals and where there is feedback to individual practitioners as to how their care compares to that outlined in guidelines. Other features associated with successful guidelines are when there is simultaneous production of patient specific materials and when guidelines are adapted and adopted at a local level, within a district, in an emergency department, in a hospital or in an individual practice [7]. For these reasons many parts of the country have found it advantageous to launch local asthma task forces which can look at the problems in their area and adapt the organizational parts of the guidelines to their locality so that there is a

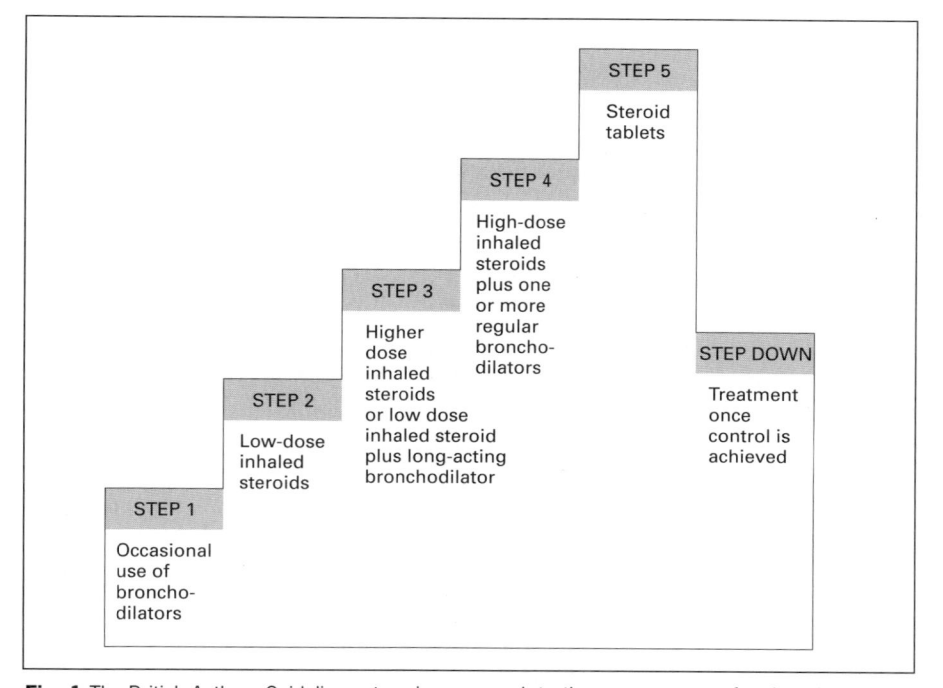

Fig. 1 The British Asthma Guidelines stepwise approach to the management of asthma in adults.

sense of ownership and relevance. The National Asthma Campaign has published a book *Purchasing and Providing Good Asthma Care*, which contains advice for local asthma task forces.

Communication and compliance

As a result of health professional education and introduction of guidelines and audit, it may be possible to ensure that the health professional writes the correct prescription, but unless this is delivered in the correct manner then the patient may, for a variety of reasons, choose not to take the medication [8]. Factors associated with the likelihood of non-compliance are listed in Table 2. Many of these are not

Table 2 Factors associated with non-compliance.

Drug factors	Patient/physician factors
Problems with inhalers	Misunderstanding
Complicated regimens	Lack of information
	Youth
	Cultural misconceptions
	Inappropriate expectations
	Unexpressed fears or concerns
	Attitudes towards ill health
	Poor communication

disease-specific and are common to any long-term condition. However, as we become better scientists, we continually need to reinforce to ourselves and our colleagues the absolute importance of good communication as a prerequisite for good compliance.

Patient satisfaction with the communication aspects of the consultation and the health professional's approach is an essential foundation for subsequent good compliance (Table 3). We need to recognize that each patient brings to this common

Table 3 Good communication is an essential prerequisite for good compliance and involves a sender, a message and a recipient. However, it is important to realize that the recipient (the patient) is also a sender and the doctor must appreciate the circular nature of this model and hear the patient's messages.

Sender	Message	Recipient
Doctor	The diagnosis	Assess beliefs
Nurse	The treatments	Clarify information needs
Educator	Inhaler techniques	Explain rationale
Books	Monitoring	Explore barriers
Audio tapes	Signs of loss of control	Negotiate goals
Video tapes	What to do if it worsens	Help cost/benefit balance
TV programmes	Information about support groups	Enlist family and friends
		Follow-up

condition of asthma a different personality, past life experiences and expectations of both the condition and its treatment. We need to elicit this information and be aware that any unexpressed fears will act as a barrier to subsequent educational efforts. If a patient comes to see the doctor hoping that the doctor will tell him or her what to avoid to make the asthma go away, but the doctor fails to perceive that that was the patient's desire and instead writes a prescription for steroids, telling the patient the drugs will need to be taken for a long time, then the patient is unlikely to leave the surgery feeling satisfied, and is unlikely to comply with the treatment. We therefore need to elicit from our patients their understanding of the condition, their expectations and their fears. One such barrier is that of steroid phobia which, while well known to doctors, is rarely aired during a consultation. It is clearly good practice to ask always at the time of issuing a prescription how the patient feels about their treatment, and to invite questions, but this is especially important when prescribing steroids. Any fears may be elicited by the use of open-ended questions such as 'Some people think that steroids are harmful, what do you think?' [3]. If the patient then expresses concern, it is possible to give them a rational explanation of the differences between the steroids used by athletes and those used for medicinal purposes, and to explain the differences between inhaled and oral steroids. The patient will forget some of these details after the consultation, or their new-found confidence may be shattered by doubts expressed by loved ones or friends, and it should therefore be usual practice to reinforce such explanations with written booklets, such as the *Steroids and Asthma* booklet available free from the National Asthma Campaign.

Reinforcing the spoken word

About 50% of all that is said to a patient during the consultation may be forgotten within 5 minutes of its ending. However, by the time the patient has had the same message on three occasions, or by three different routes, significant long-term retention of information can be expected. Although giving information alone is no more likely to alter a patient's behaviour than giving information to health professionals alters the health professional's behaviour, we need to recognize that lack of information or misunderstanding very frequently leads to unintentional non-compliance. Several studies have shown that the simple giving of written information describing an individual patient's medication regimen can have a significant beneficial effect on the patient's subsequent recall of that regimen and on their behaviour [9,10] yet is rarely undertaken (Table 4).

Studies in several fields have shown that compliance can be improved if the patient recognizes that within the spectrum of possible outcomes lies the risk of either hospitalization or death, and that the risk may apply to them and not just to the other person. However, appropriate use of medications is unlikely unless the patient has received an adequate explanation of the expected risk-versus-benefit of any prescription, and there has to have been adequate opportunity for the patient or parent to express any fears or concerns regarding side effects [11].

The other features likely to be associated with good compliance are a general feeling of satisfaction with the communication aspects of the doctor/patient

Table 4 National Asthma Campaign 1993. In the same survey as in Table 2, members of the National Asthma Campaign were asked what information had been given to help them manage their asthma; 1631 people responded.

Information given	Number of people
Information booklets	635 (39%)
Videos	61 (4%)
Written advice regarding medicines	441 (27%)
Demonstration of inhalers	1026 (63%)

relationship. This will be enhanced if those patients who wish it are given information that enables them to take greater responsibility for their own condition (Table 5).

Table 5 Compliance can be increased by the following parameters.

The patient believes the disease may be dangerous
The patient believes that he or she is at risk
The patient believes that the treatment is safe
The patient feels in control
There is good communication between patient and doctor

The goal: guided self-management

All of the published guidelines on asthma suggest a goal of guided self-management. Determining which patients and which parents wish to take responsibility for their own condition is an essential part of the intraconsultation negotiation, which is essential in any long-term condition.

Self-management requires that, within the context of a partnership with the doctor or nurse, a patient is given advice enabling them to adjust their own treatment in response to a variety of circumstances, with the aim of keeping themselves well. The concept does not have to be complicated, and for many patients it merely involves the patient appreciating the importance of recognizing that waking at night with asthma, or needing increased use of bronchodilators, represents deteriorating asthma and the need to seek a further consultation with the doctor. For other patients, it is appropriate to give more detailed self-management plans such that, in response to increasing symptoms, sleep disturbance, an increased need for bronchodilators or a reduction in measured peak flow, the patient takes a variety of steps of action ranging from doubling their preventive therapy through to the initiation of a course of high-dose steroid tablets or the seeking of urgent medical attention. Such self-management plans need to be written and they may be based on either symptoms or measurement of peak flow or a combination of both subjective and objective monitoring (Table 6 and Plate 11).

The effectiveness of such self-management plans has now been studied in several trials [12–15] based in several countries. In some, the benefit appears to be limited

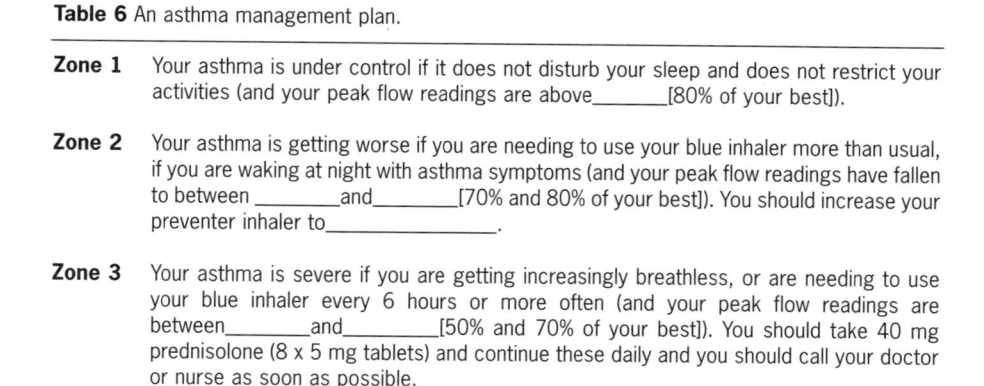

Table 6 An asthma management plan.

Zone 1	Your asthma is under control if it does not disturb your sleep and does not restrict your activities (and your peak flow readings are above_____[80% of your best]).
Zone 2	Your asthma is getting worse if you are needing to use your blue inhaler more than usual, if you are waking at night with asthma symptoms (and your peak flow readings have fallen to between_____and_____[70% and 80% of your best]). You should increase your preventer inhaler to_____.
Zone 3	Your asthma is severe if you are getting increasingly breathless, or are needing to use your blue inhaler every 6 hours or more often (and your peak flow readings are between_____and_____[50% and 70% of your best]). You should take 40 mg prednisolone (8 x 5 mg tablets) and continue these daily and you should call your doctor or nurse as soon as possible.
Zone 4	It is a medical emergency if you are continuing to get worse (and if your peak flow readings have fallen below_____[50% of your best]). You should take 40 mg prednisolone (8 x 5 mg tablets) and call an ambulance or ring your doctor **IMMEDIATELY**. Do not be afraid of causing a fuss. Your doctor or nurse will want to see you immediately so that they may adjust treatment to make you well.

to those with more severe disease, and the potential for any form of self-management plan to show benefit is less likely in an overtreated population in whom the possibility of an exacerbation is less. However, several trials on asthma control before and after administration of self-management plans have shown a benefit. More recently a number of controlled clinical trials with a lengthy period of follow-up have shown unequivocal evidence of benefit from the use of self-management plans [12,13]. Improved outcomes include reduction in symptoms, reduction in time off work, reduction in use of health service resources and improvement in peak flow readings. In two of the studies it was also interesting to note that after administration of self-management plans, and despite the fact that such plans involved the possibility of a patient taking courses of steroid tablets, there were improved outcomes and less use of steroid tablets compared to both before the introduction of the self-management plan and to the control group. The only possible explanations for this paradox are either that the lesser steps in the self-management plans (ie doubling inhaled steroids at the first sign of deterioration) works or, equally likely, that when you give control of the condition to the patient themselves they are more likely to comply with these lesser steps so that exacerbations requiring rescue courses of steroid tablets become less likely.

The way forward

Thus there is now good evidence that, in addition to good verbal communication between patients and health professionals, all patients require simple written information regarding their drug regimen. Within this they should receive information about signs that suggest that their asthma is worsening. For some patients it is then appropriate to discuss with them whether they wish to take more control of their own condition. Those who do should receive a more detailed self-management plan and be given control of their own condition in a guided way with the several zone plans (see Plate 11). There are, of course, some remaining scientific questions about the form of these plans, and some doubt remains about whether all should be based on objective recordings of peak flow, symptoms, or a combination of the two. It is also possible that the same does not apply to children as it does to adults. Sometimes health professionals remark that they do not feel that their patients would want to cope with self-management plans, and yet in the published studies where patients have been asked whether they preferred subjective or objective based plans a preference has been expressed for objective plans [16]. Even in the case of children, mothers of those old enough to record peak flow have expressed satisfaction with their ability to monitor objectively the severity of their child's condition.

Any doubts about the exact necessity for objective monitoring of peak flow should be an incentive for further research rather than an excuse to discard a tool that many believe has led to improved assessment of asthma severity. There is also an increasing awareness that some patients have an impaired ability to perceive changes in their airway calibre. Although this phenomenon has been known for many years, more recent studies in primary care among adults have shown that 60% of patients may be poor discriminators of the severity of their asthma, with some patients feeling unwell and being able to detect relatively minor falls in peak flow, while others can suffer catastrophic falls in peak flow and not perceive that deterioration [17]. Japanese workers have also suggested that such impaired perception may be more common among those requiring ventilation because of severe attacks of asthma [18].

Targeting those most at risk

For the time being, a sensible compromise would be to target our efforts and the use of education and administration of guided self-management and peak-flow monitoring on those who are most at risk. These at-risk categories are likely to include all patients who have been hospitalized, any who have had sudden severe attacks of asthma and any who are identified as poor perceivers of severity. Adolescent patients with asthma receive the double burden of a long-term condition at a time when they may have other stresses and are sometimes less willing to accept advice. It therefore seems sensible to negotiate with these adolescent asthmatic patients to see whether they wish to take more control of their condition and to use such plans. A similar educational approach is probably sensible during pregnancy, or pre-conception, because of the understandable, but mistaken, fear of pregnant patients that asthma drugs may in some way be harmful. We need to ensure that this fear does not lead to discontinuation of therapy and subsequent exacerbation of asthma, for such attacks may represent the greatest threat to the fetus.

There is increasing anecdotal evidence, and some evidence from clinical trials, that there may also be an association between depression and diminished compliance and this also requires some targeting of efforts. It is also clear from the

USA and to a lesser extent the UK that, while asthma may be slightly less common among patients who are socio-economically deprived, if these people do have asthma they are likely to suffer from it to a greater extent than more affluent patients. It is essential when planning the organization of our services that we devise ways to make our care equally accessible to all.

☐ CONCLUSION

The challenge for the future is to find out why the common condition of asthma is becoming even more common, so that we may hopefully one day prevent the onset of the condition. Until that day arrives, our challenge is to ensure that the excellent therapies already available reach the patients, and this is likely to involve production, and more especially implementation, of guidelines so that health professionals know the optimal management regimens. This involves active education, local adoption of guidelines and institution of feedback and audit. At a doctor/patient level we need to think beyond the prescription and take a more patient-centred approach, which involves giving to those patients who wish it a greater responsibility for control of their own condition. We need to recognize that, as with any long-term condition, we need to revise and reinforce our educational messages continually and to provide regular follow-up and reassurance to our patients.

REFERENCES

1   Laitenen LA, Heino M, Laitenen A, Kava T, Haahtela T. Damage of the airway epithelium and bronchial reactivity in patients with asthma. *Am Rev Respir Dis* 1985; **131**: 599–606.
2   British Thoracic Society, British Paediatric Association, Royal College of Physicians of London, The King's Fund Centre, the National Asthma Campaign, *et al*. Guidelines on the management of asthma. *Thorax* 1993; **48**: S1–S24. Summary charts. *Brit Med J* 1993; **306**: 776–82.
3   National Institutes of Health. *Global Strategy for Asthma Management and Prevention*. NHLBI Workshop report. National Heart Lung Blood Institute 1995; **95**: 3659.
4   International consensus report on the diagnosis and management of asthma. *Clin Exp Allergy* 1992; **22** (Suppl): 1–72.
5   The British Guidelines on Asthma Management: 1995 review and position statement. *Thorax* 1997; **52**(Suppl): S1–S21.
6   Grimshaw JM, Russell IT. Effect of clinical guidelines on medical practice: a systematic review of rigorous evaluations. *Lancet* 1993; **342**: 1317–22.
7   Feder G, Griffiths C, Highton C, Eldridge S, Spence M, Southgate L. Do clinical guidelines introduced with practice based education improve care of asthmatic and diabetic patients? A randomised controlled trial in general practices in east London. *Brit Med J* 1995; **311**: 1473–8.
8   Partridge MR. Asthma: lessons from patient education. *Patient Education and Counselling* 1995; **26**: 81–6.
9   Pedersen S. Ensuring compliance in children. *Eur Respir J* 1992; **5**: 143–5.
10 Rayner DK, Booth TG, Blenkinsopp A. Effects of computer-generated reminder charts on patients' compliance with drug regimens. *Brit Med J* 1993; **306**: 1158–61.
11 Evans D. To help patients control asthma the clinician must be a good listener and teacher. *Thorax* 1993; **48**: 685—7.
12 Ignacio-Garcia J, Gonzalez-Santas P. Asthma self-management education programme by home monitoring of peak expiratory flow. *Am J Respir Crit Care Med* 1995; **151**: 353–9.

13 Lahdensuo A, Haahtela T, Herrala J, Kava T, *et al*. PEF guided use of an inhaled corticosteroid is successful. Finnish Asthma Self-Management Study. *Eur Respir J* 1994; 7 (Suppl 18): P1425.
14 Grampian Asthma Study of Integrated Care (Grassic). Effectiveness of routine self-monitoring of peak flow in patients with asthma. *Brit Med J* 1994; **308**: 564–8.
15 Yoon R, McKenzie DK, Bauman A, Miles DA. Controlled trial evaluation of an asthma education programme for adults. *Thorax* 1993; **48**: 1110–16.
16 Lloyd BW, Ali MH. How useful do parents find home peak flow monitoring for children with asthma? *Brit Med J* 1992; **305**: 1128–9.
17 Kendrick AH, Higgs CMB, Whitfield MJ, Laszlo G. Accuracy of perception of severity of asthma patients treated in general practice. *Brit Med J* 1993; **307**: 422–4.
18 Kikuchi Y, Okabe S, Tamura G, *et al*. Chemo-sensitivity and perception of dyspnoea in patients with a history of near fatal asthma. *New Engl J Med* 1994; **330**: 1329–34.

The National Asthma Campaign (Providence House, Providence Place, London N1 0NT. Telephone 0171-226-2260) has available a large range of educational materials for patients and health professionals.

☐ MULTIPLE CHOICE QUESTIONS

1 Statements about asthma:
   (a) It is increasing in prevalence
   (b) It is commoner in urban areas in the UK
   (c) Airway hyper-responsiveness occurs only in asthma
   (d) It is likely to be inherited on one gene

2 Factors particularly likely to lead to non-compliance with asthma therapy:
   (a) Male sex
   (b) Steroid phobia
   (c) Poor perception of breathlessness
   (d) Adolescence
   (e) Four times daily drug regimens

3 Factors likely to be involved in the increasing prevalence of asthma:
   (a) Industrial pollution
   (b) Increased consumption of fish
   (c) Overuse of bronchodilators
   (d) Increased domestic ventilation
   (e) Changes in our genetic constitution

4 Compliance may be enhanced by:
   (a) Exploring patients' fears and concerns
   (b) Greater use of guidelines by health professionals
   (c) Giving patients control of their own condition
   (d) Group education programmes
   (e) Publicizing the fact that asthma can kill

5 Statements about asthma:
   (a) There is a close correlation between peak-flow reading and subjective perception of dyspnoea

(b) The British Guidelines on Asthma was published for the first time in 1996
(c) There is good evidence that nurses are better educators than doctors
(d) Steroid tablets should be avoided during pregnancy
(e) Self-management plans lead to improved control of asthma but greater use of steroid tablets

ANSWERS

1a True	2a False	3a False	4a True	5a False
b False	b True	b False	b ?	b False
c False	c True	c False	c True	c False
d False	d True	d False	d True	d False
	e True	e False	e True	e False

Practical problems in the management of chronic obstructive pulmonary disease

P M A Calverley

☐ INTRODUCTION

Chronic obstructive pulmonary disease (COPD) is an important cause of morbidity and mortality in developed countries. Its incidence has increased significantly in the USA, being diagnosed in 5.7% of people aged between 25 and 74. The problems rise with age and in the UK COPD accounts for approximately 10% of general practitioner (GP) consultations in men aged over 75. Although the pathophysiology is reasonably well established, attempts to provide systematic guidance about treatment are relatively recent. This review focuses on the problems in managing stable COPD but does include a brief mention of some recent changes in the care of the inpatient with an acute exacerbation.

☐ DEFINING CHRONIC OBSTRUCTIVE PULMONARY DISEASE

Many terms have been used to describe what we now consider to be COPD, with chronic bronchitis being favoured in the UK and emphysema in the USA. Although the former is diagnosed epidemiologically and the latter pathologically, careful longitudinal pathological studies have shown substantial overlap between the two conditions. COPD is the resulting, rather cumbersome, compromise term which includes both specific clinical features, ie cough, sputum, breathlessness, and pathological changes occurring within the small airways and alveoli. The important additional component of COPD is the emphasis on the presence of airflow limitation defined physiologically [1,2]. This has been repeatedly shown to be the most important prognostic variable. The clinical and physiological features of COPD do not change greatly over time, unlike asthma, but some bronchodilator reversibility is present. Representative current definitions are given in Table 1.

☐ DIAGNOSIS AND TREATMENT OF COPD

What diagnostic test to do?

Key features in the diagnostic analysis of the COPD patient are shown in Table 2. Spirometry remains the most useful diagnostic aid after a good clinical history and examination have been performed. Although cough is the earliest feature of the disease, persisting breathlessness in a patient aged over 40 who is a cigarette smoker strongly suggests COPD. This is uncommon in younger patients although, when typical features of COPD are present, α-1-antitrypsin deficiency should be considered. The principal differential diagnoses in most patients remain chronic

Table 1 Several current definitions of chronic obstructive pulmonary disease.

European Respiratory Society [1]	A disorder characterized by reduced maximum expiratory flow and slow forced emptying of the lungs: features that do not change markedly over several months
American Thoracic Society [2]	A disease state characterized by the presence of airflow obstruction due to chronic bronchitis or emphysema. The airflow obstruction is generally progressive, may be accompanied by airway hyper-reactivity and may be partially reversible
British Thoracic Society [3]	A chronic, slowly progressive disorder characterized by airways obstruction (reduced FEV_1 and FEV_1/VC ratio) which does not change markedly over several months. Most of the lung function impairment is fixed, although some reversibility can be produced by bronchodilator (or other) therapy

FEV_1 = forced expiratory volume in 1 second; VC = vital capacity

Table 2 Key features in the diagnostic analysis of COPD patients.

Clinical	Slowly progressive symptoms Persistent symptoms Age greater than 40 years, smoker, 'recurrent chest infections'
Spirometric	Absolute reduction in FEV_1 Abnormal FEV_1/VC ratio, ie less than 75% Limited bronchodilator reversibility, eg <500 ml post-nebulizer Negative corticosteroid trial
Radiographic	Chest X-ray excluding alternative diagnoses Computerized tomography (CT) scan useful in assessing bullae and emphysema distribution
Other	α-1-Antitrypsin level in blood; check in those with strong family history, early onset severe disease

pulmonary oedema and bronchiectasis, which are relatively easier to separate from COPD than are bronchiolitis obliterans or chronic asthma. The differentiation of COPD from chronic asthma is often blurred and depends on an arbitrary assumption about how much bronchodilatation is compatible with asthma or COPD. Such changes are relatively unimportant since the management plan adopted is very similar and dictated by the severity of the persisting airways obstruction.

All patients need a chest X-ray to exclude other pathology, eg bronchial tumour, and to identify bullous lung disease. The exact protocol used for bronchodilator reversibility testing is debated, but usually involves measuring lung function before and after either high-dose nebulized bronchodilators or a combination of β-agonist and an anticholinergic administered via a metered dose inhaler under supervision. Defining the baseline spirometry as a percentage of predicted values provides a useful pointer to subsequent management, while a substantial response to a bronchodilator, eg an absolute change in FEV_1 of 500 ml or more, suggests that the diagnosis is more likely to be chronic asthma. Bronchodilator responses are often expressed as a percentage change from baseline, usually 15%, but must include an absolute change of at least 200 ml when the FEV_1 is low. Approximately 30% of patients fail to show any bronchodilator response when tested in this way, but repeat testing will reduce the number of negative responses [4,5]. Some groups express bronchodilator response as the absolute change in FEV_1 divided by the predicted FEV_1 and report that a change of more than 9% represents a biologically meaningful effect. Whether this approach adds to further management is unclear. Most groups agree that the use of a single peak-flow value to assess COPD severity is undesirable and is certainly less sensitive than using spirometry.

Unlike in other countries, many UK physicians conduct a formal trial of oral corticosteroids, measuring lung function before and after an arbitrary period of treatment, usually 30 mg of prednisolone a day for two weeks. In an unselected population, approximately 20% of severe (FEV_1 <1.2 l) patients will show a significant (see above) change in FEV_1, but a meta-analysis of the wider population suggests that the true change may be approximately 10% [4,6] (Fig. 1). Trials using inhaled rather than oral corticosteroids have reported greater response rate after 6 weeks of treatment, but these employed more end-points than just a change in FEV_1.

Other lung function tests, such as flow volume loops, lung volumes and gas transfer factors contribute additional information but are not essential to patient management, while CT and radioisotope studies are usually restricted to diagnostically difficult cases or to the surgical assessment of bullous disease.

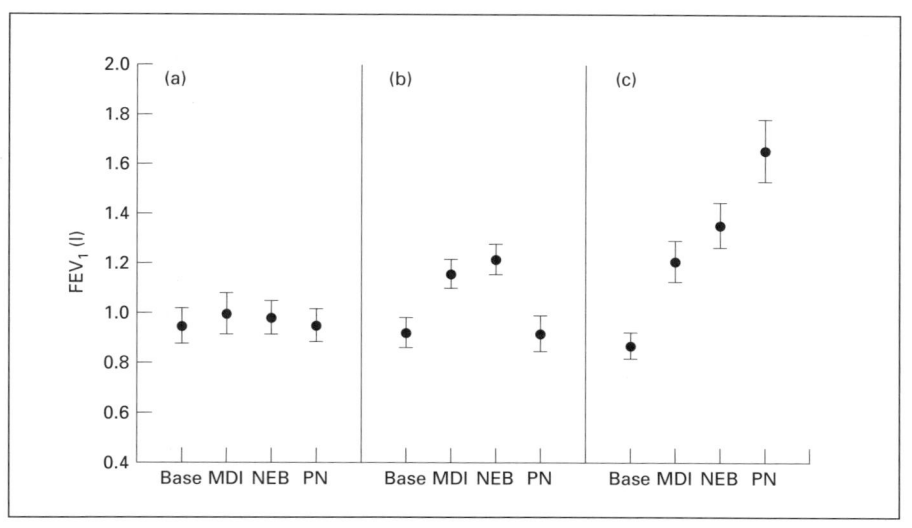

Fig. 1 The response to salbutamol given by metered dose inhaler (MDI 400 mcg) or nebulizer (NEB) and to 2 weeks of oral prednisolone (PN) in 127 patients with COPD. Of these patients: (a) 35% showed no bronchodilator response to any of the drugs; (b) 45% were reversible to salbutamol but not prednisolone; (c) 20% showed reversibility to both salbutamol and prednisolone. In patients who showed a response to salbutamol, the response was significantly greater after the nebulizer than after the metered dose inhaler. (Modified from Nisar et al. [4].)

Whose advice to follow?

Several different national/international sets of guidelines for COPD management have now been published [1,2]. They reflect the different target audiences to which they are addressed, varying from respiratory specialists in rehabilitation hospitals through to GPs. The European Respiratory Society guidelines address a range of problems in COPD with equal weight being given to severe and mild disease. Management suggestions are largely reduced to a series of algorithms with suggestions for optimum treatment and key decision points. The American Thoracic Society guidelines are longer, but include much more practical detail about specific management issues. However, they are difficult to use without reading the entire document each time a problem arises. The more recent guidelines subdivide COPD by severity of the airways obstruction and this approach is being adopted in the forthcoming British Thoracic Society recommendations [3]. Unfortunately, there is significant disagreement about where to separate mild, moderate and severe disease. Despite these differences in approach, there is a broad consensus about the treatments to be used and the fact that treatment is generally cumulative and not associated with steps down, as in asthma. The principal components of these schemes are seen in Fig. 2.

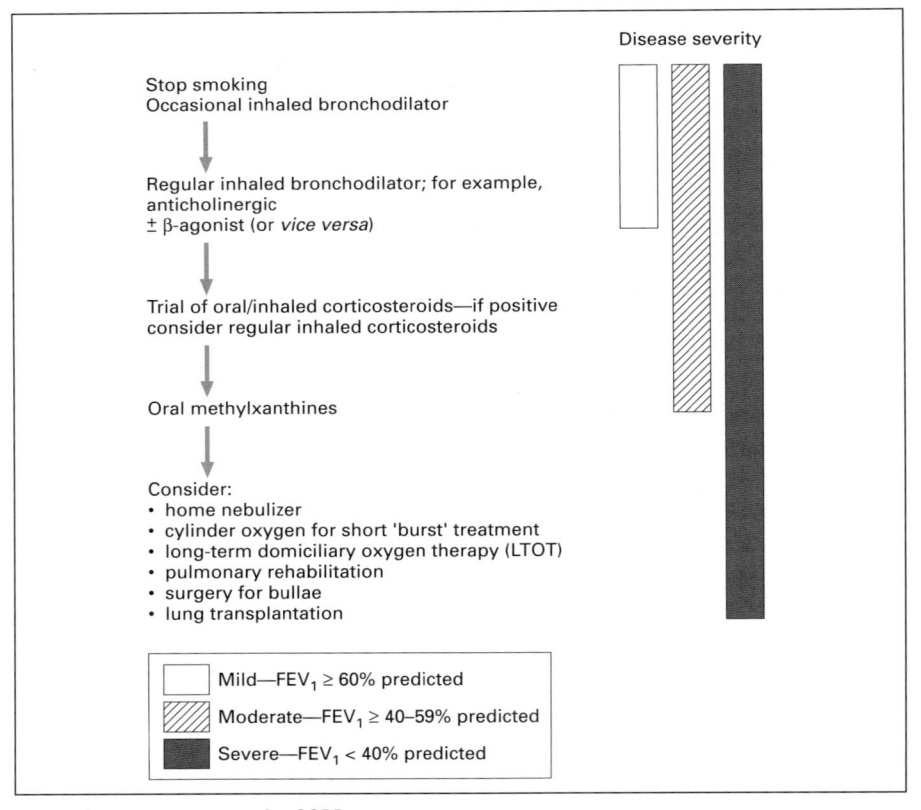

Fig. 2 Stepwise treatment for COPD.

Is it worth trying to stop smoking?

Cigarette smoking is undoubtedly the cause of most of the small airway and alveolar damage that characterizes COPD. Although difficult, stopping smoking is possible for individuals, but would be made much easier by government action to restrict tobacco advertising and increase the cost of cigarettes beyond the rate of inflation [7]. Stopping smoking is worthwhile as illustrated by the recent Lung Health Study of 5881 patients followed for five years [8]. They were randomized to intensive smoking advice or normal advice. Those in the intensive group, who underwent counselling for smoking cessation and used nicotine chewing gum, showed a substantially greater sustained quit rate (25%) than did those offered normal treatment [8]. Even chance encounters can produce a small, but useful, increase in the quit rate, it being 3% for GPs and 8% in hospital chest clinics [7].

Which bronchodilator drug?

As already noted, bronchodilator responsiveness expressed as an increase in FEV_1 is very frequent in COPD. In fact, there are data using more sensitive tests, such as airways resistance, that show that relaxation of airway smooth muscle by any bronchodilator is likely to produce some improvement compared with placebo. A small change in airway calibre when the baseline FEV_1 is low would produce a proportionately larger change in airways resistance at that lung volume than a similar change in airways dimension when the resting dimensions are higher (see Fig 3). Thus bronchodilator response of 200–300 ml can produce very important functional improvements in patients with more advanced COPD.

The principal drugs used are inhaled β-agonists, eg salbutamol, and inhaled anticholinergics, eg ipratropium. Their relative mechanisms of action are now better understood [9] and are illustrated in Fig. 4. Most β-agonists have a relatively rapid onset of action with bronchodilatation lasting 4 to 6 h. They exhibit dose-dependent improvements in both FEV_1 and corridor walking distance. Unfortunately, there are similar dose-dependent increases in side effects, such as palpitations and tremor, although their extent varies with the patient [10]. Anticholinergic drugs are slightly slower in onset of action, but their effect lasts for between 6 and 9 h and when given three times daily can provide sustained bronchodilatation. They have a more bitter 'flavour' than β-agonists, but are relatively free from side effects. They appear to be more potent than β-agonists in COPD but fixed-dose combinations may offer the opportunity of maximizing bronchodilatation without increasing side effects, a factor that could improve compliance. As with other inhaled treatments, inhaler technique must be assessed and alternative formulations, eg dry powder or via a spacer, should be used when the patient cannot activate a metered dose inhaler correctly.

Data about longer acting β-agonists such as salmeterol are only just emerging. Initial studies confirm that salmeterol has a similar extended effect in COPD to that seen in asthma, and at least one abstract has suggested that it can produce worthwhile improvements in quality of life. Another novel drug, tiotropium, is a very

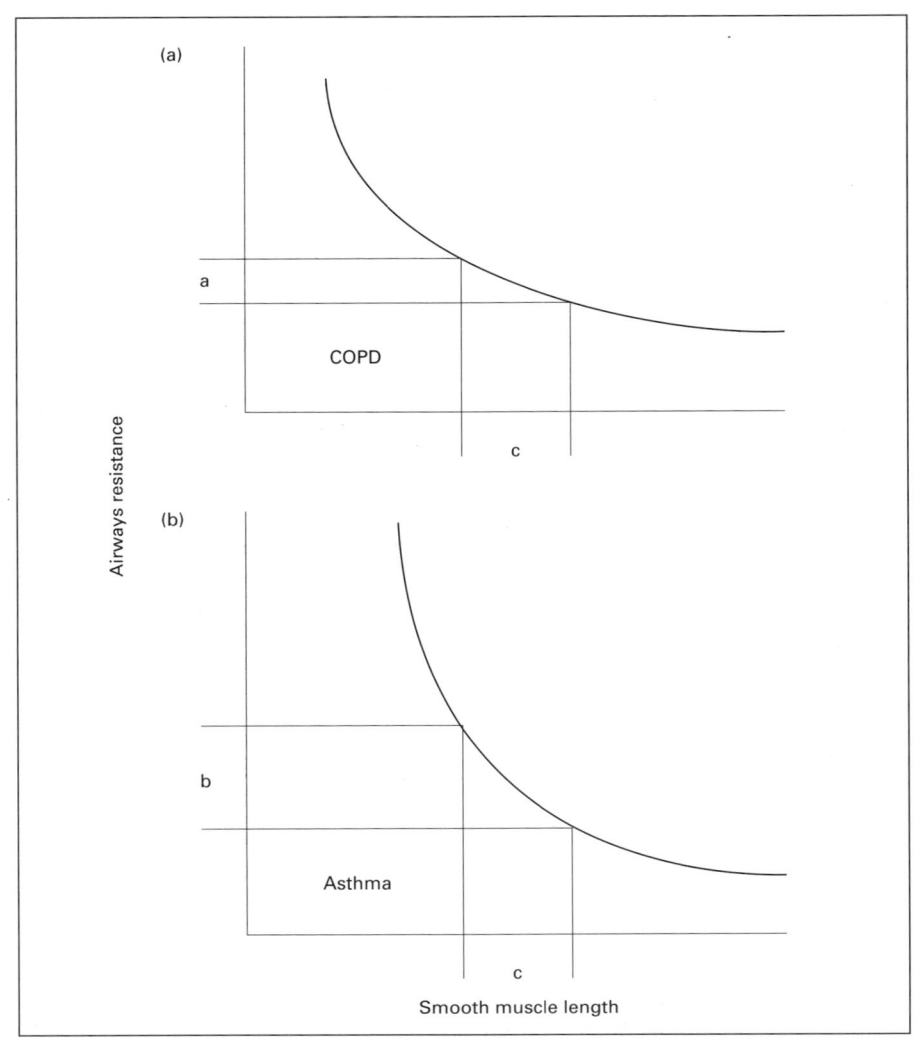

Fig. 3 Schematic relationships between airways smooth muscle length and airways resistance. This relationship is influenced both by the point on the hyperbola where a change in smooth muscle length occurs and the shape of this relationship. In (a) a typical relationship is shown for COPD. For a given change in smooth muscle length c, airways resistance changes by an amount a. (b) In asthma the same change in smooth muscle length produces a much greater change, b, in airways resistance. Drugs that change the shape of the relationship from the COPD curve (a) to the asthmatic (b) curve may include corticosteroids. Drugs such as anticholinergics shift the relationship to the right along any given curve without changing its shape. Thus, for the same amount of smooth muscle relaxation when on the steep part of the curve, a greater change in airways resistance occurs. This may explain why some people with COPD show only small changes in FEV_1 but larger changes in airways resistance and functional performance.

long-acting anticholinergic agent that has just entered clinical trials and may prove to be equivalent to or even more potent than salmeterol in the COPD patient.

Requests for nebulized bronchodilators seem to rise in inverse proportion to the

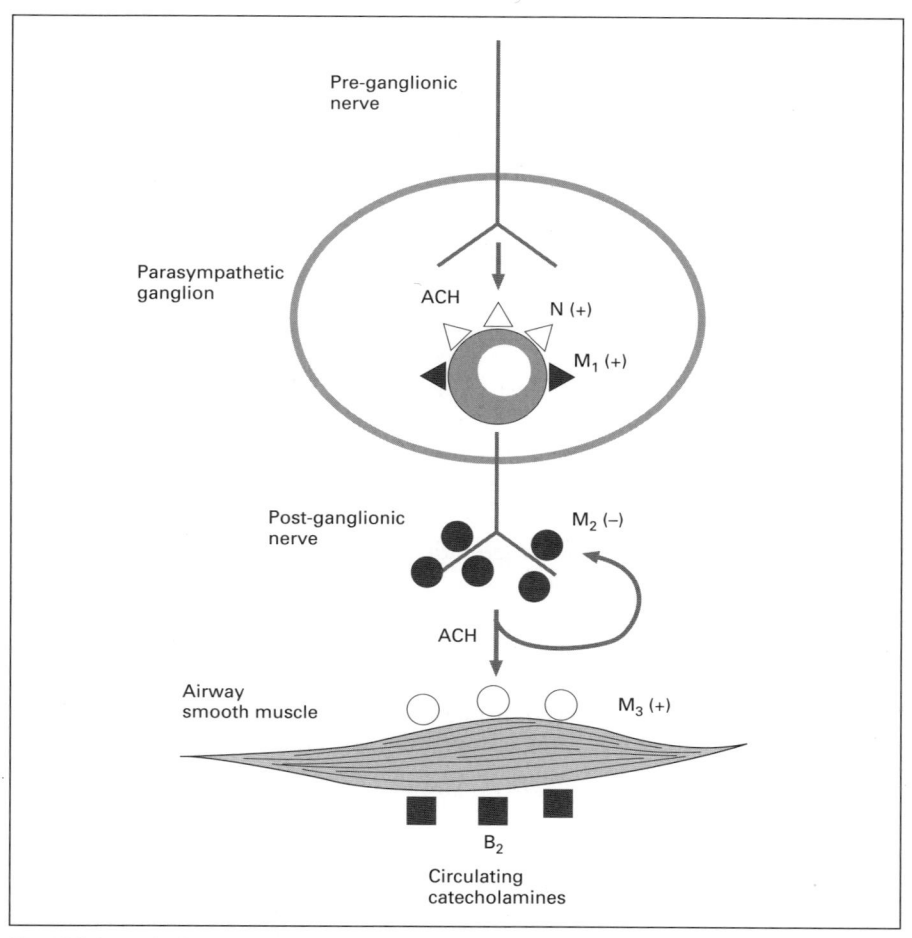

Fig. 4 Schematic diagram of the receptor subtypes relevant to airway smooth muscle contraction. The airways are innervated only by parasympathetic nerves; acetylcholine (ACH) release from the pre-ganglionic nerve stimulates nicotinic (N) receptors. This can be facilitated by stimulation of muscarinic M_1 receptors. Muscarinic M_2 receptors at the post-ganglionic nerve ending stimulate re-uptake of ACH and so limit persistent stimulation of muscarinic M_3 receptors that cause airway smooth muscle contraction. Ipratropium bromide blocks all three types of receptors. Airway smooth muscle relaxes when β-2 receptors are stimulated. This occurs in response to circulated catecholamines and provides functional antagonism to neurally mediated ACH release. Inhaled β-agonists such as salbutamol have the same effect. (From Barnes et al [9].)

degree of initial bronchodilator reversibility! Their use is contentious but the soon to be published British Thoracic Society guidelines [3] provide an empirical approach to their prescription. They advise that prescription should be confined to patients showing a significant increase in mean peak expiratory flow (PEF) from baseline when recorded over at least one week. Local availability of nebulized solutions depends on purchaser choice, but the major costs are in the drugs nebulized, not the equipment.

All oral bronchodilators are slow-acting and have more side effects whether β-agonists or theophyllines are considered. Theophylline is still widely used in COPD, but its benefits are more likely to be due to bronchodilatation than any proposed anti-inflammatory effect. Some subjects do show improved walking distances and quality of life as well as reduced lung volumes when treated with relatively high doses of theophyllines. However, many do not, and the risk of inducing ventricular tachyrhythmias or convulsions due to toxicity makes theophyllines a cheap but hazardous alternative to inhaled treatment. For this reason, many people confine them to third-line therapy.

Recent investigations have found evidence of eosinophils and lymphocytes in both bronchial biopsies and broncho-alveolar lavage from stable COPD patients [11]. These data provide scientific justification for the frequent empirical practice of prescribing inhaled corticosteroids, but clinical data to support this approach are still sketchy. In a mixed group of patients with mild COPD and asthma, Dutch workers have shown significant reductions in bronchial reactivity and an increase in FEV_1 over a year's follow-up compared to placebo, a change more likely to occur in atopic patients. Our own data suggest that patients responding to oral corticosteroids have a better survival over 5 years than those who respond to bronchodilators but not oral prednisolone. Whether these findings can be extrapolated to all patients is now under study in four large multicentres, due to report towards the end of this decade. Until clear evidence is available, our practice is to restrict prescription of inhaled corticosteroids (usually beclomethasone 500 mg twice daily) to patients exhibiting positive spirometric response after oral corticosteroid assessment.

When should non-drug therapy be considered?

Patients with mild to moderate COPD can usually be managed by stopping smoking and by bronchodilator treatment with or without inhaled corticosteroids. There is probably a role for pulmonary rehabilitation programmes for patients whose FEV_1 lies between 50% and 30% of predicted values, although whether they have value in the extremely disabled patient, ie FEV_1 less than 30% of predicted value, is contentious. Pulmonary rehabilitation programmes are still rudimentary in the UK, but are recognized to be of substantial value elsewhere. The randomized control trials of Goldstein et al. on hospital-based treatment [12] and Wijkstra et al. on rehabilitation in the home [13] confirm this benefit. The key components of the rehabilitation programme are listed in Table 3. Changes in exercise capacity relate to improvements in respiratory muscle function in these studies, but are not so closely related to changes in reported quality of life. This may have relevance when assessing the value of nebulizer treatment in the home. Even when formal rehabilitation programmes are not available, there is a need to assess the severe patient for treatment with domiciliary oxygen. It is 15 years since the North American and British MRC trials confirmed that oxygen treatment for 15 h a day or more had a significant survival benefit compared to no treatment in COPD patients with chronic hypoxaemia and a history of cor pulmonale (Fig. 5). International guidelines about

Table 3 Components of a hospital/outpatient based pulmonary rehabilitation programme. The exact details will depend on resources available and type of patients recruited.

Assessment	Physiological, eg FEV$_1$, maximum inspiratory pressures
	Functional, eg symptoms, walking distance
	Psychosocial, eg quality of life
Education	Goals of the programme
	Disease related, ie what is COPD
	How/when to seek help
	Smoking cessation
Action	Drug treatment (including compliance/technique)
	Physical therapy/exercise training/respiratory muscle training
	Oxygen therapy (home, portable)
	Nutrition, dietary changes
Follow-up	

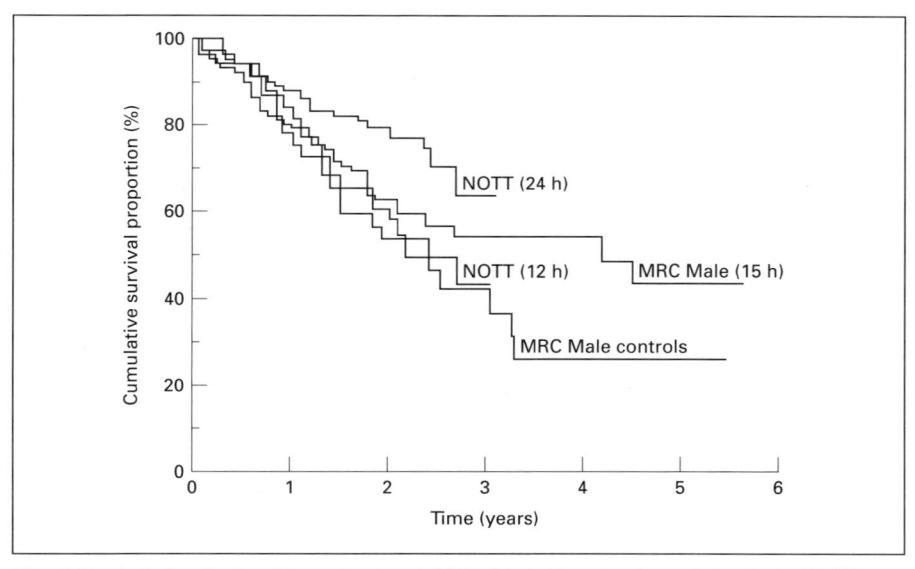

Fig. 5 Survival of patients with previously established hypoxic cor pulmonale treated with different durations of home oxygen therapy, including a group who did not receive this treatment. Combined results from British MRC and Canadian NOTT (Nocturnal Oxygen Therapy Trial Group) studies. These data provide the scientific basis for continuous oxygen treatment by oxygen concentrator.

oxygen prescription differ in specifics, but all have agreed that a sustained Pa,O_2 of less than 7.3 kPa when clinically stable is an indication for domiciliary oxygen. The role of portable oxygen, which increases exercise tolerance in most patients without necessarily changing the quality of life, is much less settled. The commonest reason for prescribing oxygen in the UK is as an intermittent treatment for breathlessness, an indication that is much less well established in terms of either short-term or long-term benefits.

Can surgery help?

Surgery for emphysematous bullae which exhibit compression of the adjacent lung on plain X-ray and CT and which are not contributing to gas-exchange function on a ventilation perfusion scan, can produce sustained improvements in exercise tolerance and even resting spirometry. Sadly, such patients are relatively infrequent, but the recent development of lung volume reduction surgery or pneumectomy by Cooper and coworkers has given hope that similar benefits will be possible in many moderate to severe COPD patients with emphysema [14]. The key features in patients selected are the presence of increased functional residual capacity and CT evidence of diffuse bullous disease in the absence of hypercapnia or bronchiectasis. Long-term follow-up data on the patients treated with this newly developed procedure are eagerly awaited. Lung transplantation, preferably a single-lung procedure, is still restricted to the most disabled patients with a life expectancy of 3 years or less. It produces substantial symptomatic benefit, but progress in this field is still limited by the onset of obliterative bronchiolitis in the transplanted lung, probably reflecting a chronic rejection process.

New treatment of acute exacerbations

A detailed review of the treatment of acute exacerbations of COPD is beyond this article, but the general steps in patient management are listed in Table 4. Controlled oxygen, preferably via Venturi mask, should be monitored by regular blood gas measurements in these patients. Patients need supervision to ensure that they continue to keep their mask on, a simple point that is often forgotten. A combination of β-agonists and anticholinergic nebulizer treatment is usually given, although both drugs may not be needed throughout the exacerbation. Antibiotics are restricted to those patients with purulent sputum, fever or evidence of pneumonia, while the role of oral corticosteroids is still poorly defined. Good prospective data

Table 4 Management of an exacerbation of COPD in hospital.

Assessment	Clinical: eg evidence of infection, accessory muscle use Blood gases: on air, oxygen; state Fi,O_2 Chest X-ray: look for pneumonia, pneumothorax, pulmonary oedema, etc Sputum/blood culture Haematology/biochemistry
Treatment	Controlled O_2 via mask/cannulae Antibiotics to cover *H. influenzae*, *Strep. pneumoniae* Nebulized β-agonists with anticholinergic +/– i.v. theophylline Corticosteroids role unclear
Respiratory failure	$Pa,O_2 < 7.3$ kPa and $Pa,CO_2 > 6.0$ kPa Low pH (<7.26) more important than high Pa,CO_2 Add respiratory stimulant, eg doxapram, or commence nasal intermittent positive pressure ventilation (IPPV) Consider IPPV in ITU – ethics important, so senior physician to decide

about the use of a ventilatory stimulant, doxapram, are still not available and this approach may fall into disuse with the more widespread application of nasal intermittent positive pressure ventilation (IPPV). The report by Brochard and colleagues [15] has shown that mortality and hospital stay can be reduced among patients treated in this way. The decision to institute IPPV in the intensive therapy unit (ITU) still needs input from senior medical staff, taking into consideration the potential reversible factors available and whether or not the patient has had an appropriate prior assessment. The wishes of both patient and family are important. The unusually pessimistic view taken by many UK intensivists about the prognosis and potential difficulties in weaning COPD is still far too prevalent and does not accord with the data.

☐ CONCLUSIONS

Managing COPD throws up many practical difficulties for which solutions are available. Many of these treatments must remain provisional and subject to review as new data come along. Nonetheless, worthwhile improvement in the COPD patient can be produced and neither patient nor doctor should be too pessimistic about the long-term outcome of this common illness.

REFERENCES

1. Siafakas NM, Vermeire P, Pride NB, Paoletti P, *et al.* European Respiratory Society: consensus statement. Optimal assessment and management of chronic obstructive pulmonary disease (COPD). *Eur Respir J* 1995; **8**: 1398–420.
2. American Thoracic Society. Standard for the diagnosis and care of patients with chronic obstructive pulmonary disease. *Am J Respir Crit Care Med* 1995; **152**: S77–S120.
3. British Thoracic Society. Guidelines for the management of chronic obstructive pulmonary disease. *Thorax* 1997; **52**(Suppl).
4. Nisar M, Walshaw MJ, Earis JE, Pearson MG, Calverley PMA. Assessment of reversibility of airway obstruction in patients with chronic obstructive airways disease. *Thorax* 1990; **45**: 190–4.
5. Anthonisen NR, Wright EC, IPPB Trial Group. Bronchodilator response in chronic obstructive pulmonary disease. *Am Rev Respir Dis* 1986; **133**: 814–9.
6. Callahan CM, Dittus RS, Katz BP. Oral corticosteroid therapy for patients with stable chronic obstructive pulmonary disease. *Ann Intern Med* 1991; **114**: 216–23.
7. Foulds J, Jarvis MJ. Smoking cessation and prevention. In: Calverley PMA, Pride NB, eds. *Chronic Obstructive Pulmonary Disease*. London: Chapman and Hall, 1995: 373–90.
8. Anthonisen NR, Connett JE, Kiley JP, *et al.* Effects of smoking intervention and the use of an inhaled anti-cholinergic bronchodilator in the rate of decline of FEV_1. The Lung Health Study. *J Am Med Assoc* 1994; **272**: 1497–505.
9. Barnes PJ. Bronchodilators: basic pharmacology. In: Calverley PMA, Pride NB, eds. *Chronic Obstructive Pulmonary Disease*. London: Chapman and Hall, 1995: 391–417.
10. Calverley PMA. Symptomatic bronchodilator treatment. In: Calverley PMA, Pride NB, eds. *Chronic Obstructive Pulmonary Disease*. London: Chapman and Hall, 1995: 419–45.
11. Ollerenshaw SL, Woolcock AJ. Characteristics of the inflammation in biopsies from large airways of subjects with asthma and subjects with chronic airflow limitation. *Am Rev Respir Dis* 1992; **145**: 922–7.
12. Goldstein RS, Gort EH, Stubbing D, Avendano MA, Guyatt GH. Randomised controlled trial of respiratory rehabilitation. *Lancet* 1994; **344**: 1394–7.

13 Wijkstra PJ, van Altena R, Kraan J, et al. Quality of life in patients with chronic obstructive pulmonary disease improves after rehabilitation at home. *Eur Respir J* 1994; 7: 269–73.
14 Cooper JD, Trulock EP, Triantafillou AN, Patterson GA, Pohl MS, et al. Bilateral pneumectomy (volume reduction) for chronic obstructive pulmonary disease. *J Thorac Cardiovasc Surg* 1995; 109: 106–19.
15 Brochard L, Mancebo J, Wysocki M, Lofaso F, Conti G, et al. Non-invasive ventilation for acute exacerbations of chronic obstructive pulmonary disease. *New Engl J Med* 1995; 333: 817–22.

☐ MULTIPLE CHOICE QUESTIONS

1   Bronchodilator reversibility in COPD:
    (a) Is an infrequent finding
    (b) Is present when the FEV_1 increases by 15% and 200 ml
    (c) Varies from day to day
    (d) Is best assessed by using a peak-flow meter
    (e) Suggests chronic asthma when the FEV_1 increases by more than 500 ml

2   Anticholinergic bronchodilator drugs:
    (a) Can be safely combined with β-agonists
    (b) Are generally less effective than β-agonists in treating stable COPD
    (c) Are associated with tachycardia and prostatic symptoms
    (d) Are effective for 6–8 h post-inhalation
    (e) Block muscarinic receptors at the motor end-plate

3   Pulmonary rehabilitation:
    (a) Has not yet been shown to be effective in placebo-controlled trials
    (b) Usually involves a quality-of-life assessment
    (c) Should include an assessment of inhaler technique
    (d) Is relatively expensive to provide
    (e) Involves whole-body exercise training supervised by a physiotherapist

4   Oral corticosteroids:
    (a) Are indicated in patients showing a significant increase in FEV_1 after 2 weeks of treatment
    (b) Produce sustained bronchodilatation in 10–20% of COPD patients
    (c) Produce significant increases in FEV_1 during exacerbations only in patients with audible wheeze
    (d) Can improve patient mood without changing lung function
    (e) Should be given in high doses for 2 weeks to test for an objective improvement in lung function

5   Domiciliary oxygen:
    (a) Is one of the two treatments that can prolong life in COPD
    (b) Should be given when the Pa,O_2 is less than 7.3 kPa at discharge from hospital
    (c) When given during exercise increases walking distance

(d) When given regularly during exercise, can improve quality of life
(e) Should be prescribed for 15 hours or more a day when the blood gas criteria are met.

ANSWERS

1a False	2a True	3a False	4a False	5a True
b True	b False	b True	b True	b False
c True	c False	c True	c False	c True
d False	d True	d False	d True	d False
e True	e True	e True	e True	e True

Tuberculosis

J Moore-Gillon

☐ INTRODUCTION

One of the health issues prominent in the broadcast and written media of the mid- to late-1990s has been the resurgence of tuberculosis (TB). Although many of the newspaper articles and television documentaries have undoubtedly been excessively alarmist, things do have to be taken seriously when even the *Lancet* can carry a leading article entitled 'Is Africa lost?' and the World Health Organization designates TB as 'a global health emergency'. Predictions in the 1960s that TB would be eradicated in developed countries by 1990, and worldwide by the turn of the century, have proved disastrously wrong. This chapter examines the reasons for the increase in TB, outlines recent advances in diagnosis and management, describes some of the pitfalls for practising clinicians, and sums up the prospects for the future.

☐ CURRENT SITUATION

It is estimated that about 1.7 billion individuals – a third of the earth's population – are infected with TB. The majority of these are individuals in whom the primary infection has been overcome by immune defences. Viable bacteria may, however, remain dormant for years or even decades in old, apparently healed, tuberculous lesions, and may thus reactivate to produce progressive post-primary disease if at any time the host defences become weakened. Disease in such individuals, along with those who develop progressive disease straight after their primary infection, accounts for the 6 to 8 million new cases of active TB each year, the 20 million or so currently ill with tuberculosis, and the 3 to 4 million deaths annually.

After decades of decline, the incidence of TB has increased in most countries over the past few years. In Europe, the absolute increases have been modest and the upward trend may be levelling off. Even these increases acquire much greater significance, however, when it is realized that they have occurred against a background of an expected continuing decrease; there is thus a substantial excess of cases of TB over those that should have occurred had the preceding downward trend been maintained.

☐ INCREASE IN TUBERCULOSIS

Factors other than AIDS (acquired immune deficiency syndrome)

In developed countries, tuberculosis rates began declining a hundred years before the introduction in the 1950s of effective drug treatment. This decline can be attributed to modest improvements in housing, public health, nutrition and measures to limit the spread of disease from infected individuals. Experience in the UK mirrors that in other European countries, with the steady decline in tuberculosis being halted and reversed on three occasions: after World Wars 1 and 2, and now. A feature common to the first two was that previously relatively settled communities experienced increased nutritional deprivation and poorer housing conditions, and delivery of health care was either disrupted or devoted to alternative challenges. In many countries, there was mass movement of displaced populations. An individual who is poorly nourished and perhaps co-infected with parasites and other diseases is less likely to mount a satisfactory immune response to the TB bacillus. Newly infected individuals may therefore not progress satisfactorily to healed, quiescent TB but will instead develop active, progressive disease; furthermore, quiescent lesions in individuals infected at some time in the past may reactivate. This active, infectious disease is more likely to be transmitted to others in crowded rooms, tents or refugee camps than in less deprived conditions, and those exposed to the infection will have similar problems in mounting an adequate host response.

Many of the features common to the earlier periods of increase in TB are present again today. In the former Soviet Union, a decline in living standards for many and a breakdown in the health services previously present probably account for much of the current rapid increase in TB. Political instability and its consequences lead to increases in TB in villages and camps, whether these are in former Yugoslavia, Kurdistan, or sub-Saharan Africa [1]. The movement of large numbers of people, as refugees or other migrants, from areas of high TB incidence to relatively low-incidence countries has been suggested to account for the rise in TB in the latter. While it is certainly a contributory factor, it is unlikely to be the whole answer. In the UK, the rise is most marked in areas of social deprivation and it is suggested that this is attributable to an increase in TB in the long-established population as well as to recent arrivals from high-incidence countries [2].

Impact of AIDS

A crucial difference between earlier periods of increased TB incidence and the present one is the impact of acquired immunodeficiency due to infection with HIV (human immunodeficiency virus) [3,4]. The World Health Organization estimates that not only will the total number of TB deaths increase each year but that an increasing proportion of these deaths will be in individuals with TB/HIV co-infection (Table 1). In HIV-positive individuals, tuberculosis at any site (including pulmonary) is now accepted as an AIDS-defining diagnosis.

In any population, the scale of the problem due to TB and AIDS co-infection will

Table 1 World Health Organization estimates of deaths from tuberculosis.

Year	Total TB deaths	HIV attributable (%)
1990	2.5 million	4.5
1995	3.0 million	8.9
2000	3.5 million	14.2

depend on how common TB is, how common HIV infection is and, of course, the degree to which these subgroups of the population overlap. AIDS is thus a major factor in the increase in tuberculosis in many parts of sub-Saharan Africa and, to a growing extent, in south east Asia. In the USA, the impact on *national* tuberculosis rates is far smaller, but it is very marked in some more localized areas such as New York city, where the relatively high incidence of HIV infection co-exists with the relatively high rates of TB expected in a socio-economically deprived inner city population with a substantial proportion of recent migrants. In Europe, including the UK, the impact of HIV infection on overall TB rates is very limited, although for that small segment of the population that *is* HIV-positive TB is a common and significant hazard.

HIV infection predisposes to the reactivation of disease in an individual previously infected with TB. Similarly, an HIV-positive individual newly infected with TB is more likely to progress to clinically evident active disease than a fully immunocompetent individual. Reactivation of old disease has been thought to be overwhelmingly the more important of these two, but recent molecular epidemiology studies (see below) are making it apparent that newly acquired infection is probably much more common than previously realized.

The special problems of treating TB in HIV-positive patients are summarized in Table 2. It should be noted that HIV infection is not of itself a risk factor for multi-drug resistant tuberculosis, but that some circumstances predispose to both problems. In African countries where HIV infection is very common, for instance, most people with TB may not have access to a full course of multiple drug TB therapy and suboptimal treatment encourages the development of drug resistance. Similarly, intravenous drug abusers, at high risk of HIV infection, may be less likely than non-drug abusers to comply with a long and complex chemotherapy regime.

Finally, it should be remembered that the HIV/TB interaction may not be all one-way traffic; there is increasing evidence that infection of HIV-positive individuals with tuberculosis may influence the rate of progression of the underlying disorder.

☐ MOLECULAR BIOLOGY

Molecular biology is often regarded as immensely exciting by the scientists concerned, but dull and irrelevant by practising clinicians. When advances in basic

Table 2 Problems encountered in managing TB/HIV co-infection.

Atypical clinical presentation
Widely disseminated disease
Difficulty in interpreting tuberculin test
Confusion with other mycobacterial infections
Increased rate of drug-resistant organisms
Increased rate of adverse drug reaction
Problems with drug absorption
Increased relapse rate with non-rifampicin regimes

science do occur, their effect on clinical practice, if any, may be delayed by many years. Nothing could be further from the situation in tuberculosis, where an increasing understanding of the tubercle bacillus is already having a major impact, even on aspects of the disease as apparently far removed from the laboratory bench as epidemiology.

Microbe virulence and host immune response

The molecular mechanisms determining virulence are becoming clearer, along with the ways in which the host's immune response is programmed to respond to the presence of mycobacteria [5,6]. If the predominant route of T-cell maturation is the TH1 pathway, cells carrying bacilli are recognized and lysed. This is a predominantly protective mechanism. If TH2 maturation is dominant, however, there is widespread necrosis of tissues containing mycobacteria. It has been suggested that modulation of this potentially harmful immune response by another related bacterium *Mycobacterium vaccae* could be beneficial in patients critically ill with tuberculosis, or in whom multi-drug resistance makes treatment particularly difficult; the results of clinical trials are awaited. Unravelling the details of the immune response may, moreover, clarify the role of BCG (bacille Calmette-Guérin) vaccination and offer prospects for the development of more effective vaccines [7].

Diagnosing tuberculosis

Confirmation of the diagnosis of TB can be one of the major problems in managing the disease. When bacteria are copious, as they may be in cavitating pulmonary disease, direct microscopy of sputum leads to their rapid detection and a *presumptive* diagnosis. When they are scant in number, often in pulmonary disease, and frequently in pleural effusions, cerebrospinal fluid and lymph nodes, culture may take weeks and, indeed, may never be positive. The polymerase chain reaction (PCR) is now widely used in medicine to detect tiny quantities of nucleic acid, and in tuberculosis the technique can be applied to clinical specimens to detect mycobacterial DNA or RNA. The drawback of PCR is that it may even be too sensitive, detecting mycobacterial material from an old, clinically 'healed' case, when no active disease is present. Further work is under way to overcome these problems [8,9].

Molecular fingerprinting

Within any one species of microorganism, differing strains may be recognized by differences in their DNA. Strain differences are due in large part to the mobility of certain elements of the DNA: between one bacterium and another, within a bacterium from one DNA site to another (transposition), and by inversion of a sequence of DNA. In the TB bacillus, the second of these mechanisms leads to the movement and reduplication of 'insertion sequences' within the DNA. The bacterial phenotype is unaffected, since such sequences code only for their own transposition. Many such insertion sequences (IS) have been identified, that designated IS 6110 being the best studied.

Mycobacterial DNA from a cultured specimen can be treated with enzymes that cleave the molecule at certain chemical points to produce so-called restriction fragments. Restriction fragment length polymorphism (RFLP) can be identified by Southern blot analysis using probes for DNA sequences such as IS 6110. Most strains of tuberculosis contain eight or more copies of IS 6110, and the number of copies and their position within the DNA molecule can be used to 'fingerprint' the strain. Further differentiation between strains, particularly where there are only a small number of copies of IS 6110, can be undertaken using gene probes for other insertion sequences. The clinical impact of such information is already immensely important. Suspected nosocomial spread of infection within a hospital or institution can be confirmed or refuted. Apparently unrelated cases may be linked to a common source of infection. Many cases of TB which would in the past have been attributed to reactivation of old disease can now be shown to be exogenous reinfection [10].

Identifying drug resistance

The problem with conventional fingerprinting is that it requires large quantities of DNA, obtained from cultured specimens and thus inevitably imposing delay. As already noted, PCR can be used to multiply up minute quantities of mycobacterial DNA or RNA so that it can be detected. A combination of PCR with RFLP and related identification techniques would be a dramatic step forward, and one that is being tentatively taken even now with the development of new techniques. This is of special importance because of current progress being made in elucidating the molecular mechanisms of drug resistance, which are now well understood for several antituberculous drugs [11]. Rifampicin, for instance, binds to the DNA-dependent RNA polymerase, and prevents the transcription of mycobacterial DNA. A single-step mutation in a gene (known as rpoB) encoding part of this RNA polymerase confers a high degree of rifampicin resistance. Techniques for rapid detection of the presence of this mutation, and those associated with resistance to other drugs, are moving from the research laboratory to the clinical application.

The way forward

After 40 years, during which a clinician caring for a patient with TB would notice little change in the speed or nature of the information emerging from the laboratory, things are changing. Molecular biology can influence clinical practice now, and even more in the *very* near future. Soon we could and should be able to send a clinical specimen to the laboratory and within hours a report should return confirming the presence and precise identity of a mycobacterial species, the 'family history' of the infecting organism and its relationship to other isolates, and, crucially, its drug sensitivity. This future does depend, though, on whether we are willing or indeed able to pay for it.

☐ CLINICAL PROBLEMS IN DIAGNOSIS AND MANAGEMENT

Part of the fascination and challenge of tuberculosis for the clinician is its protean manifestations; sadly, it is exactly that attribute which is the setting for unnecessary suffering and even death.

Making the diagnosis

In developed countries, failure to suspect the diagnosis until too late (or even not at all) is probably the most common cause of mortality from TB in immunocompetent individuals, a situation all the more likely when the perceptions of public and health care professionals are of TB as a disease of the past. In the UK, such mistakes are a particular risk in areas of the country where relatively little TB is seen, and also when junior medical staff who trained in low-incidence areas move to high-incidence districts.

Most microbiology laboratories will *only* look for tuberculosis if specifically

Table 3 Clinical problems in the diagnosis of tuberculosis.

Cryptic disseminated (miliary) tuberculosis
Unexplained weight loss or fever. Patient often assumed to have malignant disease

Bone and joint tuberculosis
Lytic bony lesions and pain assumed to be malignant
Joint disease assumed to be pyogenic infection or inflammatory
Back pain mistakenly thought to be degenerative
Osteomyelitis misdiagnosed as staphylococcal
Cutaneous ulcers or sinuses with underlying TB of bone or joint

Respiratory tuberculosis
Unexplained respiratory failure (miliary disease with normal X-ray)
Clinical and radiological confusion with lung cancer
Acute presentation mistaken for lobar pneumonia
Unexplained pleural effusion
Failure to diagnose in pregnancy if X-ray not performed

Central nervous tuberculosis
Symptoms of TB meningitis attributed to 'tension headache' or depression
Tuberculoma mistaken for neoplastic space-occupying lesion

Abdominal tuberculosis
Unexplained abdominal pain or ascites
Abnormal liver biochemistry or hepatic granulomata on biopsy
Intestinal obstruction
Misdiagnosis as Crohn's disease

Renal tract tuberculosis
Unexplained 'sterile pyuria'
Tuberculous interstitial nephritis causing renal failure
Obstruction due to ureteric or bladder TB

Lymph node tuberculosis
Mistaken for lymphoma or metastatic carcinoma
May be hot and tender, simulating pyogenic infection

requested to do so. Routine requests for culture and sensitivity of sputum and other specimens will not lead to a diagnosis of TB. No laboratory, furthermore, can come to a diagnosis on a specimen it has never received; portions of excised lymph nodes, synovial biopsies, bone biopsies for apparent osteomyelitis etc should *always* be sent for TB culture as well as histology.

Table 3 and Figs 1–8 demonstrate just a few of the pitfalls in establishing a diagnosis of tuberculosis. A high index of suspicion for TB is plainly vital. Perhaps the most common potentially avoidable mistake is where an everyday symptom (such as low back pain) is not diagnosed as tuberculous because a history of systemic symptoms typical of TB (malaise, weight loss, fevers, night sweats) is either not elicited or is ignored. Note, however, that the absence of such symptoms is not a reliable indication that TB is not present. Consider TB when there is no clear diagnosis in a patient presenting with odd symptoms, signs or investigations, just as was the case with syphilis in the past. Medical students apparently used to be taught 'If it's bizarre, do a WR'. A 1990s equivalent is, perhaps, 'If it's puzzling me, I should think of TB'.

Treatment

The apparent simplicity of antituberculous chemotherapy ('Three drugs for two months, two drugs for four more') is misleading. Drug reactions are common, and problems with compliance very common indeed. The incidence of drug-resistant organisms is rising worldwide. Although cases of multi-drug resistance in the UK are at present measured in scores rather than hundreds or thousands, single-drug resistance rates are as high as 10% in some areas. Failure to respond to treatment is still, however, more usually due to non-compliance than drug resistance. Problems like continuing enlargement of lymph nodes and persistent fever, even when on apparently appropriate therapy, test the nerves of those unfamiliar with treating TB.

Whatever the organ affected, the treatment of TB should always be supervised by a clinician who deals with the disease regularly. In most hospitals this will be the respiratory medicine specialist, and in some an infectious diseases specialist. Where the organ or part affected is not the lung, 'shared care' is appropriate. Failure to adhere to these principles has been shown to increase morbidity, mortality and relapse rates.

☐ THE FUTURE

The rise in tuberculosis has in many developed countries stimulated renewed clinical and research interest and, crucially, the allocation of funds to tuberculosis control measures. In consequence, TB rates are levelling off and perhaps dropping even in countries with a moderately large AIDS problem, like the USA. Prospects for the developing world are far more gloomy.

Key needs for the immediate future are more rapid diagnosis of TB and determination of drug sensitivity. These are readily achievable given the will and the finance. The development of new, safe and highly effective drugs is eminently

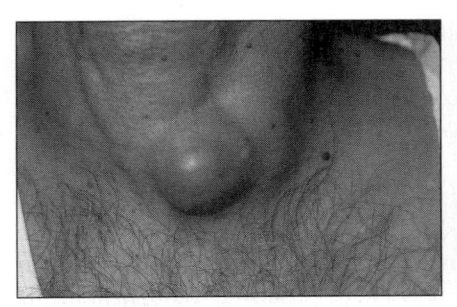

Fig. 1 Tuberculous nodes can be red, hot and exquisitely tender.

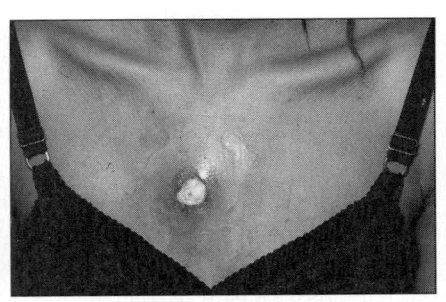

Fig. 2 This ulcer was enlarging for 6 months before underlying tuberculous osteomyelitis of the sternum was diagnosed.

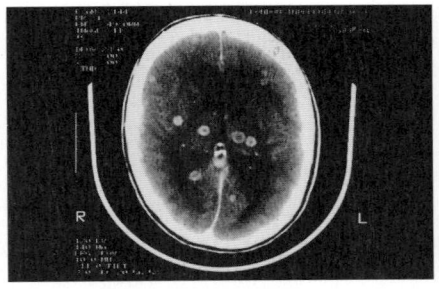

Fig. 3 Contrast-enhanced brain computerized tomography (CT) scan. The ring shadows are multiple tuberculomata. The patient's symptoms had been attributed to 'overwork'.

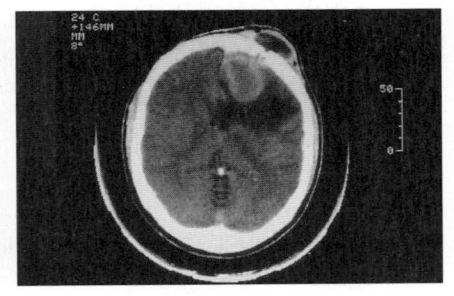

Fig. 4 Attempted excision of a 'sebaceous cyst of the forehead' was abandoned due to its extent. The CT scan shows a tuberculous lesion affecting the frontal lobe of the brain.

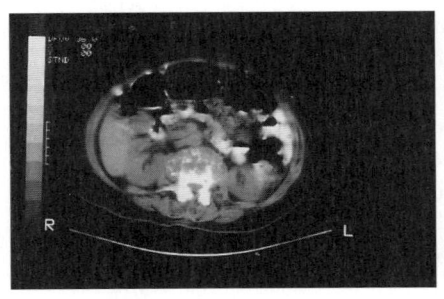

Fig. 5 CT scan of lumbar spine showing gross vertebral destruction by TB. The patient presented with paraplegia after a year's back pain.

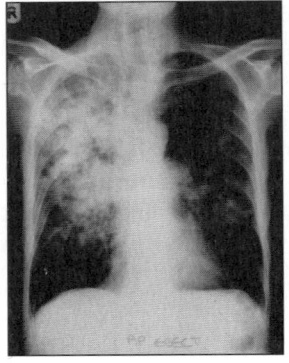

Fig. 6 The patient's symptoms of TB (haemoptysis, pain, weight loss) were identical to those of a relative with lung cancer. He delayed seeking medical advice, and died 12 hours after eventual admission to hospital.

possible, but they will probably be unaffordable by the countries that need them most. Prerequisites for the eventual eradication of TB would seem to be global political stability and a cure for AIDS; these may take a little time to achieve, but

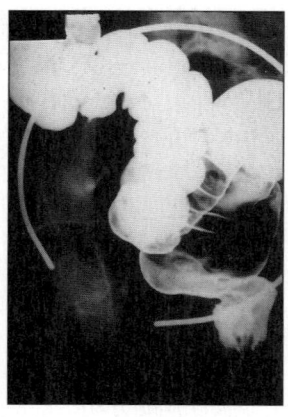

Fig. 7 Barium enema showing tuberculous ulcers in the colon in a patient thought to have inflammatory bowel disease.

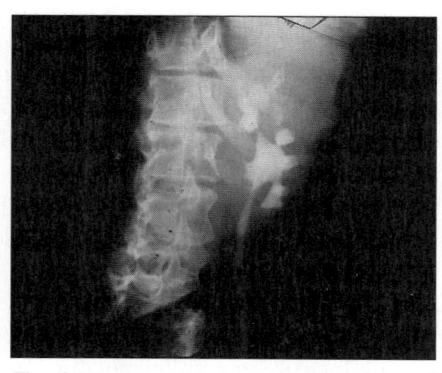

Fig. 8 Intravenous urogram showing distorted calyces in active renal tuberculosis confirmed on culture. No urinary symptoms, but patient systemically unwell.

hope springs eternal. In the meantime, it should be achievable to ensure that when confronted with a clinical problem we ask ourselves 'Could this possibly be tuberculosis?'.

REFERENCES

1. Trkanjec Z, Puljic I, Tekavec J. Tuberculosis in refugees. *Lancet* 1994; **343**: 1640.
2. Bhatti N, Law MR, Morris JK, Halliday R, Moore-Gillon J. Increasing incidence of tuberculosis in England and Wales: a study of the likely causes. *Brit Med J* 1995; **310**: 967–9.
3. Drobniewski FA, Pozniak AL, Uttley AH. Tuberculosis and AIDS. *J Med Microbiol* 1995; **43**: 85–91.
4. Shafer RW, Edlin BR. Tuberculosis in patients infected with human immunodeficiency virus: perspective on the last decade. *Clin Infect Dis* 1996; **22**: 683–704.
5. Costello AM, Rook G. Tuberculosis in children. *Curr Opin Pediatr* 1995; **7**: 6–12.
6. Grange JM, Stanford JL, Rook GA. Tuberculosis and cancer: parallels in host responses and therapeutic approaches? *Lancet* 1995; **345**: 1350–2.
7. Roche PW, Triccas JA, Winter N. BCG vaccination against tuberculosis: past disappointments and future hopes. *Trends Microbiol* 1995; **3**: 397–401.
8. Marshall BG, Shaw RJ. New technology in the diagnosis of tuberculosis. *Brit J Hosp Med* 1996; **55**: 491–4.
9. Richeldi L, Barnini S, Saltini C. Molecular diagnosis of tuberculosis. *Eur Respir J* 1995; **20**: 689s–700s.
10. van Soolingen D, Hermans PW. Epidemiology of tuberculosis by DNA fingerprinting. *Eur Respir J* 1995; **20**: 649s–656s.
11. Heym B, Philipp W, Cole ST. Mechanisms of drug resistance in *Mycobacterium tuberculosis*. *Curr Top Microbiol Immunol* 1996; **215**: 49–69.

FURTHER READING

Davies PDO, ed. *Clinical Tuberculosis*. London: Chapman and Hall, 1994.

MULTIPLE CHOICE QUESTIONS

1. In HIV-positive individuals with TB:
   (a) Drug reactions are more common than in HIV-negative patients
   (b) The clinical presentation is usually typical of tuberculosis
   (c) Multiple drug resistance is more common
   (d) The tuberculin test may remain positive
   (e) Pulmonary TB is not an AIDS-defining diagnosis

2. In the UK:
   (a) Increased TB rates are largely due to increases in AIDS
   (b) Increases are uniformly distributed across the country
   (c) Increases can be wholly explained by patterns of immigration
   (d) The rate of drug-resistant TB is rising
   (e) Multiply resistant strains of TB are rare

3. In tuberculosis:
   (a) Demonstration of mycobacterial DNA by the polymerase chain reaction indicates active disease
   (b) Failure to respond to therapy is usually due to drug resistance
   (c) Lymph nodes may enlarge during therapy
   (d) Absence of systemic symptoms makes the diagnosis very unlikely
   (e) Respiratory failure may occur with a normal chest X-ray

4. Tubercle bacilli:
   (a) Are usually present in large numbers in tuberculous pleural effusions
   (b) Are often scanty and hard to identify in tuberculous lymph nodes
   (c) Acquire rifampicin resistance by plasmid transfer
   (d) Infect about 10% of the world's population
   (e) May be present in apparently healed tuberculous lesions

5. Factors associated with increased tuberculosis rates in a population include:
   (a) Poor nutrition
   (b) Overcrowding
   (c) High average income
   (d) Warm climate
   (e) High rates of intravenous drug abuse

ANSWERS

	1	2	3	4	5
a	True	False	False	False	True
b	False	False	False	True	True
c	True	False	True	False	False
d	True	True	False	False	False
e	False	True	True	True	True

Guidelines and the management of community acquired pneumonia

J T Macfarlane

☐ INTRODUCTION

All practising clinicians will be aware that pneumonia remains a common problem on medical wards. Pneumonia accounts for between 2.5% and 7% of all adult medical admissions, with a mortality of around 10%. The impact on hospital services is considerable as up to 10% of hospital admissions for pneumonia require intensive care management and 10% of medical admissions to an intensive care unit (ICU) are for community acquired pneumonia (CAP). What is seen in hospital is the tip of the iceberg, as community studies have demonstrated that 80% of CAP cases are managed at home by general practitioners [1].

Over the past 15 years there has been a considerable expansion in our knowledge of CAP, helped by numerous studies from around the world which have clarified the aetiology and outcome of CAP and allowed the development of guidelines for management. This review highlights some of these issues.

☐ AETIOLOGY OF COMMUNITY ACQUIRED PNEUMONIA

The results of worldwide studies of many thousands of adults hospitalized with CAP can be used to produce an overview of the spectrum of pathogens involved (Fig. 1). However, this overview conceals considerable variation within different studies [2] (Fig. 2). Numerous factors affect the reported frequency of pathogens in different pneumonia studies, including the population studied or excluded, geographical, epidemiological and seasonal factors, the clinical and laboratory methods used to identify pathogens, the completeness of investigations and specimen collection and the criteria used to define presence of specific infections. An example of the last factor is the definition used for pneumococcal infection. The frequency of reported pneumococcal infection is consistently higher in those studies that have included testing for pneumococcal capsular antigen (PCA) in respiratory secretions, serum, pleural fluid and urine (Fig. 3). Evidence supports the inclusion of PCA detection in the identification of pneumococcal infection.

The variable incidence of *Mycoplasma pneumoniae* infection in different studies is partially explained by the epidemic nature of community infection with peaks of activity occurring every 3 or 4 years. Studies performed during an epidemic period not surprisingly find it to be the second most common identified pathogen (after pneumococcal infection), but it is uncommon at other times (Fig. 4).

☐ MANAGEMENT OF COMMUNITY ACQUIRED PNEUMONIA

The correct management of CAP involves diagnosing the pneumonia, considering

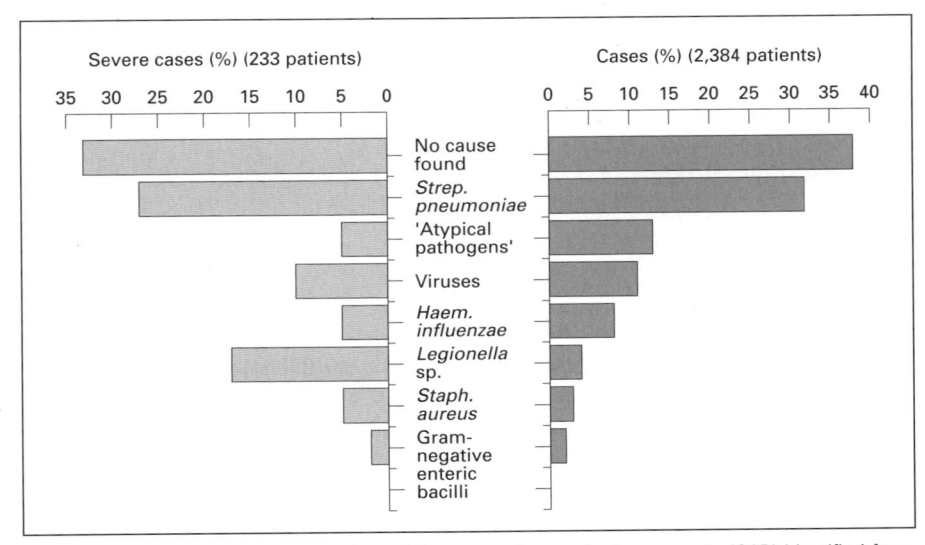

Fig. 1 Spectrum of pathogens causing adult community acquired pneumonia (CAP) identified from numerous studies throughout the world in the past 15 years. For comparison, the pathogens identified as a cause of severe CAP, requiring ICU admission, are shown from several European studies.

clues to likely aetiology and assessing severity. The initial management should be tailored to the severity, likely pathogens and underlying host factors. Investigations are used to help with all three of these steps (Fig. 5).

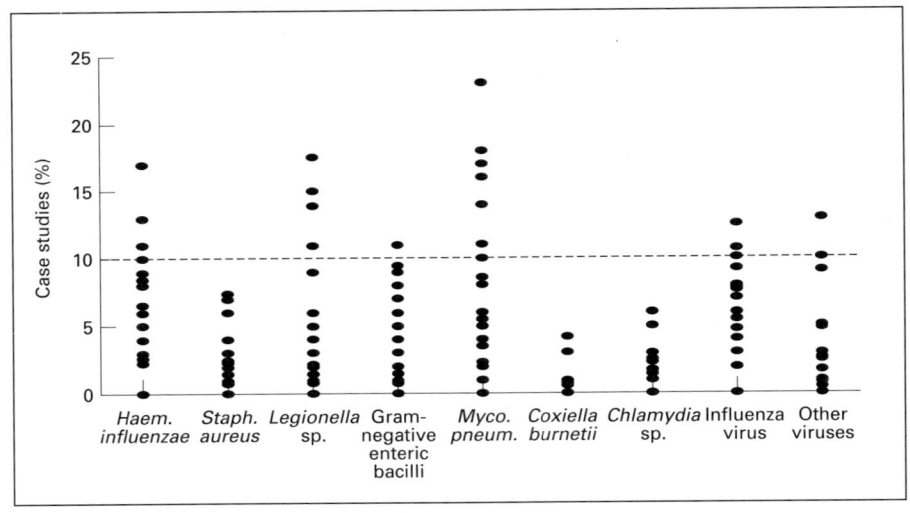

Fig. 2 The incidence of different pathogens causing adult CAP found in 26 studies worldwide demonstrating the wide variation in reported frequency from the different studies. (From Macfarlane [2].)

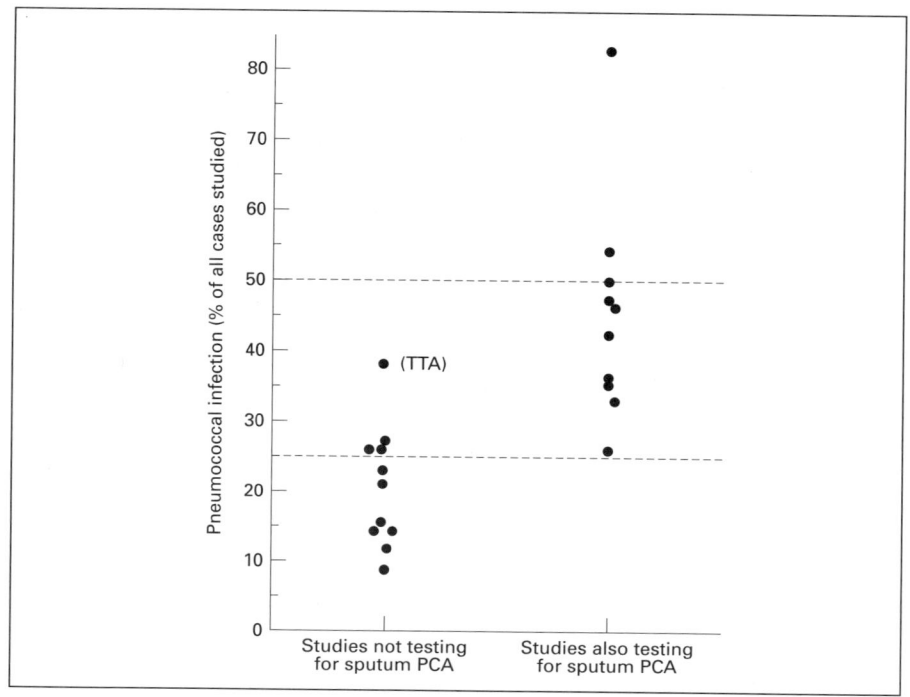

Fig. 3 Incidence of pneumococcal infection reported from 22 studies of adult CAP demonstrating that studies which have included the testing for pneumococcal capsular antigen (PCA) report a higher incidence of pneumococcal infection. (TTA, one study that used transtracheal aspiration for obtaining lower respiratory secretions.) (From Macfarlane [2].)

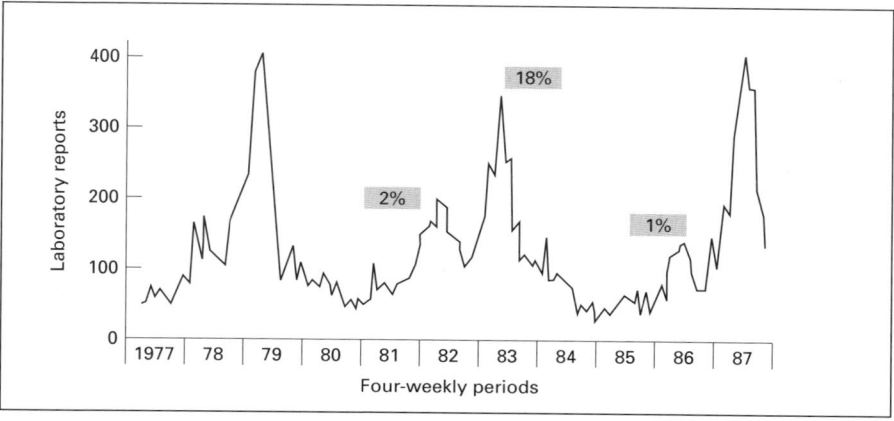

Fig. 4 The relationship between incidence of *Mycoplasma pneumoniae* (% figures shown in bars) reported from three clinical studies of adult CAP in the UK and the laboratory reports to the Communicable Disease Surveillance Centre (CDSC), London, for England and Wales between 1977 and 1987. Mycoplasma infection was identified frequently during epidemic periods but was an uncommon cause of CAP during non-epidemic periods.

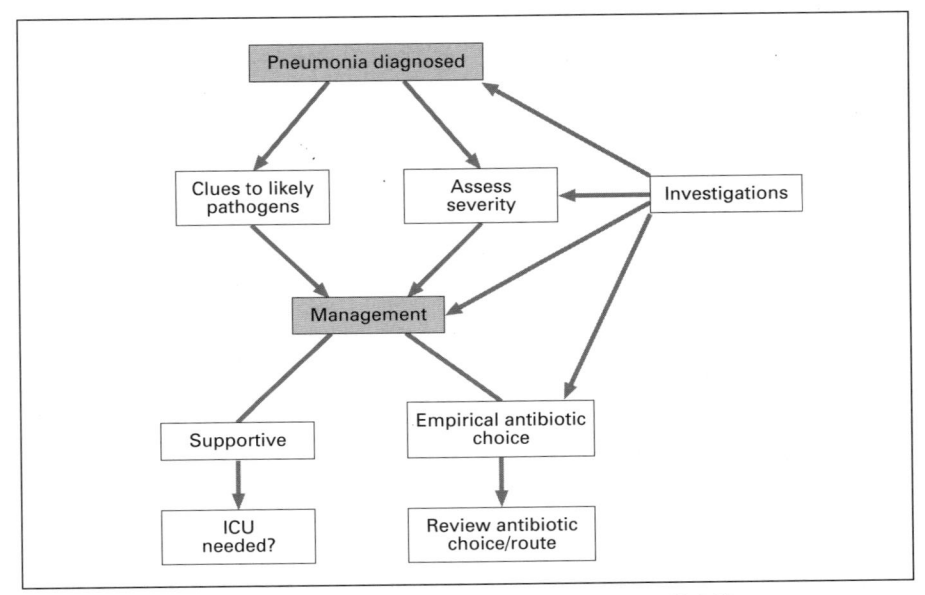

Fig. 5 Steps to consider when planning the management of a patient with CAP.

Clues to likely pathogens

The cause of pneumonia cannot be reliably predicted from the clinical, laboratory and radiographic features when the patient is first assessed. There are numerous clues that the clinician can use when considering the aetiology of the infection and planning initial, empirical antibiotic management (Fig. 6). Generally bacterial infections, such as pneumococcal, staphylococcal and legionella infections, will be associated with a short history, features of multisystem involvement or septicaemia and a raised white cell count with a neutrophilia, less so for legionella infection. Mycoplasma infection more commonly affects younger adults with a longer clinical history, lack of response to β-lactam antibiotics, less multisystem involvement and little effect on the white cell count.

The recognition that the clinician usually has to decide on initial management empirically without laboratory support has resulted in the development of guidelines.

Guidelines for the management of CAP

Guidelines have been published from Britain [3], USA [4], Canada [5], France [6], Spain [7] and Italy [8] following either a Consensus Conference or a Working Party of the National Thoracic Specialty Group. Many factors will influence the production of local or national guidelines, not least the results of geographically relevant studies of CAP aetiology and also the acceptability of either a pragmatic or defensive initial management strategy. Although the guidelines have varied

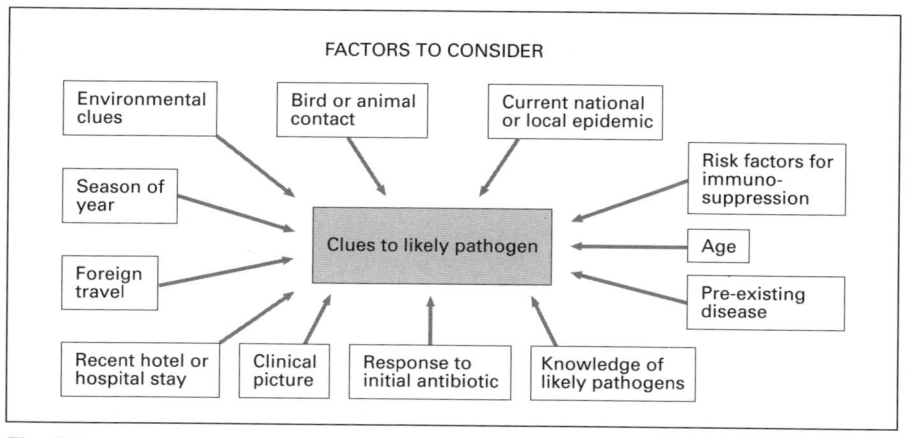

Fig. 6 Factors to consider when assessing the possible aetiological cause of CAP when the patient first presents.

considerably in the depth and detail of their considerations regarding CAP, the broad conclusions regarding empirical management have many similarities.

The majority of the guidelines, excluding those from the British Thoracic Society (BTS), group the patients into four categories: (1) patients managed in the community (not considered further here); (2) previous well patients with non-severe infection; (3) patients with pre-existing disease or the 'elderly', with non-severe infection; and (4) patients with severe infections.

Non-severe CAP in previously well adults

In this group the most common infections include those due to *Strep. pneumoniae* and mycoplasma. For this reason, macrolides (such as erythromycin) feature in all the guidelines. An aminopenicillin, such as amoxycillin, is also recommended as a first-line choice in European guidelines (providing excellent cover against the most common pathogen – *Strep. pneumoniae*). Unlike in North America, tetracyclines are not popular choices in Europe. Paradoxically, this has resulted in a fall in the incidence of resistant pneumococci in some areas, making tetracyclines a possible first-line choice again in the future.

Non-severe CAP in adults with underlying disease

The guidelines, with the exception of the BTS, all recommend a different management approach for those adults with comorbid or underlying chronic disease. The argument is that the spectrum of likely pathogens is wider in this group because of reduced defences, increased susceptibility and exposure to other pathogens (eg while visiting or staying in a hospital environment) and altered endogenous microbiological flora related to increased use of antibiotics. As a consequence, bacteria such as *Haemophilus influenzae*, *Staphylococcus aureus*, *Moraxella catarrhalis* and

Gram-negative enteric bacilli (GNEB) must be considered, including β-lactamase-producing strains. For this reason, second and third generation cephalosporins, a β-lactam antibiotic combined with a β-lactamase inhibitor (eg co-amoxiclav) or co-trimoxazole are recommended, with the optional addition of a macrolide to cover legionella infection.

Non-severe CAP in the elderly

The guidelines from USA, Canada and France identify age as an independent factor that should affect management. Age has been shown to have a minor effect on mortality from pneumonia, independent of underlying chronic disease. It is hard to dissect out the relative contributions of age and underlying chronic disease to the aetiology of CAP. Data from USA and Canada suggest an increased incidence of GNEB, particularly in residents of nursing homes (who are likely to have underlying chronic disease), whereas studies from Britain report GNEB infection rarely in the elderly admitted with CAP. Consequently, for British practice, it seems appropriate to regard the likely pathogens in the previously well, elderly patient with CAP as similar to those in younger adults (except that atypical pathogens such as *Mycoplasma pneumoniae* are less frequent). In the elderly patient with underlying disease there will be a rising frequency of other bacteria including *H. influenzae* (particularly in those with chronic lung disease), *Staph. aureus*, GNEB and possibly anaerobes in those with increasing debility, comorbid illness and prior exposure to antibiotics.

These recommendations demonstrate some of the inherent weaknesses of guidelines, placing broad patient groups together and suggesting 'defensive' therapy to cover every likely eventuality in every patient. Such an approach may be appropriate in patients seriously ill due to the severity of their infection or its impact on severe underlying disease, but less so in the majority of cases with mild to moderate infection.

In practice it is likely that the majority of patients with mild or moderate underlying chronic disease or increasing age, admitted from their own home to hospital in Britain with CAP, will have one of the common infections, such as *Strep. pneumoniae* or *H. influenzae*. These are likely to respond to an aminopenicillin, thus making this a reasonable and pragmatic first choice in many cases.

Severe CAP

The mortality of severe CAP is high and the early recognition of severe infection is an essential part of management.

Recognition of severe CAP. Numerous studies have identified features on hospital admission associated with a poor prognosis [9] (Fig. 7). The presence of at least two out of four simple clinical features (confusion, respiratory rate >30/min, diastolic blood pressure <60 mm Hg, blood urea >7 mmol/l) appears to be a specific but not sensitive indicator of poor prognosis or death.

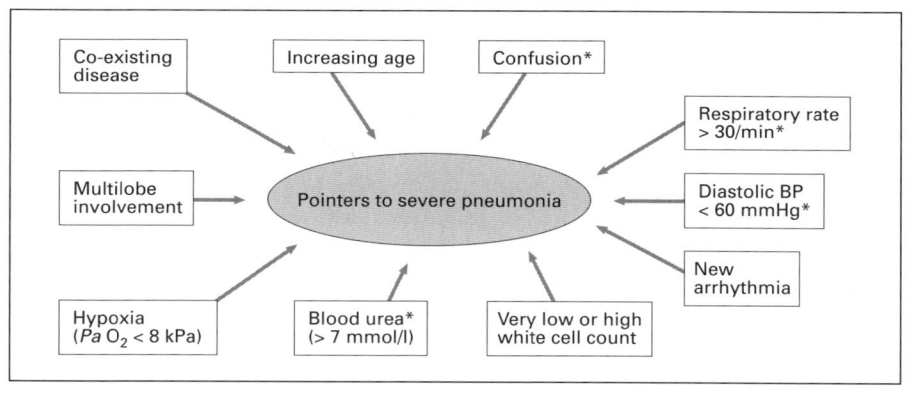

Fig. 7 Simple factors that are helpful for assessing severity of CAP when the patient first presents. These relate to host factors, clinical features and initial laboratory investigations.
*Mortality substantially increased in the presence of two or more of these factors.

Factors shown: Co-existing disease; Increasing age; Confusion*; Respiratory rate > 30/min*; Multilobe involvement; Diastolic BP < 60 mmHg*; Hypoxia ($PaO_2 < 8$ kPa); Blood urea* (> 7 mmol/l); Very low or high white cell count; New arrhythmia — all pointing to "Pointers to severe pneumonia".

Aetiology of severe CAP. Although pneumococcal infection remains the most common cause, legionella and staphylococcal infections become much more important in the severe group (see Fig. 1). Initial antibiotic therapy must cover all likely pathogens, pending laboratory results.

Antibiotic management for severe CAP. Different national guidelines are remarkably consistent in the recommendations for empirical antibiotic management, to cover the likely pathogens (Table 1). All recommend a macrolide together with a β-lactamase stable β-lactam antibiotic such as a second or third generation cephalosporin. North American guidelines also recommend including cover for pseudomonal infection. Primary pseudomonal pneumonia is extremely uncommon as a cause of CAP in European studies. Antibiotics are adjusted depending on the progress of the patient and microbiological findings.

Table 1 A summary of recommendations for initial antibiotic therapy for severe CAP, taken from different national guidelines. Parenteral administration of antibiotics is recommended initially.

National guidelines	Macrolide (M) plus cephalosporin (C)	Comments
Canadian Consensus	M + 3rd C*	*Advised antipseudomonal cover. Add aminoglycoside
American Thoracic Society		
British Thoracic Society	M + 2nd/3rd C	
Spanish Thoracic Society	M + 3rd C	
French Consensus	M + 3rd C	Alternatives include quinolone + co-amoxiclav

2nd/3rd = second or third generation cephalosporin
*North American guidelines also recommend cover for pseudomonal infection but this is extremely uncommon as a cause of CAP in European studies

Supportive management of severe CAP. The general management of the patient is very important. In one study of preventable deaths from pneumonia, inadequacies of oxygenation, fluid management and investigations were cited as the cause in over half of the cases. Ideally all patients identified as having severe CAP should be managed on a high dependency unit or ICU. Assisted ventilation can be life-saving for advancing respiratory failure and around 50% of patients requiring assisted ventilation survive, emphasizing its value. Patients who are transferred to an intensive treatment unit unexpectedly, following a cardiorespiratory arrest, do less well.

Investigation of CAP

Investigations are performed for a number of different reasons including assessing the severity of infection and its impact on underlying disease, to identify the cause of the infection and for epidemiological reasons (eg identifying an epidemic and screening for antibiotic resistance). Some guidelines comment on the appropriateness of different investigations. Those recommended as necessary for all cases of CAP include chest radiograph, routine haematology and biochemistry tests, blood culture, culture of any pleural fluid and assessment of arterial oxygenation (Table 2). The value of more detailed microbiological tests, including sputum Gram stain and culture, viral and atypical serology, detection of bacterial antigens and invasive tests, is debatable for most patients and they should be reserved for patients with severe or deteriorating disease. The identification of a predominant pathogen in sputum or respiratory secretions by Gram stain is a highly specific, but insensitive investigation and should be remembered as a simple, rapid and valuable investigation for patients with severe pneumonia (see Plate 12).

Table 2 Recommendations for investigations for patients admitted to hospital with CAP, taken from British Thoracic Society and American Thoracic Society guidelines.

Investigations	British Thoracic Society	American Thoracic Society
Chest X-ray	+	+
Routine blood tests	+	+
Arterial oxygen saturation	+	+
Blood culture	+	+
Sample any pleural fluid	+	+
Sputum culture	+	–/+
Sputum Gram stain	+*	–/+*
Viral/legionella serology	+*	–
Pneumococcal antigen detection	+*	–
Invasive tests	+*	Occasionally*

*If severe

Problem of antibiotic resistance among respiratory pathogens

Ampicillin-resistant *Haemophilus influenzae* (ARHI) has been recognized as a problem for several years owing mostly to β-lactamase production. The isolation of ARHI is more common in patients who have recently received aminopenicillins and the incidence is higher where antibiotic prescription policies are lax, eg Spain. The incidence of ARHI in Britain (up to 14%) is such that it need not influence initial antibiotic policy, but the presence of ARHI should be considered in patients at risk of *H. influenzae* infection (eg those with chronic lung disease) who have not improved with aminopenicillin therapy.

The majority of *Moraxella catarrhalis* strains are also ampicillin-resistant but as this is a rare cause of CAP it has little relevance to this discussion.

The more worrying situation is the emergence of penicillin-resistant *Strep. pneumoniae* strains (PRSP). It is thought that pneumococci capture DNA from environmental streptococci, resulting in remodelling of the genes that encode for penicillin binding proteins. Pneumococcal serotypes 6, 14, 15, 19 and 23 are usually involved. Genetic transformation to other serotypes has also been reported and geographical spread of PRSP can easily occur through travel and transfer of carriage of PRSP, particularly among children. Excess antibiotic use in a community selects out increasingly resistant strains. Most experience is reported from Spain [11] and USA [12], where incidence of PRSP has been recently reported as 35% (including 15% high resistance) and 25% (7% highly resistant) respectively. Experience from Spain over the past 10 years has supported the conclusion that current PRSP levels are not associated with increased mortality for pneumococcal pneumonia and that high-dose penicillin remains appropriate for cases with intermediate penicillin resistance and cephalosporins, such as cefotaxime and ceftriaxone, used for those with highly resistant strains (ie minimum inhibitory concentration >2 mmol/l). The emergence of PRSP is another strong argument for considering preventive pneumococcal vaccine in those at increased risk of pneumococcal infection.

Management subsequent to hospital admission

Invariably initial antibiotic management will be empirical [13], pending the results of any laboratory investigations and initial patient progress. All too often there is a delay in simplifying antibiotic therapy either by changing from parenteral to oral medication or reducing therapy in patients initially assessed as having severe infection but who subsequently rapidly improve. Parenteral can be changed to oral therapy 24 h after the fever has settled. Often initial oral therapy is quite adequate in patients with non-severe infection.

☐ CONCLUSION

Guidelines are useful in reminding us of a logical approach to the common problem of CAP. Guidelines must be tailored to local and national circumstances and not extrapolated from those of other countries. Recommendations for the management of CAP can be encompassed by 'ten simple commandments' and hospitals should be encouraged to develop their own protocols. These 'commandments' can be summarized as follows:

All infections

- ☐ Only a few pathogens are involved
- ☐ Always cover *Strep. pneumoniae* – the most common cause
- ☐ Cover mycoplasma during epidemics, *Staph. aureus* in flu season
- ☐ Consider epidemiology, patient's age and prior health
- ☐ Do not delay starting antibiotics

Severe infections

- ☐ Identify severe infection early
- ☐ Establish aetiology quickly
- ☐ Adequate oxygen and hydration essential
- ☐ Transfer high-risk patients early to intensive treatment unit
- ☐ Initial antibiotics must cover all the likely pathogens

A simplified flow diagram can be produced which summarizes one approach to antibiotic management suitable for clinicians in UK practice (Fig. 8).

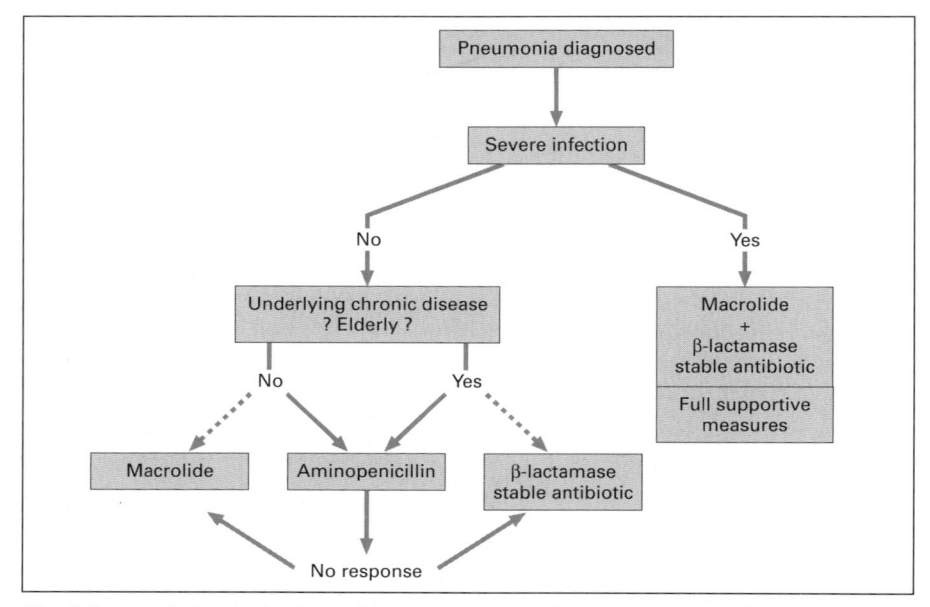

Fig. 8 Proposed strategy for the antibiotic management of an adult admitted to hospital with CAP. For many patients with non-severe infection, an aminopenicillin remains an appropriate, initial choice.

REFERENCES

1. Woodhead MA, Macfarlane JT, McCracken JS, Rose DH, Finch RG. Prospective study of the aetiology and outcome of pneumonia in the community. *Lancet* 1987; i: 671–4.
2. Macfarlane JT. An overview of community acquired pneumonia with lessons learned from the British Thoracic Society study. *Semin Respir Infect* 1994; **9**: 153–65.
3. British Thoracic Society. Guidelines for the management of community-acquired pneumonia in adults admitted to hospital. *Brit J Hosp Med* 1993; **49**: 346–50.
4. American Thoracic Society. Guidelines for the initial management of adults with community-acquired pneumonia: diagnosis, assessment of severity, and initial antimicrobial therapy. *Am Rev Respir Dis* 1993; **148**: 1418–26.
5. Mandell LA, Niederman MS. The Canadian Community Acquired Pneumonia Consensus Group. Antimicrobial treatment of community acquired pneumonia in adults: a conference report. *Can J Infect Dis* 1993; **4**: 25–8.
6. Société de Pathologie Infectieuse de Langue Française. Infections des voies respiratoires. Conférence de consensus en thérapeutique anti-infectieuse. *Med Mal Infect* 1991; **21** (Suppl): 1–8.
7. Sociedad Española de Neumologia y Cirurgia Toracica (SEPAR). Normativa sobre diagnostico y tratamiento de las neumonias. Barcelona: Ediciones Doyma, 1992.
8. Gialdroni Grassi G, Bianchi L. Guidelines for the management of community-acquired pneumonia in adults. *Monaldi Arch Chest Dis* 1995; **50**: 21–7.
9. Woodhead MA. Management of pneumonia. *Respir Med* 1992; **86**: 459–69.
10. Macfarlane JT, Finch RG, Cotton RE. In: *Colour Atlas of Respiratory Infections*. London: Chapman and Hall, 1993.
11. Pallares R, Linares J, Vadillo M, Gabellos C, Manresa F, Viladrich PF, Martin R, Gudiol F. Resistance to penicillin and cephalosporin and mortality from severe pneumococcal pneumonia in Barcelona, Spain. *New Engl J Med* 1995; **333**: 474–80.
12. Hofmann J, Cetron MS, Farley MM, Baughman WS, Facklam RR, Elliott JA, Deaver KA, Breiman RF. The prevalence of drug-resistant *Streptococcus pneumoniae* in Atlanta. *New Engl J Med* 1995; **333**: 481–6.
13. Torres A, Ausina V. Empirical treatment of nonsevere community-acquired pneumonia: still a difficult issue. *Eur Respir J* 1995; **8**: 1996–8.

☐ MULTIPLE CHOICE QUESTIONS

1. Aetiology of community acquired pneumonia in adults:
   (a) Pneumococcal infection is no longer the commonest cause of CAP
   (b) *Mycoplasma pneumoniae* infection occurs in epidemics every 3 or 4 years and usually affects younger adults
   (c) Pneumonia caused by Gram-negative enteric bacilli is common and must always be considered in adults presenting with CAP
   (d) Legionella infections are the second most common cause of CAP in adults
   (e) Legionella infections are the second most common cause of severe CAP in most studies

2. Antibiotic resistance to respiratory pathogens:
   (a) Penicillin-resistant pneumococci are rare throughout the world
   (b) Ampicillin-resistant *Haemophilus influenzae* is caused by a change in the penicillin binding protein on the capsule of non-capsulated strains
   (c) The incidence of ampicillin-resistant *Haemophilus influenzae* is now over 50% in Britain
   (d) *Moraxella catarrhalis* remains invariably sensitive to ampicillin in Britain
   (e) Patients with pneumonia caused by penicillin-resistant pneumococci of intermediate resistance must not be treated with penicillin

3   Antibiotic therapy for initial management of adult CAP:
    (a) A penicillin or aminopenicillin can no longer be regarded as appropriate initial choice for CAP in Europe
    (b) The best initial therapy for patients with severe CAP is an amino glycoside together with metronidazole
    (c) Macrolides should always be considered as one of the appropriate initial antibiotics for severe CAP
    (d) Initial macrolide therapy is particularly appropriate for the elderly patient presenting with non-severe CAP
    (e) Pneumococcal vaccine is only recommended for patients with sickle cell disease or asplenia

4   Assessment of severe pneumonia on hospital admission:
    (a) Low blood pressure is an important pointer to severe infection
    (b) Serum urea and electrolytes are of little value in assessing pneumonia severity
    (c) The white cell count may give an indication of the aetiology of pneumonia but not of the severity
    (d) The chest X-ray pattern is not helpful for assessing either aetiology or severity
    (e) The most important pointers to severity of infection include the presence of confusion, tachypnoea, hypotension and raised blood urea

5   Investigation of CAP:
    (a) All patients with CAP should have full investigations to assess the likely cause
    (b) Blood cultures are only recommended for those patients with severe infection or who do not improve following antibiotics
    (c) The assessment of oxygen saturation or arterial oxygen tension is only indicated in patients with severe pneumonia admitted to an intensive care unit
    (d) The detection of pneumococcal capsular antigen adds little to the ability to identify pneumococcal infection
    (e) Pleural fluid should not be sampled in a patient with pneumonia
    (f) Invasive investigations are never indicated in a patient with CAP

ANSWERS

1a False	2a False	3a False	4a True	5a False
b True	b False	b False	b False	b False
c False	c False	c True	c False	c False
d False	d False	d False	d False	d False
e True	e False	e False	e True	e False
				f False

Practical approach to sleep disordered breathing

J R Stradling

☐ INTRODUCTION

Our understanding of obstructive sleep apnoea (OSA) and its variants continues to progress at a considerable rate. Much of what was written 10 years ago is now regarded as too simplistic and dogmatic. In this era of guidelines and protocols there is a problem for rapidly evolving specialties: on the one hand, if such guidelines are laid down then progress is inhibited because of adherence to out-of-date approaches; on the other hand, if guidelines cannot be drawn up then health purchasers wonder whether *anyone* knows what they are doing and use this as an excuse not to assess the value of what is going on. The investigation and management of sleep apnoea and its variants have suffered in this way, perhaps due to the honesty of the practitioners involved who have not tried to oversell their own particular approach to the problem. Some health authorities deny the value of diagnosing and treating sleep apnoea on the basis of reviews by individuals with no relevant clinical experience and no dimly remembered undergraduate experience either. The real point, often lost in these theoretical and evidence-based approaches, is that, when a treatment is so obviously effective, many clinicians are not prepared to perform 'perfect' placebo-controlled trials, an approach easily understood when speaking to patients with sleep apnoea who use nasal continuous positive airway pressure (CPAP) treatment every night, and in some cases have done so for over ten years. There *are* now good trials demonstrating excellent treatment benefits in sleep apnoea, but many health authorities use the 'last in, first out' approach to purchasing rather than anything more sophisticated. The following text is an attempt to describe a pragmatic and economical approach to the management of OSA and its variants, based on over ten years experience and a current referral rate of more than 20 patients a week, four or five of whom start nasal CPAP treatment.

☐ AETIOLOGY AND PREVALENCE

Although it was thought originally that sleep apnoea was something you either did or did not have, it is now clear that this is not so. Sleep apnoea should be viewed more like hypertension, a condition that exists as a continuum, which at milder levels may not require treatment. In addition, the presence of symptoms and consequences greatly influences treatment decisions. With the onset of sleep there is withdrawal of upper airway muscle tone, just as there is in the rest of the skeletal muscles in the body. Normally this leads to a minor narrowing of the upper airway, which does not restrict airflow. If there is greater narrowing, then inspiratory airflow may be limited, with or without an associated noise – snoring. Snoring is a marker of inspiratory airflow limitation in the pharynx. Initially the body may perfectly compensate for this upper airway loading by increasing inspiratory effort and hence maintaining gas exchange. At some point this increased effort acts as an arousal stimulus, which briefly wakes the subject (Fig. 1), thus restoring tone to the upper airway muscles and reversing the narrowing. Recurrent 'snoring-induced

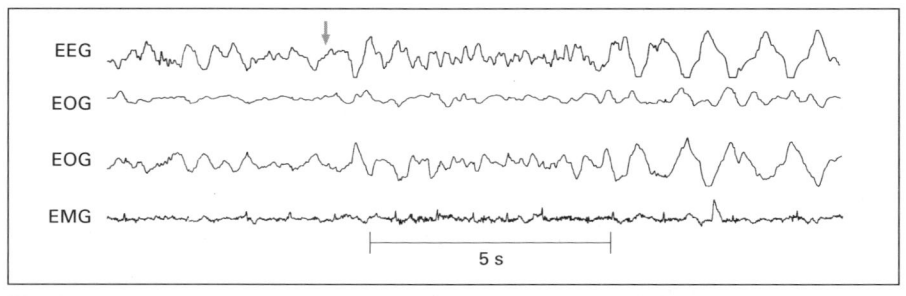

Fig. 1 Polysomnographic recording of sleep showing an electroencephalogram (EEG), two electro-oculograms (EOG) and an electromyogram (EMG). This 15-s tracing taken during slow-wave sleep shows one microarousal lasting only 5 s. There is a transient increase in the frequency of the EEG waves and a small rise in EMG tone measured sub-mentally. Hundreds of these microarousals per night can be present in patients with sleep-related breathing disorders, which leads to excessive daytime sleepiness.

arousals' have only recently been recognized as a variant of classic sleep apnoea in which complete collapse of the upper airway occurs during sleep. This means that within a population there exists a range of upper airway narrowing with sleep. This varies from virtually none (someone who probably never snores), through minor narrowing (occasional snorer), moderate narrowing (regular snorer), substantial narrowing (regular snorer with arousals), and severe narrowing with complete collapse (classic sleep apnoea). Not only does this spectrum exist, but individuals will move within it, both on a night-to-night basis (changing sleep posture, alcohol consumption, nasal blockage), and over a longer time-scale (due to body weight changes, for example). Along this spectrum there comes a point when the degree of sleep disruption leads to noticeable daytime symptoms, usually excessive sleepiness. However, whether the patient is aware of this, or complains of it, will depend on the interaction of many different factors. For example, hypersomnolence may be blamed simply on getting older, or because of increased pressures at work. Individuals may make up for quality by increasing quantity, such as having to sleep for more hours, particularly at weekends. The type of job may bring out differences, for example a boring sedentary job requiring great vigilance will be affected first, compared to an interesting job requiring constant physical activity.

This variability in the amount of sleep apnoea and its impact means that defining the syndrome is difficult. One can either simply measure a physiological variable (such as apnoeas) and define a threshold, or one can try to assess the impact of the physiological variable as well. Many physicians in this area now accept that a combination of appropriate symptoms and some appropriate measure of nocturnal physiological abnormality is the correct way to diagnose and define the condition. A recent review on the epidemiology of sleep apnoea expands these points and concludes that the prevalence of symptomatic sleep apnoea, worthy of treatment with nasal CPAP, is probably between 0.5% and 2% of middle-aged men.

The factors that push individuals along the spectrum towards symptomatic disease are mainly obesity, the shape of the lower face, or both. The effect of obesity is to load the upper airway by mass loading and perhaps also by infiltrating pharyngeal tissues and reducing dilator efficacy. For this reason, neck circumference is a better predictor of sleep apnoea than general obesity. The pharyngeal dilator muscles are working harder than normal during the day to fend off this extra loading, but cannot maintain this extra activity during sleep. The other important factor that narrows the airway is retrognathia. Most studies have found retropositioning of both maxilla and mandible in patients with sleep apnoea, particularly those who are not that overweight. This facial structure may be the result of external factors during early childhood (nasal blockage, large tonsils) or may be inherited. Other acquired factors such as hypothyroidism and acromegaly are also important and probably influence upper airway muscle function as well as anatomical shape.

Important aspects of the above can be summarized as follows:

- Continuously variable severity from trivial snoring to severe sleep apnoea
- Snoring is a marker of upper airway narrowing during sleep
- Recurrent sleep fragmentation is the cause of the dominant symptom, excessive sleepiness
- The relationship between sleep fragmentation and sleepiness is not close
- Obesity and differences in facial morphology are the main causes of sleep apnoea
- 0.5–2% of middle-aged men would benefit from treatment

TYPES OF PATIENT

Patients referred to our sleep laboratory tend to fall into only a few categories. The majority are heavy snorers who have presented mainly because of the social problem of snoring. Many of these come via the ear, nose and throat (ENT) surgeons. Snoring can be a very disabling symptom leading to separate bedrooms, ridicule, embarrassment in hotels when neighbours insist on changing rooms, reluctance to fall asleep on public transport etc. The unhappiness from snoring is often much worse than other non-life-threatening conditions treated by the National Health Service (NHS). On questioning, a proportion of these snorers turn out to have symptoms of significant sleep apnoea and are grateful when identified and treated. Those who, on questioning them and their partners, are apparently just snorers may need a sleep study for two main reasons. First, the snoring may not be anything like as bad as suggested. Snoring is very much in the ear of the listener as well as the pharynx of the snorer. Complaints of snoring can be a marker of marital disharmony, rather than its cause, and be an apparently legitimate reason for leaving the marital bed. Thus, before instigating all but the simplest treatment, we insist on some evidence of snoring, either from the original sleep study or from home recordings using a voice activated tape recorder and tie-clip microphone mounted on a headband about 3 inches above the nose. It is remarkable how often couples cannot get recordings of snoring following complaints of being kept awake all night by it. The second reason to do a sleep study on snorers, even with no complaints of daytime sleepiness, is if a significant operation is planned by the ENT surgeons such as uvulopalatopharyngoplasty (UPPP). This operation is extremely poor at helping sleep apnoea and indeed may be harmful by preventing easy use of nasal CPAP at a later date. Thus if the sleep study reveals sleep apnoea, which usually means there is obstruction behind the tongue in addition to any higher up, removing the palate and 'redundant' tissue in the oropharynx is unlikely to be very helpful. Such patients are a problem because they often do not have symptoms bad enough to justify a trial of nasal CPAP, but really want something done about their snoring. This group are likely to respond to a mandibular repositioning device worn just at night, but this approach is in its infancy in the UK.

Clinic assessment of a patient complaining of snoring is relatively simple and centres on establishing why snoring is present and if any of the causes might be reversible. Most studies on snoring show that obesity, nasal congestion, smoking, alcohol in the evening, residual tonsils and retrognathia are the most common causes of snoring. Thus simple advice on weight reduction, nasal decongestion (nasal steroids and elevating the head of the bed a few inches), stopping smoking and alcohol avoidance may be all that is required. Very recent onset of snoring raises the suspicion of hypothyroidism, and the menopause is often when women snore for the first time. Thus reduced snoring can be one of the benefits of hormone replacement therapy.

☐ SLEEP STUDIES

The usefulness of sleep studies depends much more on the skill of the interpreter than on the actual equipment used. If one were setting out to provide an echocardiography service the first step would be to get training and then worry about the equipment. Our unit is constantly asked what is the ideal system (or minimal requirement) for doing sleep studies, and much less often where can some time be spent learning how to interpret the signals.

As will be apparent from the earlier section, there are two important aspects to a sleep study designed to identify significant sleep apnoea. First, it must identify sleep disruption in some way, since it is this that leads to the dominant symptom of hypersomnolence. Previously this was done very badly by using epoch-based sleep scoring of the EEG, a process designed to paint a very broad picture of the sleep architecture. Indeed the majority of the microarousals associated with sleep-related breathing disorders are not recognized by this old approach. Unfortunately counting often hundreds of microarousals (Fig. 1) from raw EEG tracings is an incredibly laborious procedure only undertaken by the richest laboratories. New computerized analysis of microarousals using neural network, fast Fourier or autoregressive techniques may be useful developments. However, sleep disturbance can be inferred from signals other than EEG. For example, body movements correlate very well with arousals and can be measured with simple techniques such as wrist-worn actigraphs, special bed sensors, or video-derived systems using image analysis. An alternative approach is to use autonomic markers of arousal such as heart rate or rises in blood pressure (Fig. 2). An arousal begins in the brain stem and passes up to the cortex through well-mapped pathways. In the process, the cardiovascular centres are

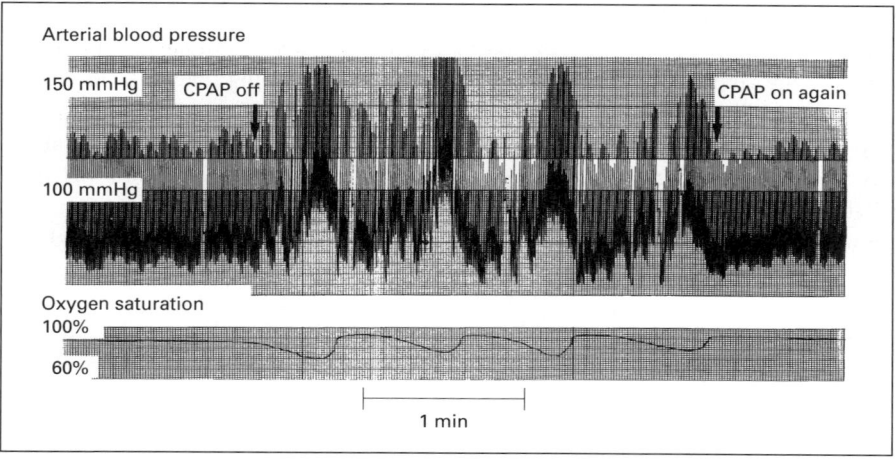

Fig. 2 Beat-to-beat arterial blood pressure tracing (Finapres device) from a patient with obstructive sleep apnoea while on nasal CPAP treatment. After the first minute the pressure is lowered to a sub-therapeutic level and the sleep apnoea returns. Note the surges in blood pressure with arousal from each apnoeic event, and the increased respiratory swings in blood pressure (pulsus paradoxus) between the arousals when the patient is struggling to breathe against a collapsed pharynx. These abnormal blood pressure swings are instantly abolished when a therapeutic pressure is reintroduced.

activated which suppress the baroreceptor reflex and enhance the chemoreceptor reflex. It is possible for these centres to register an arousing stimulus that does not penetrate to the cortex. For example, the cortical EEG response to recurrent noises usually habituates, whereas the autonomic response does not, presumably implying a mechanism for limiting cortical arousal to incoming stimuli. It has been shown that rises in blood pressure and heart rate accurately reflect the recurrent arousals due to both respiratory and non-respiratory sleep disorders. Thus any system that registers arousals will help differentiate simple snoring without sleep disturbance from snoring or sleep apnoea with sleep disturbance. There is no evidence that conventional EEG analysis is any better than these simpler techniques at recognizing those microarousals that produce symptoms. The important point for the clinician is to learn how to read the chosen system's output of the data.

The second important aspect of a respiratory sleep study is to identify if there are respiratory events that produce any increased frequency of arousals. The old approach using apnoeas, hypopnoeas and hypoxic dips measured by oximetry certainly identified the severe end of the spectrum, but failed to identify the 'snoring-induced arousal' or 'upper airway resistance syndrome' (Fig. 3). Not only can obstructive events occur without significant hypoxia, but there are also many non-obstructive causes of hypoxia at night. Since it is usually increased inspiratory effort that arouses the patient, techniques to measure or infer this are required. Some laboratories routinely use oesophageal balloons in sleep studies to detect increasing inspiratory effort as this approach is the gold standard. However, it is very labour intensive and uncomfortable. Snoring itself is an indirect marker of upper airway narrowing although significant narrowing can occur without noise generation, particularly after a UPPP. Other techniques used include measuring the inspiratory depression of the skin in the suprasternal notch, ribcage/abdominal paradox (out-of-phase movements in response to upper airway loading; Fig. 4), increased oscillations in a cardioballistogram, and identifying inspiratory airflow limitation (Fig. 5). This latter technique shows great promise, and analysis of the inspiratory flow profile has been used to control automatically the pressure delivered by a CPAP machine to abolish significant upper airway narrowing. An approach that our laboratory has investigated is the measurement of pulsus paradoxus on a beat-to-beat arterial blood pressure tracing. Because the heart and great blood vessels are in

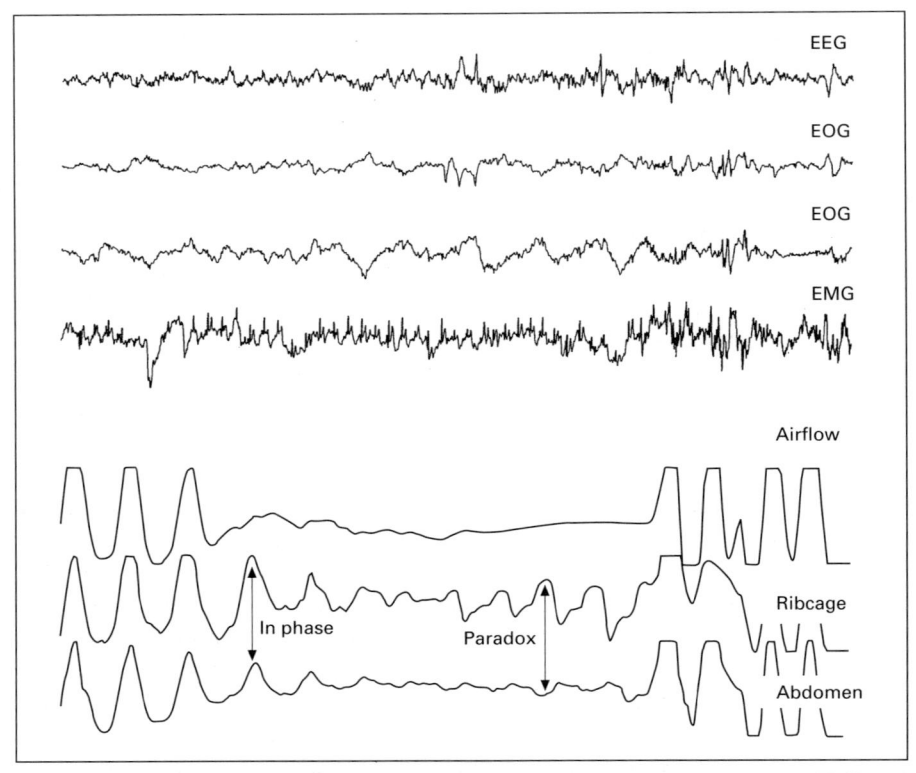

Fig. 3 Polysomnographic recording of sleep (EEG, two EOG, eye movements, and EMG) and respiratory channels. This event is an obstructive apnoea with more than 10 s of absent airflow at the nose and mouth with continuing respiratory efforts, evident on the ribcage and abdominal movement sensors.

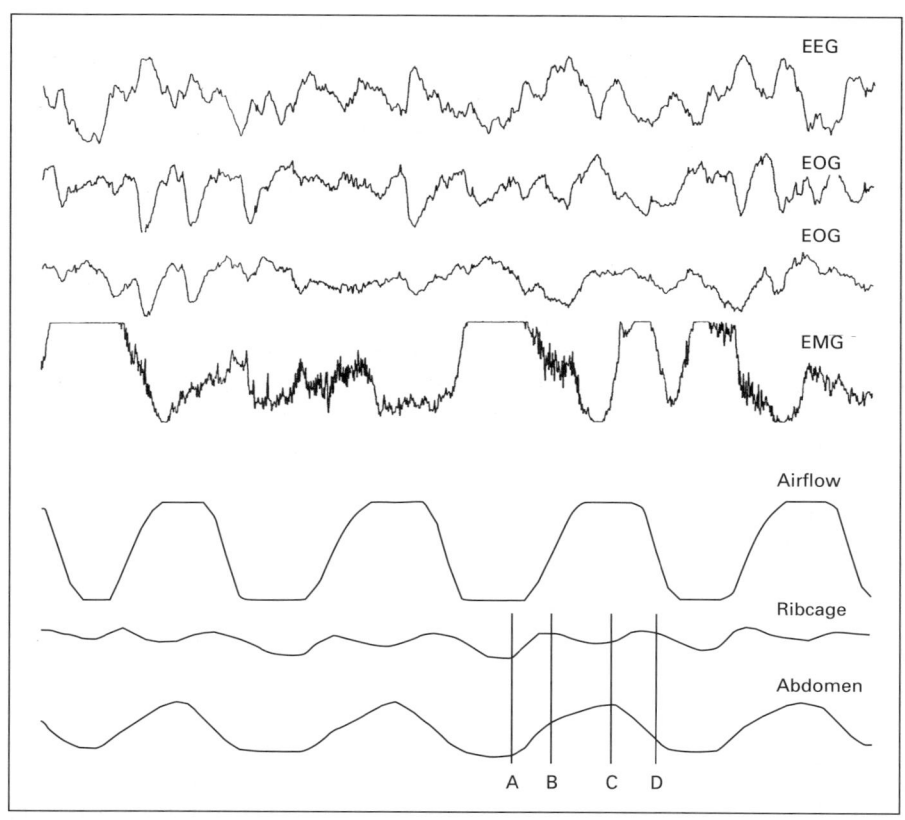

Fig. 4 Polysomnographic recording of sleep and respiratory channels. During this tracing the patient has upper airway narrowing sufficient to 'load' inspiration and produce respiratory paradox. At A, a breath in begins with synchronous outward ribcage and abdominal movements; at B, increased inspiratory effort by the diaphragm, due to upper airway loading, actually sucks in the ribcage wall while the abdominal wall continues to move out; at C, inspiratory effort ceases, the abdominal wall returns in again while the ribcage springs out; at D, both compartments are now passively returning to their end expiratory positions.

the chest, any reductions in intrathoracic pressure are reflected in the peripheral arterial circulation since it acts as a manometer line to the thoracic cavity. The Finapres device (Ohmeda, Colorado) is a non-invasive photoplethysmographic volume clamp technique that produces a tracing virtually identical to an intra-arterial line. The respiratory oscillations in systolic blood pressure are easy to measure and correlate well with swings in intra-oesophageal pressure (Figs. 3 and 6). The Finapres device is not suitable for home sleep studies, but beat-to-beat changes in blood pressure can be inferred from changes in pulse transit time; this is the time taken from the opening of the aortic valve to the arrival of the pulse pressure wave (or shock wave) at a peripheral artery (usually the finger). As the blood pressure rises the arterial wall tenses and the pulse wave travels faster, and of course vice versa. Respiratory swings in pulse transit time – measured more conveniently from the

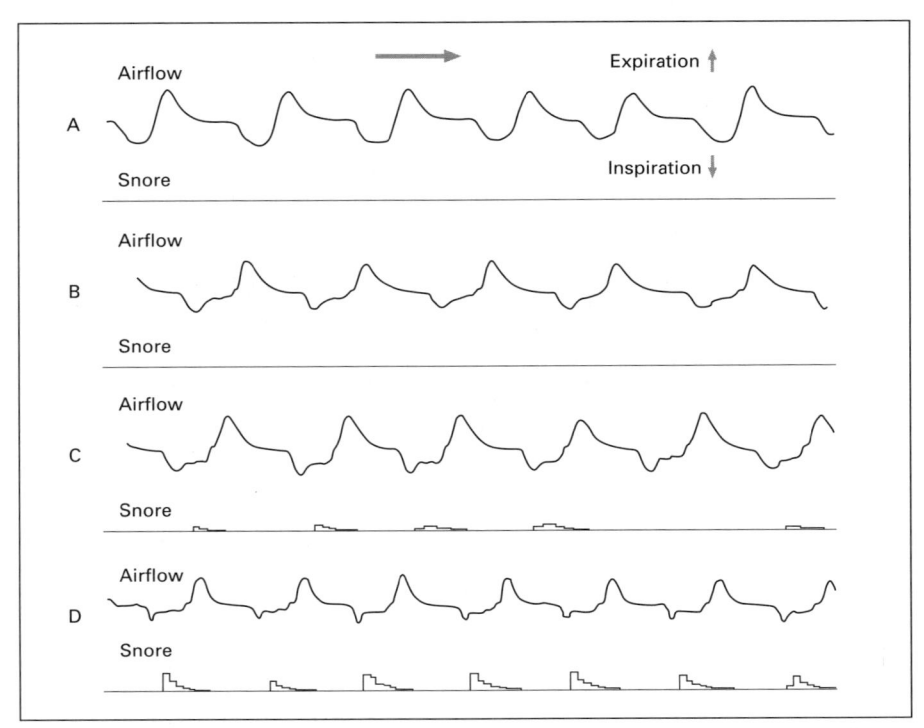

Fig. 5 Four 20-s tracings of airflow and snoring from different times during a sleep study. A, normal, non-inspiratory flow limited, breathing with no snoring. Note the nice rounded inspiratory waveform (downwards). B, early inspiratory flow limitation with still no snoring. Note the scalloping of the latter part of the inspiratory waveform compared to A. C, Slightly more severe airflow limitation with the appearance of snoring. D, Severe flow limitation and snoring. Note the long horizontal plateau on the inspiratory waveform clearly indicating flow limitation.

electrocardiogram (ECG) R-wave to the arrival of the pulse at the finger (measured optically) – have also been shown to reflect the degree of inspiratory effort (Fig. 7). If increased upper airway narrowing has impaired gas exchange then there will be a fall in oxygen saturation. Finger oximetry is a useful tool but it should be remembered that there can be significant respiratory events provoking arousal without any fall in oxygen saturation.

There are many systems on the market that combine a selection of the signals and derivatives referred to above. For example, the MESAM system (Madaus, Freiburg, Germany) records heart rate (marker of arousal), snoring (marker of upper airway narrowing), and oxygen saturation (marker of severe upper airway narrowing). This device is in use in many laboratories. There are systems (for example DENSA, Clwyd, Wales) using movement sensors (for arousals) plus ribcage/abdominal sensors to record apnoeas/hypopnoeas and respiratory paradox, with arousals inferred from the sudden lessening of paradox as the upper airway reopens. Our system in regular use (VISI Lab, Stowood Scientific Systems, Oxford) is based on oximetry and video recordings; the video signal is digitally processed to measure

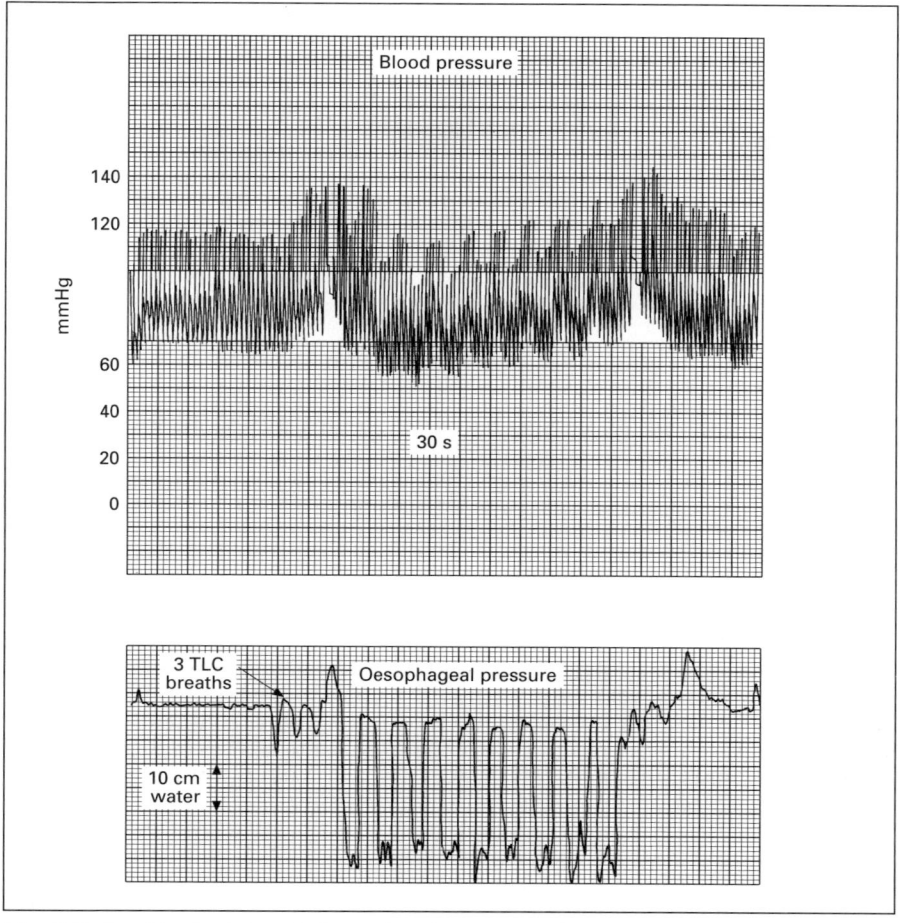

Fig. 6 During this simulation of obstructive sleep apnoea there are nine obstructed inspiratory efforts with pleural pressures developed of about 30 cm H_2O below atmospheric (measured with an oesophageal balloon). Note how the beat-to-beat blood pressure tracing (Finapres device) reflects these large inspiratory efforts.

movement (arousals), the audio channel provides snoring (upper airway narrowing), and the oximeter provides both heart rate (arousals) and oxygen saturation (severe upper airway narrowing) (Fig. 8).

The way these systems should be used is not to place great emphasis on numbers of events generated by analysis algorithms, but to use them to answer the question 'Does this study reveal a possible cause for the patient's symptoms?'. We do not know enough about the pathophysiology of sleep apnoea and its variants to state that particular events are more significant than others. Thus the sleep study should be used in a qualitative way to identify patients that might benefit from the available treatments (Table 1). Currently this requires experience, and no amount of expense on equipment can replace it.

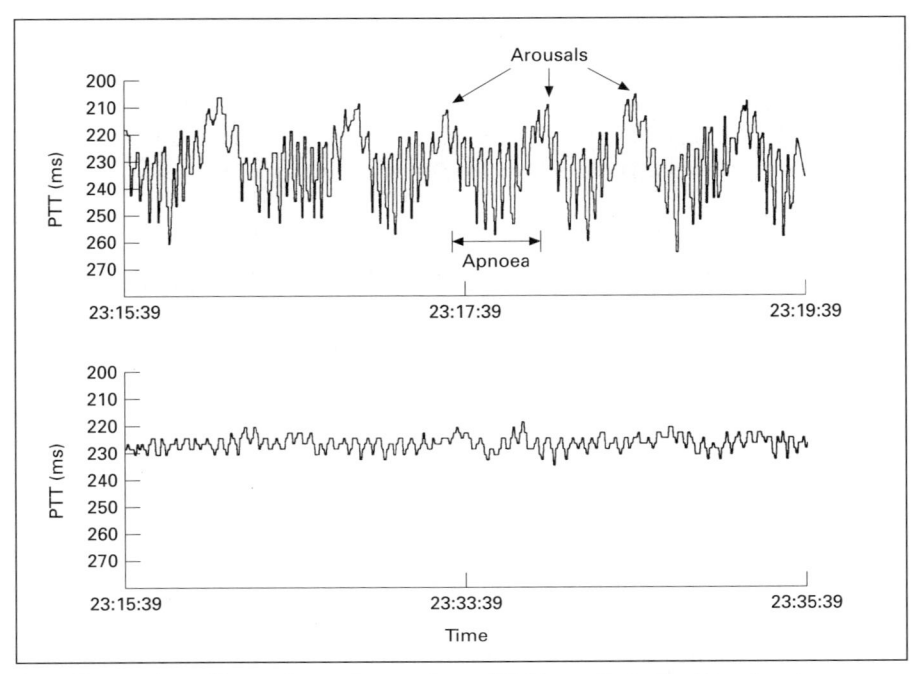

Fig. 7 Two tracings of beat-to-beat pulse transit time (PTT) in a patient with obstructive sleep apnoea before and during treatment with nasal CPAP. The PTT tracing is inverted to reflect correctly rises and falls in blood pressure. Note in the top tracing during sleep apnoea there are the arousal related rises in blood pressure and the inspiratory related falls. In the tracing taken on nasal CPAP not only have the arousal peaks been abolished, but the respiratory swings are much smaller, reflecting the reduction in inspiratory effort now that the upper airway is well open.

Table 1 Use of sleep studies to assess sleep arousal and increased respiratory effort.

Sleep studies need to document sleep fragmentation/recurrent arousals
- ☐ eg body movements
- ☐ autonomic markers: heart rate, blood pressure, skin resistance
- ☐ abrupt reduction in airway narrowing: from airflow limitation, ribcage/abdominal paradox
- ☐ sophisticated detection of EEG microarousals

Sleep studies need to document increased respiratory effort (from upper airway narrowing)
- ☐ eg snoring
- ☐ pleural pressure monitoring (oesophageal balloons)
- ☐ ribcage/abdominal paradox
- ☐ inspiratory airflow limitation
- ☐ systemic blood pressure respiratory oscillations (pulsus paradoxus)

☐ TREATMENT

Treating OSA needs to be tailored to severity. For mild disease, weight loss, reduction in alcohol intake, improving nasal patency and learning to lie on one's side may be all that is required. For more moderate disease the above may work, but

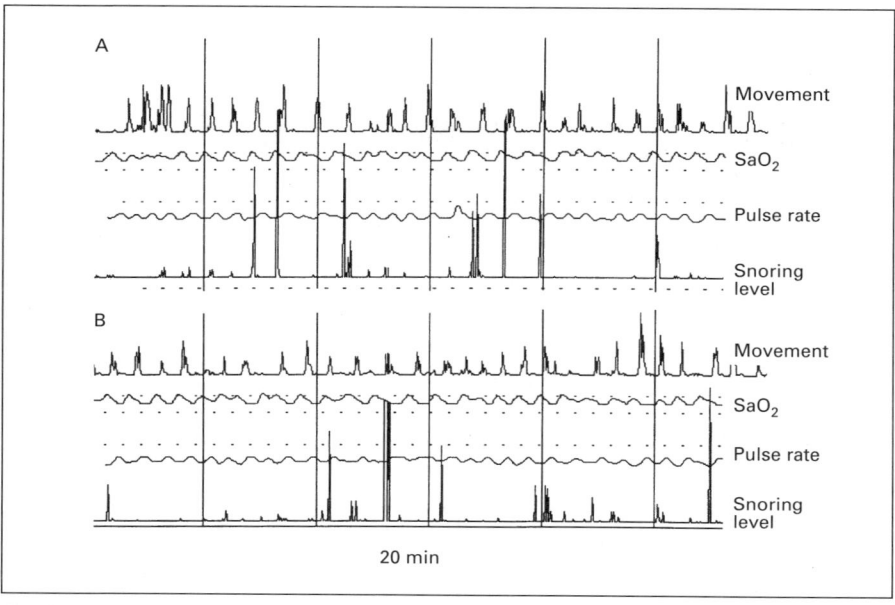

Fig. 8 Two sequential tracings (A and B) from a man with obstructive sleep apnoea. The top channel is body movement derived from digital processing of the video signal. The second channel is oxygen saturation from a pulse oximeter, the third is pulse rate from the oximeter, and the fourth is low-frequency noise from a microphone above the head representing snoring. Movement and pulse rate increases are surrogate markers of arousal, snoring is a surrogate marker of upper airway obstruction, and SaO_2 indicates hypoventilation. In this patient the diagnosis could be nothing other than obstructive sleep apnoea; central sleep apnoea would have no snoring but otherwise be similar, and periodic movements of the legs would again produce nothing on the snoring channel but would also show a flat oximetry line.

tonsillectomy, or the wearing of a mandibular repositioning device at night, may be appropriate. For more severe disease (the definition of severity is discussed below) the use of nasal CPAP treatment is currently regarded as the most effective.

The *purpose* of treatment for OSA is under debate. At one extreme there is the argument that, because of an apparent increased risk of cardiovascular disease in these patients, they should all be treated with the most effective treatment, usually nasal CPAP, whether or not they have symptoms. The other extreme argues that since increased cardiovascular risk has not been proven, and the most effective treatments are difficult to use, management of these patients should be entirely symptom-led with no consideration of the potential long-term complications of OSA.

In our view, to put a truly asymptomatic patient with OSA on to nasal CPAP (currently the best treatment) is likely to be doomed to failure. Nasal CPAP is a difficult treatment to get used to and to tolerate night after night. The compliance of such a patient will be very poor, as it is with the treatment of other asymptomatic problems, such as hypertension. To expect an asymptomatic man aged 40 to wear a mask over his nose every night for the rest of his life, for the distant benefit of a reduction in cardiovascular death expectation of about 5% in 20 years or so, is simply to fail to understand human nature. Thus to use criteria derived from a sleep study to initiate a prescription for nasal CPAP will also fail because of the very poor relationship between the findings on a one-night sleep study and the patient's symptoms. As mentioned earlier, reliance on a measure such as the apnoea index will miss patients who will benefit from treatment, and will lead to the offer of treatment to those who have no intention of using it.

This has led to a pragmatic approach to the provision of nasal CPAP in our unit. The decision to prescribe nasal CPAP is a clinical one based both on symptoms and the result of the sleep study. The essential question asked is 'Does the patient have anything on the sleep study that is likely to be nasal CPAP responsive, and are his symptoms bad enough such that the patient is prepared to have a trial of nasal CPAP?'. This means that we would offer a trial of nasal CPAP to a patient prepared to try it, who had extreme sleepiness, even if there was only heavy snoring on the sleep study with some evidence of sleep disturbance. This would be a qualitative decision, not a quantitative one. On the other hand, if a patient was not sleepy (genuinely so) then the sleep study would have to show bad sleep apnoea to make us try and persuade an individual to try nasal CPAP. This clearly leaves grey areas, but this is the state we are in given the clinical situation. Our experience is that most patients either are using, and want to keep, their nasal CPAP machines at the end of a 4 to 6 week trial or not (verified from the time counters built into most nasal CPAP machines). Unless nasal CPAP is producing a placebo effect, then the patient's view of the matter is likely to be the best judge of future long-term use. Since we rely on symptom improvement to guide us (Fig. 9), it is clearly important to set up nasal CPAP as best possible to maximize the response. In our view this requires a considerable amount of education and support of the patient starting before trying nasal CPAP in hospital. Carefully worded information and a professionally produced training video have helped in this respect. Recently we tried setting up patients in an afternoon session with the first night at home, but this proved far less satisfactory than spending the first night in hospital. There is also a need for support during the trial period to make sure they do not give up for the wrong reasons. We provide intensive support to make sure that problems such as nasal blockage, rhinorrhoea, nasal bridge ulceration, air leaks, mouth leaks and many others are dealt with as quickly as possible. In addition, there is a patient support group with phone numbers that patients can call to talk to an experienced user in their area. There are also partner support numbers. It seems that this level of support produces a high level of acceptance of nasal CPAP (about 85%).

Finally, it is important not to say to a patient that they must use their machine all night and every night. Most will not do so because, as with every other treatment that requires patient motivation, only the amount necessary to control symptoms to the patient's satisfaction is likely to be used. No one with psoriasis uses their creams and ointments to remove every last plaque, and very few patients with OSA want to use nasal CPAP during every sleeping hour. Because we are treating symptoms, the patient may well be happy with 3 h of good sleep a night, or only five nights a week. Units that suggest full usage find that the patients mislead them about the hours

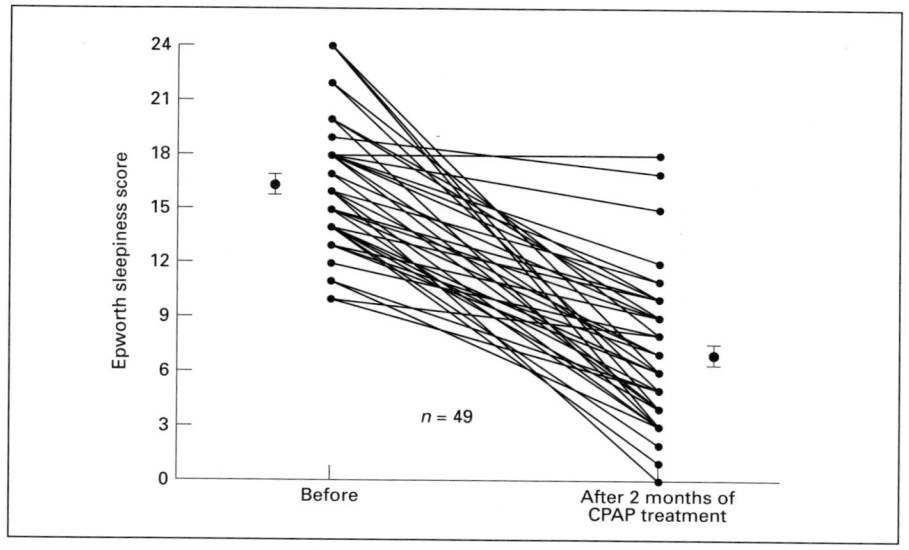

Fig. 9 The Epworth sleepiness score is a simple questionnaire-derived index of excessive daytime hypersomnolence. Most patients with obstructive sleep apnoea or snoring induced arousals, who will benefit from nasal CPAP treatment, have scores over 12 or 13 (normal values are usually less than 10). Following successful treatment, the daytime sleepiness score reflects the improved sleep quality; failure of the score to fall usually means the patient has not been able to use the treatment for some reason, or that the sleepiness was not due to sleep apnoea.

used (compared to the built-in timers) whereas in our unit they do not, since there is no pressure to do so.

Following successful institution of nasal CPAP there is no need for repeat sleep studies unless something changes. For example, the sleepiness may return and the continuing adequacy of the chosen nasal CPAP pressure needs to be checked. Following weight loss it may be possible significantly to lower the required pressure, or come off nasal CPAP altogether. If the patient is happy and asymptomatic, then all should be well since this was the purpose of the original exercise.

☐ CONCLUSION

This account of the management and approach to patients with sleep fragmentation due to upper airway narrowing during sleep has been necessarily didactic and pragmatic. In an ideal world one might run a more sophisticated programme but I doubt it would bring much extra benefit to the patients. In a world of rationed health care it is the clinician's duty to ensure that he is providing as cost-effective a service as possible.

FURTHER READING

Ferguson KA, Fleetham JA. Sleep-related breathing disorders: 4 – Consequences of sleep-disordered breathing. *Thorax* 1995; **50**: 998–1004.

Gleeson K, Zwillich CW, White DP. The influence of increasing ventilatory effort on arousal from sleep. *Am Rev Respir Dis* 1990; **142**: 295–300.

Stradling JR. *Handbook of Sleep-related Breathing Disorders*. Oxford: Oxford University Press, 1993.

Stradling JR. Obstructive sleep apnoea: definitions, epidemiology and natural history. *Thorax* 1995; **50**: 683–9.

Guilleminault C, Stoohs R, Duncan S. Snoring (I). Daytime sleepiness in regular heavy snorers. *Chest* 1991; **99**: 40–8.

Douglas NJ. Sleep-related breathing disorders: 3 – How to reach a diagnosis in patients who may have the sleep apnoea/hypopnoea syndrome. *Thorax* 1995; **50**: 883–6.

Grunstein RR. Sleep-related breathing disorders: 5 – Nasal continuous positive airway pressure treatment for obstructive sleep apnoea. *Thorax* 1995; **50**: 1106–13.

White DP. Sleep-related breathing disorders: 2 – Pathophysiology of obstructive sleep apnoea. *Thorax* 1995; **50**: 797–804.

Gaultier C. Sleep-related breathing disorders: 6 – Obstructive sleep apnoea in infants and children: established facts and unsettled issues. *Thorax* 1995; **50**: 1204–10.

Davies RJO, Belt PJ, Robert SJ, Ali NJ, Stradling JR. Arterial blood pressure responses to graded transient arousal from sleep in normal humans. *J Appl Physiol* 1993; **74**: 1123–30.

Pitson D, Sandell A, van de Hoot R, Stradling JR. Pulse transit time as a measure of respiratory effort in patients with obstructive sleep apnoea. *Eur Respir J* 1995; **8**: 1669–74.

☐ MULTIPLE CHOICE QUESTIONS

1 In most cases of sleep apnoea, likely contributory causes are:
   (a) Neck obesity
   (b) Abnormal hypothalamic activity
   (c) Narrow retroglossal space due to relative retrognathia
   (d) Poor respiratory drive
   (e) Spasm of pharyngeal constrictors

2 Snoring:
   (a) Is only likely to cause daytime hypersomnolence if it causes recurrent arousals
   (b) Is mainly due to vibration of the soft palate so surgical removal of the palate will cure snoring
   (c) Only occurs when the mouth falls open
   (d) Complaints about a partner's snoring may be the result rather than the cause of marital disharmony
   (e) Is a proven cause of heart attacks and strokes

3 Simple advice to patients with snoring or mild sleep apnoea should include:
   (a) Reduce or stop evening alcohol
   (b) Tape the mouth closed at night
   (c) Improve nasal patency as much as possible
   (d) Stop smoking
   (e) Reduce weight

4 Upper airway narrowing and/or increased inspiratory effort during sleep can be inferred from:

(a) Increasing respiratory swings on an oesophageal pressure tracing
(b) Flow limitation on an inspiratory flow tracing
(c) Nocturnal falls in oxygen saturation
(d) Increasing paradoxical movement of the ribcage and abdominal wall during a series of inspirations
(e) Increased respiratory swings in systolic blood pressure on a beat-to-beat tracing

5   Nasal CPAP for patients with obstructive sleep apnoea:
(a) Should always be used whenever asleep to derive symptomatic benefit
(b) Should only be prescribed when the sleep study shows significant sleep apnoea
(c) Can cause nasal bridge ulceration
(d) Is an easy treatment for the patient to master
(e) All patients successfully established on CPAP need regular monitoring with sleep studies thereafter

ANSWERS

1a True	2a True	3a True	4a True	5a False
b False	b False	b False	b True	b False
c True	c False	c True	c False	c True
d False	d True	d True	d True	d False
e False	e False	e True	e True	e False

New approaches to lung cancer

S G Spiro

☐ INTRODUCTION

Lung cancer continues to be the greatest source of morbidity and mortality of all cancers in the western world, and its impact in the developing world is rapidly being understood. Approximately 30% of all male cancer deaths in Europe are due to lung cancer, and in women it is, in many countries, a more frequent cause of death than breast cancer.

While greater insights into the molecular biology of lung cancer provide some hope for better therapeutic approaches, these advances have not to date been reflected in greater survival statistics. Advances in treatment have been painfully slow and have involved rationalization of the treatments we have and how to apply them rather than major new options.

It is becoming apparent that the disease is increasingly affecting the ageing population. Those over 70, while bearing a disproportionately high burden of malignant disease, have traditionally been underutilized as receivers of innovative therapies, and are commonly excluded from clinical trials. As a community, the elderly have a poor record of survival from cancer and are rarely treated with curative intent. Table 1 shows the incidence of lung cancer with increasing age in the European Community. It is clear, therefore, that this large and frailer section of society needs to be included in the planning of treatments, and special assessment of treatment tolerance, toxicity and quality of life need to be included as the elderly may withstand treatment less robustly than their younger counterparts.

Table 1 Mortality for major cancer sites by age and sex, expressed as the crude rate (average rate per 100 000). (From European Community data 1980–84.)

	Age (years)		
	0–44	45–64	65
Male			
All cancers	16.4	354	1568
Lung cancer	2.2	118	436
Colon cancer	0.6	17	106
Female			
All cancers	16.3	229	838
Breast cancer	0.6	21	60
Lung cancer	4.3	60	118

☐ SCREENING

Although the cause of the great majority of lung cancers is known to be cigarette smoking (small cell, squamous cell and at least some adenocarcinomas), and high-risk populations are easy to identify, screening has failed to be a sensitive cost-effective tool. Three large prospective studies, using either the chest X-ray alone or in combination with sputum cytology, showed no improvement from a control population in cancer-related mortality. Although the interventions identified more tumours of favourable stage and there was an apparent prolongation of survival, this was due to a lead-time bias as the tumour was identified while clinically occult; the natural history of the tumour was not affected. In short, cancers are too far advanced and 'established' by the time of detection (see Fig. 1).

The scientific goal is to detect the disease further back on its developmental curve. To date, no candidates have emerged as sensitive detectors. Studies of tumour markers associated with lung cancer (Table 2) have proven them to be too insensitive and non-specific. They are certainly not sensitive enough to be a successful therapeutic marker [1]. Research continues in this field, but tumour markers currently add little to physical examination and conventional staging methods.

☐ STAGING

The clinical staging of lung cancer was revised in 1986 and is summarized in Table 3. This revision has attempted to widen the scope for inclusion of resectability. Patients with clinical stage I, II and IIIa disease are now considered surgical candidates. The

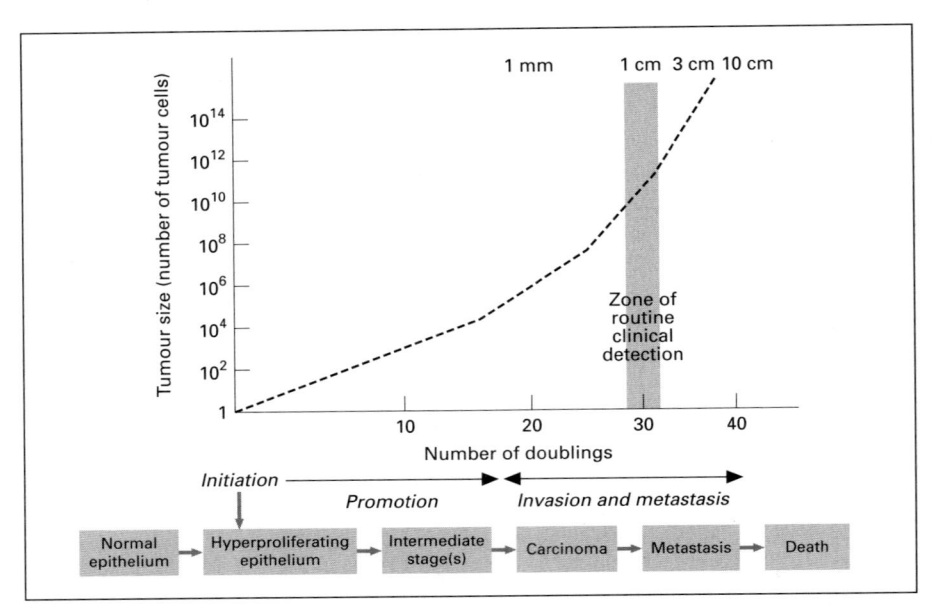

Fig. 1 The progression of lung cancer. The relation of tumour doubling, tumour size and progression to death. (Adapted from [9].)

Table 2 Tumour markers in lung cancer.

Carcinoembryonic antigen (CEA)	Neuron-specific molecule (NSE)
Tissue polypeptide antigen (TPA)	Creatinine-phosphokinase-BB (CPK-BB)
Squamous cell carcinoma antigen (SCC-Ag)	Chromogronin A (ChrA)
CYFRA 21.1	Soluble interleukin-2 receptor (SIL-2R)
Neural cell adhesion molecule (NCAM)	

Table 3 Definitions for staging bronchogenic carcinoma (American Joint Committee on Cancer Staging 1986).

T0: No evidence of primary tumour.

TX: Tumour proven by the presence of malignant cells in bronchopulmonary secretions but not visualized roentgenographically or bronchoscopically, or any tumour that cannot be assessed.

TIS: Carcinoma *in situ*.

T1: A tumour that is 3 cm in greatest diameter, surrounded by lung or visceral pleura, and without evidence of invasion proximal to a lobar bronchus at bronchoscopy.

T2: A tumour that is 3 cm in greatest diameter, or a tumour of any size that either invades the visceral pleura or has associated atelectasis or obstructive pneumonitis extending to the hilar region. At bronchoscopy, the proximal extent of demonstrable tumour must be within a lobar bronchus or at least 2 cm distal to the carina. Any associated atelectasis or obstructive pneumonitis must involve less than an entire lung.

T3: A tumour of any size with direct extension into the chest wall (including superior sulcus tumours), mediastinal pleura or pericardium without involving the heart, great vessels, trachea, oesophagus or vertebral body, or a tumour in the main bronchus within 2 cm of the carina without involving the carina.

T4: A tumour of any size with invasion of the mediastinum or involving the heart, great vessels, trachea, oesophagus, vertebral body or carina as presence of malignant pleural effusion.

N0: No demonstrable metastasis to regional lymph nodes.

N1: Metastasis to lymph nodes in the peribronchial or the ipsilateral hilar region, or both, including direct extension.

N2: Metastasis to ipsilateral mediastinal lymph nodes and subcarinal lymph nodes.

N3: Metastasis to contralateral mediastinal lymph nodes, contralateral hilar lymph nodes, ipsilateral or contralateral sclera or supraclavicular lymph nodes.

M0: No (known) distant metastasis.

M1: Distant metastasis such as in scalene, cervical, or contralateral hilar lymph nodes, brain, bones, liver or contralateral lung.

Summary staging

Stage I (operable)	T1	N0	M0
	T2	N0	M0
Stage II (operable)	T1	N1	M0
	T2	N1	M0
Stage IIIa (operable)	T3	N0	M0
	T3	N1	M0
	T1–3	N2	M0
Stage IIIb (inoperable)	Any T	N3	M0
	T4	Any N	M0
Stage IV (inoperable)	Any T	Any N	M1

major change from the previous classification is the inclusion (as stage IIIa) of patients with tumour extending directly into the chest wall, the mediastinum or pleura, and if the tumour is within 2 cm of the carina. All these changes reflect improvement in surgical skill and technology rather than improved disease detection. In all, approximately 75% of patients considered to have undergone a curative resection will die of their disease within the following 5 years. This is due to failure to detect small tumour deposits either within or outside the thorax at the time of surgery. In fact, the failure of computerized tomography (CT), isotope bone scanning and ultrasonography to detect metastases of <1 cm in size have led to the abandonment of these investigations in patients who are physically well at the time of diagnosis and where symptoms are those only due to the presence of the primary tumour (eg cough, wheeze, haemoptysis). In 'fit' patients without any non-specific or organ-specific symptoms, preoperative staging can be limited to a CT scan of the thorax as abdominal scans, brain scans and bone scans will identify a metastasis too rarely to make these investigations cost-effective.

Recently, however, whole body fluoro-2-deoxyglucose positron emission tomography (PET) in patients with lung cancer has shown much greater sensitivity and accuracy for identifying metastases than CT. One study of 34 'operable' patients with non-small cell lung cancer (NSCLC) found that PET scans identified unsuspected malignant lesions in ten patients and management changes were made in 14, including six who became unresectable [2]. Another study, also in a small number of patients (30) with clinical stage I NSCLC, compared CT to PET. Although neither CT nor PET scanning identified all patients with metastatic mediastinal nodes, PET was better. The sensitivity, specificity, accuracy, positive predictive value and negative predictive value for imaging of mediastinal metastases with PET were 78%, 81%, 80%, 64% and 82% respectively, and for thoracic CT scan the same variables were 56%, 86%, 77%, 63% and 87% [3]. Clearly, PET scanning is a useful and potentially important staging technique, but its cost and availability are major limiting factors.

☐ SMALL CELL LUNG CANCER

The treatment of small cell lung cancer remains an area of intense research – the tumour is so sensitive to cytotoxic chemotherapy, yet death results in the great majority of patients due to the emergence of resistant tumour. Most of the newer approaches to treatment of this cell type are based on combinations of cytotoxic chemotherapeutic drugs. Cyclophosphamide, cisplatin, etoposide, adriamycin and the vinca alkaloids remain the most commonly used drugs, usually in a three or four drug regimen. With these agents, at least 50% of patients presenting with limited disease (LD), ie disease confined to the ipsilateral hemithorax, should achieve a complete clinical and radiological response; the figure for extensive disease (ED) patients is 20–30%.

Attempts to intensify treatment by means of either alternating schedules of active drugs, dose escalation regimens, re-induction or late intensification chemotherapy have made little impact [4]. Maintenance chemotherapy in patients who are established in complete response also does not appear to confer a survival benefit.

It has become clear, however, that short courses of conventional dose-combination chemotherapy (four to six courses) will be as effective as more prolonged courses of treatment, thus saving patients unnecessarily prolonged treatment with days in hospital and potentially additional toxicity and morbidity. It is now generally recommended that six courses of combination chemotherapy will suffice and produce survival data similar to those achieved by longer or more intensive treatment, ie limited disease 12–15 months median survival and extensive disease 6–10 months medial survival.

The use of pre-treatment prognostic variables based on simple measures, such as performance status and biochemical laboratory values (sodium, albumin, alkaline phosphatase, liver transaminases) will identify patients with a good prognosis from those with a poor or intermediate prognosis [5]. This allows selection of patients likely to do well (ie 20% 4-year survival) and these patients may receive more intensive treatment regimens in clinical trials in an attempt to improve their survival prospects further. New approaches to overcome the development of tumour resistance include changing the scheduling of chemotherapy. Our group attempted weekly dosing versus the standard 3 weekly courses in more than 400 patients with no survival advantage for the weekly regimen but poorer quality of life. Biological response modifiers have also been extensively assessed. Haemopoietic growth factors, in particular granulocyte-macrophage colony-stimulating factor (GM-CSF) and granulocyte colony-stimulating factor (G-CSF), decrease the period of neutropenia and sepsis following chemotherapy. Attempts to use these agents to intensify the administration of chemotherapy, as opposed to preventing toxicity from conventional doses, do not look as promising and may even be associated with greater toxicity than patients not receiving the GM-CSF in some controlled studies.

Other useful agents include recombinant human erythropoietin, which may delay the anaemia associated with chemotherapy in these patients [6].

☐ NON-SMALL CELL LUNG CANCER

For patients with NSCLC, the intervention most likely to effect cure is surgery. However, this option is only available to a minority of patients who present with lung cancer. Recently, it has become apparent that some combinations of chemotherapy are more effective than those evaluated in the 1970s and 1980s with very little evidence of activity. Single agent response rates of 20% have been documented for several drugs (Table 4). Combinations of mitomycin C, ifosfamide and cisplatin have a response rate (ie >50% reduction in tumour size) in excess of 50% for patients with LD. Other active combinations include mitomycin C, cisplatin and a vinca alkaloid, or just cisplatin and a vinca alkaloid. These combinations, together with the emergence of some promising new agents, have led to a major effort to discover if the addition of chemotherapy to standard treatment such as surgery, radiotherapy or just best supportive care can improve median survival and also cure rates.

The greatest effort has been made in patients with disease confined to one hemithorax, but too advanced for curative resection. Most of these subjects have N2 disease – mediastinal nodal involvement, either just visible on CT or confirmed at

Table 4 Active cytotoxic agents in non-small cell lung cancer. (From Smit and Postmus [11].)

Drug	Response rate (%)	No. of assessable patients
Cisplatin	21	568
Ifosfamide	25	460
Vindesine	18	449
Vinblastine	28	38
Vinorelbine	20	634
Mitomycin C	18	115
Etoposide	9	278
4-Epirubicin	25	131
Gemcitabine	21	211
Camptothecin-11	28	107
Taxol	22	49
Taxotere	31	51

mediastinoscopy. Pilot studies have shown that preoperative chemotherapy, sometimes with the addition of radiotherapy, has rendered up to 60% of locally advanced cases of NSCLC operable, with median survival data of around 18 months – approximately twice that expected for non-surgical therapy. The 5 year survival rates have varied with one study returning a 37% figure [7]. In some studies, tumours have completely resolved at resection and some radiological partial responses have been shown pathologically to be complete responses on post-resection examination. Most of the data accumulated to date have come from uncontrolled studies. Two controlled studies are now available of neoadjuvant chemotherapy followed by surgery versus surgery alone. Both are of small numbers and are open to criticism, but both showed a significant survival advantage for the neoadjuvant arm [8]. Considerably more data are required before this approach should become accepted practice.

A comprehensive meta-analysis of 52 randomized clinical trials comparing the addition of chemotherapy to surgery, radiotherapy or best supportive care has shown a trend to improved survival with modern (cisplatin-containing) chemotherapy with surgery and radiotherapy. Controlled trials of chemotherapy and surgery versus surgery alone gave a hazard ratio of 0.87, ie a 13% reduction in the risk of death, equivalent to an absolute survival benefit of 5% at 5 years for the addition of chemotherapy (Figs 2 and 3). Trials comparing radical radiotherapy with radical radiotherapy and chemotherapy also gave a hazard ratio of 0.87, with an absolute benefit for the addition of chemotherapy of 4% at 2 years [10]. In trials examining the possible benefits of adding chemotherapy to best supportive care versus best supportive care alone, the hazard ratio for the addition of chemotherapy was 0.73, a 27% reduction in the risk of death and a 10% improvement in survival at 1 year (Figs 4 and 5). The essential drug(s) to achieve these benefits could not be identified from these data. However, the result offers some hope of progress, suggesting chemotherapy may have a role in treating NSCLC. No data are available

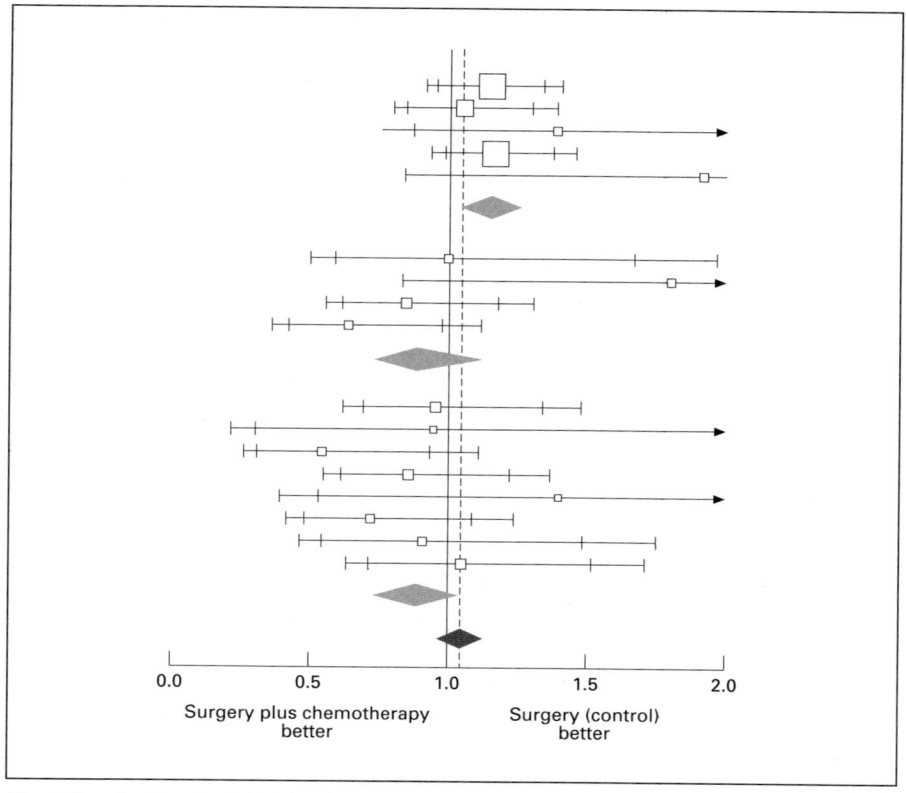

Fig. 2 Results of controlled trials of surgery plus chemotherapy versus surgery alone. Each individual trial is represented by a square, the centre of which denotes the hazard ratio for that trial, where horizontal bars denote the 99% confidence interval and the inner bars the 95% confidence interval. The size of the square is proportional to the amount of information in that trial. The black diamond gives the overall hazard ratio when the results of all trials are combined, the centre of which denotes the hazard ratio and the extremities the 95% confidence intervals. The shaded diamonds represent the hazard ratio for the various specified categories of chemotherapy. (From NSCLC Collaborative Group [10] with permission.)

on the effects of chemotherapy on quality of life, particularly for patients receiving best supportive care, ie those with advanced incurable disease. Prospective studies on the possible benefits of chemotherapy in NSCLC are now in progress. New chemotherapeutic agents, including gemcitabine, taxols and camptothecin, are being assessed (Table 4). They all have modest but acceptable activity, but whether they will be even more effective in combination with other agents remains to be evaluated.

Progress in the management of lung cancer remains slow; clearly efforts should intensify around prevention. We are failing dramatically to make any impact whatsoever on the smoking epidemic in the Far East, South America and southern Europe, which continues unabated. Last year, the number of children aged under 15 years who smoke went up yet again in the UK.

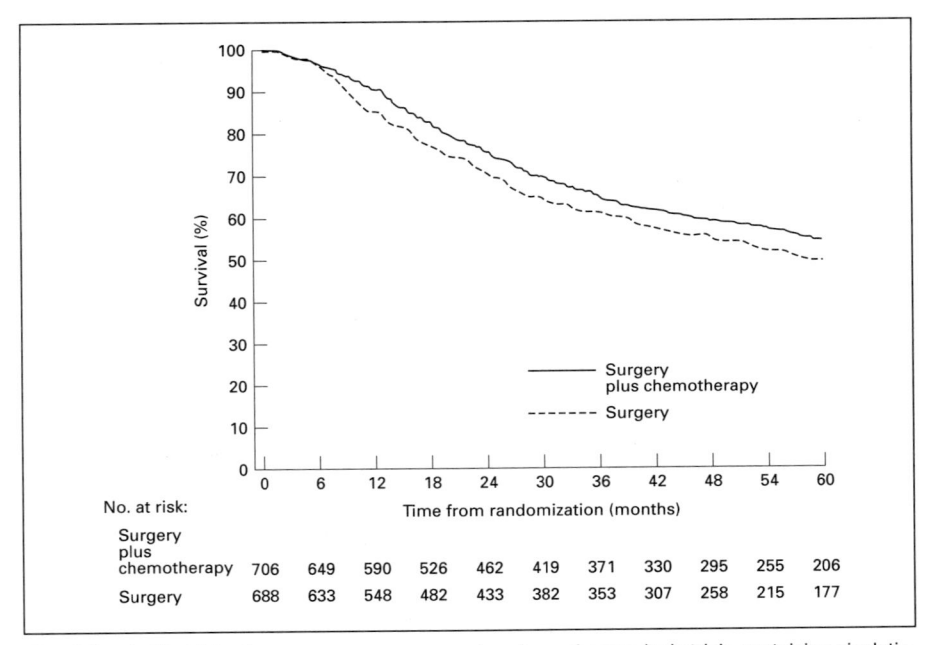

Fig. 3 Survival in trials of surgery versus surgery plus chemotherapy (only trials containing cisplatin-based regimens). (From NSCLC Collaborative Group [10] with permission.)

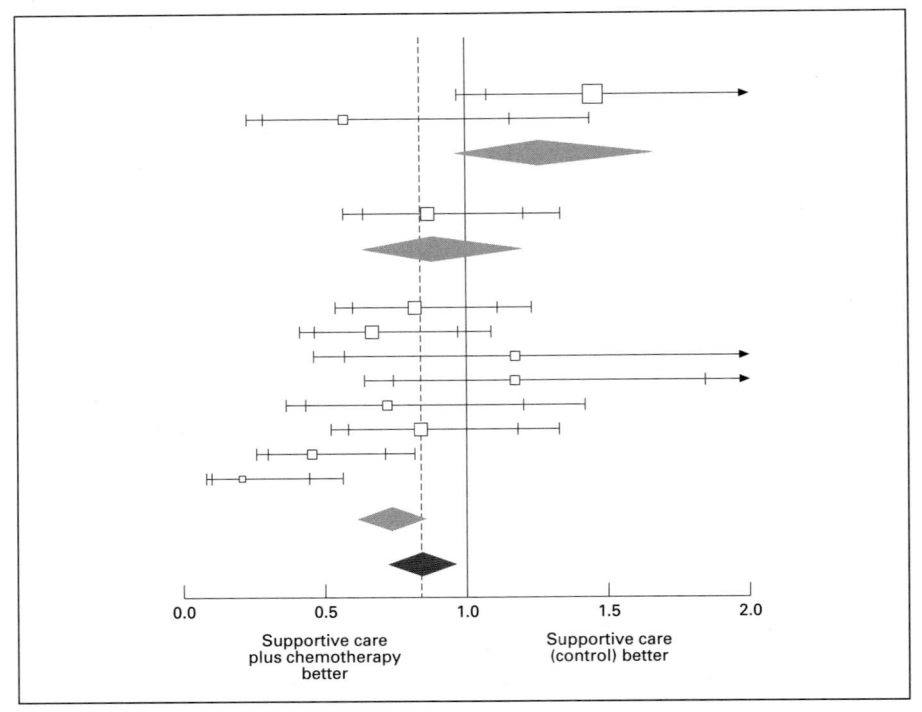

Fig. 4 Results of trials of supportive care plus chemotherapy versus supportive care (see Fig. 2 legend for symbols and conventions). (From NSCLC Collaborative Group [10] with permission.)

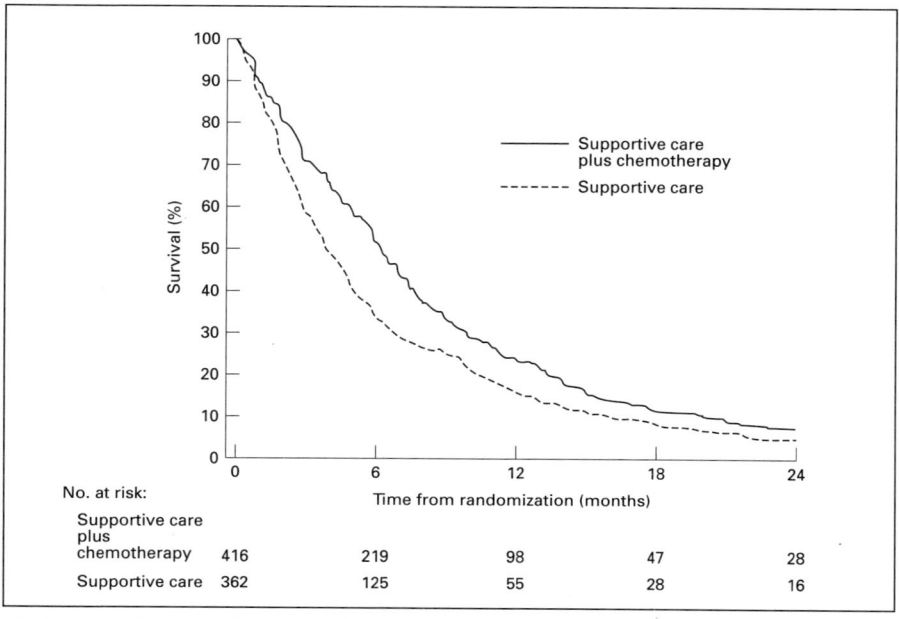

Fig. 5 Survival in trials of best supportive care plus chemotherapy versus supportive care (only trials containing cisplatin regimens). (From NSCLC Collaborative Group [10] with permission.)

REFERENCES

1. Ferrigno D, Buccheri G. Clinical application of serum markers for lung cancer. *Resp Med* 1995; **89**: 587–97.
2. Lewis P, Griffin S, Marsden P, et al. Whole body ^{18}F-fluoro-deoxyglucose positron emission tomography in pre-operative evaluation of lung cancer. *Lancet* 1994; **344**: 1265–6.
3. Chin R, Ward R, Keyes JW, et al. Mediastinal staging of non-small cell lung cancer with positron emission tomography. *Am J Respir Crit Care Med* 1995; **152**: 2090–6.
4. Spiro SG. Bronchial tumours. In: Brewis RAL, Corrin B, Geddes DM, Gibson GJ, eds. *Respiratory Medicine.* London: WB Saunders, 1995: 924–61.
5. Souhami RL, Bradbury I, Geddes DM, et al. Prognostic significance of laboratory parameters measured at diagnosis in small cell carcinoma of the lung. *Cancer Res* 1985; **45**: 2878–83.
6. De Campus E, Radford J, Steward W, et al. Clinical and *in vitro* effects of recombinant human erythropoietin in patients receiving intensive chemotherapy for small cell lung cancer. *J Clin Oncol* 1995; **13**: 1623–31.
7. Cameron R, Ginsberg RJ. Induction (pre-operative) therapy and surgery for locally advanced stage IIIa (N2) non-small cell lung cancer. In: Carney DN, ed. *Lung Cancer.* London: Arnold, 1995: 78–95.
8. Milroy R, Macbeth F. Neo-adjuvant chemotherapy in stage IIIa non-small cell lung cancer. *Thorax* 1995; **50**: 525–30.
9. Carney DN, ed. *Lung Cancer.* London: Arnold, 1995.
10. Non-Small Cell Lung Cancer Collaborative Group. Chemotherapy in non-small cell lung cancer: a meta-analysis using updated data on individual patients from 52 randomised clinical trials. *Brit Med J* 1995; **311**: 899–909.
11. Smit EF, Postmus PE. Chemotherapy of non-small cell lung cancer. In: Carney DN, ed. *Lung Cancer.* London: Arnold, 1995: 98–113.

MULTIPLE CHOICE QUESTIONS

1. In the staging of lung cancer, patients are still considered potentially curable if:
   (a) The chest wall is involved by the primary tumour
   (b) A Pancoast tumour has invaded a vertebral body
   (c) Contralateral mediastinal nodes (N3) are involved
   (d) The T stage is III
   (e) The trachea is involved

2. Screening for lung cancer in high-risk populations:
   (a) Has an advantage for chest X-ray and sputum examination over chest X-ray alone
   (b) Identifies tumours at an earlier stage than when they usually present
   (c) Has shown no long-term survival benefit for the earlier discovery of the disease
   (d) Has no overall advantage and has been abandoned

3. Chemotherapy in non-small cell lung cancer:
   (a) Can produce partial response in up to 50% of patients with combination chemotherapy
   (b) Is now generally recommended as an adjunct before surgery
   (c) Is not recommended outside clinical trials
   (d) Is much less active than for small cell lung cancer

4. In small cell lung cancer, important prognostic features are:
   (a) A normal haemoglobin
   (b) Male gender
   (c) High performance status
   (d) Normal serum sodium, alkaline phosphatase and albumin

5. Chemotherapy in small cell lung cancer:
   (a) Should obtain a complete response in 50% of patients presenting with limited disease
   (b) Has a high response rate in patients who have relapsed after prior chemotherapy
   (c) Is more effective if given as early or late course intensification
   (d) Is associated with better survival if maintenance chemotherapy is given once an initial response has been achieved

ANSWERS

1a True	2a False	3a True	4a False	5a True
b False	b True	b False	b False	b False
c True	c True	c True	c True	c False
d True	d True	d True	d True	d False
e False				

Advances in the drug therapies of rheumatoid arthritis

S Jawed, I C Chikanza and D R Blake

☐ INTRODUCTION

Rheumatoid arthritis (RA) is a multisystem autoimmune disease that usually takes the form of a chronic synovitis that progressively destroys bone and cartilage leading to an increased morbidity and mortality in affected individuals. Patients often manage satisfactory symptom control but suppression of underlying inflammation and therefore joint destruction remains unsatisfactory. In this brief review we discuss present and future drug treatments for RA.

☐ PATHOGENESIS OF RHEUMATOID ARTHRITIS

The initial trigger for RA remains unknown. Aetiological factors that have stimulated greatest interest are listed in Table 1. Once the disease process is triggered, there follows a cascade of macrophage and T cell activation [1], inflammatory cell influx, cytokine release, cell proliferation and progressive tissue destruction (Fig. 1). T cells then appear to become anergic. The cause for the subsequent switch from acute to chronic inflammation remains subject to debate, but leading contenders are listed in Table 2. The increased understanding of the inflammatory cascade and its key players has allowed the development of many new potential therapeutic agents. The greatest challenge to the success of new therapies

Table 1 Aetiology of RA.

Viruses	Parvovirus B19, Epstein-Barr virus (EBV)
Bacteria	*Proteus mirabilis, Yersinia*
Genetic	12% concordance in monozygous twins

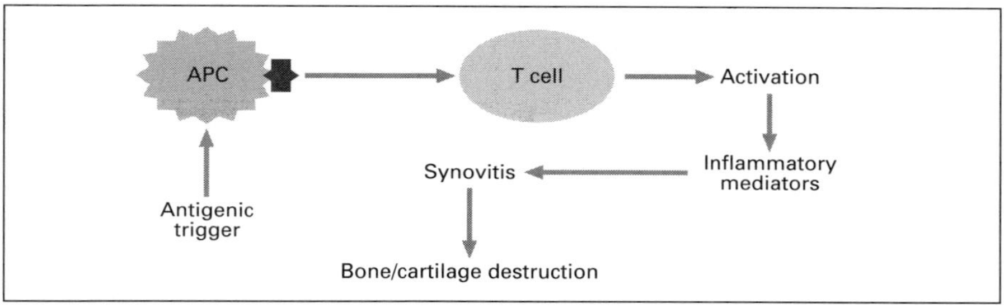

Fig. 1 Pathogenesis of rheumatoid arthritis

Table 2 Causes for chronicity of RA.

Genetic predisposition
Hypoxia reperfusion injury
Hypothalamic pituitary axis dysfunction
Macrophage/fibroblast 'activation'
Neuronal damage

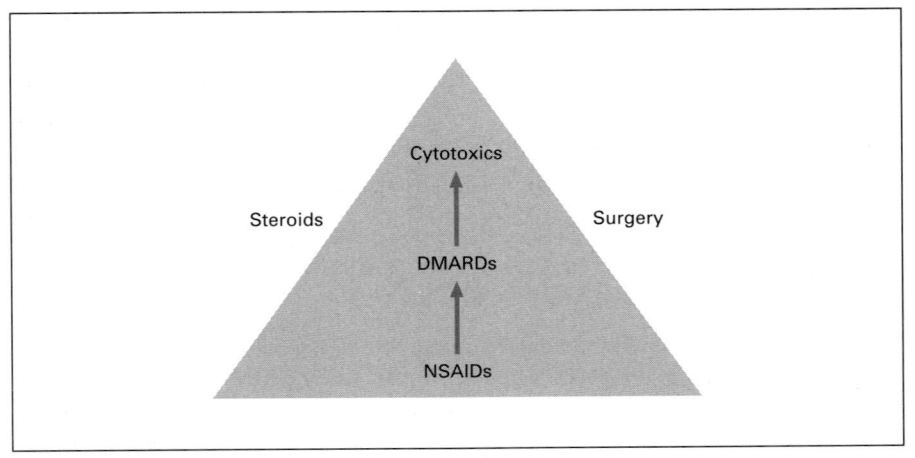

Fig. 2 Pyramid of rheumatoid arthritis treatment

will not only be their ability to inhibit the inflammatory process but their ability to reduce joint destruction and thereby improve long-term outcome in RA patients.

CURRENT THERAPIES

The traditional treatment principles of RA (Fig. 2) are now being questioned. Long-term outcome studies have failed to show effective disease control and hence prevention of joint destruction and disability in the majority of patients. However, recently published research suggests that this failure of current drugs may be due to the use of potentially effective drugs too late in the disease process. Evidence is accumulating that early and aggressive disease suppression is the most likely route to a favourable outcome [2]. The majority of patients who develop erosive and destructive RA begin to show radiological evidence of joint destruction within 2 years of disease onset. A window of opportunity may exist early in the disease process when 'switching off' the inflammatory process will have its maximum impact on long-term outcome. However, at an early stage in the disease process the diagnosis may not be clear and the patients who require long-term treatment may not be easy to identify. Therefore, it is crucial that patients are referred to a specialist rheumatologist at this stage to allow the patients to be treated appropriately in a multidisciplinary setting.

Disease modifying agents of rheumatoid disease (DMARDs) revisited

Corticosteroids

Although steroids are undoubtedly effective in suppressing inflammation, their use is limited by their side effects, in particular osteoporosis. Steroids are not historically regarded as DMARDs, but a recent study has questioned this belief. A recent report of an Arthritis and Rheumatism Council study showed that, in patients with early RA, 2 years of low-dose prednisolone reduced the rate of radiologically detected disease progression [3]. Interestingly, the anti-inflammatory effect was lost in 3–6 months but the anti-erosive effect continued, suggesting the existence of different mechanisms for inflammation and bone erosion in RA. The issue of osteoporosis was not addressed in this study and routine bone densitometry measurements were not made. This is of critical importance as bone mineral loss occurs rapidly at the beginning of steroid treatment. Active synovitis can cause both local and systemic osteoporosis. The routine use of steroids in early RA is not practised by the authors and remains a controversial issue at present. If patients do receive steroid therapy, then a concurrent 'bone-sparing' agent such as a bisphosphonate should be considered.

DMARDs

The majority of patients with RA are at some time treated with DMARDs. Most patients will have been given one or more agents, often moving down the list of DMARDs after episodes of loss of efficacy or adverse events. For the most part, their mode of action remains unknown and evidence that they improve long-term outcome has not always been very convincing. However, a recent study demonstrates a high risk of relapse if DMARDs are discontinued. The commonly prescribed DMARDs and their side effects are listed in Table 3. Gold and penicillamine are older treatments of RA. They have an efficacy comparable to newer agents but have a slow onset of action and a high incidence of adverse events. Antimalarials (A) are less effective than gold and penicillamine but are also less toxic. Sulphasalazine (S) and methotrexate (M) are now established as the most widely prescribed second-line agents in clinical practice. They have a relatively rapid onset of action and a low incidence of serious adverse events. Weekly low-dose methotrexate has revolutionized DMARD therapy. It is effective in up to 70% of patients with up to 50% of patients tolerating treatment for over 5 years. Azathioprine and

Table 3 Side effects of DMARDs.

Gold	Rashes, mouth ulcers, diarrhoea, glomerulonephritis
Penicillamine	Rashes, taste loss, mouth ulcers, agranulocytosis, thrombocytopenia
Antimalarials	Headache, retinal damage, corneal opacities, alopecia
Azathioprine	Nausea, diarrhoea, agranulocytosis, thrombocytopenia
Sulphasalazine	Nausea, vomiting, haematological abnormalities, azoospermia, lupus-like syndrome
Methotrexate	Nausea, marrow suppression, hepatic fibrosis, pneumonitis, lung fibrosis

cyclophosphamide are comparable in efficacy to gold. However, cyclophosphamide is rarely used due to its toxicity.

Combination DMARD therapy

Combination therapy with DMARDs has long been used in clinical practice but data to support its use have been scarce. O'Dell *et al.* [4] recently published (in abstract form) the results of a 2-year randomized controlled study on combination DMARD therapy. In this study patients were treated with different combinations of up to three DMARDs (MSA, SA or M alone). The combination of methotrexate, sulphasalazine and hydroxychloroquine not only showed greater efficacy than dual or monotherapy but also showed a much greater tolerance with fewer adverse events. From the emerging data it would seem that combination therapy provides a sensible treatment strategy in patients not responding to monotherapy. It will have an important role in the future management of RA.

Cyclosporin A

Cyclosporin A is an established immunosuppressive agent used in transplant medicine which specifically targets T cells. Despite being extremely effective at preventing allograft rejection, its efficacy at low doses in RA is barely comparable to other DMARDs. The risk of nephrotoxicity in RA patients is also a major concern, which will need to be fully evaluated before cyclosporin A can be used in routine clinical practice. It is unlikely to have a role in the treatment of established disease but may have greater efficacy in early RA when the T cell might be playing a significant role in disease pathogenesis.

☐ NOVEL THERAPIES UNDERGOING EVALUATION

The advance in the understanding of the mediators of inflammation has allowed the development of a whole host of new therapies. The majority of new therapies can be divided into those that target cytokines or those that target activated T cells. These therapies are based on the concept that if cytokines or T cells play a role in the disease process then their inhibition will cause disease suppression.

Cytokines are soluble molecules that control cellular communications and mediate the inflammatory response. Cytokines are produced by a variety of cells including macrophages, fibroblasts and lymphocytes. Some are pro-inflammatory (TNFα, IL1, IL6, IL8, IL12 and GM-CSF) and others anti-inflammatory (IL4, IL10 and TGFβ). As more and more cytokines are being characterized, therapeutic agents to inhibit their actions are being developed. Some of the cytokines targeted in RA are shown in Fig. 3. Macrophage- and fibroblast-derived cytokines have been found in abundance in inflamed joints but suprisingly T cell derived cytokines have been difficult to find. We can neatly divide most future therapies into those that are directed against macrophage/fibroblast cytokines, T cells and their cytokines or cytokine products.

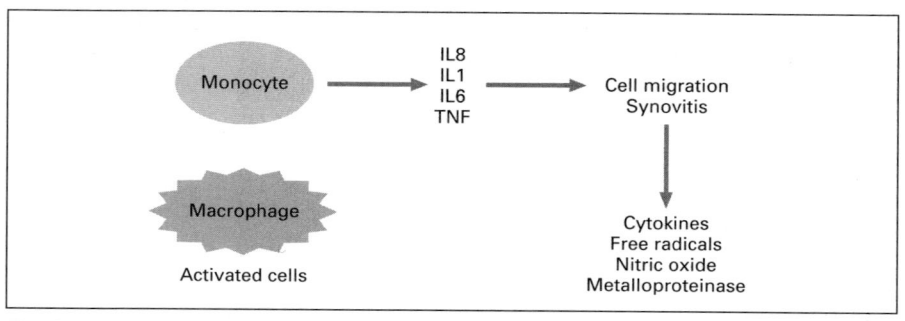

Fig. 3 Potential therapeutic targets in rheumatoid arthritis

Agents directed against macrophage/fibroblast cytokines
Monoclonal antibodies (MoA)
Following the use of MoA in transplant medicine their use is now being evaluated in the treatment of RA. Experience so far has mainly been with monoclonal antibodies targeted against TNFα, T cell epitopes and other receptor–ligand interactions. The important results to date are discussed below.

Anti-TNFα MoA. There is some evidence that TNFα is an important inflammatory mediator in RA [5]. Following encouraging results regarding the safety profile and efficacy of the monoclonal chimeric anti-TNFα antibody cA2 in open trials, a 4-week randomized double-blind placebo-controlled trial was undertaken [6]. The results and major adverse events of this study are summarized in Fig. 4. Elliott concluded from this study that specific cytokine blockade can rapidly suppress inflammation for a short time, but the mode of action was not clear and long-term adverse effects remain unknown.

Anti-IL6 MoA. This treatment (also in a small open study) has shown a transitory improvement in some patients. Somewhat surprisingly the IL6 levels actually increased in four patients with no increase in disease activity.

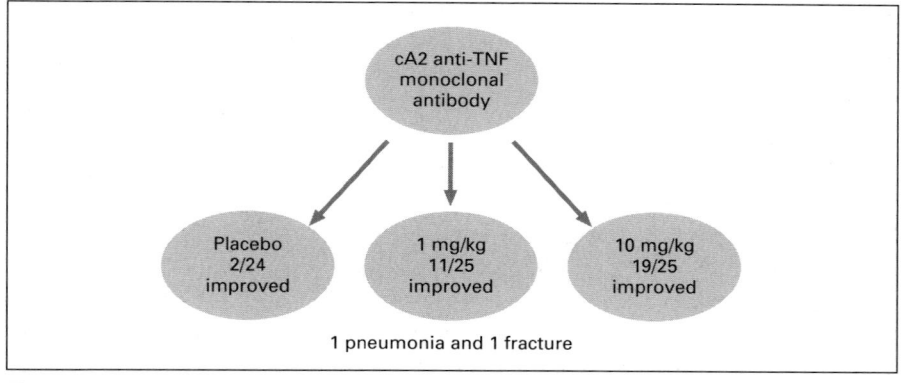

Fig. 4 Four week trial of anti-TNF treatment

Overall it would seem that MoA offer a brief respite during active disease although, apart from anti-TNFα treatment, the results of clinical trials have been disappointing. The side effects experienced with these biologic agents are listed in Table 4.

Table 4 Side effects of monoclonal antibody (MoA) therapy.

Fever, chills, anaphylaxis
Nausea, diarrhoea
Myalgia
Hypotension, seizures
Risk of infection
Carcinogenesis
Human anti-mouse antibodies
Anti-nuclear antibodies

Importantly, patients receiving MoA develop human anti-mouse antibodies that may cause resistance to future treatment and may even be pro-inflammatory. The need for randomized controlled trials and evaluation of long-term toxicity of MoAs is critical if they are to be used in routine clinical practice. The effects of long-term cytokine suppression also need to be studied.

TNFα soluble receptor (TNFsR)

TNFsR is a specific inhibitor of TNFα. Two recent studies published in abstract form have shown a modest improvement in RA patients treated with TNFsR infusions. One of the difficulties has been the extremely short circulating half-life of TNFsR and an immunoconjugate with a longer half-life is being developed for further studies.

IL1 receptor antagonist protein (IRAP)

IL1 is a major pro-inflammatory cytokine which is increased in RA along with its inhibitory receptor protein, IRAP. There is evidence that IRAP production relative to IL1β is defective in RA. An analogue of this protein has shown promising results in animal models of arthritis, but open trials have been less convincing with an increased incidence of infections noted. It also has a very short half-life and is required in great excess of IL1 to cause any inhibition. A European multicentre trial is currently underway and results are awaited.

Tenidap

Tenidap is currently being evaluated as a drug that not only inhibits cyclo-oxygenase but also reduces circulating cytokines IL1, IL6 and TNFα [7]. A 1-year trial is currently underway which has shown encouraging results at an interim analysis. Its long-term acceptance as an effective treatment for RA will require evidence that it improves long-term outcome.

☐ THERAPIES DIRECTED AGAINST THE ACTIVATED T CELL

Monoclonal antibodies

Several open studies using anti-CD4 MoA have shown potential in the treatment of refractory RA with clinical and biochemical improvement demonstrated in many patients. Most patients have shown CD4 depletion and there has been one death due to infection. However, a recent randomized placebo-controlled trial [8] using the anti-CD4 MoA (cM-T412) showed no benefit in patients with active RA after an initial 6 weeks of treatment in 60 patients or after a further 9 months of treatment in 30 of those patients. CAMPATH-IH is a 'humanized' MoA directed against the glycopeptide CD52 which is highly expressed on lymphocytes and macrophages. Despite impressive early *in vivo* experimental results, its use in clinical trials has been disappointing with two deaths recorded due to infection. Anti-CD5 immunoconjugate and anti-CD7 MoA have been unimpressive in clinical trials so far. Anti-IL2 MoA has shown an improvement in more than 50% of patients in a small open study. Further studies are underway. These disappointing results suggest a limited role for the T cell in established RA.

T cell vaccination

Vaccination with attenuated autoimmune T cells has been effective in treating a variety of animal models of autoimmune disease. In RA, activated and attenuated synovial T cells are inoculated into patients, who should then develop an immune response against these cells. As RA is a chronic disease there should be scope for treating all patients. However, the few clinical studies so far in RA patients have failed to show a significant benefit. The major antigenic component of the activated T cell is its receptor, and studies using T cell receptor peptides for vaccination are being tested in animal models of autoimmune disease. These have not yet reached human studies. Although work in this field is progressing it is still in the very early stages of development. The presence of an unknown triggering antigen in RA will also hinder progress.

Oral antigens (collagen II and heat shock proteins)

Experimental autoimmune arthritis has been prevented by oral vaccination with a peptide fragment of type II collagen in several animal studies. From this encouraging experimental work, several open trials in human autoimmune diseases have been undertaken. A variety of oral collagens have now been tested. In one open study complete remission was reported in four out of the 28 RA patients treated. However, the results in larger studies of RA patients have been disappointing, and it is unlikely that oral collagens have a future in the treatment of RA.

☐ BLOCKING THE PRODUCTS OF CYTOKINE ACTION

Non-steroidal anti-inflammatory drugs

Non-steroidal anti-inflammatory drugs (NSAIDs) have long remained the cornerstone of RA treatment. Although they usually produce symptomatic relief through an anti-inflammatory and analgesic effect, they can also cause potentially fatal side effects (Table 5). Despite an improvement in the gastroprotective agents available, there is still a considerable morbidity and mortality from NSAID-induced side effects. NSAIDs produce their therapeutic effect by inhibiting cyclo-oxygenase (COX) and reducing prostaglandin production (Fig. 5). A recent breakthrough in this field has been the identification of two forms of COX. Constitutively expressed COX-1 is important in circumstances where prostaglandins have a protective effect (gastric mucus and renal blood flow) and cytokine-inducible COX-2 is implicated in the production of pro-inflammatory prostanoids [9]. NSAIDs produce their effect by inhibiting both enzymes, but research is now underway to develop anti-inflammatory drugs that selectively inhibit COX-2 activity. It is not anticipated that such drugs will exhibit greater efficacy as many available agents suppress COX-2 adequately.

Matrix metalloproteinase inhibitors

Matrix metalloproteinases (MMPs) are enzymes that have the ability to degrade bone and collagen. Their levels have been shown to be increased in active RA and their release can be stimulated by pro-inflammatory cytokines such as TNFα. MMP inhibitors have already shown encouraging results in attenuating animal models of arthritis in a number of reports. Trials in humans are now being designed.

Table 5 Side effects of NSAIDs.

Gastrointestinal	Nausea, dyspepsia, peptic ulceration
Allergic reactions	Bronchospasm, angio-oedema rashes
Renal	Papillary necrosis, interstitial nephritis
Blood	Agranulocytosis, aplastic anaemia, thrombocytopenia
Cardiovascular	Fluid retention, heart failure
Central nervous system	Headache, vertigo, confusion

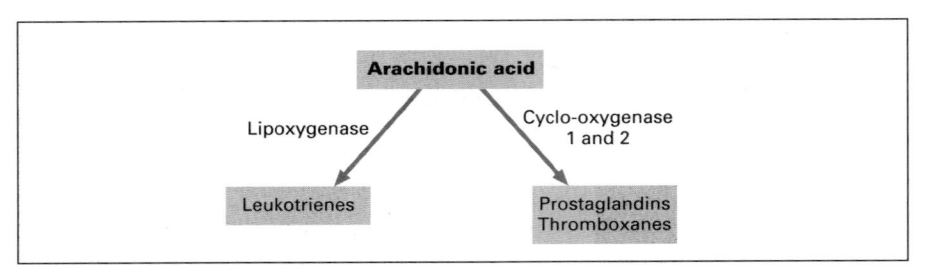

Fig. 5 Arachidonic acid metabolism

MoA to intercellular adhesion molecules (anti-ICAM 1)

Adhesion molecules produced as a result of cytokine stimulation have been successfully targeted in animal models of arthritis. Anti-ICAM 1 has now undergone a phase I/II open study with clinical improvement in some patients. Several patients experienced cutaneous anergy. The disadvantages of MoA treatment are listed in Table 6.

Table 6 Disadvantages of MoA treatment.

Improvement is short-lived
Intravenous administration
Repetitive treatments required
Long period of monitoring for side effects
Resistance to treatment may develop
Cost

☐ THERAPIES ON THE HORIZON

From the evidence given above, it seems unlikely that the T cell plays a significant role in established RA as therapies directed against it have failed to show any significant clinical benefit. It appears that once the inflammatory process has been triggered, the process continues independent of antigen presentation with an imbalance between pro- and anti-inflammatory cytokines being observed. In RA macrophages, fibroblasts and possibly specialized synoviocytes may have developed a certain autonomy resulting in an 'auto-inflammatory' system.

Bioreductive cytotoxic agents

In RA the inflamed synovium is chronically hypoxic [10]. This hypoxic environment of RA stimulates macrophages and fibroblasts to produce cytokines and suppresses T cell activation rendering it anergic. This would neatly explain the cytokine profile seen in RA and the results observed with various new therapies. Bioreductive agents are compounds that are inert until they reach hypoxic tissue where they are metabolized and become cytotoxic. They have already stimulated enormous interest in the field of oncology, where they are used to target hypoxic tumour cells. In RA bioreductive cytotoxic agents could in theory selectively target hypoxic synovium and induce a chemical synovectomy independent of underlying immune mechanisms. These would clearly be an ideal therapy in established RA.

Gene therapy

Gene therapy has made enormous advances in the last decade, with around a hundred clinical trials currently in progress. The potential exists to treat inherited genetic defects and genetically normal individuals with chronic conditions. Genetic treatment will hopefully be long-lasting and cost-effective. Vectors (usually retroviruses) can be used to insert genetic material into patients to stimulate anti-inflammatory mediators. RA is an ideal disease to treat with gene therapy as it offers direct access via the intra-articular route to the diseased tissue, eg delivering the potentially anti-arthritic IRAP gene to synovial lining cells. Promising results have already been seen in the rabbit model using the IRAP gene. However, treatment of a polyarticular disease will be more difficult. Several animal studies are currently underway and it should not be long before we see human studies.

Nitric oxide synthase inhibitors

Nitric oxide (NO) is a free radical gas that is the previously described endothelium-derived relaxing factor. NO is synthesized from L-arginine by nitric oxide synthase (NOS). NO has a role in the pathophysiology of a wide range of biological processes, including immunity and inflammation. The effects of NO on osteoblasts, osteoclasts and chondrocytes are still not clear, with some conflicting results, but there is some *in vitro* evidence that NO stimulates bone resorption [11]. Several animal studies using NOS inhibitors have shown a reduction in the severity of experimentally induced arthritis. There seems a possibility that NOS inhibitors might prevent joint destruction in RA. A major problem will be trying to target the joint without having any effect on constitutive NO. A selective inhibitor of inducible NO is required.

Inhibitors of cytokine production

Selective inhibition of cytokine production remains an attractive option for the treatment of inflammatory diseases (Table 7). A number of therapeutic agents are

Table 7 Targets for cytokine inhibition.

Inhibit cytokine production
Inhibit cytokine action
Inhibit signal transduction
Stimulate anti-inflammatory cytokines
Block consequences of cytokines

now being developed which will inhibit cytokine processing and release. Many different areas in the genetic pathway are being targeted. For example, anti-sense oligonucleotide drugs are agents that can selectively block gene transcription. Other compounds which target cytokine transcription, specific gene promoters, nuclear transcription factors or post-translational processing are being investigated [12].

☐ CONCLUSIONS

The key points in this chapter can be summarized as follows:

- RA requires specialist management in a clinical setting
- RA should be treated early and aggressively to prevent disability
- Combination DMARD therapy may be more effective than monotherapy
- Persistent RA may be a T cell independent process propagated by cytokines derived from macrophages and monocytes
- The hypoxic environment in RA augments this cytokine profile

REFERENCES

1. Panayi GS. The immunopathogenesis of rheumatoid arthritis. *Brit J Rheumatol* 1993; **32** (Suppl 1): 4–14.
2. Emery P, ed. Management of early inflammatory arthritis. In: *Baillière's Clinical Rheumatology*. Baillière Tindall, 1992; **6**(2): 251–61.
3. Kirwan JR. The effect of glucocorticoids on joint destruction in rheumatoid arthritis. The Arthritis and Rheumatism Council Low-Dose Glucocorticoid Study Group. *New Engl J Med* 1995; **333**: 142–6.
4. O'Dell J, Haire C, Erikson N, et al. The efficacy of triple DMARD therapy for rheumatoid arthritis. *Arthritis Rheum* 1994; **37**: S295.
5. Maini RN, Elliott M, Brennan FM, Williams RO, Feldmann M. Targeting TNF alpha for the therapy of rheumatoid arthritis. *Clin Exp Rheumatol* 1994; **12**(Suppl 11): S63–6.
6. Elliott MJ, Maini RN, Feldmann M, et al. Randomised double-blind comparison of chimeric monoclonal antibody to tumour necrosis factor alpha(cA2) versus placebo in RA. *Lancet* 1994; **344**: 1105–10.
7. Madhok R. Tenidap. *Lancet* 1995; **346**: 481–5.
8. van der Lubbe PA, Dijkmans BAC, Markusse HM, Nassander U, Breedveld FC. A randomised, double-blind, placebo-controlled study of CD4 monoclonal therapy in early rheumatoid arthritis. *Arthritis Rheum* 1995; **38**: 1097–106.
9. Seibert K, Masferrer J, Zhang Y, et al. Mediation of inflammation by cyclooxygenase-2. *Agents Actions Suppl* 1995; **46**: 41–50.
10. Stevens CR, Williams RB, Farrell AJ, Blake DR. Hypoxia and inflammatory synovitis: observations and speculation. *Ann Rheum Dis* 1991; **50**: 124–32.
11. Farrell AJ, Blake DR. Nitric oxide. *Ann Rheum Dis* 1996; **55**: 7–20.
12. Firestein GS. Cytokine networks in rheumatoid arthritis: implications for therapy. *Agents Actions Suppl* 1995; **47**: 37–51.

☐ MULTIPLE CHOICE QUESTIONS

1 Corticosteroids:
   (a) Should be prescribed for all RA patients
   (b) Should never be prescribed in RA
   (c) Have no anti-inflammatory effect
   (d) Cause osteoporosis only after long-term treatment
   (e) Require concomitant treatment with a 'bone sparing agent'

2 DMARDs may cause:
   (a) Thrombocytopenia
   (b) Skin rashes
   (c) Lung cancer
   (d) Azoospermia
   (e) Pericarditis

3   The following are pro-inflammatory cytokines:
    (a) IL4
    (b) IL1
    (c) TGFβ
    (d) IL6
    (e) TNFα

4   Tenidap:
    (a) Is a DMARD
    (b) Inhibits IL4
    (c) Inhibits cyclo-oxygenase
    (d) Stimulates TGFβ
    (e) Inhibits IL1

5   In rheumatoid arthritis:
    (a) T cell vaccination is effective
    (b) Cytokines are increased
    (c) Monoclonal antibodies are a safe therapy
    (d) Gene therapy is effective
    (e) The synovium is hypoxic

ANSWERS

1a False	2a True	3a False	4a False	5a False
b False	b True	b True	b False	b True
c False	c False	c False	c True	c False
d False	d True	d True	d False	d False
e True	e False	e True	e True	e True

Scleroderma spectrum disorders

C M Black

☐ INTRODUCTION – THE SPECTRUM

Scleroderma spectrum disorders include: Raynaud's (primary and secondary); systemic sclerosis with its two major subgroups: diffuse and limited; localized scleroderma (divided into morphea, linear and *en coup de sabre*); scleroderma occurring in childhood; environmentally induced scleroderma-like diseases; overlap syndromes; undifferentiated autoimmune rheumatic diseases; and localized fibroses (Table 1).

Most of the scleroderma spectrum disorders can develop at any stage of life, although scleroderma occurring in childhood is different from that in the adult, with the localized forms of scleroderma predominating. Most of these disorders show female predominance, although environmentally induced disease, except for that associated with the toxic oil syndrome, occurs mainly in males in association with chemical exposure. The disease we call systemic sclerosis has also been confused with other diseases that have cutaneous features resembling it, eg scleroedema, primary amyloidosis and scleromyxoedema. The first clinical task is therefore to classify the condition as each clinical grouping will have its own features, pattern of progression, prognosis and treatment possibilities [1].

Table 1 Spectrum of scleroderma and scleroderma-like syndromes.

Raynaud's phenomenon	Primary Raynaud's Secondary Raynaud's
Scleroderma—localized	Morphea (plaque, guttate, generalized) Linear *En coup de sabre*
Scleroderma—systemic	Limited cutaneous systemic sclerosis Diffuse cutaneous systemic sclerosis Scleroderma sine scleroderma
Juvenile onset scleroderma	Localized (morphea, linear, *en coup de sabre*) Systemic sclerosis
Chemically induced	Environmental/occupational Drugs
Scleroderma-like diseases	Metabolic, eg carcinoid syndrome, scleromyxoedema Immunological/inflammatory, eg eosinophilic fasciitis, overlap syndromes Localized systemic sclerosis and visceral diseases, eg infiltrating cardiomyopathy, sarcoidosis

LOCALIZED SCLERODERMA

Scleroderma is a word meaning 'hard skin' and at one end of the spectrum is localized disease (morphea and linear scleroderma), where dermal inflammation and fibrosis are prominent with a virtual absence of vascular pathology [2]. These syndromes are almost never associated with systemic involvement but may demonstrate abnormal autoimmune serology and inflammatory histology. Sometimes localized scleroderma and eosinophilic fasciitis, a rare connective tissue disorder, merge or overlap, appearing either together or sequentially. Juveniles may develop any form of scleroderma, but fortunately there is a predilection for these localized forms, in which the skin, subcutaneous fascia, muscle and bone are the main organs to be attacked. The extent of fibrosis and atrophy are the major problems and severe growth defects can occur, which in adult life may require extensive plastic surgery, orthopaedic surgery, or in extreme cases amputation. There is no consensus of opinion as to how to treat these excessively uncommon disorders in childhood. Clinical experience would indicate that therapy is often inadequate, lagging behind disease activity and possibly not continued for long enough. A summary of localized disease is found in Table 2 [3].

ENVIRONMENTAL FACTORS

The range of known agents that can induce a systemic sclerosis-like disease is large and growing (Table 3) [1]. Although it must be noted that, in formal epidemiological studies, no excess has been found, it is almost certain that sporadic cases can follow certain occupational exposures, but both the absolute and the attributable risks are low. Major histocompatibility complex (MHC) associations have been reported with some environmentally induced cases; for example, vinyl chloride disease (VCD) is primarily associated with DR4 and DR3 which is a marker of severity. Toxic oil syndrome is characterized by a raised incidence of DR4. The newest arrivals to the group of environmentally induced scleroderma-like syndromes are the eosinophilic myalgic syndrome associated with the oral ingestion of an essential amino acid L-tryptophan and an ongoing interest in the possible association between disease development and silicone breast implants. Much of the work in this area has been generated by the need to obtain accurate data because of the considerable litigation, particularly in the USA. To date, none of the available studies has demonstrated a statistical association between augmentation mammoplasty with silicone gel-filled prostheses, scleroderma or other autoimmune disorders.

RAYNAUD'S PHENOMENON

Raynaud's phenomenon is now best classified as either primary or secondary (the terms Raynaud's disease and Raynaud's syndrome should be abandoned and replaced by these more accurate simple descriptive terms) [4]. The overall prevalence of this phenomenon in the population has been variably assessed as between 3% and 10% of adults worldwide. The prevalence varies somewhat

Table 2 Localized scleroderma in adults and children. (From Black and Denton [3] by permission of Oxford University Press.)

Pattern of disease	Clinical features	Treatment	Prognosis
Localized morphea	One or a few circumscribed sclerotic plaques with hypo- or hyperpigmentation and an inflamed violaceous border	Often unnecessary Serial measurement to assess progress	Good prognosis, lesions less active within 3 years but pigmentary changes often persist
Generalized morphea	Widespread pruritic lesions, often symmetrical and following the distribution of superficial veins	Suppress inflammation with oral or i.v. steroids Maintenance treatment with D-penicillamine (at least 500 mg/day). Methotrexate and systemic or intralesional interferon may be effective, and cyclosporin has been used in refractory cases	Internal organ pathology very rare. Raynaud's seldom associated. Generally improves within 5 years of onset although textural and pigmentary changes can remain
Linear scleroderma	Sclerotic areas occurring in linear distribution often on limbs and asymmetrical. In childhood can lead to serious growth defect of affected limbs. Careful, serial measurement of muscle bulk and limb length is essential	Suppression of inflammation with oral or i.v. steroids. Maintenance treatment with D-penicillamine or methotrexate Physiotherapy and appropriate regular exercise to minimize growth defect in childhood onset form	Long-term effects of childhood onset form minimized by effective suppression of inflammatory process, and by good physiotherapy. Ultimately the disease tends to resolve, but it can remain active for many years
En coup de sabre	Linear scleroderma affecting the face and scalp, involving underlying subcutaneous tissues, muscles periosteum and bone. Underlying cerebral abnormalities have been reported	Therapeutic options as for scleroderma, systemic sclerosis only for active inflammatory lesions	Scarring, growth defects and alopecia persist but inflammatory component settles

depending on climate, skin colour, ethnic background and occupational exposure to vibrating machines. Raynaud's phenomenon can be a forerunner of one of the autoimmune rheumatic diseases and important clues to Raynaud's secondary to scleroderma are listed in Table 4. Two inexpensive, non-invasive procedures are good predictors for patients in the Raynaud's group who will develop systemic sclerosis in

Table 3 Chemical agents implicated in the development of scleroderma. (From Black and Stephens [1] by permission of Oxford University Press.)

Organic chemicals	Silica	Drugs

Aliphatic hydrocarbons
  Chlorinated
    vinyl chloride
    trichlorethylene
    perchlorethylene
  Non-chlorinated
    naphtha-n-hexane
 	
Aromatic hydrocarbons
  Benzene
  Toluene
  Xylene
  Mixtures, eg diesel fuel,
    white spirit
	Stone masons
	Coal miners
	Gold miners
	Foundry workers
	
	Toxic oil (aniline-treated rapeseed oil)
	Epoxy resins
	Foam insulation (urea-formaldehyde)
	Metaphenylene diamine (biogenic amine)
	Augmentation mammoplasty (silicone,
	    paraffin)
		Bleomycin
		L-5-Hydroxytryptophan
		Appetite suppressants
		  diethylpropion
		    hydrochloride
		  mazindol
		  fenfluramine
		Pentazocine
		Carbidopa
		Cocaine
		Amide-type local
		  anaesthetics

Table 4 Raynaud's phenomenon: factors useful in predicting outcome.

Good	Bad
Teenage and early 20s onset	Infancy and childhood onset
Stable symptoms	Later onset 35 years +
Familial Raynaud's	Increasingly severe symptoms
Normal capillaries	Male with no family history or environmental exposure
No antinuclear antibodies	Abnormal capillaries
	Disease-specific antinuclear antibodies

the future. These tests, serum autoantibody determination and nailfold capillary microscopy, should be performed in all Raynaud's patients. Autoantibody production is an early and almost universal feature of scleroderma patients. About 97% of patients with scleroderma have detectable antinuclear antibodies when HEp_2 lines are used as the detection tissue. In a prospective study of primary Raynaud's and undifferentiated autoimmune rheumatic diseases, Kallenberg [5], using the immunoblot method, found that the presence of antinuclear antibodies at the time of entry into the study was associated with the evolution of an autoimmune rheumatic disease, usually scleroderma. Furthermore, in those who initially presented with Raynaud's disease alone, anticentromere antibody had a predictive value for the development of limited cutaneous scleroderma (sensitivity 6%, specificity 98%), Scl-70 for diffuse cutaneous systemic sclerosis (sensitivity 38%, specificity 100%).

    Direct observation of nailfold capillary beds dates back almost 70 years and was introduced by German investigators. Recent refinements in techniques have permitted permanent photographic recording of a row of horizontal capillary loops at the nailfold, just proximal to the cuticle. The characteristic pattern of enlargement and loss which is seen in patients with a connective tissue disorder is a useful diagnostic tool. It appears early in the disease and is remarkably constant over time (Fig. 1). Autoantibody detection and nailfold capillaroscopy together detect more

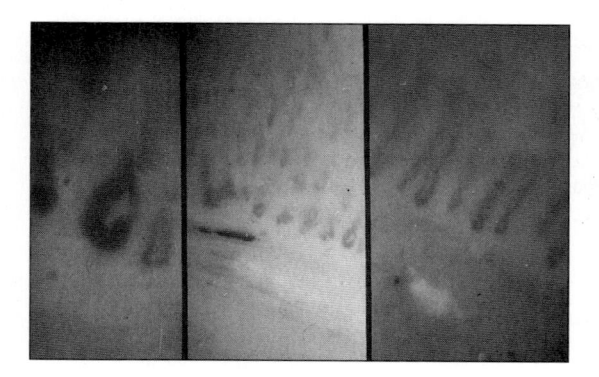

Fig. 1 Nailfold capillary photography. Left: normal regularly formed capillary loops. Centre: capillary loops in scleroderma; the outlines are fainter and less regular and there is subcuticular capillary haemorrhage. Right: capillary loops are large and of a bizarre shape.

than 90% of patients destined to have generalized systemic sclerosis. Of the 3–10% of the population with Raynaud's, up to 15% are positive for one or both procedures. These recent observations are now leading to a reduction in the number of patients diagnosed with true primary Raynaud's and an increase in the number of potential autoimmune rheumatic disease patients. There is no evidence that symptomatic treatment of Raynaud's phenomenon in any way influences the evolution of systemic sclerosis. However, once the mechanisms of vascular damage and fibrosis are better understood, the predictive power of these two tests possibly coupled with other serological or genetic markers ought to allow for a more preventive approach. The number of autoantibody targets identified in systemic sclerosis (SSc) patients continues to grow (Table 5); the major ones are topoisomerase-1, centromeric proteins and ribonucleic acid (RNA) polymerases I, II and III. Anti-RNA polymerase antibodies are the latest scleroderma-specific antibodies to be described. Disease-specific antibodies segregate with the different subsets of systemic sclerosis and particular organ involvement.

☐ SYSTEMIC SCLEROSIS

The prevalence and impact of systemic sclerosis (scleroderma; SSc) makes it the most important of the 'scleroderma spectrum' disorders. It is a multisystem disease predominantly affecting females and of unknown cause. Understanding and managing the disease are made possible by a combination of accurate subsetting, including recognition of the Raynaud's population at risk, staging the subsets and monitoring the internal organs by relevant investigations at appropriate intervals. Therapy may then be matched as closely as possible to the current knowledge of the pathogenic process. Such knowledge is still in its infancy and until a better

Table 5 Autoantibodies in scleroderma.

Antigen	Molecular identity	Immunofluorescence pattern	disease subtype frequency
Kinetochore centromere	17, 80, 140 kDa proteins at inner and outer kinetochore	Centromere	70–80% in limited cutaneous systemic sclerosis 9–29% with primary biliary cirrhosis
Scleroderma-70 (topoisomerase)	100 kDa protein degrades >70 kDa	Nuclear (diffuse fine speckles)	Up to 40% with diffuse cutaneous systemic sclerosis 10–15% limited
RNA polymerase I, II, III	Complex of 13 proteins 12.5–210 kDa	Nucleolar (punctate)	23% especially diffuse; high prevalence of renal involvement
Fibrillarin	34 kDa protein – component of U3 ribonucleoprotein	Nucleolar (clumpy)	6% (immunofluorescence) 60% by fibrillarin fusion protein assay; clinical association uncertain ? less articular disease
PM-Scl	Complex of 11 proteins 20–110 kDa	Nucleolar (homogeneous)	3% high prevalence of myositis
To or Th	40 kDa protein associated with 7–2 and 8–2 kDa ribonucleic acids	Nucleolar (homogeneous)	rare – lc systemic sclerosis
Mitochondrial M2	70 kDa protein-dihydrolipoamide acyltransferase	Cytoplasmic (rod-like)	25% of CREST (95% primary biliary cirrhosis)

CREST – calcinosis, Raynaud's, esophagus, sclerodactyly, telangiectasiae

understanding of pathogenesis is achieved the aim of therapy is to halt disease progression and prevent further extension. The major pathological processes occurring in scleroderma are increased deposition of extracellular matrix in the skin and internal organs [6], apparently resulting from disruption of the normal steady-state turnover of connective tissue and regulated repair, vascular change and immune cell activation (Fig. 2) [3]. It is thought that these processes are closely related. Currently, the most favoured explanation for them indicates widespread intimal vascular damage, and/or activation occurring as a result of immune or non-immune mediated events, which result in increased vascular permeability and leucocyte/endothelial adhesions with subsequent leucocyte migration into the interstitium. Either concomitantly with, or following on from, these inflammatory events, mediators are released and there is an expansion of fibrogenic clones of tissue fibroblasts which seem to accompany clinical progression. Ultimately, these cells appear to behave relatively autonomously. One of their hallmarks is an

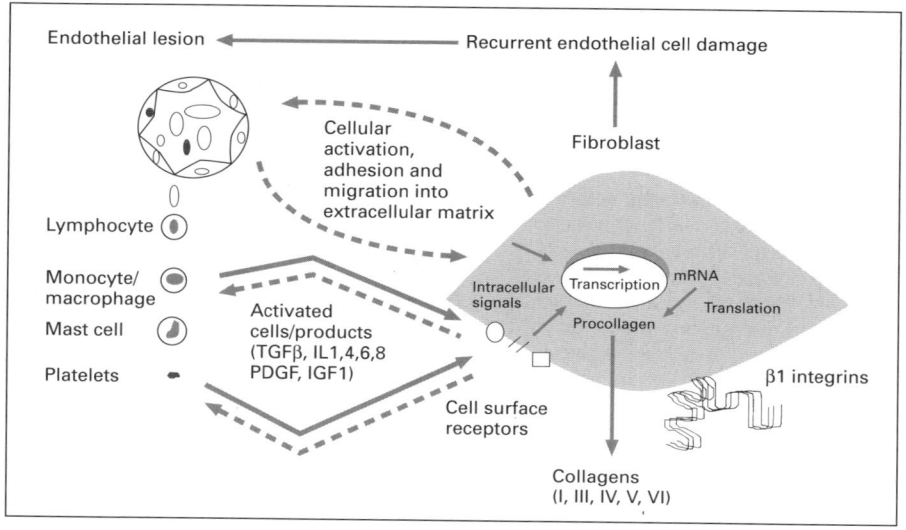

Fig. 2 Interactions between endothelial cells, leucocytes and fibroblasts in scleroderma pathogenesis. (From Black and Denton [3] by permission of Oxford University Press.)

overexpression of genes encoding extracellular matrix components. The ultimate clinical outcome of these processes is organ dysfunction.

Classification

Classification of systemic sclerosis is difficult and a number of different systems have been proposed. Currently, the most widely used classification defines two subsets based on the extent of skin involvement, together with a number of reliable clinical, laboratory and natural history associations. The two subset model divides the disease into limited cutaneous systemic sclerosis (lcSSc) and diffuse cutaneous systemic sclerosis (dcSSc) and for completeness the 'pre-scleroderma' group and the rare scleroderma sine scleroderma have been included in Table 6. Over 60% of scleroderma patients fall into the subset lcSSc where visceral involvement is a late event and tends to occur 10–30 years after the onset of Raynaud's. The term lcSSc is preferable to CREST because cutaneous manifestations often extend beyond sclerodactyly, and the late onset of pulmonary hypertension and/or gut disease makes CREST an inadequate descriptive term for many patients in this group. The more serious form of the disease (dcSSc) is usually much more rapid in onset, with organ failure often present within 5 years of the first symptoms, and renal crisis being a definite risk within the first 3 years. This classification is simple and will almost certainly be changed and developed as knowledge of the pathogenesis of the disorder advances and the ever increasing number of autoantibodies are matched to clinical subsets. The antibody profile currently permits the association of scleroderma-70 with pulmonary fibrosis, polymerase I and III with renal disease, and a useful negative association of anticentromere antibodies with pulmonary

Table 6 Classification of the systemic sclerosis subsets.

Pre-Scleroderma
Raynaud's phenomenon plus nailfold capillary changes, disease-specific circulating antinuclear antibodies (topoisomerase-1, anti-centromere, RNA polymerases I, II, III), and digital ischaemic changes.

Diffuse cutaneous systemic sclerosis (dcSSc)
Onset of skin changes (puffy or hidebound) within 1 year of onset of Raynaud's
Truncal and acral skin involvement
Presence of tendon friction rubs
Early and significant incidence of interstitial lung disease, oliguric renal failure, diffuse gastrointestinal disease, and myocardial involvement
Nailfold capillary dilatation and drop-out
Anti-topoisomerase-1 (anti-topo) antibodies (30% of patients), RNA polymerase antibodies I, II, III (20–25%)

Limited cutaneous systemic sclerosis (lcSSc)
Raynaud's for years (occasionally decades)
Skin involvement limited to hands, face, feet and forearms (acral)
A significant (10–15 years) late incidence of pulmonary hypertension, with or without interstitial lung disease, skin calcifications, telangiectasia and gastrointestinal involvement
A high incidence of ACA (70–80%)
Dilated nailfold capillary loops, usually without capillary drop-out

Scleroderma sine scleroderma
Raynaud's +/−
No skin involvement
Presentation with pulmonary fibrosis, scleroderma renal crisis, cardiac disease, gastrointestinal disease
Antinuclear antibodies may be present (anti-topo, ACA, nucleolar)

---

fibrosis and renal scleroderma. An example of the power of autoantibody analysis is given in Fig. 3.

Subsetting

Disease staging within a subset is equally important as it helps us approach the patient's course prognosis and treatment requirements in a logical manner. The typical natural history for development of visceral complications in dcSSc and lcSSc is shown in Fig. 4 [7]. There is variability in the pace of the disease within each subset and, whereas some patients with diffuse disease develop extensive internal organ involvement within 2 to 4 years, others have widespread skin disease and minimal internal organ dysfunction. In the lcSSc group some 10% of the group will develop pulmonary hypertension, whereas others will have no more than severe Raynaud's, ulcers and oesophageal dysmotility. Therefore not only is there disease heterogeneity but differential progression within a subset. Not withstanding these problems, it is useful to stage the disease, because it permits the doctor, the patient and his or her family to anticipate certain developments which will concentrate attention on early detection and correct management of complications. The investigation of patients

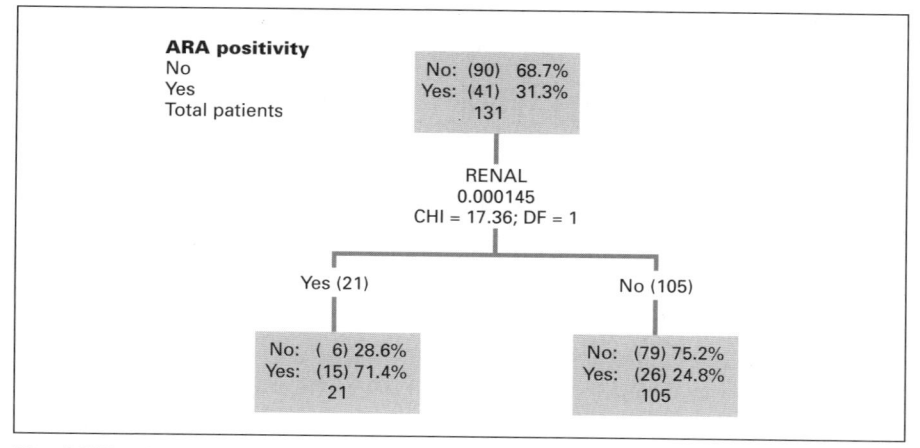

Fig. 3 RNA polymerase AB and renal disease.

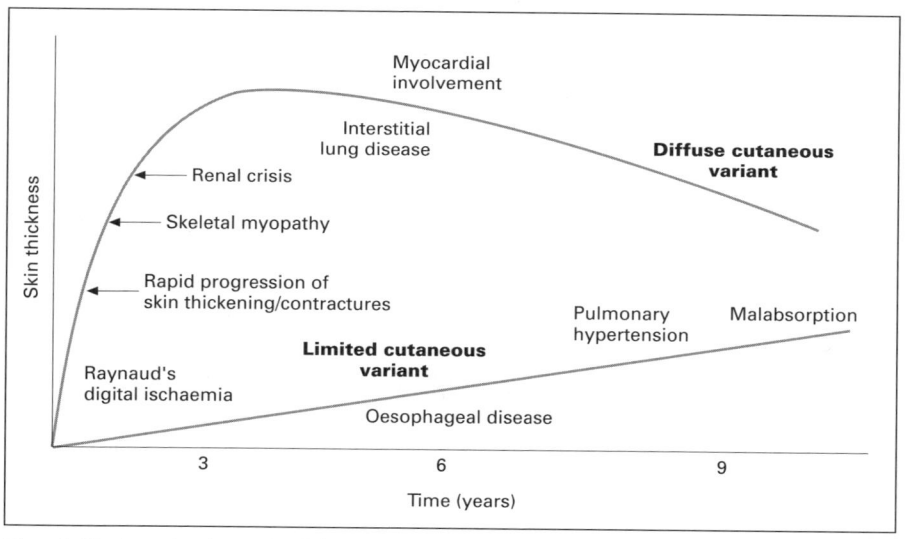

Fig. 4 Staging: development of internal organ complications in limited and diffuse cutaneous systemic sclerosis. (From Medsger [7] with permission.)

with systemic sclerosis should be adapted to the subset and stage of the individual patient's disease.

☐ ORGAN INVOLVEMENT

William Osler stated, many years ago, that 'patients with scleroderma are prone to succumb to pulmonary complaints or to nephritis'. This is still true today, although with the improved management of hypertensive renal crisis (Fig. 5) lung disease is now the major cause of death [8]. The long-term dangers of internal organ

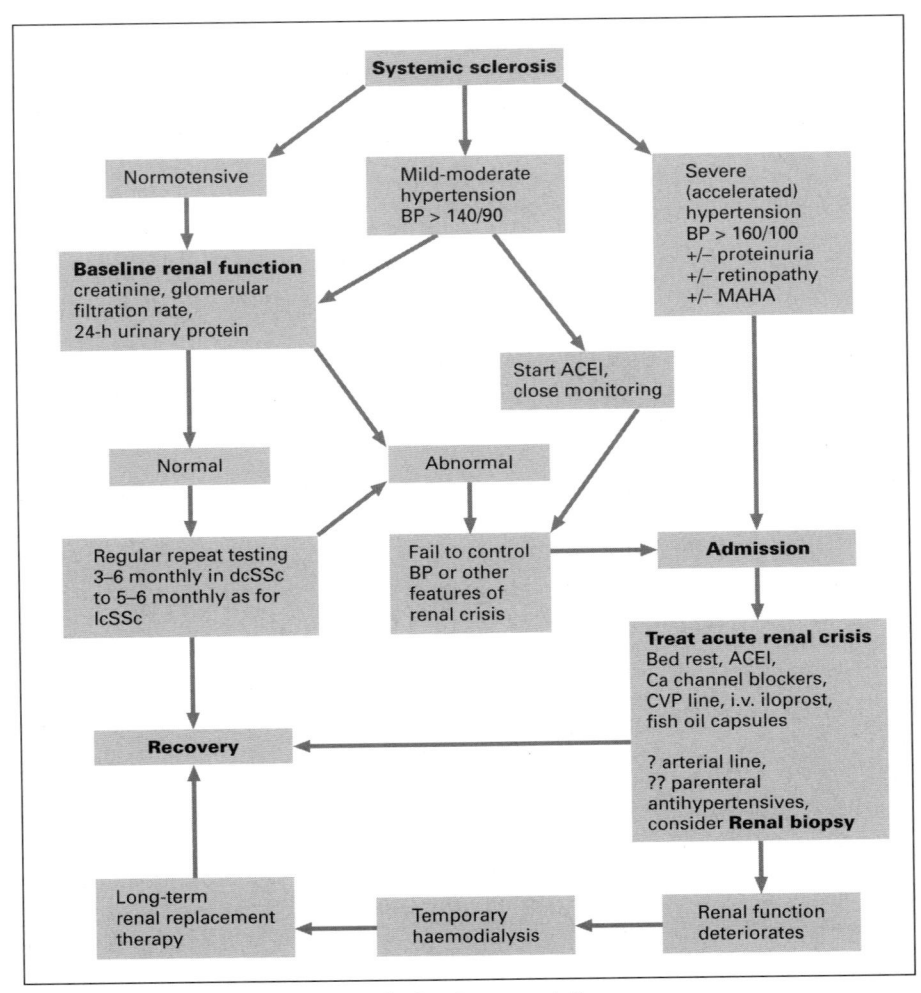

Fig. 5 Algorithm for the management of scleroderma renal disease.

involvement necessitate the earliest possible recognition of organ based pathology. The investigation and management of lung disease have improved considerably, reflecting recent advances in investigation and treatment, and these will be discussed in some detail [9–11].

Lung disease

The two major clinical manifestations of lung involvement are fibrosing alveolitis and pulmonary vascular disease. Pulmonary fibrosis occurs in more than 75% of patients with SSc, and pulmonary vascular disease in approximately 15%. Postmortem reports have always yielded higher percentages than clinical studies. In the past 5 years there have been improvements in the early diagnosis and management of interstitial lung disease. There are now predictors of involvement and tools for early diagnosis, predictors of histological type, prognosis, and therefore survival, and predictors of progression. The investigation of pulmonary hypertension is not so well advanced, but the group at risk can be broadly identified, if not yet precisely targeted, and non-invasive serial monitoring can identify early rises in pulmonary artery pressure [12].

Interstitial lung disease

Interstitial lung disease often develops insidiously, but once established into a reticular pattern is irreversible with present-day therapy. Early diagnosis is therefore vital and genetic markers and autoantibodies may help to identify this group at presentation. The presence of the genetic markers DR3/DR52a and antibodies to topoisomerase-1 (Scl-70) in a patient with scleroderma denote a 16.7 relative risk of developing interstitial lung disease. The chest radiograph is an insensitive indicator of fibrosing alveolitis, and should be used only as an initial screen or to exclude infection or aspiration secondary to oesophageal abnormalities. When used, a high KV film should be requested. There are many symptomatic patients (often mildly so) with normal chest radiographs, and lung function tests have, until recently, been used as the discriminating tests. The single-breath diffusion test (DLCO) is abnormal in over 70% of patients with dcSSc, including asymptomatic patients with no complaints and an unremarkable chest radiograph. A reduction in DLCO is the earliest proven functional abnormality in patients with SSc who develop interstitial lung disease. Lung function tests which show normal volumes but reduced gas transfer in the face of normal imaging are suggestive of pure pulmonary vascular disease. Measurement of the alveolar-arterial oxygen difference during exercise also appears to be a sensitive indicator of lung disease in SSc.

The application of thin (3 mm) section (high-resolution) computerized tomography (CT) scanning of the lungs (Table 7) over the past 5 years has revolutionized the approach to diffuse lung diseases and has revealed the character and distribution of fine structural abnormalities not visible on chest radiograph. It is important to perform prone as well as supine scans, particularly in more subtle cases, to exclude the contribution of gravity to the radiographic appearances due to vascular and interstitial pooling in the dependent areas. Using this technique, the earliest detectable abnormality is usually a narrow, often ill-defined, subpleural crescent of increased density in the posterior segments of the lower lobes (Fig. 6). When more extensive, the shadowing often takes on a more characteristic

Table 7 Role of high-resolution computerized tomography (HRCT).

Improves the sensitivity of diagnosis
Predicts relative degree of cellularity and fibrosis within the lung
Improves the assessment of treatment response and prognosis
Identifies change in disease extent not identifiable using other tools
Does not indicate progression

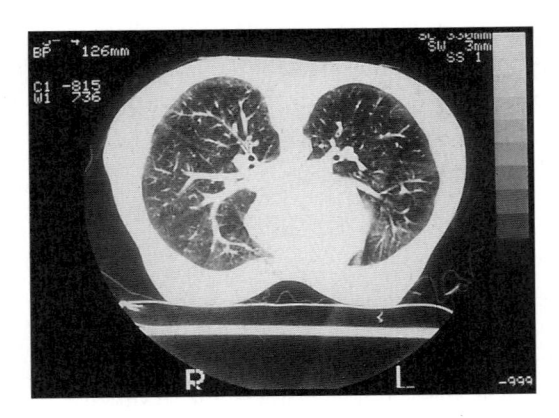

Fig. 6 Early interstitial lung disease. The scan shows a subpleural crescent of increased density.

reticulonodular appearance yet frequently retains a subpleural distribution. It also becomes associated with fine honeycomb air spaces and ultimately larger cystic air spaces – an appearance that mirrors the macroscopic appearance. A semi-quantitative comparison of the predictive value of these CT appearances to mirror biopsy evidence of an inflammatory alveolitis has been performed, and a 'ground glass' pattern of opacification on CT is associated with a predominantly cellular biopsy, whereas an abnormal reticular pattern was found in patients whose subsequent lung biopsy confirms a particularly fibrotic disease process.

In addition to identifying early disease, high-resolution CT scanning can identify a pattern of disease that predicts a better response to therapy and a better prognosis and therefore survival. Furthermore, the extent of disease present, defined by CT within the lavage lobe, correlates with the predominant type of inflammatory cell obtained by bronchoalveolar lavage of that same lobe: lymphocytes are present in excess before CT identifies disease; eosinophils appear as the lung becomes abnormal; neutrophils are found in greatest abundance when at least 50% of the lavage lobe is involved in the disease process, ie the predominant type of inflammatory cell traffic into the lungs depends on disease extent. This would suggest that different inflammatory cells are involved in different stages of disease pathogenesis. The extent of lung involved on CT can also be used in therapeutic studies to give a more sensitive measure of change than other parameters. The value of bronchoalveolar lavage prognostically has been demonstrated in several studies and it has been shown that scleroderma patients with persistent alveolitis have greater deterioration in their pulmonary function than alveolitis-negative patients with systemic sclerosis. Bronchoalveolar lavage is not, however, a test that can be easily repeated on a regular basis – it is not 'patient friendly'.

The role of ^{99}Tc-labelled diethylenetriamine penta-acetic acid (DTPA) in the management of systemic sclerosis has been the subject of extensive study and has been shown to be of value, particularly as a marker of stability or progression [10]. It identifies early disease and also identifies a group of patients whose disease will run a more stable non-progressive course, ie those with normal clearance. The speed of clearance of the isotope depends on the integrity of the epithelial barrier and therefore anything that disrupts this, either inflammation or fibrosis, will increase the rate of clearance, eg smoking. In systemic sclerosis, clearance of DTPA may be abnormal even when chest radiography and pulmonary function tests are normal. In established disease, clearance is enhanced compared with normal individuals. Rate and pattern of clearance can predict subsequent changes in pulmonary function tests. Moreover, patients whose clearance is persistently abnormal are more likely to have a deterioration in pulmonary function test at follow-up after the DTPA measurements. In contrast, persistently normal DTPA clearance rates predict stable disease and therefore provide a good prognostic index. Significant improvement in pulmonary function tests occurred in 75% patients whose clearance returned to the normal range, whereas similar improvements were not seen in patients whose clearance remained normal or abnormally fast. Using these tools for diagnosis and serial monitoring, an algorithm can be drawn up for the investigation and treatment of fibrotic lung disease (Fig. 7).

Pulmonary hypertension

Pulmonary vascular disease is a more deadly complication of systemic sclerosis with no drugs as yet known to influence its ultimate outcome. Pulmonary hypertension

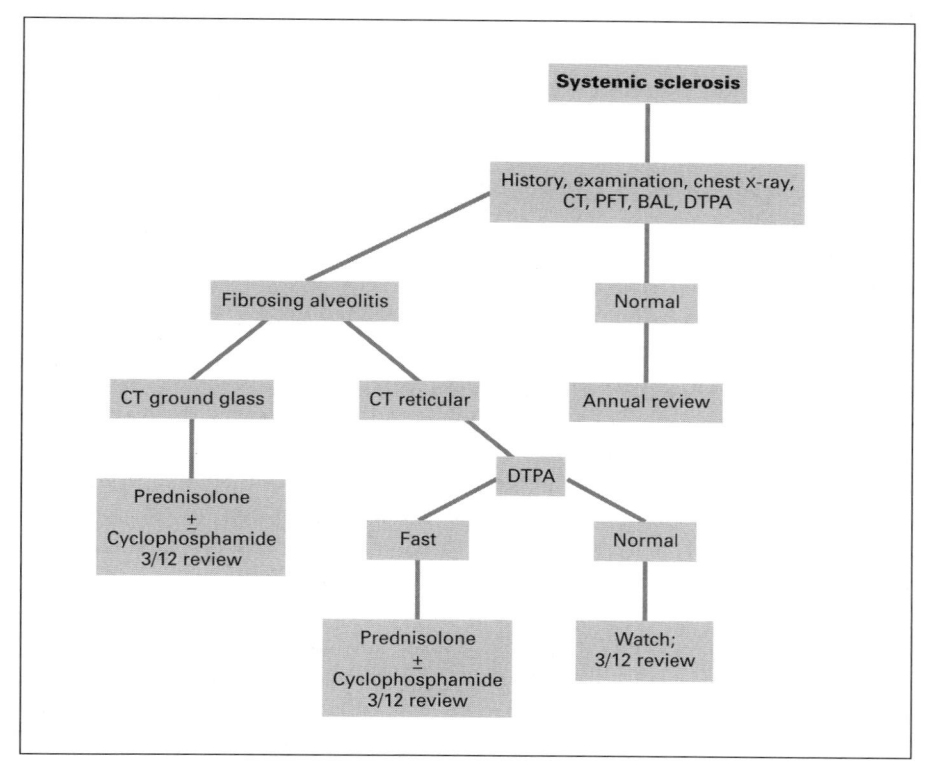

Fig. 7 Algorithm for the investigation and treatment of fibrotic lung disease. BAL, bronchoalveolar lavage; PFT, pulmonary function tests.

occurs in both the limited (lcSSc) and diffuse (dcSSc) cutaneous subsets of the disease. The major focus of interest is, however, isolated pulmonary hypertension which occurs in the absence of significant pulmonary fibrosis. This is the pattern of pulmonary disease that occurs most commonly in limited SSc. Unless screened prospectively, pulmonary hypertension will be picked up late when the patient is symptomatic either with breathlessness or cardiac failure. The defining test for pulmonary vascular disease is cardiac catheterization. It is obviously not practical to carry this out in a large series or to carry it out prospectively on a serial basis. Screening tests based on clinical examination, electrocardiograph (ECG) and X-ray findings are insensitive and will only pick up established disease. Lung function tests can be helpful and a reduction in carbon monoxide transfer factor in the absence of substantially reduced lung volumes raises the strong possibility of pulmonary vascular disease. More specific diagnostic tests are therefore needed and currently the most useful non-invasive technique available is echo-Doppler. This approach has proven reliable in practice and has been used to provide an estimate of pulmonary artery pressure in a variety of chronic lung diseases. The use of this modality should help to identify pulmonary hypertension in connective tissue diseases, and hopefully lead to earlier diagnosis of mild cases of pulmonary hypertension in SSc when the condition would be expected to be most amenable to treatment. A recent study (accepted for publication [16]) compared the information obtained by echo-cardiographic assessment with that from right-heart catheterization in 33 SSc patients in whom clinical assessment including ECG, chest X-ray, lung function tests and high-resolution CT had raised strong suspicion of pulmonary hypertension. The mean (SD) interval between echocardiography and right-heart catheterization was 1.8 (2.3) months. Twenty-one patients (64%) had pulmonary hypertension (pulmonary artery systolic pressure ≥30mmHg) on right-heart catheterization, and echocardiography correctly identified 19 of these (sensitivity 90%). Of the 12 patients without pulmonary hypertension on right-heart catheterization, nine were correctly identified by echocardiography (specificity 75%). The five incorrectly classified patients all had pulmonary artery systolic pressure in the borderline normal/abnormal range. Doppler estimation of pulmonary artery systolic pressure was possible in 20 patients (61%) and correlated highly with right-heart catheterization values ($r = 0.83$, $p < 0.001$), with a sensitivity for the diagnosis of pulmonary hypertension of 100%. We conclude from this study that echo-cardiography is a sensitive and specific method for determining the presence or absence of significant pulmonary vascular disease in SSc. The non-invasive nature of this test, compared with right-heart catheterization, makes it particularly appropriate in this group of patients, in whom screening might lead to earlier identification of this potentially fatal complication, and allow response to therapy to be more readily evaluated. Our current practice is to perform echo-Dopplers and lung function tests annually on all patients with lcSSc and a disease duration of more than 5 years and to increase this to more frequent observations if required. Possible therapies for pulmonary hypertension are listed in Table 8. Therapy to date has been disappointing, but in most cases it has been introduced at a late stage. The introduction of life-long anticoagulation or prostacyclin infusions has yet to be

Table 8 Pulmonary hypertension.

Therapies currently in use	Therapies under consideration
Oral vasodilators	Oral Iloprost
Nifedipine	Inhaled – PEI$_2$, Iloprost
Diltiazem	ET-1 receptor antagonists
Captopril	L-Arginine
Anticoagulation	
Warfarin	
Intravenous therapy	
Prostacyclin PEI$_2$	
Prostacyclin analogue Iloprost	

evaluated in early disease. These therapies are of reported value in primary pulmonary hypertension [13] and 24 h ambulatory prostacyclin has just received FDA approval for primary pulmonary hypertension. The introduction of these other therapies when there may be a reversible component to the hypertension is an exciting opportunity in this lethal complication.

An approach to therapy of systemic sclerosis is summarized in Tables 9–11. At present there is no cure for scleroderma, but there are therapies available that can offer partial relief, control end organ damage and improve quality of life for the scleroderma patient [14,15]. The choice and evaluation of any treatment regimen is not easy. This is because:

- ☐ The disorder is heterogeneous
- ☐ Its extent, severity and rate of progression are highly variable
- ☐ There is a tendency towards spontaneous stabilization and/or regression after a few years, particularly within the more benign and numerically larger lcSSc subset
- ☐ The disease is complex and the relationship between immune dysfunction, vascular damage and fibrosis speculative
- ☐ There is a paucity of both clinical and laboratory features for ascertaining improvement (or deterioration) in the disease, especially with respect to visceral change.

The ideal group to target and treat would be the 'at risk' patients, those in the pre-sclerotic state. Many such patients can now be identified by circulating antibodies, cytokine production and nailfold changes. Unfortunately, adequate preventive therapy is still wanting. An extension of this idea, and one that has been discussed with relevance to the lung, is the earliest possible diagnosis of internal organ involvement so that containment therapy may be attempted.

Table 9 Treatment options for Raynaud's phenomenon (RP).

Treatment	Examples	Comments
Simple measures		
Non-drug	Hand warmers Protective clothing	Universally helpful; also useful to minimize cold exposure and ambient temperature changes in work environment
Pharmacological	Evening primrose oil Fish oil capsules	Evening primrose oil has been shown effective in controlled clinical trial
Oral vasodilators		
Calcium channel blockers	Nifedipine retard Nicardipine Felodipine Amlodipine	Responses often idiosyncratic; therefore best to try several drugs in rotation to find most effective
5-Hydroxytryptamine	Ketanserin	Only available on named-patient basis but shown to be effective in clinical trials
ACE inhibitors	Captopril Enalapril	In Raynaud's secondary to dcSSc may protect from hypertensive renal crisis
Topical vasodilators	GTN patches	Shown to be effective in short-term use but often cause headaches
Parenteral vasodilators	Carboprostacyclin (Iloprost) Prostaglandin E1	Effective and reasonably tolerated. Given for severe frequent attacks of RP, digital ulceration or gangrene and prior to digital surgery
Antibiotics	Flucloxacillin Erythromycin	Important in secondary infection in RP. Prolonged oral administration may be necessary
Surgical procedures		
Lumbar sympathectomy	Chemical or operative	For severe RP of lower limbs
Digital sympathectomy (radical microarteriolysis)		Useful treatment for isolated ischaemia of one or two digits
Debridement Amputation	Surgical or auto-amputation	Such surgery should be conservative to allow maximum possibility of spontaneous healing

Table 10 Immunomodulatory therapies for systemic sclerosis.

Treatment	Mechanisms of action	Comments	Efficacy in clinical trials
Selective immunosuppression			
Cyclosporin-A	Inhibits T-helper cell actions by reducing IL-2 release	Reported beneficial effects on skin sclerosis may be confounded, increased incidence of renal crisis	Yes (two open studies) (1990, 1994)
Anti-thymocyte globulin Anti-lymphocyte globulin pilot	Temporary suppression of cell-mediated immunity	Possible benefit for skin sclerosis although controlled trial of ATG confirms considerable therapy-associated morbidity	Yes (open study) (1993) Possible benefit in placebo-controlled study (1993)
Photopheresis	Extracorporeal photo-activated 8-methoxy-psoralen inhibits activated T-cells	Benefit has been reported but good placebo-controlled clinical trial is needed	No (open study) (1993) Yes (open study) (1993) Yes (controlled trial comparing with D-penicillamine therapy) (1992) Multicentre placebo-controlled trial currently in progress
Plasmapheresis	Removes circulating immune mediators	Equivocal results but anecdotal benefit	Possible benefit (open study) (1991)
Pooled human gammaglobulin	Possible inhibition of lymphocyte function via regulatory idiotype cross-reactivity		Not formally evaluated
Non-selective immunosuppression			
Methotrexate	Folic acid antagonist	Currently under formal evaluation in dcSSc	Yes (open study) (1993) Controlled trial in progress
Cyclophosphamide, chlorambucil, azathioprine	Alkylating agent suppressing production of immunocompetent leucocytes	Anecdotal benefit reported in open studies but controlled trial of chlorambucil failed to show superiority over placebo. Cyclophosphamide often combined with corticosteroids	Yes (cyclophosphamide in SSc lung fibrosis – open study) (1994) No (chlorambucil, controlled trial) (1994)

Table 11 Anti-fibrotic therapies for systemic sclerosis.

Treatment	Mechanisms of action	Comments	Efficacy in clinical trials
Colchicine	Inhibition of collagen production by disrupting microtubule formation in fibroblast cytoskeleton. Possible enhancement of collagenase activity	Currently not widely used	Equivocal results in open trials. No controlled studies
D-Penicillamine	Inhibits formation of stable collagen cross-links by forming complex with hydroxylysine aldehyde and lysine groups on collagen precursors	Widely used in UK, doses above 750 mg daily probably needed for any benefit. Open studies have shown beneficial effects on lung skin and kidney disease in SSc. Placebo-controlled trial currently underway in USA	No (controlled trial) (1992). Yes (two open studies) (1990, 1991). Multicentre trial underway in USA
Interferon-α	Inhibits collagen production by dermal SSc fibroblasts *in vitro*, at transcriptional level. May also eliminate high high collagen producing fibroblast sub-populations	Efficacy has been confirmed in open studies and a placebo-controlled trial is currently underway in UK. Benefits must be balanced; considerable morbidity of IFN administration	Yes (open study) (1992). Ongoing UK controlled trial
Interferon-γ	As above	Considerable support for use from open studies and *in vitro* properties	Yes (three open studies) (1992, 1992, 1993)

REFERENCES

1. Black CM, Stephens CO. Systemic sclerosis (scleroderma) and related disorders. In: Maddison PJ, Isenberg DA, Woo P, Glass DN, eds. *Oxford Textbook of Rheumatology* 1993: 2: 771–89.
2. Guitart J, Micali G, Solomon LM. Localized scleroderma. In: Clements PJ, Furst DE, eds. *Systemic Sclerosis*. Baltimore: Williams and Wilkins, 1996; 4: 65–80.
3. Black CM, Denton CP. Scleroderma and related disorders in adults and children. In: *Oxford Textbook of Rheumatology*, in press.
4. Wigley FM. Raynaud's phenomenon. *Curr Opin Rheumatol* 1993; 5: 773–84.
5. Kallenberg CGM, Wouda AA, Hoet MH, Van Venrooij WJ. Development of connective tissue disease in patients presenting with Raynaud's phenomenon: a six-year follow-up with

emphasis on the predictive value of antinuclear antibodies as detected by immunoblotting. *Ann Rheum Dis* 1988; **47**: 634–41.
6   Black CM. The aetiopathogenesis of systemic sclerosis: thick skin–thin hypotheses. *J Roy Coll Physicians* 1995; **29**: 119–30.
7   Medsger TA. Systemic sclerosis (scleroderma), localized forms of scleroderma, and calcinosis. In: McCarty DJ, Koopman WJ, eds. *Arthritis and Allied Conditions*, 12th edn. London: Lea and Febiger, 1993.
8   Lee P, Langevitz P, Alerdice CA, Aubrey M, Baer PA, Baron M, *et al.* Mortality in systemic sclerosis (scleroderma). *Quart J Med* 1992; **298**: 139–48.
9   du Bois RM. Diffuse lung disease: combined clinical and laboratory studies. *J Roy Coll Physicians* 1994; **28**: 338–46.
10 Harrison NK, Glanville AR, Strickland B, Haslam PL, Corin B, Addis BJ, *et al.* Pulmonary involvement in systemic sclerosis: the detection of early changes by thin section CT scan, bronchoalveolar lavage and 99mTc-DTPA clearance. *Resp Med* 1989; **83**: 403–14.
11 Wells AU, Hansell DM, Corrin B, Harrison NK, Goldstraw P, Black CM, du Bois RM. High resolution computed tomography as a predictor of lung histology in systemic sclerosis. *Thorax* 1992; **47**: 738–42.
12 Stupi AM, Steen VD, Owens G, Barnes EL, Rodnan GP, Medsger TA, Jr. Pulmonary hypertension in the CREST syndrome variant of systemic sclerosis. *Arthritis Rheum* 1986; **29**: 515–24.
13 Barst RJ, Rubin LJ, Long WA, McGoon MD, Rich S, Badesch DB, *et al.* A comparison of continuous intravenous epoprostenol (prostacyclin) with conventional therapy for primary pulmonary hypertension. *New Engl J Med* 1996; **334**: 296–301.
14 Pope J. Treatment of systemic sclerosis. *Curr Opin Rheumatol* 1993; **5**: 792–801.
15 Clements PJ, Furst DE, eds. *Systemic Sclerosis*. Baltimore: Williams and Wilkins, 1996.
16 Denton CP, Cailes OB, Phillips GD, Wells AU, Black CM, du Bois RM. Comparison of Doppler echocardiography and right-heart catheterization to assess pulmonary hypertension in systemic sclerosis. *Brit J Rheumatol* 1997; **36** (in press).

☐ MULTIPLE CHOICE QUESTIONS

1   Lung disease in SSc:
    (a) HRCT is a more sensitive test for interstitial lung disease than a single breath diffusing test
    (b) A reticular pattern on HRCT is associated with reversible disease
    (c) A 'ground-glass' appearance on HRCT is equivalent to 'inflammatory alveolitis' on open lung biopsy
    (d) HRCT is better than a DTPA scan at predicting progression of interstitial lung disease
    (e) Lymphocytes are the most frequent cell type found at bronchoalevolar lavage in SSc
    (f) Methotrexate is the treatment choice for interstitial lung disease in SSc

2   Lung disease in SSc:
    (a) The genetic marker DR4 and the anticentromere antibody are useful predictors of diffuse lung disease
    (b) CXR is a useful screening test for interstitial lung disease
    (c) Pulmonary hypertension is associated primarily with diffuse cutaneous SSc
    (d) Pulmonary hypertension is associated with RNA polymerase antibodies
    (e) Captopril is a good treatment for pulmonary hypertension in SSc

3 Spectrum of scleroderma:
   (a) Childhood scleroderma can cause major growth defects
   (b) Localized scleroderma can cause major growth defects
   (c) Diffuse lung disease is found predominantly in patients with limited cutaneous SSc
   (d) Renal disease occurs late on in diffuse cutaneous SSc
   (e) Renal disease is the major cause of death in SSc

4 Antinuclear antibodies associated with systemic sclerosis:
   (a) Jo-1
   (b) Anticentromere
   (c) Ku
   (d) ANCA
   (e) RNA polymerase III

5 Raynaud's phenomenon:
   (a) Nailfold capillary changes are associated with primary Raynaud's
   (b) Antibodies to Scl-70 are found in primary Raynaud's
   (c) Raynaud's phenomenon can precede SSc by 15 years
   (d) Young females with Raynaud's are more likely to have secondary Raynaud's than middle aged males
   (e) Abnormal nailfold capillaries and positive autoantibody detects 90% of patients destined to develop SSc

ANSWERS

1a True	2a False	3a False	4a False	5a False
b False	b False	b True	b True	b False
c True	c False	c False	c True	c True
d False	d False	d False	d False	d True
e False	e False	e False	e True	e True
f False				

The antiphospholipid syndrome

D D'Cruz and G R V Hughes

☐ INTRODUCTION

The antiphospholipid syndrome is a striking clinical constellation of widespread arterial and venous thromboses (Fig. 1), together with recurrent foetal losses. In 1983 to 1986 this clinical constellation was associated with antibodies directed against phospholipids [1]. Since its original description, the clinical spectrum of this syndrome has broadened considerably [2] to include features such as livedo reticularis (Fig. 2), pulmonary hypertension, valvular heart disease, transient ischaemic attacks, epilepsy and transverse myelopathy (Table 1). Although originally described in association with systemic lupus erythematosus (SLE), the syndrome may be seen in the absence of a connective tissue disease – the so-called primary antiphospholipid syndrome.

☐ FEATURES OF THE ANTIPHOSPHOLIPID SYNDROME

Clinical features

Thrombosis, both venous and arterial, remains the hallmark of the antiphospholipid syndrome. Vesssels of all sizes have been involved, ranging from small vessels in the skin to the aortic arch. More subtle features include recurrent migraine, transient ischaemic attacks with visual disturbances and/or dysarthria and a previous history of chorea. Much more seriously however, accelerated valvular heart failure, particularly of the mitral valve, has been described [3].

Neurological features

It is likely that the antiphospholipid syndrome will assume great importance among neurologists. Cerebral ischaemia, ranging from transient ischaemia to infarction, is commonly seen and, in some untreated patients, recurrent cerebral infarcts have led to multi-infarct dementia. Epilepsy [4], chorea and movement disorders [2] have

Table 1 Clinical features of the antiphospholipid syndrome.

Thrombosis	Heart valve disease
Recurrent foetal losses	Transverse myelopathy
Thrombocytopenia	Pulmonary hypertension
Livedo reticularis	Adrenal infarction
Labile hypertension	Skin necrosis
Epilepsy	Ocular ischaemia
Accelerated atherosclerosis	Chorea

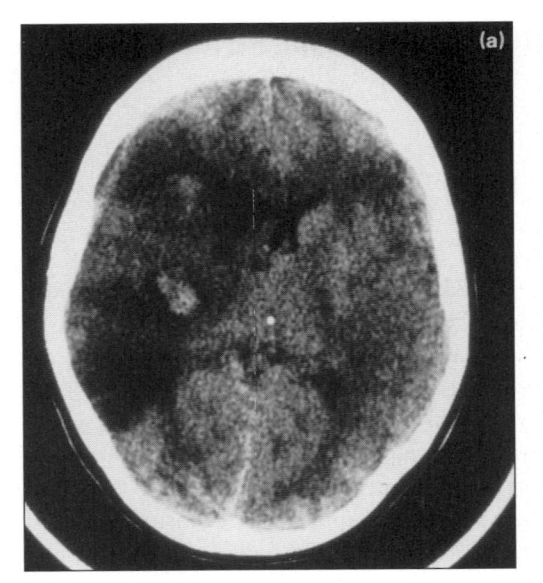

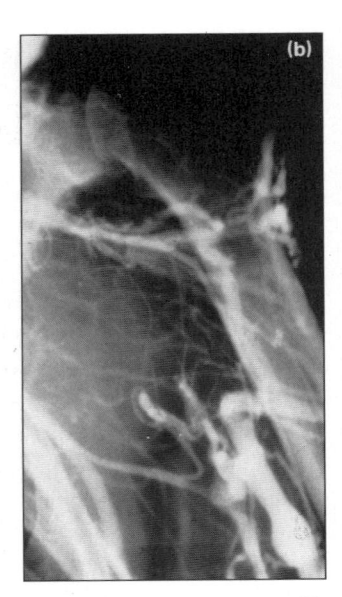

Fig. 1 (a) Computerized tomography (CT) scan showing extensive cerebral infarctions with haemorrhagic areas within the infarcts. (b) Venogram showing an axillary vein thrombosis.

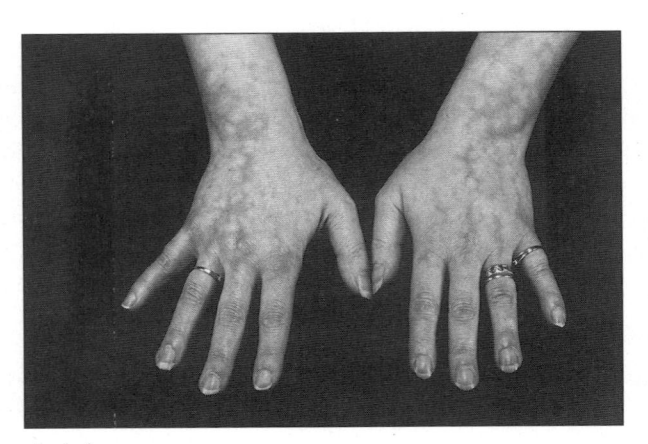

Fig. 2 Livedo reticularis.

been associated with antiphospholipid antibodies and a reasonable hypothesis would include small vessel thromboses or emboli resulting in these clinical features. Of great interest is the clinical observation that some patients with epilepsy and chorea improve strikingly following anticoagulation. Transverse myelitis (Fig. 3) is an uncommon manifestation of SLE that is closely associated with the presence of antiphospholipid antibodies [5]. Studies of unselected stroke populations have shown a relatively low prevalence of antiphospholipid antibodies but in 'young' stroke patients this rises to 18% [6] compared to a prevalence of about 30% in patients with SLE.

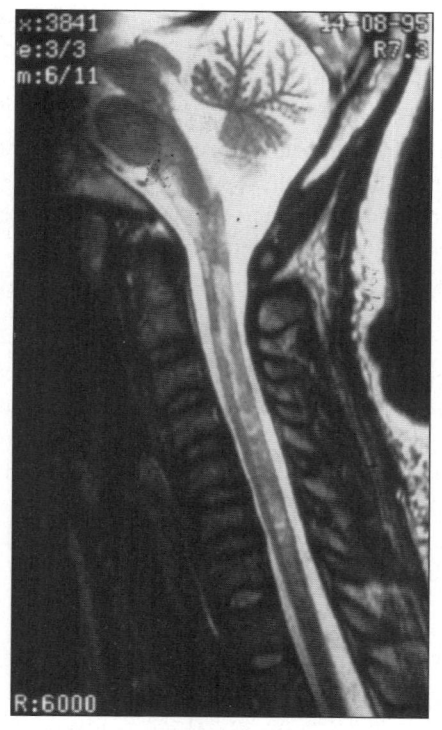

Fig. 3 Transverse myelitis in SLE and the antiphospholipid syndrome. Magnetic resonance imaging (MRI) scan (T2 weighted) showing extensive areas of high signal within the cervical cord.

Cardiovascular medicine

In an unselected population of young survivors of myocardial infarction, one-fifth of patients had antiphospholipid antibodies (reviewed in [2]). Pulmonary hypertension, with or without associated pulmonary emboli, is closely associated with the antiphospholipid syndrome and the association with valvular disease, in particular mitral valve disease, is striking. In one study [3], 38% of patients with antiphospholipid antibodies and SLE had valve abnormalities ranging from mild lesions found on echocardiography to acute fulminating valve degeneration requiring replacement surgery. Occasionally, large intracardiac thromboses have been found mimicking atrial myxomas. Splinter haemorrhages, possibly with clubbing, are clinically associated with this combination of valvular disease and antiphospholipid antibodies where blood cultures are repeatedly negative.

Obstetric features

Patients often suffer recurrent spontaneous abortions and this is a very consistent feature of the antiphospholipid syndrome. Retardation of intrauterine growth and late pregnancy losses are common and the overall loss rate during pregnancy may be as high as 81% [7]. The most likely mechanism of pregnancy loss is placental vessel thrombosis and ischaemia, which almost certainly starts from the earliest time in pregnancy. Doppler ultrasound studies of the placental and uterine vessels have proved useful in detecting reduced flow and may predict intrauterine growth retardation and early delivery [7]. A number of patients present with lupus and the antiphospholipid syndrome following a pregnancy loss and some centres advocate routine antiphospholipid antibody testing in these women. Our own policy is to offer the antiphospholipid test even to patients who have suffered a single miscarriage since the assay is reliable and relatively cheap.

Nephrology

Renal vein thromboses are well described in the antiphospholipid syndrome. Glomerular thrombosis may be an important indicator of future glomerulosclerosis in SLE. In addition, an acute microangiopathy in pregnant lupus patients, manifested by acute renal failure and hypertension, has been associated with antiphospholipid antibodies [reviewed in 2]. Malignant hypertension can certainly be a difficult clinical problem in these patients and even when it is not severe, hypertension can be labile and difficult to control.

Other clinical features

Thrombocytopenia is often seen in association with this syndrome. A certain proportion of patients with idiopathic thrombocytopenic purpura have antiphospholipid antibodies, suggesting that these patients are a subset with a specific identifiable aetiology of their low platelet count. Autoimmune haemolytic anaemia has also been noted, and this is perhaps not surprising given that antiphospholipid antibodies are directed against cell membranes.

Livedo reticularis is a prominent feature in many patients and is often a good clinical marker for the antiphospholipid syndrome. Other manifestations include widespread skin necrosis, skin ulcers and nodules.

Gut ischaemia and hepatic venous thromboses are clearly described in SLE and it has been claimed that the antiphospholipid syndrome is the second most common cause of the Budd-Chiari syndrome [8].

There have been a number of case reports of Addison's disease resulting from adrenal thrombosis. In other patients, avascular necrosis may be a complication of ischaemia of the femoral head. More recently, a catastrophic antiphospholipid syndrome has been described with severe widespread thrombosis associated with cardiovascular collapse, adult respiratory distress syndrome and multiple organ involvement. It is usually fatal (reviewed in [2]).

☐ PRIMARY ANTIPHOSPHOLIPID SYNDROME

In 1989 it became clear that the antiphospholipid syndrome can occur in its own right in patients without evidence of a connective tissue disease [9]. In these patients there is a female to male ratio of 2 : 1 compared to 9 : 1 in SLE. Interestingly, at long-term follow-up only a tiny minority of these patients went on to develop SLE, strongly suggesting that this is a separate syndrome in its own right (reviewed in [2]).

Genetic associations

The epidemiology of the antiphospholipid syndrome is still being investigated and it is unclear whether other risk factors such as the oral contraceptive, smoking or dietary intake can add to the risk of thrombosis in these patients. Certainly, thrombosis-prone families exist and human leucocyte antigen (HLA) studies have suggested an association between antiphospholipid antibodies and HLA DR7, DR4 and DQ7 and DR53 (reviewed in [2]).

Mechanisms of thrombosis

Antibodies against phospholipid are heterogeneous, but negatively charged phospholipids are the predominant antigens. Monoclonal antibodies, both human and animal, have suggested that antibodies react predominantly to phospholipids in their hexagonal but not the lamellar phase.

Wide disturbances of function have been described in endothelial cells, platelet membranes and in the clotting cascade, particularly with components such as protein C and protein S, though this area of research has been complex with conflicting results.

β2-Glycoprotein 1 cofactor

In 1990 three groups noted that purified immunoglobulin G (IgG) anticardiolipin antibodies failed to bind cardiolipin, but that binding was restored when a serum source was present in the system. It was clear that a cofactor was required for the binding of anticardiolipin antibodies; this cofactor proved to be β2-glycoprotein 1 (β2-GP1) (Fig. 4), an apolipoprotein with anticoagulant properties *in vitro*. A variety of studies have shown that β2-GP1 is an absolute requirement for binding of both the anticardiolipin antibodies and the lupus anticoagulant (Fig. 5). Animal studies have provided interesting insights into the function of β2-GP1 in that immunization of normal mice with a mixture of cardiolipin and β2-GP1 results in high titres of antiphospholipid antibodies, whereas cardiolipin alone is relatively non-immunogenic (reviewed in [2]).

Recently, it has been demonstrated that domain V is a crucial area of the cofactor molecule and contains a phospholipid binding site between residues 281 to 288 (Fig. 6). A reasonable hypothesis is that when β2-GP1 binds to cardiolipin the cofactor molecule undergoes a conformational change that exposes epitopes that are immunogenic. This has been supported by elegant studies in Harris' laboratories [10].

The full-blown clinical features of the antiphospholipid syndrome, including thrombosis, are primarily seen in the autoimmune connective tissue diseases where β2-GP1 is absolutely required for the binding of antiphospholipid antibodies. There

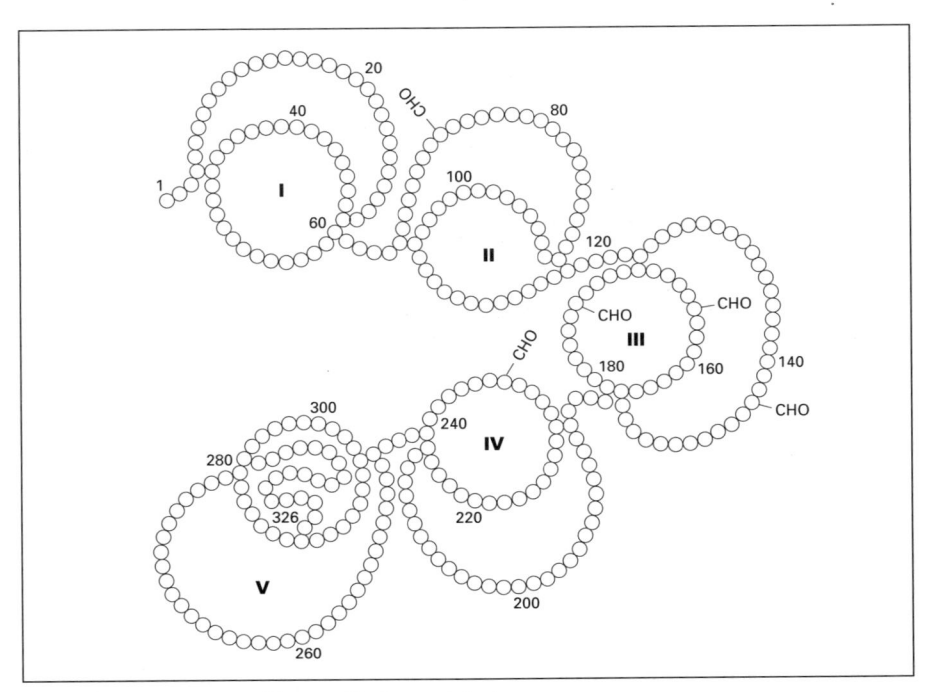

Fig. 4 Primary structure of human β2-glycoprotein 1.

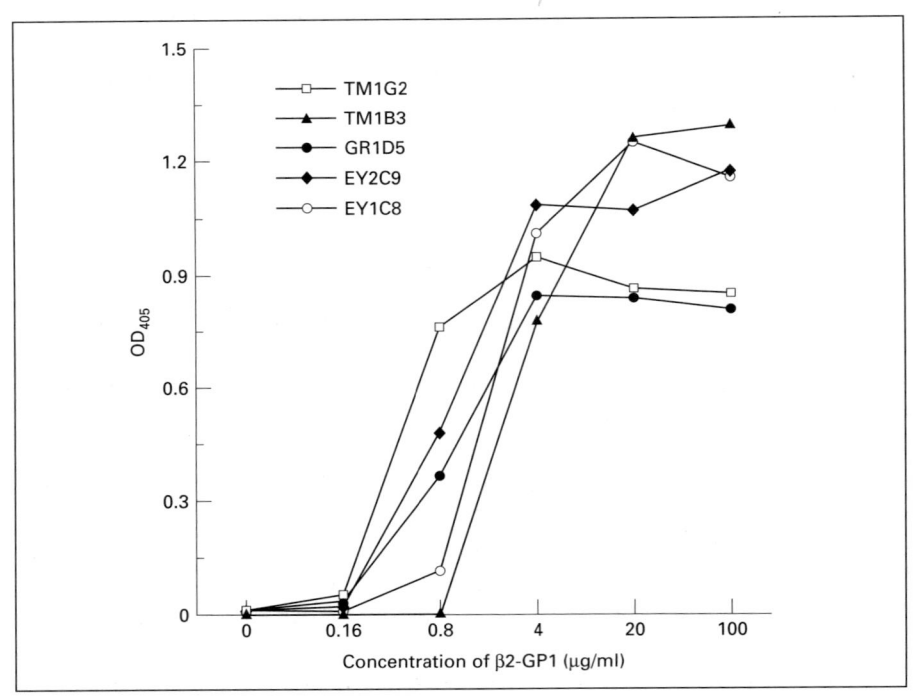

Fig. 5 Dose-dependent binding of human monoclonal anticardiolipin antibodies demonstrating absolute dependence on β2-GP1 for binding.

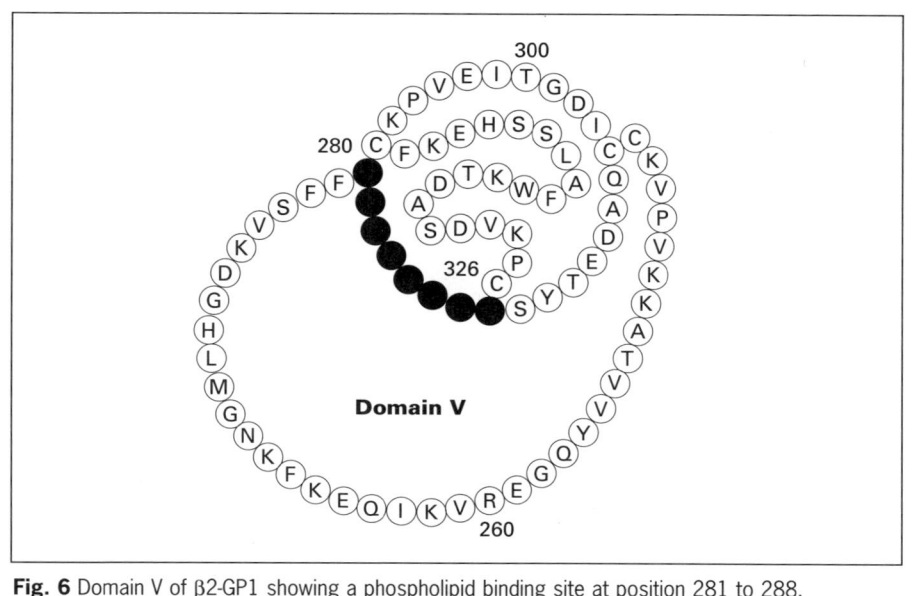

Fig. 6 Domain V of β2-GP1 showing a phospholipid binding site at position 281 to 288.

is however a significant proportion of patients, particularly with infections such as syphilis and human immunodeficiency virus (HIV) disease, where high titres of antiphospholipid antibodies are seen. Curiously, these antibodies do not require the β2-GP1 cofactor for binding, and moreover these patients do not suffer thromboses despite relatively high levels of antibodies. There is thus a clear clinical demarcation between cofactor-dependent and cofactor-independent antiphospholipid antibodies and disease.

☐ TREATMENT

Thrombosis

Until recently a wide variety of therapeutic regimens have been used in the management of the antiphospholipid syndrome. It is clear now that anti-inflammatory and immunosuppressive therapies have no effect on the risk of further thrombosis. Studies by Khamashta *et al.* [11] have shown clearly that high-intensity anticoagulation maintaining an international normalized ratio (INR) of 3 or more is necessary to reduce the risk of further thrombosis (Fig. 7). The most obvious adverse effects of this therapy included bleeding episodes in 29 patients and in seven of these patients bleeding was severe. However, anticoagulation was re-introduced uneventfully at lower INRs. Despite anticoagulation, two patients died from thrombosis, underscoring the markedly prothrombotic nature of this syndrome. Anticoagulation is required long-term, probably indefinitely.

There is currently some controversy regarding patients, usually with SLE, who are found to have high levels of antiphospholipid antibodies but who have not exhibited any clinical features of the antiphospholipid syndrome. Our current policy

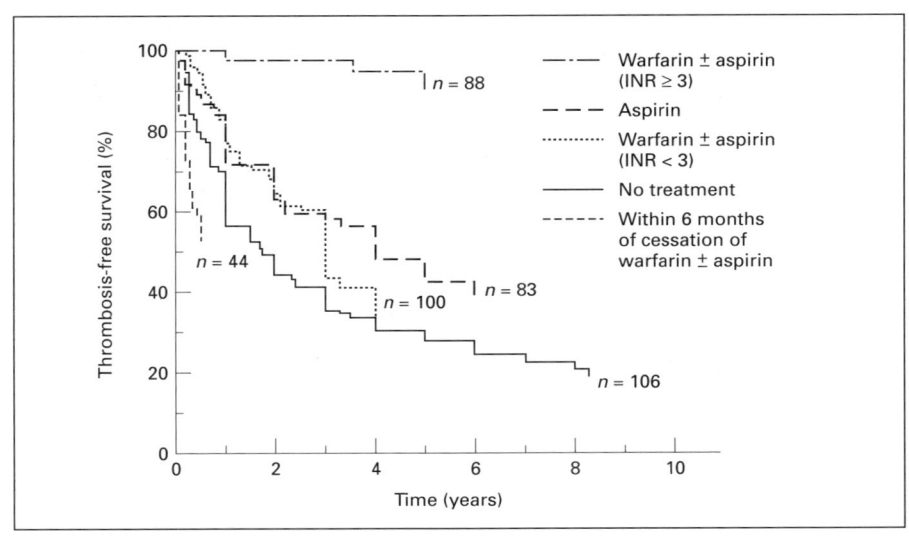

Fig. 7 Survival time analysis for patients with the antiphospholipid syndrome. Patients with INR >3 had the lowest risk for further thrombosis. Patients who stopped anticoagulation re-thrombosed within 6 months.

is to manage these patients with aspirin (75 mg daily) and/or antimalarials such as hydroxychloroquine (200 mg daily) which has a weak anticoagulant effect. However, prospective studies are required to determine the long-term risk of thrombosis in these patients.

Recurrent foetal losses

Our current policy is to manage patients with recurrent foetal losses alone with aspirin and intensive obstetric care throughout the pregnancy [7]. Doppler ultrasound studies may be useful in documenting umbilical and uterine artery flow and predicting early delivery. The critical factor, however, appears to be the level of obstetric care and it is generally sensible to manage such high-risk patients in combined rheumatology and obstetric clinics.

For those patients who have previously suffered a thrombosis, patients embarking on pregnancy are managed with heparin, preferably low-molecular-weight heparin, which is usually given once daily. Heparin may be needed throughout the pregnancy and is discontinued temporarily at the time of labour [7].

☐ FUTURE DIRECTIONS

One interesting clinical observation has been the finding of accelerated atherosclerosis in patients with SLE. The finding that antiphospholipid antibodies cross-react with oxidized low-density lipoproteins is intriguing, particularly as the latter have been shown to have a central role in the progression of atherosclerosis.

Future studies of the β2-GP1 cofactor may help to clarify whether anti-β2-GP1 antibodies rather than anticardiolipin antibodies may, in fact, be a serological marker of the antiphospholipid syndrome. Further changes in terminology in this syndrome are almost inevitable as a result of advances in understanding and it has been suggested that the syndrome be re-named eponymously to credit the original author of the syndrome [12].

REFERENCES

1. Hughes GRV, Harris EN, Gharavi AE. The anticardiolipin syndrome. *J Rheumatol* 1986; **13**: 486–9.
2. Hughes GRV. The antiphospholipid syndrome: ten years on. *Lancet* 1993; **342**: 341–4.
3. Khamashta MA, Cervera R, Asherson RA, *et al*. Association of antibodies against phospholipids with heart valve disease in systemic lupus erythematosus. *Lancet* 1990; **335**: 1541–4.
4. Herranz MT, Rivier G, Khamashta MA, Blaser KU, Hughes GRV. Association between antiphospholipid antibodies and epilepsy in patients with systemic lupus erythematosus. *Arthritis Rheum* 1994; **37**: 568–71.
5. Alarcon-Segovia D, Deleze M, Oria CV, Sanchez-Guerrero J, Gomez-Pacheco L. Antiphospholipid antibodies and the antiphospholipid syndrome in systemic lupus erythematosus: a prospective analysis of 500 consecutive patients. *Medicine* (Baltimore) 1989; **68**: 353–6.
6. Nencini P, Baruffi MC, Abbati R, Massai G, Amaducci L, Inzitari P. Lupus anticoagulant and anti-cardiolipin antibodies in young adults with cerebral ischaemia. *Stroke* 1992; **23**: 189–93.
7. Buchanan NMM, Khamashta MA, Morton KE, Kerslake S, Baguley E, Hughes GRV. A study of 100 high risk lupus pregnancies. *Am J Reprod Immunol* 1992; **28**: 192–4.
8. Pelletier S, Landi B, Piette JC, *et al*. The antiphospholipid syndrome as the second cause of non-malignant Budd-Chiari syndrome. *Arthritis Rheum* 1992: **35** (Suppl): S238.
9. Asherson RA, Khamashta MA, Ordi-Ros J, *et al*. The 'primary' antiphospholipid syndrome : major clinical and serological features. *Medicine* (Baltimore) 1989; **68**: 366–72.
10. Borchman D, Harris EN, Pierangeli SS, Lamba OP. Interactions and molecular structure of cardiolipin and β2-glycoprotein 1. *Clin Exp Immunol* 1995; **102**: 373–8.
11. Khamashta MA, Cuadrado MJ, Mujic F, Taub MA, Hunt BJ, Hughes GRV. The management of thrombosis in the antiphospholipid-antibody syndrome *New Engl J Med* 1995; **332**: 993–7.
12. Khamashta MA, Asherson RA. Hughes syndrome: antiphospholipid antibodies move closer to thrombosis in 1994. *Brit J Rheum* 1995; **34**: 493–7.

☐ MULTIPLE CHOICE QUESTIONS

1 The antiphospholipid syndrome:
  (a) Is a common complication of rheumatoid arthritis
  (b) Is associated with retardation of intrauterine foetal growth
  (c) Is only seen in patients with SLE
  (d) May occur in families
  (e) Is associated with HLA DR7

2 Clinical features of the antiphospholipid syndrome include:
  (a) Hypertension
  (b) Epilepsy
  (c) Inflammatory polyarthritis

(d) Addison's disease
  (e) Skin necrosis

3 The β2-glycoprotein 1 cofactor:
  (a) Is required for *in vitro* antiphospholipid antibody binding in patients with the antiphospholipid syndrome
  (b) Is comprised of four domains
  (c) May undergo a conformational change on binding to cardiolipin
  (d) May not be necessary for *in vitro* binding of antiphospholipid antibodies from patients with HIV disease
  (e) Has *in vitro* anticoagulant activity

4 In the antiphospholipid syndrome:
  (a) Aspirin alone effectively prevents recurrent thrombotic events
  (b) Warfarin at an INR of 2.0 provides the best protection against recurrent thrombosis
  (c) Six months anticoagulation is adequate
  (d) Immunosuppressive therapy prevents recurrent thrombosis
  (e) Epilepsy may improve with anticoagulation

5 In the management of pregnant patients with the antiphospholipid syndrome:
  (a) Aspirin may reduce the rate of recurrent miscarriages
  (b) Doppler flow studies of the umbilical artery are of no value in predicting early delivery
  (c) Low-molecular-weight heparin is useful in anticoagulation
  (d) Warfarin may be used throughout the pregnancy
  (e) Prednisolone and azathioprine therapy reduces the risk of recurrent miscarriages

ANSWERS

1a False	2a True	3a True	4a False	5a True
b True	b True	b False	b False	b False
c False	c False	c True	c False	c True
d True	d True	d True	d False	d False
e True	e True	e True	e True	e False

Management of osteoporosis in the 1990s

R W Keen and T D Spector

☐ INTRODUCTION

Osteoporosis is a systemic skeletal disease characterized by low bone mineral density (BMD), disorganized bone microarchitecture and a subsequent increased risk of fragility fracture. To date, the only cost-effective approach to managing osteoporosis is primary prevention, yet many patients will still present with established disease which only becomes apparent after a fracture is sustained. Ideal therapies should be well tolerated, available orally, increase bone mass, restore normal bone architecture and reduce the occurrence of new osteoporotic fractures. Drugs used in the treatment of osteoporosis can be broadly grouped into those that decrease bone resorption and those that increase bone formation (Table 1). Antiresorptive drugs are thought to act by decreasing the imbalance between bone formation and resorption, by decreasing the overall rate of bone turnover, or by a combination of both mechanisms. They are most effective in conditions in which bone turnover is increased, and their action is greatest on cancellous rather than cortical bone. During the first 1 to 2 years of treatment with an antiresorptive agent, bone mass increases slightly, probably as a result of the remodelling transient. Studies showing a prolonged effect on bone mass suggest, however, that these agents have a positive effect on steady-state bone balance and will favourably affect fracture incidence. Antiresorptive agents are therefore well suited for preventing osteoporosis but in theory are not ideal agents for its treatment. Bone formation agents increase both the rate at which new bone remodelling units are activated and the activity of individual osteoblasts, resulting in a sustained increase in bone mass. These agents have greater potential to increase bone mass above the fracture threshold and are theoretically preferable for the treatment of established, severe osteoporosis.

Table 1 Therapeutic agents available for the treatment of osteoporosis.

Antiresorptive agents	Bone formation	Unknown action
Oestrogen ± progestogen*	Fluoride	Vitamin D and analogues*
Bisphosphonates*	Parathyroid hormone (PTH)	Anabolic steroids*
Calcium*		Ipriflavone
Calcitonin*		

*Currently licensed in the UK

TREATMENT OF OSTEOPOROSIS

Calcium

Adequate calcium nutrition is essential for the development and maintenance of a normal skeleton. In view of its important role in bone homoeostasis, calcium supplements have been used in the treatment of osteoporosis for many years, although conflicting results have been observed between studies. Calcium appears to have little effect if given within the first 5 years of the menopause, when bone loss is predominantly due to oestrogen withdrawal. Calcium supplements have been shown to reduce ageing-associated bone loss in prospective controlled trials by up to 50% [1,2]. A retrospective case-control study has also shown a significant effect of calcium supplements on hip fracture risk [3], although data from controlled clinical trials have not yet been obtained. At present, calcium supplements are often administered as a combined therapy with other agents for the treatment of osteoporosis.

Vitamin D and its analogues

Vitamin D acts to increase calcium absorption in the gastrointestinal tract and thereby inhibits parathyroid hormone (PTH) mediated bone resorption. Supplementation with elemental calcium (1.2 g a day) and cholecalciferol (800 IU a day) has recently been shown to reduce the risk of hip fracture and other non-vertebral fractures in an elderly nursing home population [4]. Analogues of vitamin D have also been examined to see if they have increased efficacy in the treatment of mild to moderate osteoporosis [5,6]. Calcitriol (0.25 µg twice daily) reduced the rate of vertebral fractures compared to calcium (1 g) during the second (9.3 *vs* 25.0 fractures per 100 patient-years) and third years (9.9 *vs* 31.5 fractures per 100 patient-years) of the study [6]. Peripheral fractures were also reduced in the calcitriol group compared to the calcium-treated group (11 *vs* 24 fractures). Toxicity is a concern with vitamin D analogues because of hypercalcaemia and hypercalciuria, but the incidence of adverse events reported in the literature is low (< 5%). These can be minimized by monitoring calcium intake, omitting calcium supplements, measuring urinary calcium excretion, increasing water intake and administering calcitriol twice daily.

Hormone replacement therapy

Given the central role of oestrogen deficiency in the development of osteoporosis, treatment regimens to reduce fractures have focused on replacement therapy with ovarian hormones [7,8]. Several regimens and routes of administration are available and all appear capable of inhibiting bone loss, but none of these to date fully mimics the pattern of hormone release in premenopausal women. Progestogens may also effectively reduce bone loss, particularly those derived from 19-nortestosterone [9,10]. In established osteoporosis, conjugated equine oestrogens given with or without a progestogen have been shown to increase bone mass at the spine, forearm and total skeleton [8–10].

A large amount of epidemiological data support a reduction in fracture risk at hip and forearm for those treated with oestrogen and oestrogen/progestogen combinations, whereas fewer data are available for vertebral fractures. The protective effect against hip fractures is considerable, most studies showing a 50–75% reduction in risk in oestrogen users. The minimum duration of therapy required to protect against hip fracture is controversial. Cross-sectional studies suggest a duration of oestrogen therapy of 5–10 years for an effect on hip fracture, although whether this positive effect extends after the age of 75 years in past users is debatable [11]. This is of obvious importance as the incidence of hip fracture is high in women of this age, and prolonged therapy (ie lifelong) may be required to protect women fully into later life when their risk of fracture is highest. With treatment of this duration compliance will be a major issue. About 40% of women prescribed hormone replacement therapy (HRT) are not compliant at one year and in many instances the return of menstrual bleeding is cited as a major reason for discontinuing treatment. A further concern affecting long-term compliance with prolonged treatment with HRT is that the risk of breast cancer appears to be increased by 30–50% with HRT use of more than 5 years [12,13].

Recent interest has concentrated on HRT preparations that do not cause a menstrual bleed, such as the continuous combination of oestrogen and progestogen [10] and synthetic preparations [14]. However, the long-term effect of these agents on cardiovascular risk and serum lipid profiles is as yet unknown and further data are awaited. Anti-oestrogens such as raloxifine, which have positive skeletal, as well as anti-lipid and anti-breast cancer effects with little adverse effects on the endometrium, are currently under clinical investigation and may prove effective in treating established disease.

Anabolic steroids

Steroids derived from 19-norethisterone are thought to be effective in preserving BMD, by acting through a decrease in bone turnover. Their effect on bone mineral can also be explained in part by the increase in muscle mass and drop in body fat that accompanies treatment [15]. The long-term use of anabolic steroids in the treatment of osteoporosis is probably limited by their side-effects, which include an adverse effect on high-density lipoprotein cholesterol, hoarseness and virilization, which are not negated by parenteral administration.

Calcitonin

Calcitonin is an endogenous peptide of 32 amino acids which possesses anti-osteoclastic activity. In clinical practice four calcitonins (human, pig, salmon and eel) have been used in studies of osteoporosis. Parenteral administration of calcitonin is given by intramuscular injection, suppository or nasal spray.

A number of small studies have shown a positive effect of parenteral calcitonin on bone mass in postmenopausal osteoporosis, this effect being most marked at axial sites and in those with high bone turnover [3,16]. Calcitonin has also been shown to have analgesic properties, which make it suitable for use in those with pain secondary to vertebral collapse, particularly in the acute state. The physiological mechanisms underlying this action are poorly understood.

Long-term administration of intramuscular calcitonin appears safe and is not associated with any long-term side effects. The nasal spray often causes minor problems, particularly nasal irritation and discharge. One major problem, however, is that its effect appears to wane with time, the mechanism of which is unclear. Antibody formation can occur with use of non-human calcitonin and this can result in minor allergic reactions and resistance to treatment. Resistance to salmon calcitonin appears less frequent if it is given in low doses, intermittently and via the intranasal route. Problems of resistance and the costs of long-term therapy with the nasal spray are likely to limit its use to the short term.

Fluoride

Fluoride was first recognized as a stimulator of bone growth over 30 years ago and sodium fluoride (NaF) and sodium monofluorophosphate (Na_2FPO_4) are currently licensed for the treatment of osteoporosis in ten European countries.

Fluoride treatment has been shown to produce a linear increase in vertebral bone mass of 4–8% a year, although up to 40% of patients show no significant response. The effect of fluoride on new fracture frequency is controversial and depends on the dose and formulation of the fluoride salt [17–19]. Most studies have not shown increases in bone density at the cortical sites of the forearm or femoral neck, and there is concern that fluoride treatment may actually increase the risk for hip fracture. Slow-release sodium treatment has recently been shown to inhibit new vertebral fractures in patients without prevalent fractures and to increase BMD at the lumbar spine and femoral neck [20].

Fluoride salts have a narrow therapeutic window and the exact formulation and dosing schedule has yet to be determined. Impaired mineralization can occur with NaF at daily doses of 20–40 mg, although this can be overcome with concurrent administration of calcium supplements. Side effects are not uncommon, particularly gastrointestinal and lower extremity pain syndrome. The latter occurs in 15–20% of patients, is dose related, and probably represents the healing of stress microfractures. Fewer side effects are noted with use of low dosages, sustained-release preparations and with use of sodium monofluorophosphate.

Bisphosphonates

Bisphosphonates are synthetic analogues of pyrophosphate, an endogenous substance that inhibits the mineralization of bone. They contain a non-hydrolysable P-C-P bond and have two side chains, one that participates in binding to bone and one that determines the pharmacological properties of the drug.

Cyclical intermittent etidronate has been shown to increase spinal bone density by 5% during the first 2 years of treatment in two placebo-controlled studies [21,22]. Despite certain limitations regarding the power of these two studies, the combined results suggest that this regimen of etidronate therapy is effective in reducing further vertebral fractures in patients with severe osteoporosis. No clear effect was seen on bone density at the hip. Etidronate inhibits mineralization at oral doses equivalent to those for antiresorption, and the duration of treatment required in osteoporosis and the long skeletal half-life of the compounds raise the concern that osteomalacia may occur as a late complication of bisphosphonate use.

Second and third generation bisphosphonates produce little or no inhibition of mineralization at doses that show antiresorptive activity and suggest an improved safety margin. Treatment with continuous tiludronate for 6 months caused a mean increase in spinal bone mass of 1.3% which was preserved over 2 years [23]. Continuous alendronate treatment for 3 years in 994 women with postmenopausal spinal osteoporosis (BMD 2.5 standard deviations below the young adulthood peak value) caused significant increases of 2.2–8.8% at all skeletal sites, the effect being most marked at the spine [24]. The incidence of new vertebral fractures was 3.2% in the alendronate-treated group compared to 6.2% in the placebo group, a significant reduction of 48% in the risk of subsequent fracture. Although not having the power to detect a difference in non-vertebral fractures, there was a trend towards alendronate treatment reducing the incidence of fractures at the hip and wrist (9 vs 19 cases).

Parathyroid hormone

Treatment with the 1–34 fragment of PTH has been evaluated as an anabolic agent in osteoporosis. Although high plasma concentrations of PTH stimulate bone resorption, PTH may stimulate bone formation when given intermittently at low doses.

Studies indicate an increase in cancellous bone mass with treatment with PTH (1–34), although there appears to be a redistribution from cortical bone [25,26]. In an attempt to reduce this cortical loss, concurrent treatment with active vitamin D metabolites or oestrogen replacement therapy has been assessed during PTH treatment. Current data also suggest that the anabolic effect may reach a plateau after several years and the exact therapeutic regimen has still to be determined. At present no long-term data on PTH therapy and vertebral fracture incidence are available.

Ipriflavone

Flavanoids are naturally occurring plant metabolites and ipriflavone belongs to the isoflavone class, a group having weak oestrogenic properties. At present, ipriflavone is licensed for the treatment of osteoporosis in Italy, Hungary and Japan. Studies have suggested an increase in forearm bone mass and prevention of spinal bone loss, but no fracture prevention data are yet available [27].

Future agents

A growing number of new and novel treatments are emerging. Bone cells synthesize a large number of growth factors which enhance osteoblast proliferation. Various growth factors (ie insulin-like growth factors 1 and 2, transforming growth factor beta) have been isolated, and are now available as potential treatment agents. Other compounds such as strontium salts and silicon derivatives are undergoing preclinical and clinical trials and may also soon be available for the treatment of established osteoporosis.

☐ CONCLUSIONS

The incidence of osteoporosis has increased over the past 30 years, and this increase is expected to increase into the next century [28]. At present a number of different drugs can be used safely and with the expectation of preventing an initial or subsequent osteoporotic fracture. HRT remains the mainstay of treatment, although many women receive therapy for a time period that is insufficient to have any major impact on fracture risk. It is likely that 'non-bleed' preparations and raloxifene will be widely used in the future in an attempt to improve compliance, although concern will still exist about the long-term safety of these therapies. Second and third generation bisphosphonates appear good alternatives for women who are unable or unwilling to take oestrogen replacement. Data from ongoing clinical trials with these agents are eagerly awaited to assess their impact on hip-fracture prevention. Other therapies under investigation will also soon be available for clinical treatment. Exactly who will benefit from a particular therapy, the duration of treatment and the use of combinations of bone formation and antiresorptive agents are the challenges for the next decade.

REFERENCES

1   Dawson-Hughes B, Dallal GE, Krall EA, et al. A controlled trial of the effect of calcium supplementation on bone density in postmenopausal women. *New Engl J Med* 1990; **323**: 878–83.
2   Reid IA, Ames RW, Evans MC, Gamble GD, Sharpe SJ. Effect of calcium supplementation on bone loss in postmenopausal women. *New Engl J Med* 1993; **328**: 460–4.
3   Kanis JA, Johnell O, Gullberg B, et al. Evidence for efficacy of drugs affecting bone metabolism in preventing hip fracture. *Brit Med J* 1992; **305**: 1124–8.
4   Chapuy MC, Arlot ME, Delmas PD, Meunier PJ. Effect of calcium and cholecalciferol treatment for three years on hip fracture in elderly women. *Brit Med J* 1994; **308**: 1081–2.
5   Orimo H, Shiraki M, Hayashi Y, et al. Effects of 1-alpha-hydroxyvitamin D_3 on lumbar bone mineral density and vertebral fractures in patients with postmenopausal osteoporosis. *Calcific Tissue Int* 1994; **54**: 370–6.
6   Tilyard MW, Spears GFS, Thomson J, Dovey S. Treatment of postmenopausal osteoporosis with calcitriol or calcium. *New Engl J Med* 1992; **326**: 357–62.
7   Albright F, Smith PH, Richardson AM. Postmenopausal osteoporosis. *J Am Med Assoc* 1941; **116**: 2465–74.
8   Lindsay R, Tohme J. Estrogen treatment of patients with established postmenopausal osteoporosis. *Obstet Gynecol* 1990; **76**: 1–6.
9   Lindsay R, Hart DM, Purdie P, et al. Comparative effects of oestrogen and a progestogen on bone loss in postmenopausal women. *Clin Sci Mol Med* 1978; **54**: 193–5.
10   Christiansen C, Riis BJ. 17β-Estradiol and continuous norethisterone: a unique treatment for established osteoporosis in elderly women. *J Clin Endocrinol Metab* 1990; **71**: 836–41.
11   Felson DT, Zhang Y, Hannan MT, et al. The effect of postmenopausal estrogen therapy on bone density in elderly women. *New Engl J Med* 1993; **329**: 1141–6.

12 Steinberg KK, Smith SJ, Thacker SB, Stoup DF. Breast cancer risk and duration of estrogen use: the role of the study design in meta-analysis. *Epidemiology* 1994; 5: 415–21.
13 Colditz GA, Hankinson SE, Hunter DJ, et al. The use of estrogens and progestins and the risk of breast cancer in postmenopausal women. *New Engl J Med* 1995; 322: 1589–93.
14 Rymer J, Chapman MG, Fogelman I. Effect of tibolone on postmenopausal bone loss. *Osteoporosis Int* 1994; 4: 314–9.
15 Hassager C, Podenphant J, Riis BJ, et al. Changes in soft tissue body composition and plasma lipid metabolism during nandrolone decanoate therapy in postmenopausal osteoporotic women. *Metabolism* 1989; 38: 238–42.
16 Overgard K, Hansen MA, Jensen SB, Christiansen C. Effect of calcitonin given intranasally on bone mass and fracture rates in established osteoporosis: a dose-response study. *Brit Med J* 1992; 305: 556–61.
17 Mamelle M, Meunier PJ, Dusan R, et al. Risk-benefit ratio of sodium fluoride treatment in primary vertebral osteoporosis. *Lancet* 1988; ii: 361–5.
18 Buckle RM. A 3-year study of sodium fluoride treatment on vertebral fracture incidence in osteoporosis. *J Bone Miner Res* 1989; 4(**Suppl 1**): S186.
19 Riggs BL, Hodgson SF, O'Fallon WM, et al. Effect of fluoride treatment on the fracture rate in postmenopausal women with osteoporosis. *New Engl J Med* 1990; 322: 802–9.
20 Pak CYC, Sakhaee K, Adams-Huet B, Piziak V, Peterson RD, Poindexter JR. Treatment of postmenopausal osteoporosis with slow-release sodium fluoride. *Ann Intern Med* 1995; 123: 401–8.
21 Storm T, Thamsborg G, Steiniche T, et al. Effect of intermittent cyclical etidronate therapy on bone mass and fracture rate in women with postmenopausal osteoporosis. *New Engl J Med* 1990; 322: 1265–71.
22 Watts NB, Harris ST, Genant HK, et al. Intermittent cyclical etidronate treatment of postmenopausal osteoporosis. *New Engl J Med* 1990; 323: 73–9.
23 Reginster JY, Lecart MP, Deroisy R, et al. Prevention of postmenopausal bone loss by tiludronate. *Lancet* 1989; ii: 1469–71.
24 Libermann UA, Weiss SR, Broll J, et al. Effect of oral alendronate on bone mineral density and the incidence of fractures in postmenopausal osteoporosis. *New Engl J Med* 1995; **333**: 1437–43.
25 Reeve J, Meunier PJ, Parsons JA, et al. Anabolic effect of human parathyroid hormone fragment on trabecular bone in involutional osteoporosis: a multicentre trial. *Brit Med J* 1980; **280**: 1340–4.
26 Slovik DM, Neer RM, Potts JT Jr. Short-term effects of synthetic human parathyroid hormone (1–34) administration on bone mineral metabolism in osteoporotic patients. *J Clin Invest* 1981; **68**: 1261–71.
27 Brandi ML. New treatment strategies: ipriflavone, strontium, vitamin D metabolites and analogs. *Am J Med* 1993; **95**(Suppl 5A); 69S–74S.
28 United Nations. *Interpolated National Populations by Age and Sex: 1950–2025.* (1992 revision). United Nations Population Division, United Nations, New York, 1992.

☐ MULTIPLE CHOICE QUESTIONS

1 Osteoporosis is a condition in which:
   (a) The incidence has reached a plateau after a dramatic increase over the last 30 years
   (b) There is marked demineralization of bone
   (c) There is an association with hyperparathyroidism
   (d) Common fractures occur at hip, spine and wrist
   (e) Bone formation therapies are widely used

2. Bisphosphonates:
   (a) Have a strong effect on reducing fractures of the hip
   (b) Can inhibit both resorption and mineralization
   (c) Have a skeletal half-life of approximately 10 years
   (d) Are based on an endogenous pyrophosphate
   (e) Contain a hydrolysable P-C-P bond which determines the chemical properties of the drug

3. Hormone replacement therapy is:
   (a) Well tolerated for 5 years in the majority of patients
   (b) Suitable both for women with an intact uterus and for those who have undergone hysterectomy
   (c) Associated with protection from coronary heart disease
   (d) Not associated with risk of breast cancer
   (e) Sometimes obtained from horses' urine

4. Calcium and vitamin D are important for bone homoeostasis:
   (a) As calcium is able to reverse menopause-related bone loss
   (b) Because vitamin D acts to increase PTH-mediated resorption of bone
   (c) Because vitamin D has been shown to reduce the incidence of hip fractures
   (d) Although vitamin D has toxic effects in the majority of people taking supplements
   (e) Where intakes of dietary calcium should be at least 1000–1500 mg a day

5. Fluoride treatment:
   (a) Is licensed in the UK
   (b) Is associated with positive response in the majority of patients
   (c) May be associated with increase in hip fracture rate
   (d) Has a wide therapeutic safety window
   (e) Can cause mineralization defects in calcium-deficient states

ANSWERS

1a False	2a False	3a False	4a False	5a False
b False	b True	b True	b False	b False
c True	c True	c True	c True	c True
d True	d True	d False	d False	d False
e False	e False	e True	e True	e True

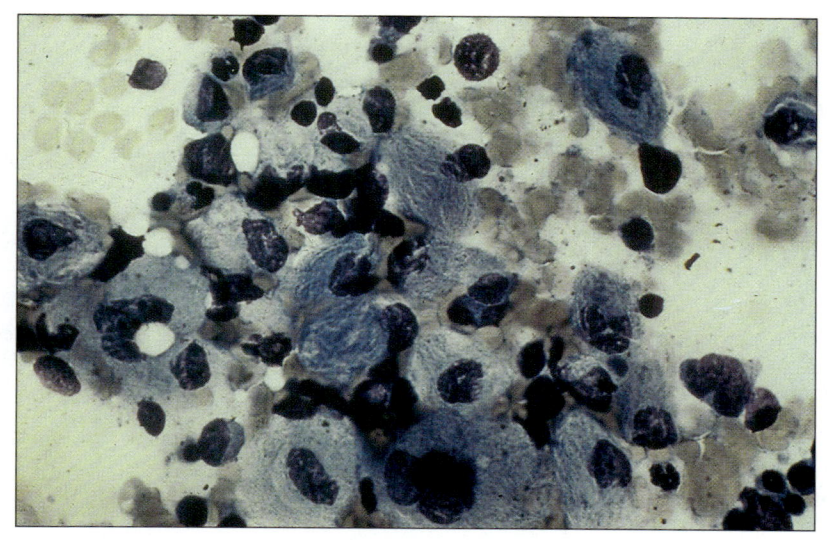

Plate 1 (Cox, p10) Photomicrograph of bone marrow aspirate specimen taken from a 23-year-old man suffering from adult Type 1 Gaucher's disease. The characteristic morphology, large histiocytes containing cellular debris and showing striations in the cytoplasm, is shown.

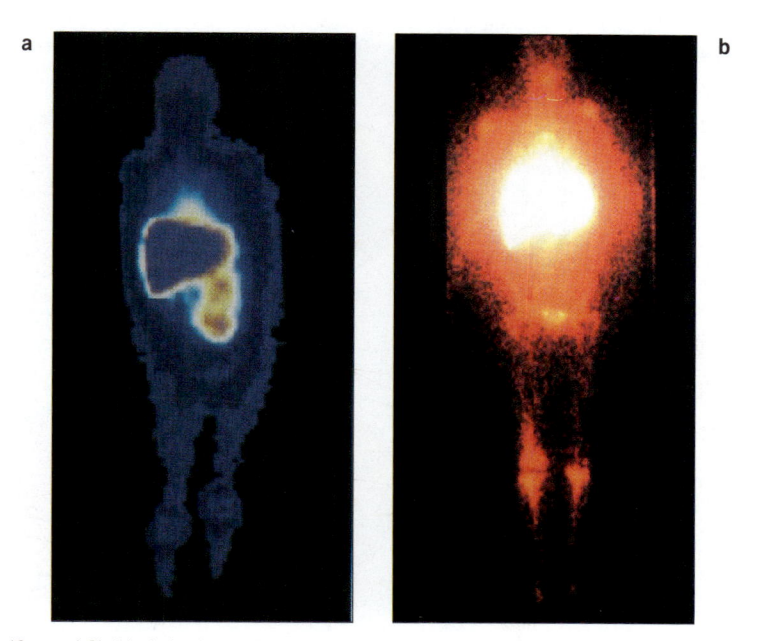

Plate 2 (Cox, p13) Whole-body γ-scintigraphy using ^{123}I-labelled mannose-terminated human glucocerebrosidase. **(a)** Anterior view 22-year-old man with hepatosplenomegaly due to non-neuronopathic Type I Gaucher's disease. Notice dramatic labelling of liver and enlarged spleen. At subsequent splenectomy for pancytopenia a massive spleen containing a large healed infarct was present corresponding to the relatively 'cold' splenic scan image. **(b)** Anterior image γ-scintigram of 23-year-old woman with Gaucher's disease diagnosed at the time of splenectomy in childhood. The patient has marked hepatic enlargement and suffers skeletal pain in the shoulders, hips and especially the right knee. In this image taken 30 min after tracer injection, note the striking localization of labelled enzyme to areas of skeletal disease. (From Mistry et al. [16], with permission.)

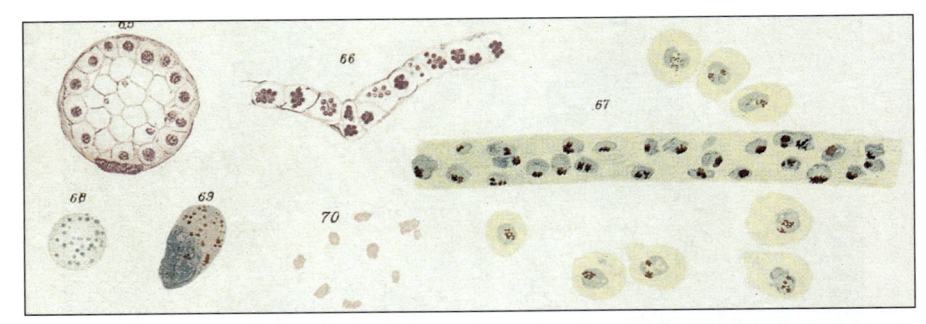

Plate 3 (Warrell, p25) Erythrocytes containing pigmented *Plasmodium falciparum* parasites in cerebral blood vessels of fatal cases of cerebral malaria as depicted by Golgi. (From Mannaberg [23].)

Plate 4 (a) (Aziz, p75) Group mean colour maps showing the scalp topography of the first negative (N1) and positive (P1) potentials recorded following oesophageal stimulation. **(b)** Group mean colour maps showing the scalp topography of the second negative (N2) and positive (P2) potentials recorded following oesophageal stimulation.

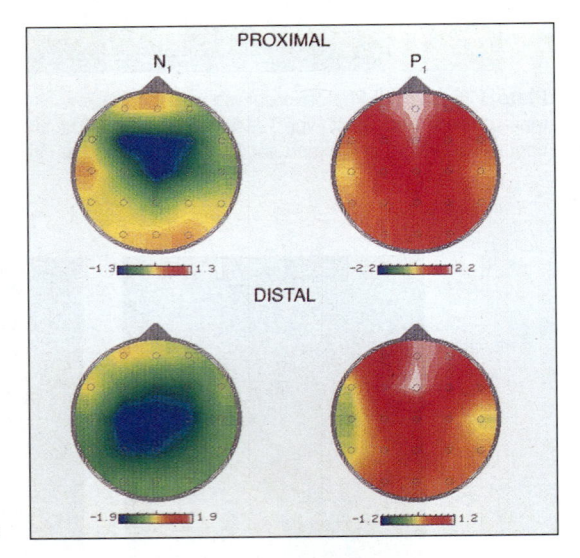

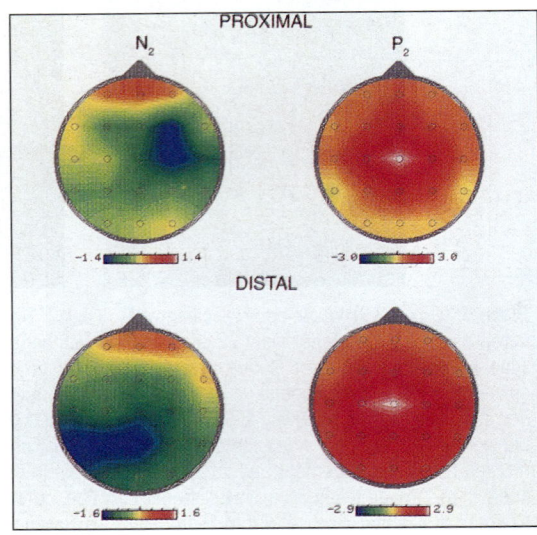

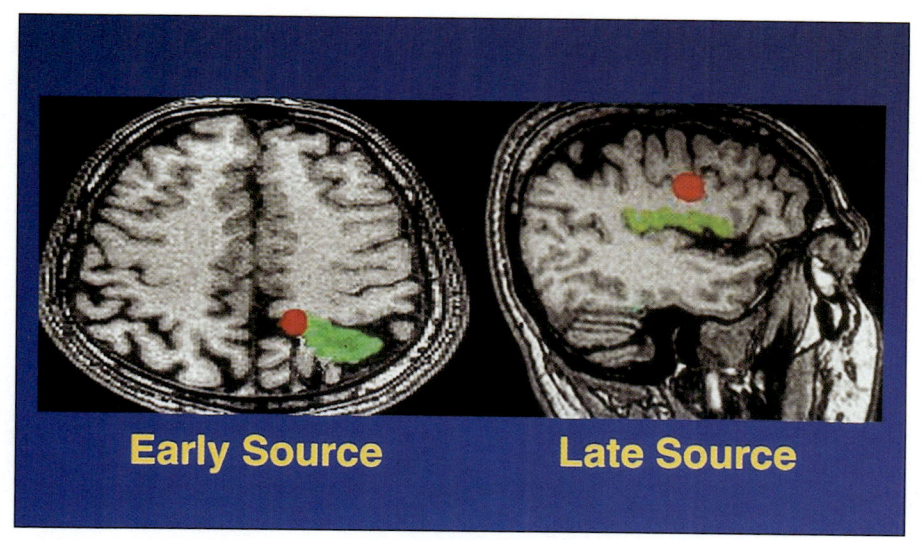

Plate 5 (Aziz, p76) Magnetic resonance scans of a healthy volunteer showing the location of the cortical sources that generate magnetic fields at short (early) and long (late) latencies following oesophageal distension. The early and the late sources, represented by the red dots, are located in the trunk area of the primary somatosensory cortex and the insular cortex, respectively. The green shaded areas for the early and the late sources represent the primary somatosensory cortex and the sylvian fissure, respectively. (By courtesy of Department of Vision Sciences, Aston University, Birmingham.)

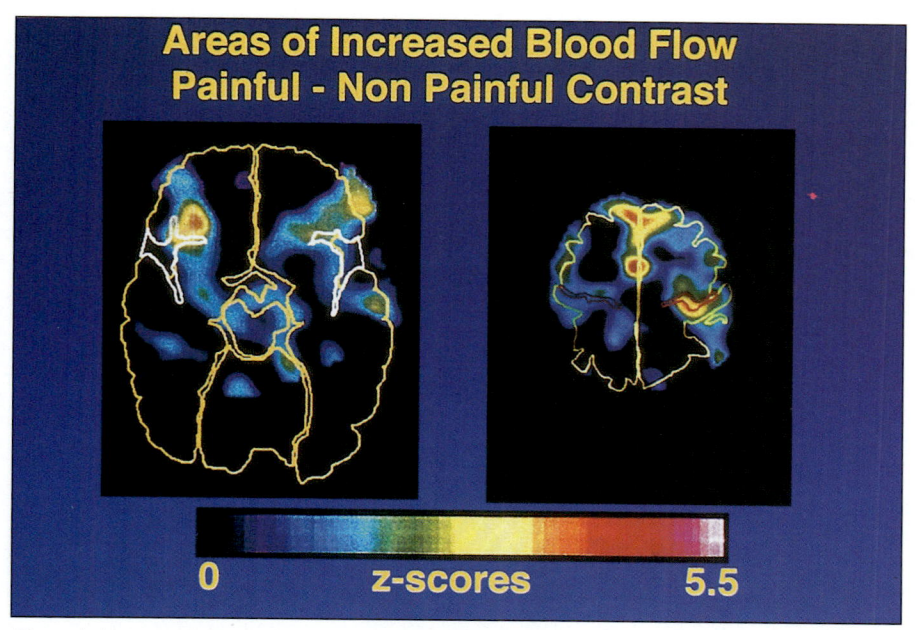

Plate 6 (Aziz, p76) Group mean positron emission tomography scans showing the areas of increased cortical blood flow when images obtained during non-painful oesophageal stimulation are subtracted from those obtained during painful oesophageal stimulation. Nociceptive oesophageal sensation appears to be processed exclusively in the right anterior insular cortex and the anterior cingulate gyri. (By courtesy of PET Centre, Uppsala University, Sweden.)

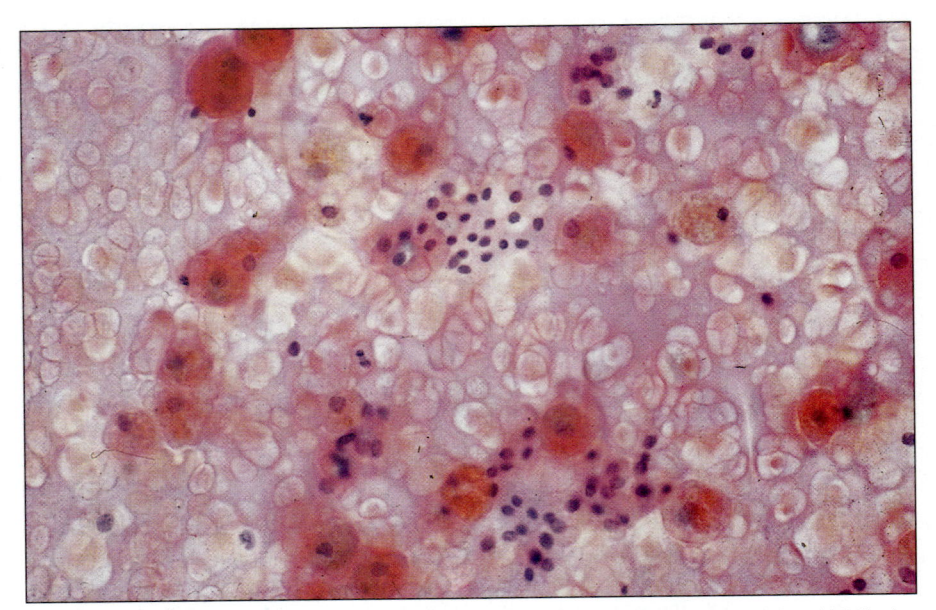

Plate 7 (Franklyn, p124) Aspirate from a colloid goitre indicating groups of normal thyroid follicular cells, and haemosiderin-laden macrophages against a background of blood and colloid.

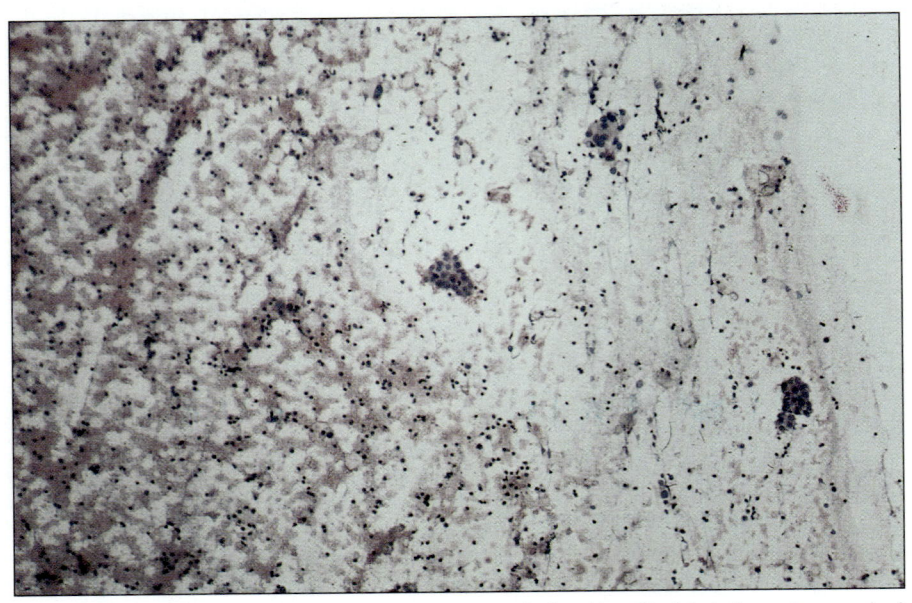

Plate 8 (Franklyn, p124) Aspirate containing normal thyroid epithelial cells and a marked lymphocytic infiltrate, indicative of Hashimoto's thyroiditis.

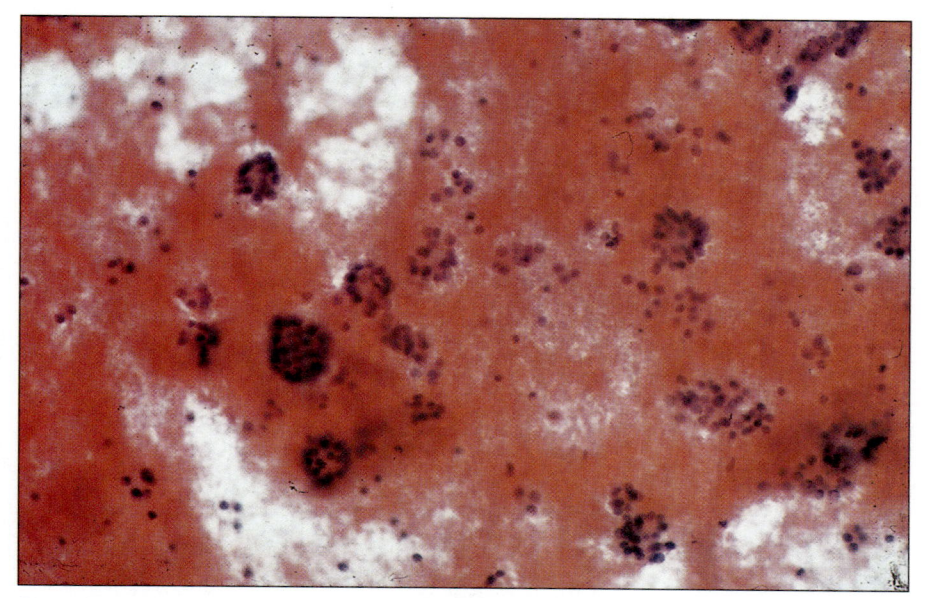

Plate 9 (Franklyn, p124) Clusters of thyroid epithelial cells indicative of a follicular neoplasm. Histology after surgical removal revealed this lesion to be a benign follicular adenoma.

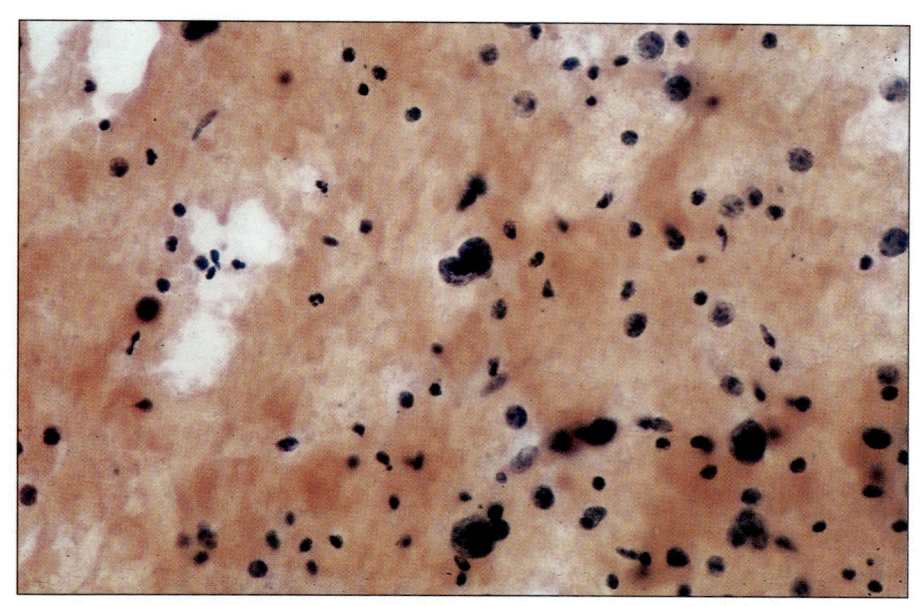

Plate 10 (Franklyn, p124) Thyroid aspirate from a patient with a poorly differentiated carcinoma including epithelial cells demonstrating marked variation in nuclear size and shape.

Plate 11 (Partridge, p190, 192) A credit-card-sized self-management plan (which is available as part of a self-management booklet from the National Asthma Campaign). On one side it is possible to base advice on self monitored peak flow, and on the reverse the plan is based on symptoms.

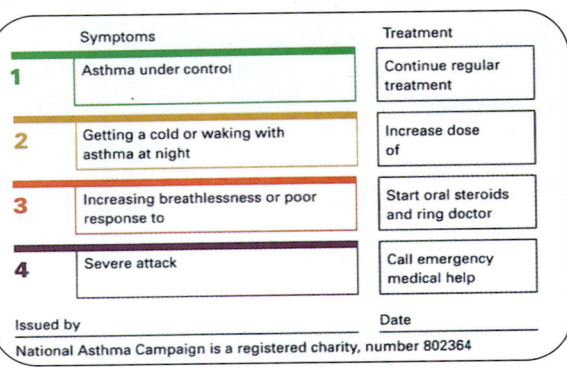

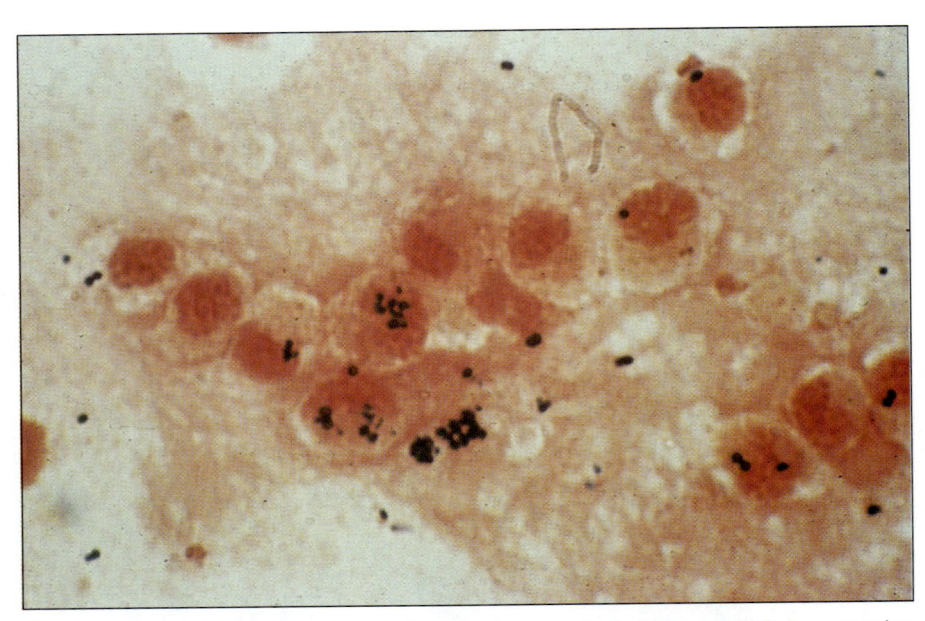

Plate 12 (Macfarlane, p228) Gram stain of sputum from a patient with severe CAP, demonstrating predominant staphylococci. The results of the Gram stain allowed early introduction of effective antistaphylococcal antibiotics for the patient, who was subsequently shown to have bacteraemic staphylococcal pneumonia. (From Macfarlane *et al.* [10], with permission.)

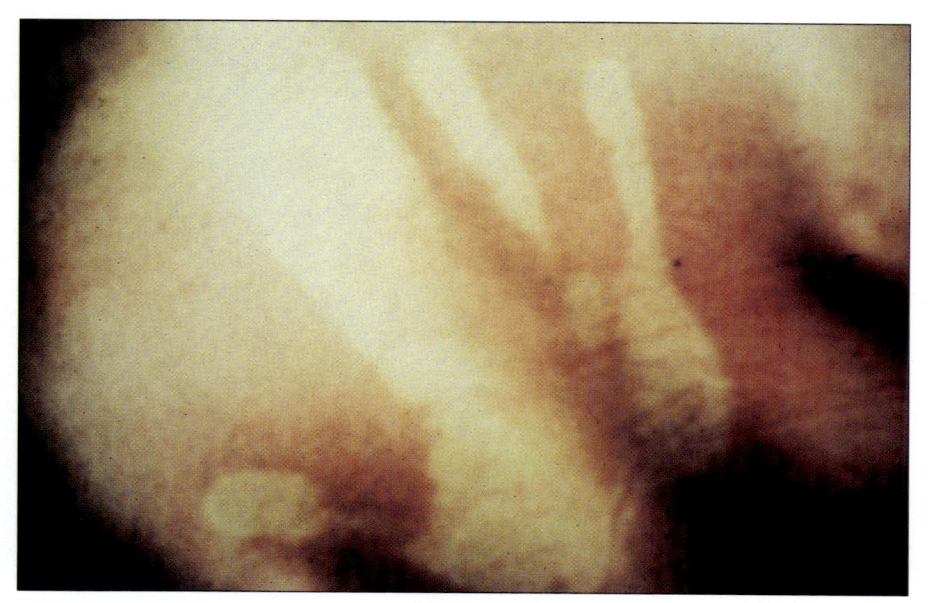

Plate 13 (Pasvol, p383–4) The characteristic blanching macular rash of dengue fever. This is probably due to vasodilation. The rash in more severe cases would also include petechiae and other signs of haemorrhage.

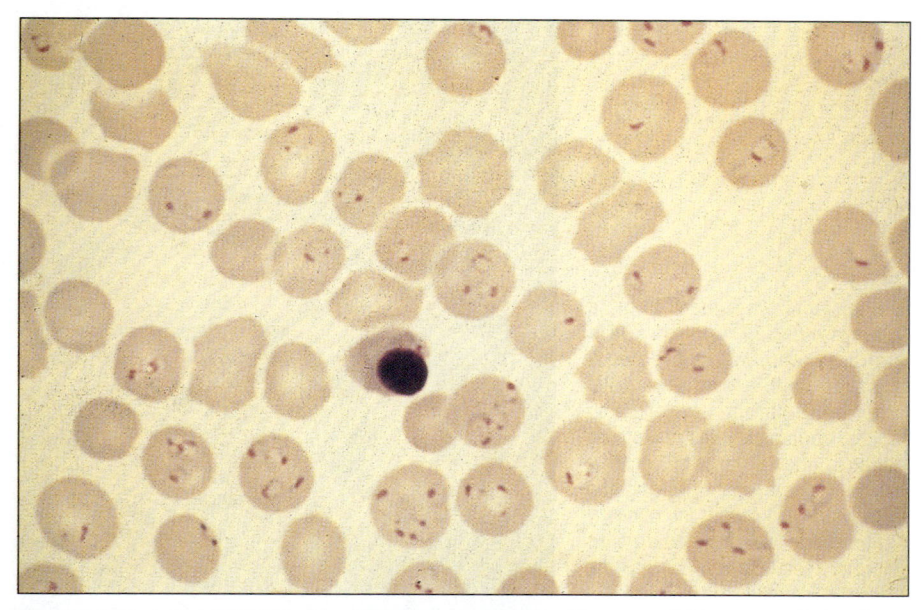

Plate 14 (Pasvol, p383) Thin blood film from a patient with severe falciparum malaria whose presentation was that of jaundice: 80% of the cells were infected. Numerous multiply infected cells are seen with small ring-stage parasites. In the centre is a nucleated erythroblast which also contains a ring form.

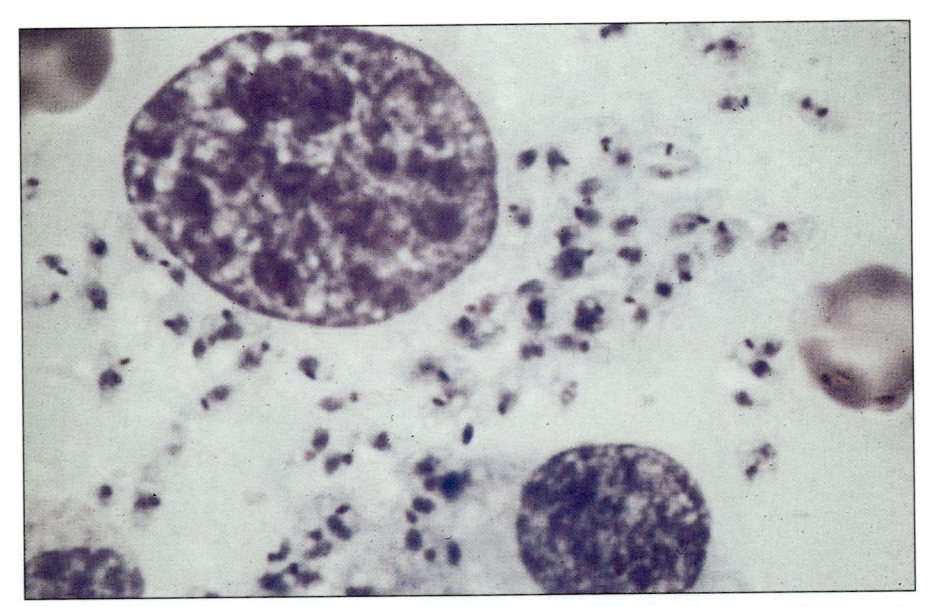

Plate 15 (Pasvol, p385) A macrophage containing typical Leishman-Donovan bodies seen in visceral leishmaniasis. Note both the nuclear and kinetoplast DNA in each organism.

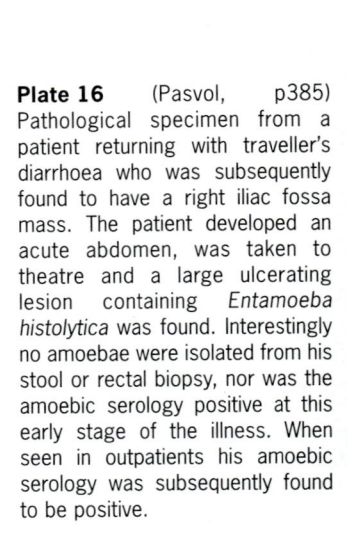

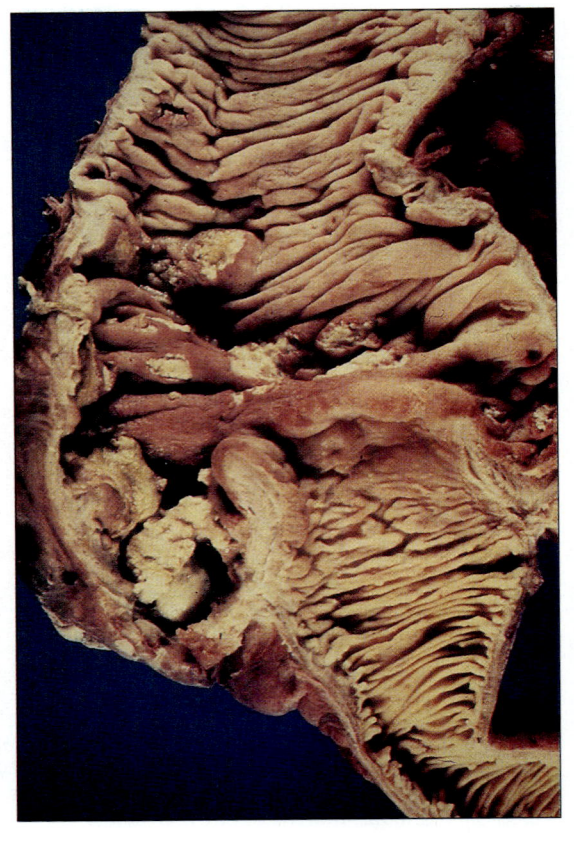

Plate 16 (Pasvol, p385) Pathological specimen from a patient returning with traveller's diarrhoea who was subsequently found to have a right iliac fossa mass. The patient developed an acute abdomen, was taken to theatre and a large ulcerating lesion containing *Entamoeba histolytica* was found. Interestingly no amoebae were isolated from his stool or rectal biopsy, nor was the amoebic serology positive at this early stage of the illness. When seen in outpatients his amoebic serology was subsequently found to be positive.

Plate 17 (Pasvol, p386) The urticarial lesions seen in Katayama fever, being the early febrile illness in schistosomal infection occurring about 4 or more weeks after exposure.

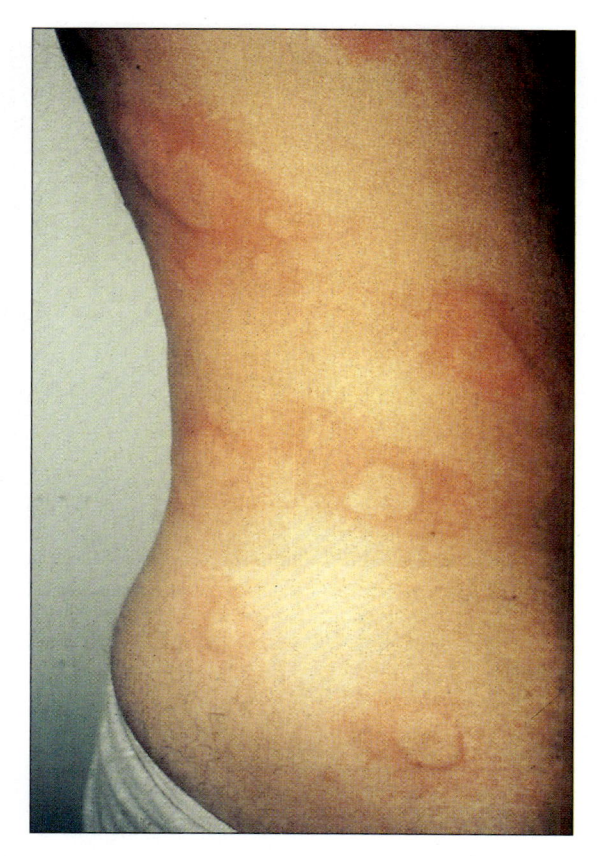

Plate 18 (Cohen, p393) Fundoscopy showing the characteristic features of Candida endophthalmitis.

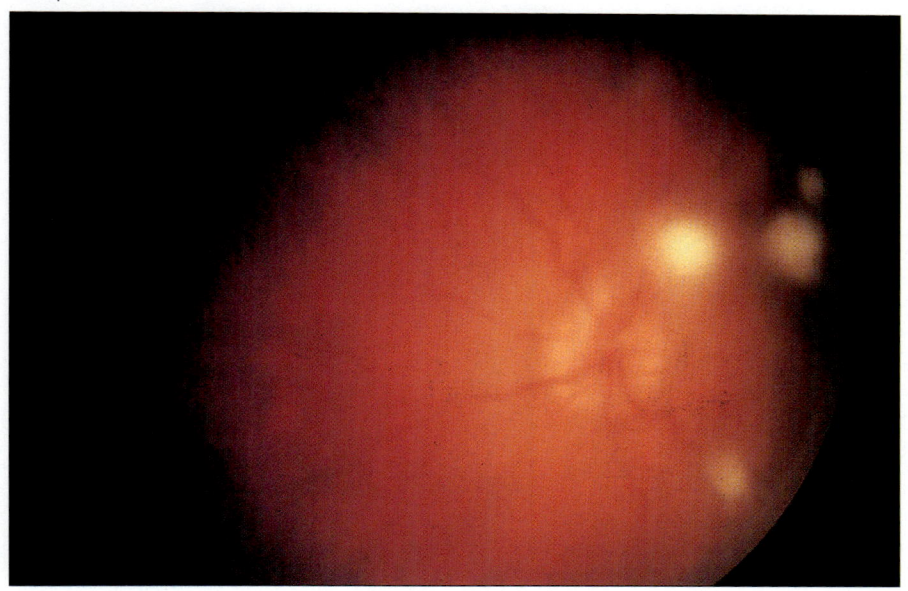

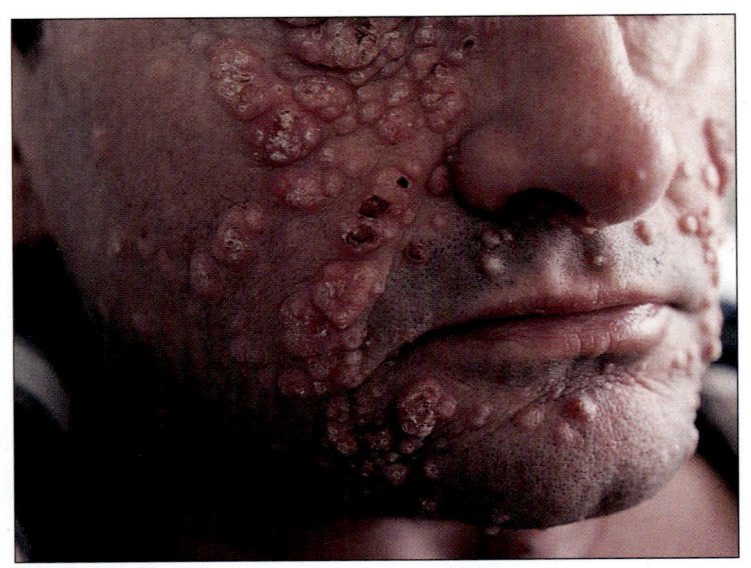

Plate 19 (Lynn, p416) This patient has severe cell-mediated immune deficiency due to AIDS. The appearances are those of molluscum contagiosum, which usually produces 2–3 mm flat lesions rather than this severe disease.

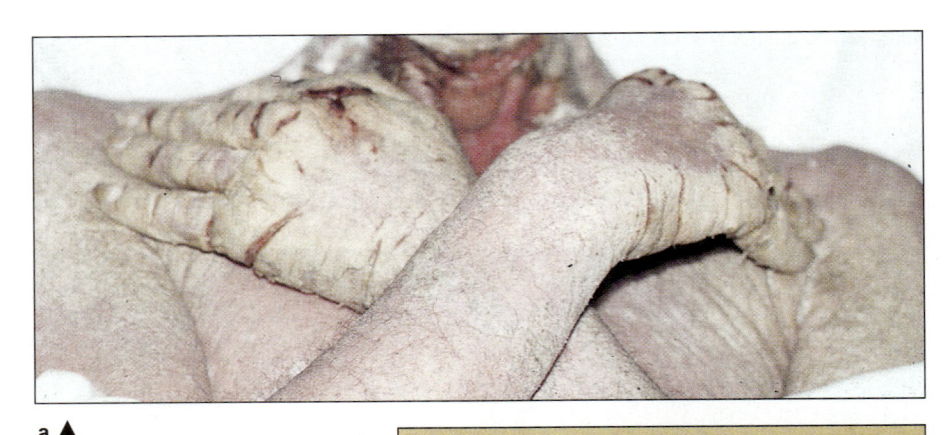

a ▲

b ▶

Plate 20 (Lynn, p416) **(a)** Severe cutaneous scabies (Norwegian variety) in a patient with AIDS. **(b)** The *Sarcoptes scabiei* mite identified from the patient's skin.

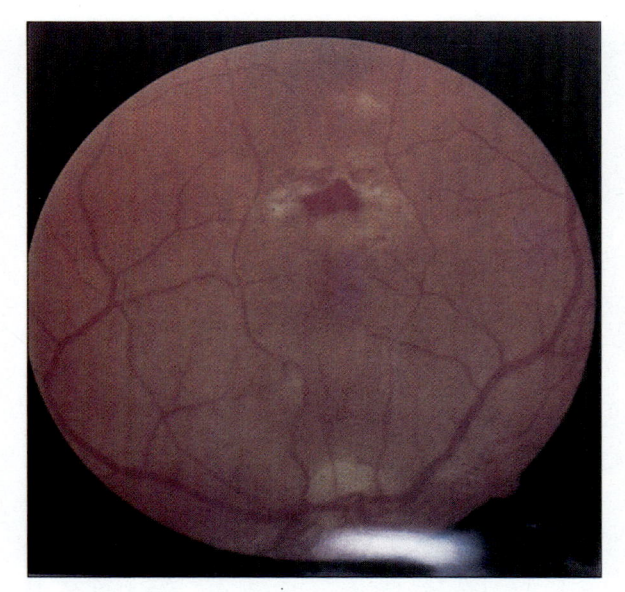

Plate 21 (Lynn, p417) Small patch of CMV retinitis showing the typical yellowish exudate with associated haemorrhage. The patient did not have any visual disturbance, but had been feeling generally unwell and tired which was resolved with anti-CMV therapy; his sight was preserved.

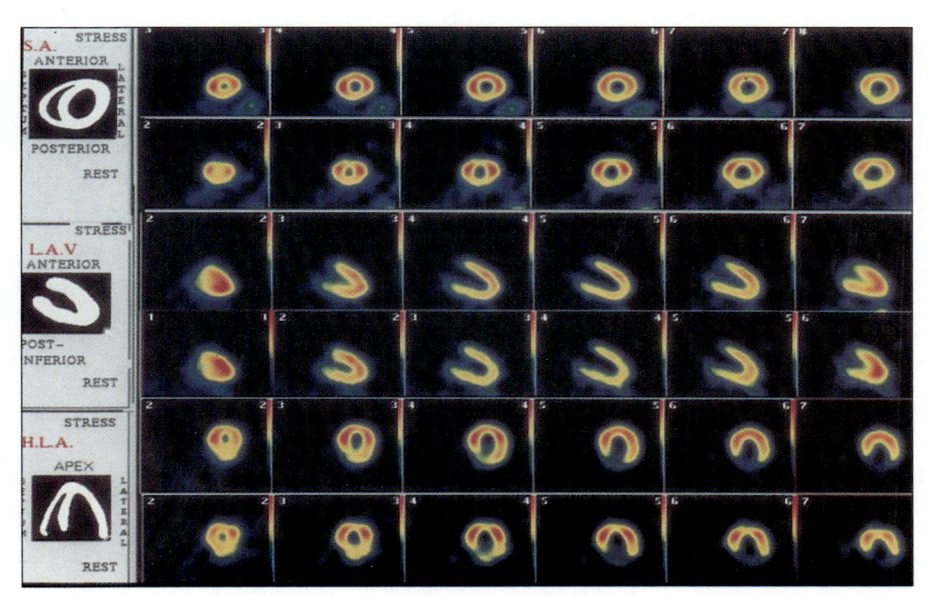

Plate 22 (Dymond, p481) Normal thallium tomogram at stress and rest in the short axis (top two horizontal panels), vertical long axis (middle two panels), and horizontal long axis (bottom two horizontal panels). Normal thallium uptake shown in yellow and red; there is symmetrical myocardial perfusion throughout. The left ventricular cavity appears as the centre of the 'doughnut' in the top two panels and in the centre of the 'horseshoe' in the middle and lower panels.

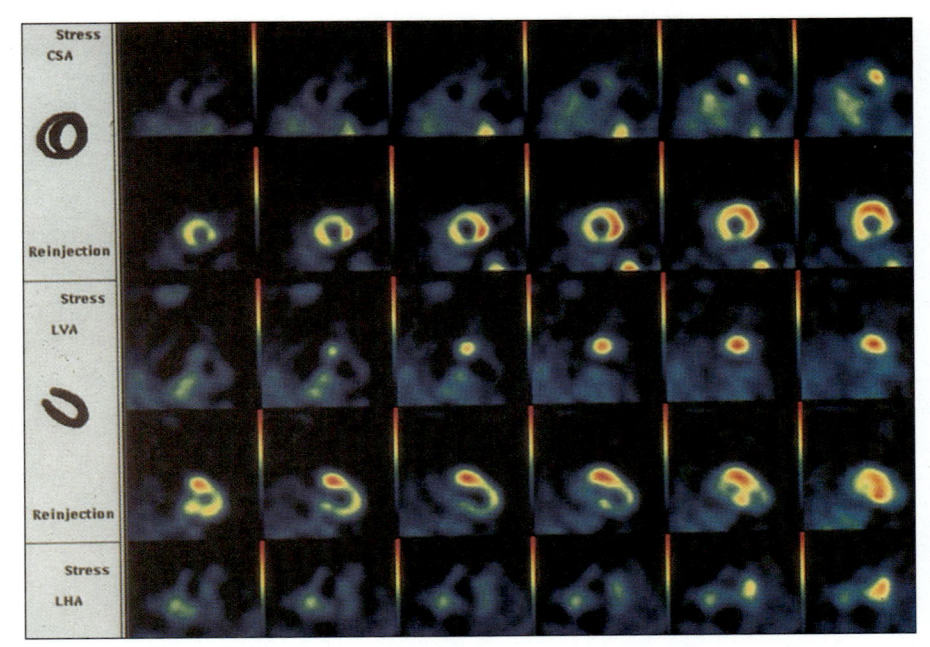

Plate 23 (Dymond, p482) Thallium tomograms in exactly the same format as in Plate 22 at stress and rest in a patient with a subtotal occlusion of the left anterior descending coronary artery. Severe global hypoperfusion is apparent in the top row of each pair of tomographic images as indicated by the prevalence of the blue colour. Flow is much improved at rest though it remains abnormal in some segments, this being particularly well seen in the fourth horizontal panel.

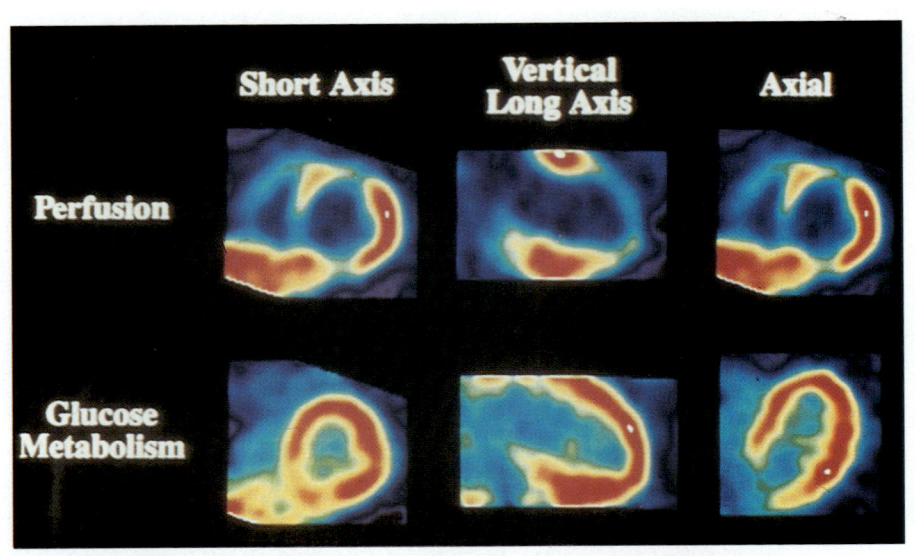

Plate 24 (Dymond, p482) Positron tomographic images of myocardial perfusion and glucose metabolism using ^{13}N-labelled ammonia and ^{18}F-labelled fluorodeoxyglucose respectively. It is apparent, particularly in the vertical long axis used, that in spite of impaired perfusion (blue colour) there is active glucose metabolism (red). This perfusion–metabolism mismatch indicates areas of myocardium that are hibernating and have switched from fatty acid metabolism to glucose metabolism. These areas may recover after revascularization.

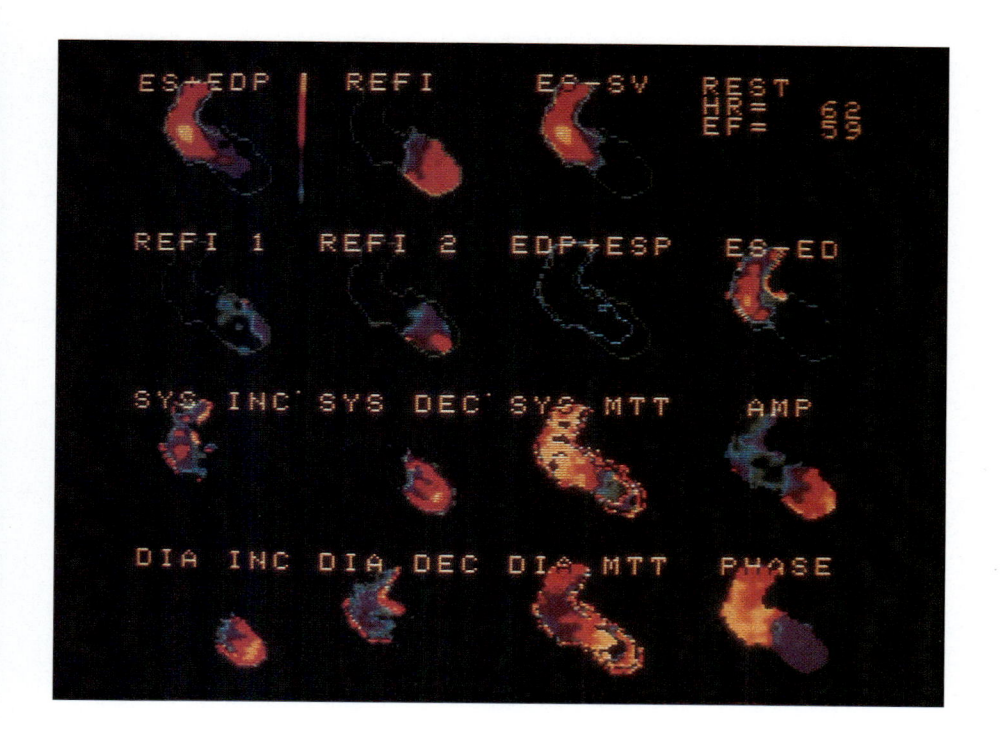

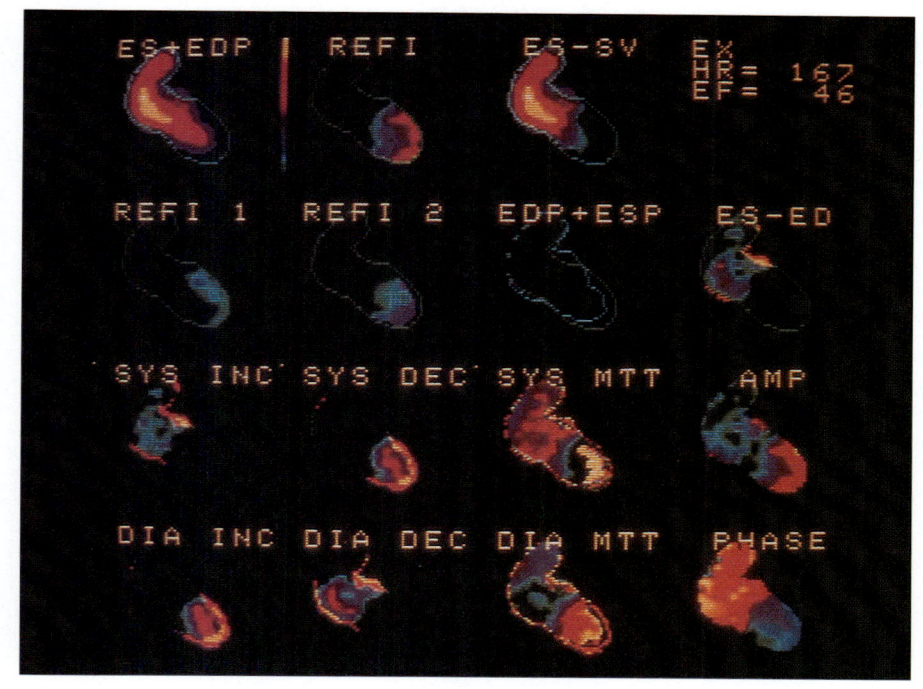

Plate 25 (Dymond, p483) First pass radionuclide angiograms at rest and with bicycle exercise in a patient with coronary artery disease. At rest ejection fraction (EF) is 59% and the images show a normal wall motion. On exercise (lower image) ejection fraction has fallen to 56% and images show marked hypokinesis particularly of the inferior wall.

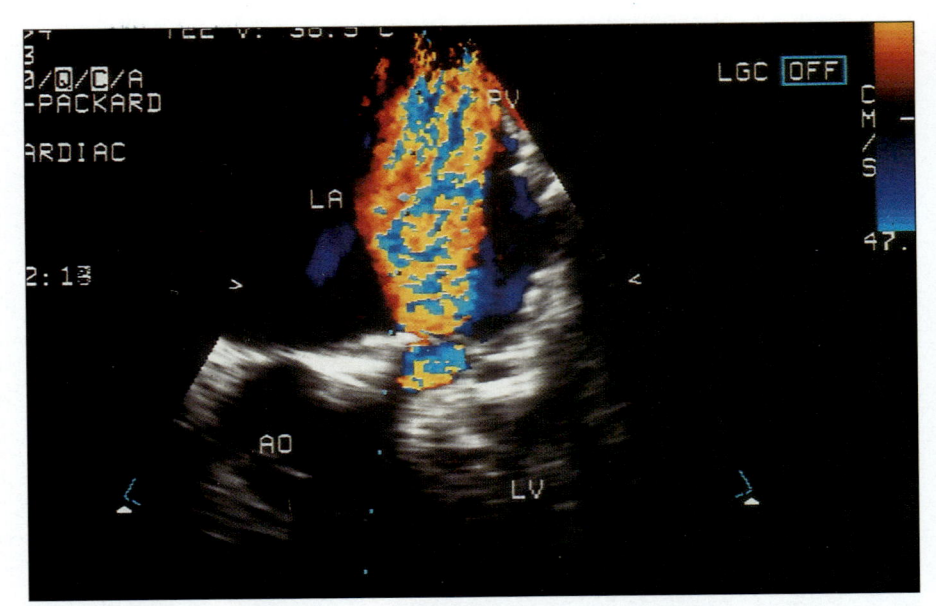

Plate 26 (Swanton, p504) Transoesophageal echocardiography. Colour Doppler imaging in severe paraprosthetic mitral regurgitation. Vertical plane. A broad regurgitant jet is shown spreading out to the back of the left atrium (LA) from the left ventricle (LV) through the lateral edge of the prosthetic valve ring. AO, aortic root.

Fibromyalgia revisited: the vicious cycle of chronic pain

P A Reilly

'There is no subject so old that something new cannot be said about it'
Dostoevsky, 1876

'Diagnosis is a system of more or less accurate guessing, in which the end-point is a name. These names applied to disease come to assume the importance of specific entities, whereas they are for the most part no more than insecure and therefore temporary conceptions'
Sir Thomas Lewis, 1944

☐ INTRODUCTION

Although the diagnostic term 'fibromyalgia' is 20 years old this year, the concept of debilitating aches and pains in the absence of recognizable pathology is not new. In a previous life it had been called 'fibrositis' by William Gowers (in 1904), and characteristic histological changes had been described by Professor Ralph Stockman in Glasgow that same year. If the condition was reborn in the 1970s in North America, it is fair to say it had a troubled early life. Particularly in the UK, fibromyalgia was thought to have little scientific validity, and was considered to be akin to diagnoses such as lumbago, gastric flu and chills in the bladder. It conjured up memories of 'fibrositis', a diagnosis much used by the lay public, but abandoned by rheumatologists getting to grips with 'real' diseases whose aetiology lay in the expanding sciences of immunology and molecular biology. As highlighted previously in a *Lancet* editorial in 1942: 'The condition referred to as fibrositis is still one of vague pathological and clinical definition; some sceptics deny its existence altogether, so that it is not surprising that the diagnosis has fallen into disrepute'. Plus ça change...

Unlike 'real' diseases such as smallpox, illnesses based on the complex interaction of the psyche, the soma and the society in which illnesses occur have a habit of being difficult to eradicate. There is no vaccine or surgical remedy for the irritable bowel syndrome, tension headaches or globus hystericus. These, and analogous conditions affecting a wide variety of body systems and bodily functions, have always been a hazard of life, the ills that flesh is heir to. Perhaps Job was patiently suffering from fibromyalgia when he complained '...the days of affliction have taken hold upon me. My bones are pierced in the night season; and my sinews take no rest' (Job 30:16–17).

The names may change to protect the innocent, but the terminology of illness changes more often than the clinical condition itself, as noted by Sir Thomas Lewis.

Perhaps nomenclature changes in an effort to adapt to the increasing sophistication of society and its members, and especially those in the medical profession. Stress must have an outlet, and we rationalize by giving it a name. Hence, ladies in a bygone age might swoon with a fit of the vapours, suffer chlorosis, endure chronic melancholia (black bile disease), have hypochondriasis (disease of the subcostal gristle) or hysteria (the dry womb moving about the body in pursuit of moisture). They might have to retire to their boudoir (from the French verb buder, to sulk). Even neurasthenia and myelasthenia, forerunners of fibromyalgia and chronic fatigue syndrome, were attributed to the stress of modern life – and that was before traffic jams, mobile 'phones and the purchaser–provider split! Whatever name has been used in the past, we should recognize that the constellation of somatic symptoms represents a failure to cope with prevailing physical, social, occupational or emotional demands.

If fibromyalgia has terminological shortcomings (fibrosis, fibrous tissue and fibroblasts being unrelated to the condition), then at least it has encouraged the application of scientific observation to the all too common problem of widespread musculoskeletal aching in the absence of overt organic pathology. Even those rheumatologists who abhor the term recognize that patients with such symptoms are often referred for diagnosis. Having satisfactorily excluded systemic lupus, myxoedema, osteomalacia, polymyalgia rheumatica and inflammatory joint disease, the doctor must ultimately deal with the patient who still has the original symptoms that prompted referral in the first place. In such circumstances, patient management becomes a matter of art rather than of science, and the most valuable management tool may well be the power of the physician to motivate a change in beliefs, attitudes and lifestyle in an unhappy, unfit individual.

☐ WHAT IS FIBROMYALGIA?

'Fibrositis does not lend itself easily to a definition that will be accepted generally, for to different people it bears varying degrees of reality'

Dr Michael Kelly, 1946

Over the past 25 years a number of different sets of diagnostic criteria have been suggested [1]. In 1990 a multicentre study was organized in North America, where much of the research was being performed [2]. A large number of potential criteria were evaluated. The two with the best combination of sensitivity and specificity, ie the most accurate for differentiating fibromyalgia from other non-specific pain problems, were the presence of widespread pain (defined as involving the axial skeleton plus two of four limb regions) and the simultaneous presence of undue tenderness at 11 of 18 sites palpated (nine symmetrical sites). As with most other criteria sets for disease, that for fibromyalgia has been derived in a circuitous fashion. The patients for inclusion were chosen on the basis that they had the problem, and further statistical evaluation of the same patients became the origin of the new classification criteria. If nothing else, the new criteria, adopted by the American College of Rheumatology, allow for comparable subjects for inclusion in research studies in all continents [2].

In addition to widespread pain and tenderness, a large number of non-criteria features are recognized. These include chronic sleep disturbance, prolonged morning stiffness, debilitating daytime fatigue, loss of functional abilities, headache, irritable bowel and bladder symptoms, Raynaud-like peripheral acrocyanosis, and modulation of pain intensity with weather, stress and exercise. Mood disturbance is common, with anxiety, panic attacks and depression predominating. Fibromyalgia therefore features dysfunction of the body and of the mind, and is an archetypal psychosomatic illness.

☐ WHAT CAUSES FIBROMYALGIA?

'...fibrositis has not a single cause, but results from the combined action of many factors, some known and others unknown'
Dr Michael Kelly, 1946

Even in the early part of the century, certain associations were recognized with the onset of fibrositis. Cold draughts, damp weather, infections such as pharyngitis, gastrointestinal disturbances and previous trauma were all implicated in the aetiology. In truth, fibromyalgia is probably the common clinical end-point of a number of different pathological processes. It may be related to a previous infection, and the clinical similarity to chronic fatigue syndrome has been noted. It can follow a frightening, but not necessarily injurious, road traffic accident, and there is overlap with post-traumatic stress disorder. It may also be a concomitant feature of other painful rheumatic conditions, including rheumatoid and osteo-arthritis, and systemic lupus erythematosus (with which it shares many non-specific complaints). Not infrequently, individuals display joint hypermobility due to one of the less severe variants of Ehlers–Danlos syndrome. Changes in weather can exacerbate the pain, as can stressful life events such as divorce and bereavement. This too was recognized by our forbears. As noted by Llewellyn and Jones, working in Bath, in 1915: 'The class of patients who come to us with such complaints are too often overworked, frequently neurotic, and nearly always, for some reason, below par.'

It is often assumed, on the basis of obvious mood disturbance, that patients with fibromyalgia have a masked depression or somatoform disorder. In fact, a huge variety of psychometric instruments have been applied to the study of fibromyalgia, with rather varied results. The Minnesota Multiphasic Personality Inventory (MMPI) cannot be relied upon to discriminate between psychogenic and organic pain, but overall conclusions from psychiatric interviews are that about one-third of patients are clinically depressed, one-third are normal, and one-third have mood states entirely appropriate to chronic pain [3]. Few actually have a somatoform disorder using Diagnostic and Statistical Manual (DSM-III) criteria. However, the higher than expected lifetime history of eating disorders, phobias and panic attacks has led to the theory that fibromyalgia is an 'affective spectrum disorder' and overlaps with many psychological and psychosomatic diagnoses [4].

What is certain is that fibromyalgia is not a muscle disease. The original observations of Stockman were discredited by Collins of the Mayo Clinic, who re-examined Stockman's original biopsies in 1942 and found them to be essentially normal. Since then there have been numerous histological, histochemical and electron micrographic studies of muscle biopsies from patients. Although abnormalities were described in open studies, blind and controlled studies were inconclusive, generally showing changes typically associated with lack of physical fitness [5,6].

☐ IS THERE AN UNDERLYING PATHOPHYSIOLOGY?

The neurobiology of pain is as complex as the clinical presentation. The thrust of recent research has drifted away from relatively simple areas such as muscle biopsies and psychometric testing. More fundamental questions are being asked about the dynamic interaction of serotonin, substance P, calcitonin gene-related peptide, endorphins, growth hormone, the hypothalamic–pituitary–adrenal axis hormones, the autonomic nervous system, and even cytokines in the onset and the perpetuation of pain [7]. The difficulty lies in relating nociception as a biochemical event to pain as a subjective experience. The relationship is not direct, but skewed by external factors such as degree of physical fitness, age, gender, culture, social circumstances and interpersonal stress.

Serotonin levels within the central nervous system are thought to be very important in the manifestations of fibromyalgia. Low levels cause loss of normal sleep patterns, depression of mood and increased sensitivity to painful stimuli, whereas serotoninergic drugs, including tricyclic agents, can lead to amelioration of symptoms.

☐ WHAT IS THE TREATMENT?

Since fibromyalgia is likely to be the common end-point of a number of differing pathologies, it follows that there is no single regime that will help all sufferers. The management has to be tailored to the individual. Most patients will be helped by the doctor recognizing the problem and being able to name it. Individuals will feel that they have been taken seriously, and not dismissed as neurotic or menopausal. Since many sufferers are unfit, a tailored regime of exercise can be recommended. Such a regime should encourage increased suppleness of muscles and ligaments, especially in the neck/shoulder and low back/pelvis regions. Weak muscles encourage poor posture, which places excessive mechanical loads on pain-sensitive ligaments. The author often recommends water-aerobics, callanetics and light weight-training. The third component of exercise should focus on cardiovascular fitness, such as brisk walking, an exercise bike or outdoor cycling, and swimming. Exercise such as yoga and t'ai chi chuan are good for mental as well as physical fitness, and are often enjoyable.

It is important that regular exercise should be enjoyable, and not viewed as a form of penance. Activities in a class or group may foster a less introspective outlook. Avoidance of stimulants should be stressed, so that late evening snacks, tobacco, caffeine and alcohol are best avoided if sleep is to be improved. Exercise can help sleep, but sometimes two or three months of a tricyclic drug is needed. In low doses, such as dothiepin 25 mg or amitryptyline 10 mg, taken one or two hours before bedtime, such 'neuropeptide modifiers' improve the quality and quantity of sleep, are non-addictive, and can break into the cycle of sleep deprivation/pain/fatigue which is so common in fibromyalgia. It is wise to tell the patient that these drugs are often used in depression, albeit in very much higher doses. If you do not, a friend or relative certainly will, and the patient will assume you have dismissed them as merely depressed yet not even had the courage to say so to their face. Of course, if clinical depression is a factor it should be treated with full doses of an appropriate antidepressant drug. Information leaflets are available from the Arthritis and Rheumatism Council, and literature can also be obtained from the Fibromyalgia Support Group. Reading about their condition can be tremendously reassuring to patients, as long as the information is factual and not skewed by a hidden agenda. Patients must not be allowed to learn new symptoms to add to their own, but learn of how others have shown successful improvement by following sensible regimes of management.

Many will explore non-traditional therapies, such as dietary modification, acupuncture, aromatherapy, homoeopathy and reflexology. They are unlikely to come to any harm, and may well benefit from feeling that they are exerting independence in managing their problem. Also, conventional medicine does not have a monopoly of answers to all ills. As Hamlet observed: 'There are more things in heaven and earth, Horatio, than are dreamt of in your philosophy.'

Of course, there are some ancient remedies which are not dissimilar to current orthodox and heterodox regimes. Massage, balneotherapy, topical oil of gaultheria and purgation with Hunyadi water move in and out of fashion, or at least some of them do!

☐ PROGNOSIS

There are few long-term follow-up studies of fibromyalgia [8–10]. The general consensus is that the outlook is not good, and that many patients have chronic symptoms of variable severity depending on concomitant life events and other unknown factors. Studies from the USA and England have painted a gloomy picture, while another from Australia was more encouraging. As with so many things, the result will depend on how much effort is put in, by both patient and doctor. In the doctor–patient relationship, well-being and optimism, just as with any other form of energy, cannot be created, but merely transferred and redistributed. In this entropy system, the doctor may well help the patient get better, only to find himself feeling rather deflated. In dealing with fibromyalgia in a conscientious fashion, perhaps only the physician can say if the end justifies the means.

REFERENCES

1   Yunus M, Masi AT, Calabro JJ, Miller KA, Feigenbaum SL. Primary fibromyalgia (fibrositis): clinical study of 50 patients with matched normal controls. *Semin Arthritis Rheum* 1981; **11**: 151–71.

2. Wolfe F, Smythe HA, Yunus MB, et al. The American College of Rheumatology 1990 criteria for the classification of fibromyalgia. Report of the Multicenter Criteria Committee. *Arthritis Rheum* 1990; **33**: 160–72.
3. Ahles TA, Yunus MB, Riley SD, Bradley JM, Masi AT. Psychological factors associated with primary fibromyalgia syndrome. *Arthritis Rheum* 1984; **27**: 1101–6.
4. Hudson JL, Hudson MS, Pliner LF, Goldenberg DL, Pope HG. Fibromyalgia and major affective disorder: a controlled phenomenology and family history study. *Am J Psychiatry* 1985; **142**: 441–6.
5. Yunus MB, Kalyan-Raman UP, Masi AT, Aldag JC. Electron microscopic studies of muscle biopsy in primary fibromyalgia syndrome: a controlled and blinded study. *J Rheumatol* 1989; **16**: 97–101.
6. Bennett RM, Clark SR, Goldberg L, et al. Aerobic fitness in patients with fibrositis: a controlled study of respiratory gas exchange and xenon-133 clearance from exercising muscle. *Arthritis Rheum* 1989; **32**: 454–60.
7. Reilly PA, Littlejohn GO. Fibrositis/fibromyalgia syndrome: the key to the puzzle of chronic pain. *Med J Aust* 1990; **152**: 226–8.
8. Felson DT, Goldenberg DL. The natural history of fibromyalgia. *Arthritis Rheum* 1986; **12**: 1522–6.
9. Ledingham J, Doherty S, Doherty M. Primary fibromyalgia syndrome: an outcome study. *Brit J Rheum* 1993; **32**: 139–42.
10. Granges G, Zilko P, Littlejohn GO. Fibromyalgia syndrome: assessment of the severity of the condition 2 years after diagnosis. *J Rheumatol* 1994; **21**: 523–9.

FURTHER READING

Wolfe F. Fibromyalgia: the clinical syndrome. *Rheum Dis Clin North Am* 1989; **15**; 1–18.

Granges G, Littlejohn GO. A comparative study of clinical signs in fibromyalgia/fibrositis syndrome, healthy and exercising subjects. *J Rheumatol* 1993; **20**: 344–51.

Carette S. Editorial: Fibromyalgia 20 years later: what have we really accomplished? *J Rheumatol* 1995; **22**: 590–3.

Management of transient ischaemic attacks: from clinical trials to individual patients

P M Rothwell and C P Warlow

'unaccustomed attacks of numbness and anaesthesia are signs of impending apoplexy'
Hippocrates *ca.* 400 BC

☐ INTRODUCTION

Hippocrates' observation that apoplexy, or major stroke, is sometimes preceded by less severe attacks of neurological symptoms is probably the first record of what we now refer to as transient ischaemic attacks (TIAs). However, it should be stated at the outset that, irrespective of treatment, only a relatively small minority of patients who suffer a TIA subsequently develop 'apoplexy'. Indeed, it is our inability to identify – and then treat – *only* these patients, and not the greater number who do not develop 'apoplexy', that colours much of the management of minor cerebral and ocular ischaemia.

Transient ischaemic attack is a rather vague term and much effort has gone into trying to develop a useful clinical definition. However, because TIAs are only a part of a spectrum of cerebral ischaemia, ranging from asymptomatic cerebral infarction to major disabling or fatal strokes, such definitions have perforce been arbitrary. Indeed, it is not entirely clear that TIA is a useful enough term to require exact definition. In reality there is very little difference between the prognosis and long-term management of what is usually regarded as a TIA and that of minor ischaemic strokes with symptoms or signs lasting up to several days, or indeed major non-disabling strokes. However, if for no other reason than that it is necessary to understand the literature, some definition of TIA must be given. In essence, a TIA is defined as an attack of focal cerebral dysfunction or monocular visual loss of vascular origin and rapid onset, which symptoms resolve completely without any permanent neurological deficit, although abnormal neurological signs may remain, and which usually lasts between a few seconds and 30 minutes, but may last up to 24 hours. For the purposes of this chapter, a term encompassing transient cerebral ischaemia, minor ischaemic stroke, major but non-disabling ischaemic stroke, transient monocular blindness (amaurosis fugax) and retinal artery occlusion would be more useful. These conditions will be referred to as non-disabling symptomatic cerebrovascular ischaemia.

☐ AETIOLOGY

Aetiology will be considered only in as much as it is likely to influence management. In the majority of cases, the precise aetiology of a non-disabling cerebrovascular ischaemic event is uncertain. Approximately 20% of events are either clinically or radiologically attributable to transient ischaemia or infarction in a small area of the deep cerebral white matter. Common sense, and a small amount of evidence, suggests that these 'lacunar' events are likely to be due to local thrombosis caused by disease of the small deep perforating arteries. Accurate diagnosis is important in that it may influence the decision whether or not to investigate or treat any possible carotid or cardiac causes of stroke. About 30% of the remaining events are associated with some stenosis of the internal carotid artery ipsilateral to the cerebral or ocular ischaemia. That *severe* carotid stenosis is likely to be of aetiological importance is demonstrated by the fact that the risk of stroke is almost abolished following successful carotid endarterectomy [1]. However, whether stroke results from reduced blood flow across the stenosis or from thrombus formation and distal embolism from the plaque surface is unknown. This is an important area for future research as elucidation of the relative importance of these two mechanisms would have important implications for treatment, in particular the likely efficacy of anticoagulation and treatment of hypertension.

A proportion of non-disabling cerebrovascular ischaemic events are due to embolism from the heart, aortic arch, and other sites of atheroma in the arteries supplying the brain. Atrial fibrillation or recent myocardial infarction should certainly prompt investigation of the heart, but investigation and management of possible embolism from aortic atheroma has not been shown to be of any value. In addition, there are several rare but treatable causes of TIA or minor stroke that should be considered if the clinical context is appropriate. These include inflammatory arterial disease (eg giant cell arteritis), haematological disorders (eg polycythaemia), specific prothrombotic states (eg deficiencies of proteins S or C, or anti-thrombin III) and arterial dissections. Optimal treatment of the last condition is unknown, but accurate diagnosis is important because dissections of the internal carotid or vertebral arteries frequently follow trauma to the neck, either accidental, in which case compensation may be available, or deliberate, in which case criminal proceedings may ensue.

☐ DIAGNOSIS

Clinical diagnosis

A detailed discussion of the diagnosis of non-disabling cerebrovascular ischaemia is not in the scope of this review, but several points should be noted. Although initial consideration might suggest that the diagnosis should be relatively straightforward, there is a wide differential diagnosis (Table 1), and considerable interobserver disagreement. Disagreement increases when observers are asked to decide whether a cerebral TIA occurred in the anterior or posterior cerebral circulation, a differentiation that is necessary to determine whether imaging of the carotid circulation is indicated. It is important, therefore, that the diagnosis is made by a neurologist or by a clinician with an interest in cerebrovascular disease. Incorrect diagnosis will lead either to inappropriate investigation and treatment or, perhaps more importantly, to delay in diagnosis of serious non-vascular pathology such as

Table 1 Differential diagnosis of transient focal cerebral symptoms and transient monocular visual loss.

Transient focal cerebral symptoms	Transient monocular visual loss
Migrainous aura	Migrainous aura
Focal epileptic seizures	Malignant hypertension
Intracranial space occupying lesion (eg tumour, subdural haematoma, arteriovenous malformation)	Papilloedema
Metabolic disturbance (eg hypoglycaemia)	Glaucoma
Multiple sclerosis	Uhthoff's phenomenon
Labyrinthine disorders	Retinal or vitreous haemorrhage
Somatization	Retinal vein thrombosis
Peripheral nerve lesions	Orbital tumour

cerebral tumour or partial epilepsy. False positive diagnoses of non-disabling cerebrovascular ischaemia will also decrease the efficacy and cost-effectiveness of preventive treatments. For example, the absolute benefit derived from carotid endarterectomy for carotid stenosis in a patient with unrelated neurological symptoms, such as non-specific dizziness, will be much less than that for truly symptomatic stenosis.

There are a number of points to remember when considering a diagnosis of TIA. In general, symptoms are usually of sudden onset and are usually negative. That is to say, they represent loss of function, eg weakness or numbness, rather than abnormal movement or tingling. In addition, as stated in their definition, TIAs are focal events. Global symptoms such as light headedness or non-specific dizziness are rarely due to focal cerebral ischaemia. TIAs rarely, if ever, cause loss of consciousness. Finally, the majority of patients with TIA have risk factors for vascular disease. Transient focal neurology in a young patient with no risk factors for vascular disease and with a normal heart is probably not a TIA.

Prognosis

The risk of stroke following TIA varies, depending on the population studied (Fig. 1). The risk is highest in community-based studies with a high proportion of elderly patients, and lowest in those patients who are referred to hospital, particularly those who are randomized in clinical trials [2]. The risk of stroke decreases steadily with time after the last TIA. On balance, the risk of stroke in the first year after a TIA is probably somewhere between 5% and 10%. About half of these strokes will be disabling. In addition, these patients are at increased risk of other vascular events. Patients presenting with symptomatic cerebrovascular ischaemia have an annual risk of myocardial infarction or non-stroke vascular death of 2–5%. Indeed, they are more likely to die as a consequence of ischaemic heart disease than cerebrovascular disease. Fortunately, many of the strategies aimed at preventing stroke also reduce the risk of cardiac death.

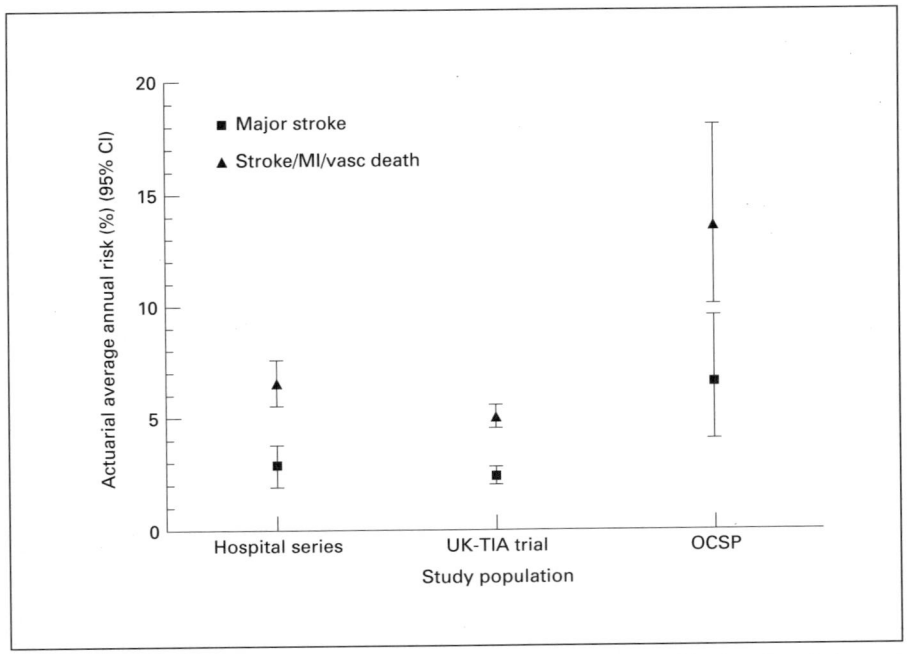

Fig. 1 The actuarial average annual risks (95% confidence interval, CI) of major stroke and stroke/myocardial infarction/vascular death (stroke/MI/vasc death) in three independent populations of patients with transient ischaemic attacks: a hospital referred population, a clinical trial population (UK-TIA trial), and a community based population (OCSP). (Further details can be found in Hankey et al. [2].)

Patients presenting with non-disabling cerebrovascular ischaemia can be stratified according to their likely risk of major ischaemic stroke on medical treatment using baseline clinical variables. If we consider the risk of carotid territory ischaemic stroke, the most important prognostic variable is the severity of any stenosis of the ipsilateral internal carotid artery (Fig. 2). Stroke risk increases with the degree of stenosis, and rises particularly sharply above 80% stenosis. The risk is approximately double that distal to an asymptomatic stenosis (Fig. 2). However, several other variables are also independent predictors of stroke risk after correction for the degree of stenosis of the symptomatic carotid artery (Table 2). In particular, the risk of stroke in patients with retinal ischaemic events is only half that in patients with cerebral ischaemic events.

Investigation

Appropriate investigation of patients presenting with non-disabling cerebrovascular ischaemic events is discussed elsewhere [3]. The most appropriate strategy for imaging and measuring the degree of carotid stenosis is subject to debate; disagreement centres on whether or not non-invasive methods are adequate or whether conventional arterial angiography is still required prior to any vascular surgery.

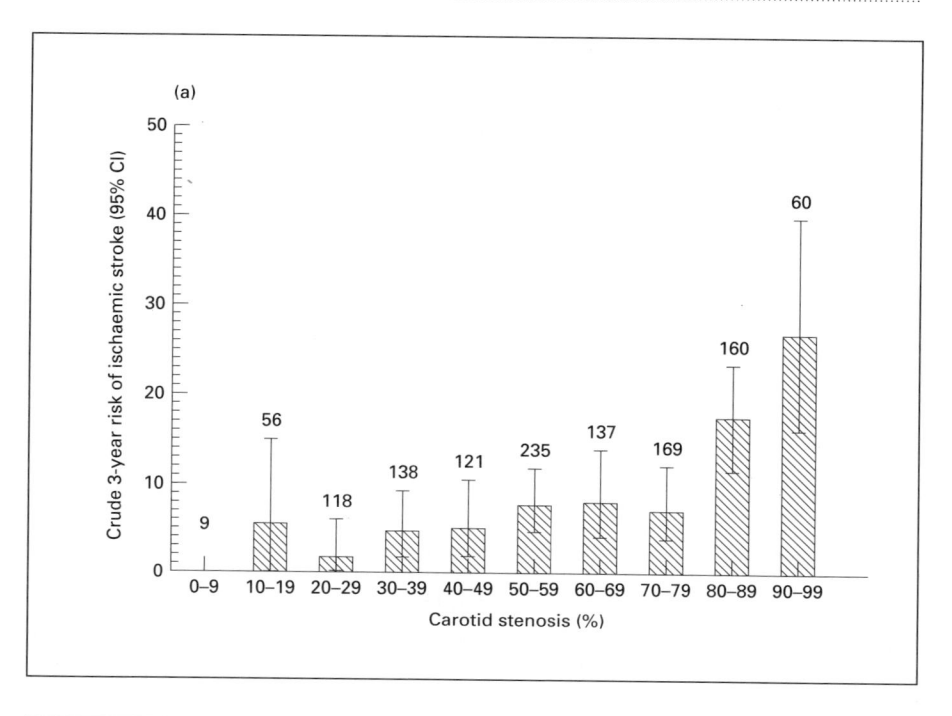

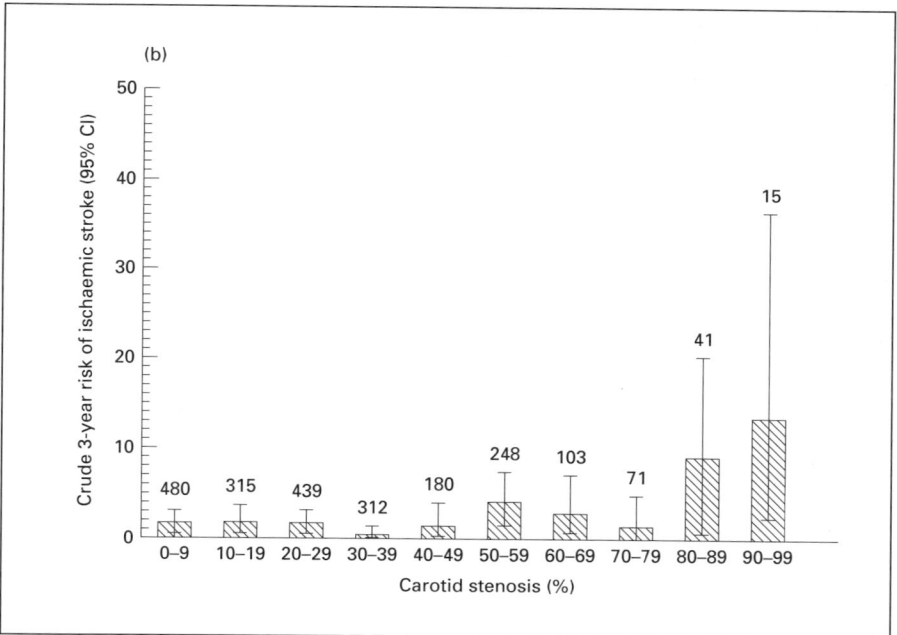

Fig. 2 The crude three-year risk (%) of ischaemic stroke according to the degree of stenosis of the ipsilateral carotid artery for: (a) events ipsilateral to the symptomatic carotid artery; (b) events ipsilateral to the asymptomatic carotid artery. Data are from The European Carotid Surgery Trial; the error bars represent the 95% confidence intervals of the risks and the number above each bar indicates the number of patients on which each estimate is based.

Table 2 A preliminary multiple-regression analysis of the baseline clinical and angiographic variables predicting carotid territory ischaemic stroke ipsilateral to the recently symptomatic carotid artery in patients randomized to medical treatment in the European Carotid Surgery Trial.

Variable	Hazard ratio (95% confidence interval)	p
Stenosis of ipsilateral internal carotid >80%	2.92 (2.05–4.16)	0.0001
Plaque surface irregularity visible on angiogram	1.88 (1.24–2.86)	0.0003
Ocular ischaemic events only	0.59 (0.40–0.89)	0.01
Myocardial infarction within past year	1.86 (1.19–2.92)	0.007
Residual neurological signs	1.71 (1.20–2.40)	0.003
Diabetes mellitus	1.97 (1.30–3.00)	0.001
Less than two months since last ischaemic event	1.82 (1.25–2.65)	0.002

☐ TREATMENT

There are several ways in which the efficacy of a treatment can be assessed (Table 3). Each involves a comparison of outcome in patients who have received the treatment with that in untreated patients. The methods differ in terms of the rigour with which the comparison is made and, consequently, the reliability of their results. For example, interpretation of studies with literature or historical controls is very difficult. Sacks et al. [4] studied six treatments, and compared the results of 56 studies, which used historical controls with the results of 50 randomized controlled trials. Treatment was found to be better than control in 80% of studies with historical controls compared with only 20% of randomized trials. The use of concurrent non-randomized controls is also open to bias which cannot necessarily be corrected by adjustment for any differences in prognostic variables between the treatment and control groups. Discussion of the management of non-disabling cerebrovascular ischaemia in this review will, therefore, be based only on data from randomized controlled trials (RCTs).

Table 3 Methods used to determine the efficacy of treatment.

Anecdote
Uncontrolled studies
Studies with literature controls
Studies with historical controls
Concurrent non-randomized controls*
Randomized controlled trials†

*The validity of this approach may be improved by correction of any differences in baseline prognosis between the treatment and control groups using a validated prognostic model
† Minimization or stratified randomization may be more appropriate in certain circumstances

Economics

Economic considerations are becoming increasingly important in decisions about how best to treat patients. Reviews of the treatment of individual patients with non-disabling cerebrovascular ischaemia will inevitably be biased in the direction of the high-risk preventive strategy rather than the population approach [5]. However, the high-risk approach does need to be considered in the context of the cost and burden of stroke in the population as a whole. Stroke is the third most common cause of death in the developed world. It is the most important single cause of disability in people living in their own home, and caring for stroke patients is estimated to account for approximately 4.3% of the National Health Service (NHS) budget and 13% of occupied inpatient bed days [6].

How much of this burden could be prevented by a high-risk secondary prevention strategy based on treating TIA patients? Only about 15% of patients who suffer an ischaemic stroke have a previous TIA, and it is unlikely that more than 25% of disabling strokes are preceded by any kind of non-disabling cerebrovascular ischaemic event. Since many of the patients who do suffer 'warning' events do not seek medical attention at the time, and the majority of preventive strategies do not reduce the risk of disabling stroke by much more than 50% in relative terms, it is unlikely that the strategy laid out below would prevent more than 5% of disabling strokes in the population as a whole. However, although in population terms treatment of patients presenting with non-disabling cerebrovascular ischaemic events is not of major importance, treatment is still very worthwhile from the point of view of the individual patient, and the high incidence of cerebrovascular disease means that such patients represent a common clinical problem. Evidence of the overall efficacy of each of the major therapeutic interventions will be reviewed briefly.

Antiplatelet agents

Data from all RCTs of antiplatelet therapy in the prevention of vascular events were combined by the Antiplatelet Trialists' Collaboration [7]. Data were obtained for 257 randomized trials involving a total of 118 958 patients. Antiplatelet treatment had no effect on non-vascular death but produced highly significant reductions in the odds of non-fatal stroke (25%), non-fatal myocardial infarction (34%) and vascular death (17%). The antiplatelet agent used in the majority of studies was aspirin. There were too few patients included in trials comparing the efficacy of different antiplatelet drugs to draw any useful conclusions. In keeping with the results of later individual trials comparing the efficacy of different doses of aspirin, the meta-analysis produced no evidence that high-dose aspirin (500–1500 mg) was any more effective than medium dose (160–325 mg) or low dose (75–150 mg) aspirin. Low dose aspirin, of course, has the advantage of a lower incidence of gastrointestinal side-effects.

Anticoagulants

Anticoagulation, usually with warfarin, is indicated when there is a definite source of cardiac embolism, eg rheumatic mitral valve disease, a prosthetic heart valve, recent myocardial infarction or dilated cardiomyopathy. In addition, warfarin has been shown to be superior to aspirin in the secondary prevention of stroke in patients with non-rheumatic atrial fibrillation, although aspirin is better than nothing [8]. Patients with recurrent TIAs refractory to treatment with aspirin are sometimes treated with an anticoagulant, although there are no data from clinical trials to support this option.

Treatment of hypertension

Observational studies have demonstrated a close relationship between blood pressure and the risk of stroke; stroke risk increases by about 2% for every 1 mmHg increase in usual diastolic blood pressure. A meta-analysis of all available data [9], and several subsequent large randomized primary prevention trials, showed that relatively small reductions in blood pressure, of the order of 5–10 mmHg in systolic pressure, reduce the risk of stroke by approximately 50%. Roughly the same relationship between blood pressure and stroke risk appears to hold in observational studies of patients who have already developed symptoms of vascular disease. However, in contrast to primary prevention, there is relatively little data on the efficacy of blood pressure lowering in the secondary prevention of stroke and other vascular events, although one RCT (PROGRESS) is ongoing. Moreover, there is a danger that treatment of hypertension might be harmful in those patients with symptomatic cerebrovascular ischaemia who have a haemodynamically significant carotid stenosis or occlusion. Thus, while moderate hypertension should probably be treated in patients with non-disabling cerebrovascular ischaemia with carotid stenosis of less than 50%, the balance of risks and benefits is unknown in patients with more severe stenosis.

Lipid lowering drugs

In contrast to hypertension, the risk of ischaemic stroke in the general population does not increase with plasma cholesterol [10]. Randomized trials of treatment with lipid lowering agents following myocardial infarction have demonstrated non-significant reductions in the risk of stroke in the treated group [11]. However, although lipid-lowering drugs do appear to lead to regression of carotid atheroma, there are no data from RCTs to support the use of these agents in the prevention of stroke in patients with symptomatic cerebrovascular disease. Nevertheless, it seems likely that patients with cerebrovascular disease will benefit, if only as a consequence of a reduction in cardiac events, while the results of an ongoing RCT are awaited (the Heart Protection Study).

Carotid endarterectomy

About 30% of patients with non-disabling cerebrovascular ischaemia have a stenosis at the bifurcation of the ipsilateral carotid artery. The stenotic plaque can be removed by a surgical procedure known as carotid endarterectomy. The operation was introduced in the 1950s and became popular in the 1970s and early 1980s, but it was not until 1991 that it was shown to be of value in patients with a recently symptomatic carotid stenosis of 70–99% [1,12] (Fig. 3a). In patients with 0–29% stenosis, the risk of stroke on medical treatment alone is low and surgery, with the associated operative risk of stroke and death, is therefore harmful [1] (Fig. 3b). There is no overall benefit or harm in patients with 30–69% stenosis [13] (Fig. 3c).

Carotid angioplasty

Angioplasty has been suggested as a potentially less costly and less uncomfortable alternative to endarterectomy in patients with carotid stenosis. However, the initial risks of the procedure and the rate of re-stenosis have yet to be defined. A large RCT of carotid angioplasty is presently ongoing (CAVATAS).

How should the results of clinical trials be applied to individual patients?

It is now widely accepted that, if at all possible, medical interventions should be tested using randomized controlled trials. However, very large trials, or meta-analyses of several smaller trials, are often necessary to define the effect of treatment with narrow confidence intervals. The results of such trials or meta-analyses are usually expressed as the overall odds or risk of outcome events in the treated group compared with controls, ie the relative treatment effect. It is often difficult, however, given the very heterogeneous population of individuals who tend to be included in megatrials and meta-analyses, to know whether the overall result can be applied with confidence to the decision whether or not to treat an individual patient. The absolute benefit a patient will derive from a treatment will of course vary, depending on their risk of a poor outcome without treatment: a 50% reduction in relative risk might be very worthwhile if the absolute risk of a poor outcome is reduced from 20% to 10%, but possibly not if it is reduced from 1% to 0.5%.

The relative treatment effect is assumed to be qualitatively, if not quantitatively, constant, and the overall reduction in relative risk to be generally applicable to all future patients who fit the criteria for trial entry [14]. This is convenient, but may not always be the case. It is quite conceivable that a treatment might be beneficial in some patients and harmful in others. For example, heterogeneity of relative treatment effect is especially likely when a treatment has an appreciable risk of serious harm. Thrombolytic therapy in acute ischaemic stroke increases early case fatality by about 10% in absolute terms, mainly as a consequence of an increased risk of intracerebral bleeding [15]. However, it decreases the risk of dependency in survivors, and may possibly reduce the overall risk of death and dependency at 6 months [15]. The increase in early case fatality with thrombolysis is present in all subgroups, and is particularly marked in patients in whom the initial neurological deficit is only 'slight' [15], the vast majority of whom would otherwise have made a full recovery. There would have been little potential for benefit in these patients, but considerable risk of harm. The overall trial result must therefore be reflecting the balance between harm in at least one identifiable group of patients and benefit in others.

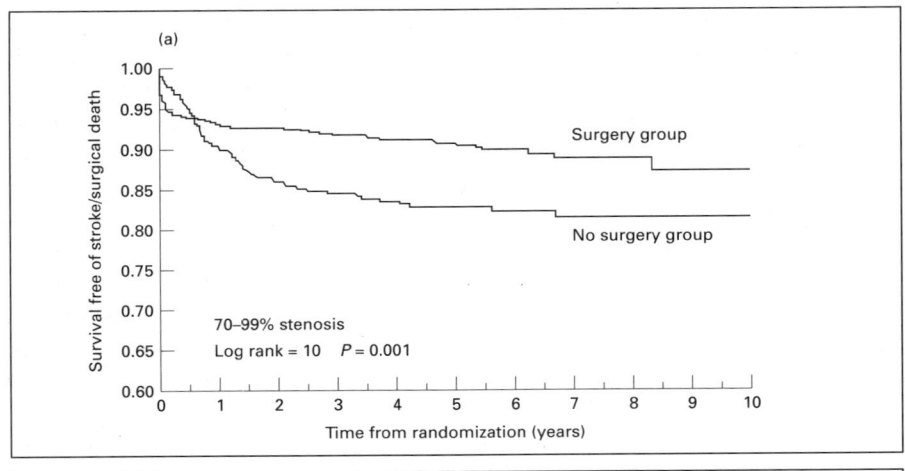

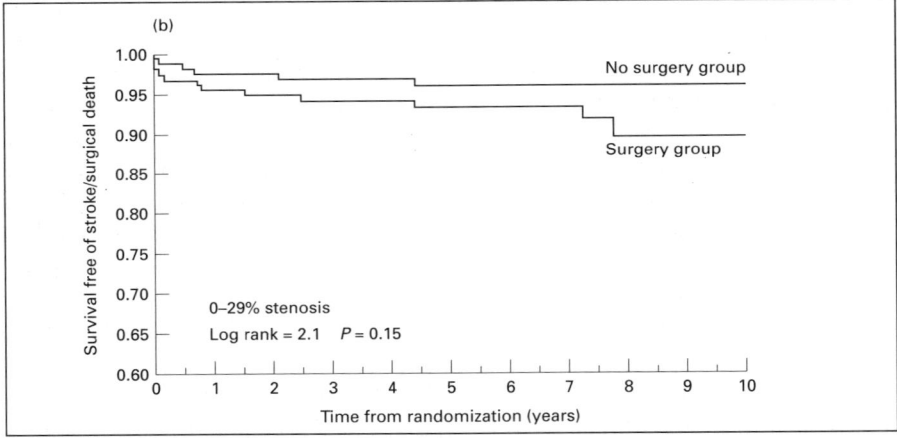

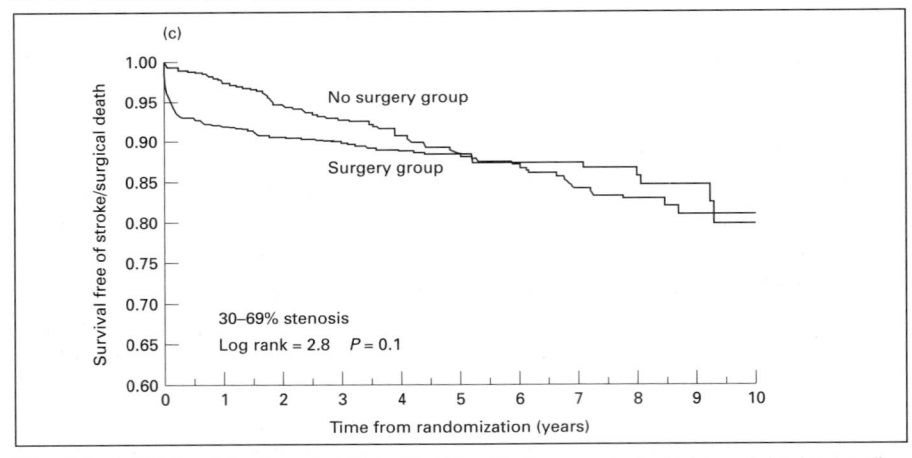

Fig. 3 Kaplan Meier plots of survival free of ipsilateral ischaemic stroke or surgical death according to treatment allocation in the European Carotid Surgery Trial (medical treatment and immediate carotid endarterectomy versus medical treatment alone) in patients with recently symptomatic carotid stenosis of: (a) 70–99%; (b) 0–29%; (c) 30–69%.

Application of the overall results of clinical trials to all patients is based on the assumption that we cannot identify in advance those patients who will do badly without treatment, and who should therefore be treated, and those patients who will do well without treatment, and who should not therefore be subjected to any risks associated with treatment. However, this negative approach may not be justified. While we cannot predict outcome with 100% accuracy, there are at least some validated prognostic models in several branches of medicine which can reliably stratify patients according to their likely level of risk of various clinical outcomes. Stratification of the results of clinical trials using such models can provide an insight into the potential unreliability of the *overall* trial results. For example, this approach proved useful in making sense of trials of bone marrow transplantation versus consolidation chemotherapy in first remission of acute leukaemia [16]. Chemotherapy is a relatively safe treatment, but is associated with a high risk of subsequent relapse, whereas bone marrow transplantation is associated with a high early mortality but a low risk of subsequent relapse in patients who survive. Consequently, there is little overall difference in disease-free survival when the treatments are compared in randomized trials. However, when prognostic models are used to stratify patients according to their risk of death without bone marrow transplantation, transplantation appears to improve survival in patients with a poor prognosis, but not in patients with a good one [16]. Similar results were reported in a meta-analysis of individual patient data from trials of coronary artery bypass grafting versus medical treatment in patients with ischaemic heart disease [17]. Bypass grafting had an associated 30-day operative case-fatality of 3.2%, but nevertheless resulted in a reduced overall case-fatality compared with medical treatment on follow-up. However, after stratification of patients according to baseline risk of death on medical treatment, using an independently derived prognostic model, it was evident that grafting was probably harmful in low-risk patients, but highly beneficial in high-risk patients. The *overall* results of the trials of bone marrow transplantation and coronary artery bypass grafting were merely reflecting the balance between benefit in some patients and harm in others.

Who benefits from carotid endarterectomy?

Carotid endarterectomy for symptomatic carotid stenosis has a 5–7% operative risk of stroke or death [18]. Despite this risk, when compared with medical treatment alone, endarterectomy reduces the overall risk of ipsilateral ischaemic stroke in patients with a recently symptomatic severe stenosis by about 50% in relative terms [1,12]. It is now widely recommended, therefore, that all such patients should be considered for surgery. However, in neither trial did more than 25% of patients randomized to medical treatment actually have a stroke on follow-up. In other words, the remaining 75% of patients who remained stroke-free could not possibly have benefited from surgery had they been randomized to endarterectomy. Indeed, given the risk of stroke or death due to the operation, they would, as a group, undoubtedly have been harmed.

The relationship between relative treatment effect and absolute baseline risk of stroke on medical treatment has been examined in the European Carotid Surgery Trial [19]. The analysis was restricted to patients with a severe carotid stenosis (70–99%) in whom, as a group, endarterectomy was found to be beneficial. The absolute risk of ischaemic stroke in the distribution of the symptomatic carotid stenosis at trial entry was predicted for all patients in both the surgery and no-surgery groups using an independently derived prognostic model based on clinical data obtained at randomization. The no-surgery and surgery groups were then divided into low-, moderate- and high-risk categories on the basis of their predicted stroke risks. These risks were then compared with the observed risk of ipsilateral ischaemic stroke during the trial in the no-surgery group and the risk of ipsilateral ischaemic stroke and perioperative stroke or death in the surgery group. The effects of relative and absolute treatment were calculated at the three different levels of baseline absolute risk by comparing the observed risk in surgery patients with the observed risk in the no-surgery patients within each predicted risk group (Table 4). In the no-surgery group, the observed stroke risk fell from 20.2% in patients predicted to be at high risk at randomization to 8.4% in those predicted to be at low risk. On the other hand, in the surgical group, the observed risk of stroke tended to fall as predicted baseline risk increased. As a result, despite significant overall benefit in patients with severe carotid stenosis as a whole, patients with a 'low' predicted stroke risk on medical treatment appeared possibly to have been harmed by endarterectomy, whereas patients at 'moderate' or 'high' risk of stroke showed clear benefit (Table 4). In other words, the overall benefit derived from endarterectomy should not be generalized to all patients because there is, in fact, an identifiable subgroup of patients with a recently symptomatic severe stenosis in whom the operation may be harmful.

Table 4 The observed stroke risk in patients with a severe (70–99%) symptomatic carotid stenosis randomized prior to 1992 in the no-surgery and surgery groups in the European Carotid Surgery Trial stratified according to predicted baseline risk of ipsilateral ischaemic stroke using data obtained at randomization. The relative and absolute reductions in ipsilateral ischaemic stroke risk following surgery and the number of patients that need to be treated to prevent one stroke are shown for each predicted risk group [19].

Predicted risk	No-surgery group			Surgery group			Relative risk reduction (95% CI)	Absolute risk reduction	Cases treated per stroke prevented
	n	Strokes	(Risk)	n	Strokes*	(Risk)			
< 10%	119	10	(8.4%)	183	18	(9.8%)	1.16 (0.6–2.4)	−1.4%	−71
10–15%	178	25	(14.0%)	273	19	(7.0%)	0.53 (0.3–0.9)	7.0%	14
> 15%	89	18	(20.2%)[†]	132	8	(6.1%)	0.34 (0.1–0.7)[‡]	14.1%	7
Total	386	53	(13.7%)	588	45	(7.7%)	0.51 (0.3–0.8)	6.0%	17

* Includes all surgery related strokes and deaths as well as all subsequent ipsilateral ischaemic strokes
[†] χ^2 for linear trend in absolute stroke risk = 6.2, $p<0.01$
[‡] Test for trend in relative risks, $p<0.01$

Prediction of the risk of stroke or death due to endarterectomy

To target a treatment most efficiently, it would be necessary to know, for each individual, the likely risk of a poor outcome with treatment as well as the risk of a poor outcome without treatment. Can we, therefore, predict the risk of stroke and death in patients who have carotid endarterectomy? Given that the risk of stroke following successful endarterectomy is low, it would seem reasonable simply to try to predict the risk of stroke or death due to endarterectomy. With this in mind, a systematic review of the literature on carotid endarterectomy published since 1980 was performed. Operative risks for endarterectomy for symptomatic or asymptomatic stenosis were identified in 126 studies [18]. Data were extracted from those studies that reported the operative risk of stroke or death according to the presence or absence of various baseline clinical and angiographic variables. For each variable a meta-analysis of all available data was performed, and the results are summarized in Fig. 4. The operative risk of stroke or death was less in patients with ocular ischaemia compared with cerebral ischaemia, but was greater in women, patients with hypertension (systolic blood pressure >180 mmHg), and patients with an occlusion of the contralateral internal carotid artery. These data demonstrate that certain baseline clinical variables do predict the risk of stroke or death due to endarterectomy, and suggest that more detailed prognostic modelling might be worthwhile.

The risk of stroke or death due to endarterectomy that an individual patient will

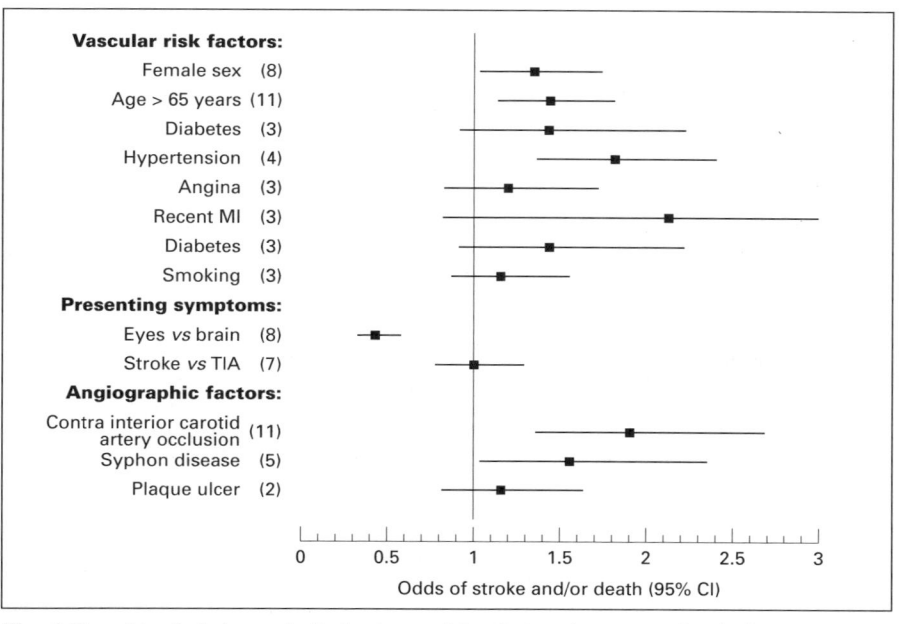

Fig. 4 The odds of stroke or death due to carotid endarterectomy according to the presence or absence of certain clinical and radiological baseline variables in a systematic review of studies published since 1980 [18]. The numbers in parentheses indicate the number of studies on which each estimate is based.

face is also likely to depend to some extent on the skills of the surgeon undertaking the operation. Although the average risk of stroke or death due to endarterectomy is between 5% and 7%, reported operative risks vary from 1% to over 20% [18]. This heterogeneity is much greater than would be expected by chance alone. However, much of this variation appears to be accounted for by differences in study authorship, studies that include a neurologist among the authors showing a significantly higher risk than studies in which all the authors are affiliated to departments of surgery, and studies in which several surgeons report their combined results having very much higher risks than studies in which a single surgeon reports his or her own performance (Fig. 5).

Pitfalls in predicting treatment effect in individual patients

One of the most frequently used approaches to improving the application of trial results to individual patients is to determine the extent to which relative treatment effect varies with the absolute risk of a poor outcome in the control group. However, there are several pitfalls which must be avoided. First, any such analysis must use relative risk rather than relative odds as the measure of treatment effect at different

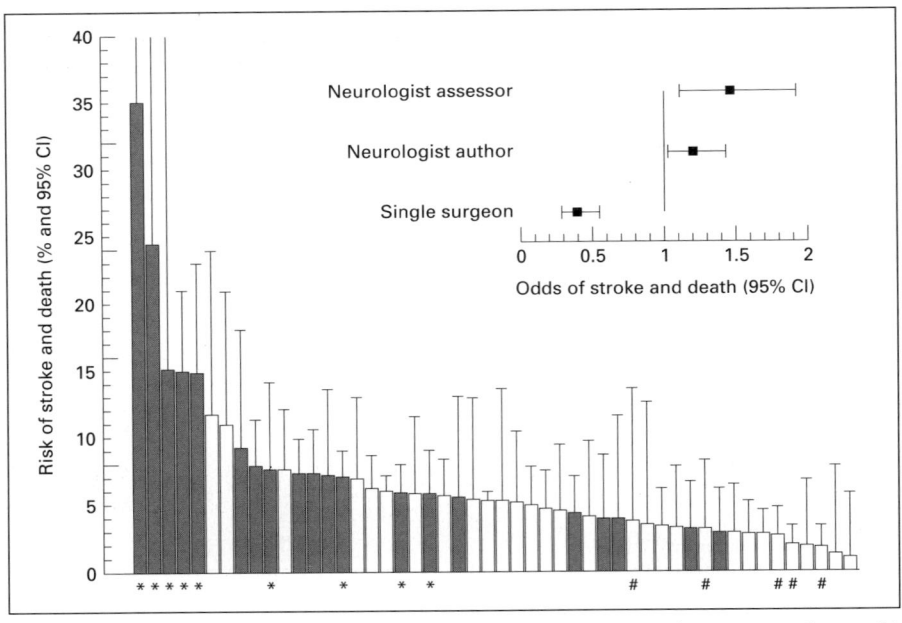

Fig. 5 The risks of stroke and death due to carotid endarterectomy for symptomatic carotid stenosis in studies that included a neurologist among the authors (shaded bars) and studies in which the authorship was comprised solely of individuals affiliated to a department of surgery (unshaded bars). Studies are further divided into those in which it was clearly stated that patients were assessed by a neurologist following surgery (denoted by *) and those studies in which a single surgeon reported his or her own results (denoted by #). Inset are the relative odds of stroke and death for these groups of studies compared with those studies with multiple authors, all of whom were affiliated to a department of surgery.

levels of baseline risk. The relative odds of the study outcome in the treatment group versus the control group will inevitably increase as the absolute risk of outcome events in the control group increases (Fig. 6). This is simply a mathematical property of the odds ratio and does not indicate any variation in the relative efficacy of treatment. A second pitfall is to use meta-analyses of different trials to examine the relationship between relative treatment effect and absolute baseline risk in the control group. Even if relative risk is used as the measure of treatment effect, the observed relationship will still be mainly artefact (Fig. 7). In all randomized trials, no matter how well conducted, some of the observed treatment effect will be due to chance. In trials in which chance results in a low risk of the study outcome in the control group, the treated group will tend, on average, to have a higher risk. In this situation, the treated group will either do worse than the control group or, if treatment is effective, the true effect will be underestimated. In contrast, if by chance the control group has a high risk of the study outcome, the baseline risk in the treated group will on average be lower, and the efficacy of treatment may be overestimated. This and other artefacts undermine the use of meta-analyses to investigate potential variation in relative treatment effect with baseline risk.

☐ CONCLUSIONS

In contrast to many areas of clinical medicine, the management of patients with non-disabling cerebrovascular ischaemia is based to a great extent on the results of

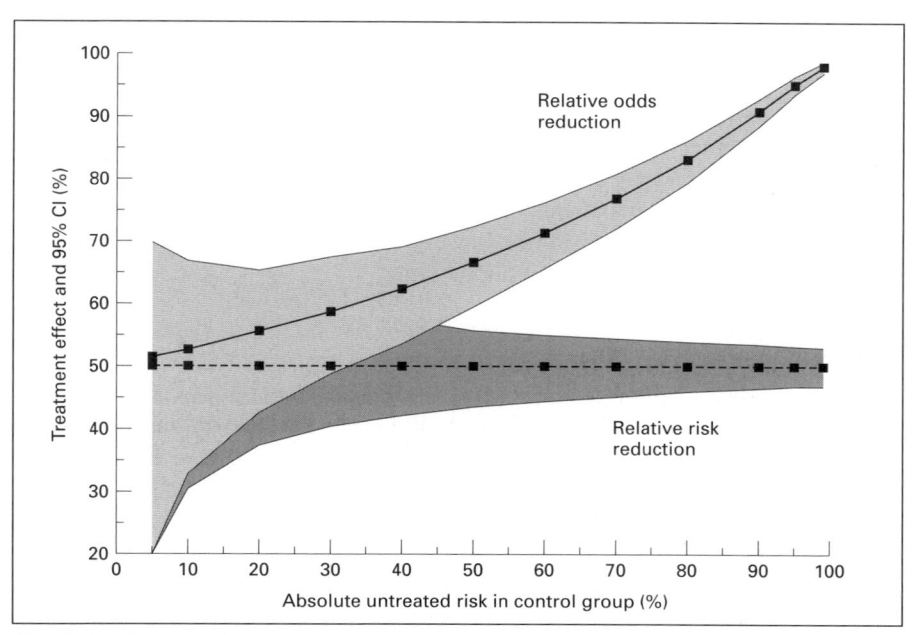

Fig. 6 Variation in relative odds reduction and 95% CI with baseline absolute risk without treatment, assuming a constant (50%) relative risk reduction. The 95% CI are based on a trial with 1000 treated patients and 1000 controls.

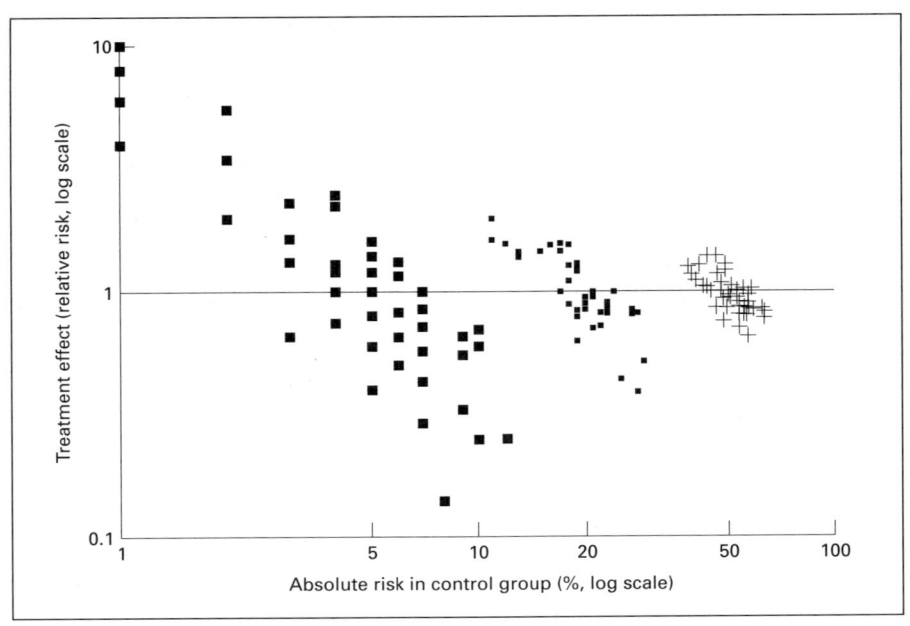

Fig. 7 A log plot of treatment effect (relative risk) against the absolute risk of trial outcome events in the control group (log scale) in three meta-analyses of 50 computer-simulated trials (100 treated patients vs 100 controls) of a treatment that has no true effect in populations with expected risks of the trial outcome event of 5%, 20% and 50%. Each point may represent more than one trial.

randomized controlled trials. Several interventions have been shown to reduce the risks of major stroke and non-stroke vascular death in these patients. The cost-effectiveness of these interventions can be improved by targeting those individuals at particularly high risk of a poor outcome without treatment, and avoiding expensive or dangerous interventions in patients who are likely to do well without treatment. This high-risk prevention strategy will not, however, prevent more than a few percent of the strokes that occur in the general population.

REFERENCES

1. European Carotid Surgery Trialists' Collaborative Group. MRC European Carotid Surgery Trial: interim results for symptomatic patients with severe (70–99%) or with mild (0–29%) carotid stenosis. *Lancet* 1991; **337**: 1235–43.
2. Hankey GJ, Dennis MS, Slattery J, Warlow CP. Why is the outcome of transient ischaemic attacks different in different groups of patients? *Brit Med J* 1993; **306**: 1107–11.
3. Hankey GJ, Warlow CP. *Transient Ischaemic Attacks of the Brain and Eye*. London: WB Saunders, 1994.
4. Sacks H, Chalmers TC, Smith H. Randomized versus historical controls for clinical trials. *Am J Med* 1982; **72**: 233.
5. Rose G. Sick individuals and sick populations. *Int J Epidemiol* 1985; **14**: 32–8.
6. Working Group of the National Medical Advisory Committee. Epidemiology and causes of stroke (chapter 3). In: *The Management of Patients with Stroke*. Edinburgh: HMSO, 1993.

7   Antiplatelet Trialists' Collaboration. Collaborative overview of randomised trials of antiplatelet therapy. I. Prevention of death, myocardial infarction and stroke by prolonged antiplatelet therapy in various categories of patients. *Brit Med J* 1994; **308**: 81–106.
8   European Atrial Fibrillation Trial Study Group. Secondary prevention in nonrheumatic atrial fibrillation transient ischaemic attack or minor stroke. *Lancet* 1993; **342**: 213–20.
9   Prospective Studies Collaboration. Cholesterol, diastolic blood pressure, and stroke: 13 000 strokes in 450 000 people in 45 prospective cohorts. *Lancet* 1995; **346**: 1647–53.
10 Collins R, Peto R, MacMahon S, *et al.* Blood pressure, stroke and coronary heart disease. Part 2. Short term reductions in blood pressure: overview of randomised drug trials in their epidemiological context. *Lancet* 1990; **335**: 827–38.
11 Scandinavian Simvastatin Survival Study Group. Randomised trial of cholesterol lowering in 4444 patients with coronary heart disease. *Lancet* 1994; **344**: 1383–9.
12 North American Symptomatic Carotid Endarterectomy Trial Collaborators. Beneficial effect of carotid endarterectomy in symptomatic patients with high-grade carotid stenosis. *New Engl J Med* 1991; **325**: 445–53.
13 European Carotid Surgery Trialists' Collaborative Group. MRC European Carotid Surgery Trial: results in patients with 30–69% stenosis. *Lancet* 1996; **347**: 1591–3.
14 Yusef S, Collins R, Peto R. Why do we need some large, simple randomized trials? *Stat Med* 1984; **3**: 409–20.
15 Multicentre Acute Stroke Trial—Italy (MAST-I) Group. Randomised controlled trial of streptokinase, aspirin, and combination of both in treatment of acute ischaemic stroke. *Lancet* 1995; **346**: 1509–14.
16 Zander AR, Keating M, Dicke K, *et al.* A comparison of marrow transplantation with chemotherapy for adults with acute leukemia of poor prognosis in first complete remission. *J Clin Oncol* 1988; **6**: 1548–57.
17 Yusef S, Zucker D, Peduzzi P, *et al.* Effect of coronary artery bypass graft surgery on survival: overview of 10-year results from randomised trials by the Coronary Artery Bypass Graft Surgery Trialists' Collaboration. *Lancet* 1994; **344**: 563–70.
18 Rothwell PM, Slattery J, Warlow CP. A systematic review of the risks of stroke and death due to endarterectomy for symptomatic carotid stenosis. *Stroke* 1996; **27**: 260–5.
19 Rothwell PM. Can overall results of clinical trials be applied to all patients? *Lancet* 1995; **345**: 1616–9.

☐ MULTIPLE CHOICE QUESTIONS

1   Symptoms suggestive of a diagnosis of transient ischaemic attack:
    (a) Loss of consciousness
    (b) Dizziness associated with perioral paraesthesia
    (c) Sudden onset weakness of left face, arm and leg
    (d) Acute confusion
    (e) Acute onset, complete loss of vision in one eye lasting for 2 minutes

2   Interventions shown in randomized controlled trials or meta-analyses definitely to reduce the risk of stroke in patients presenting with non-disabling cerebrovascular ischaemic events:
    (a) Treatment of hypertension
    (b) Carotid endarterectomy
    (c) Carotid angioplasty
    (d) Anticoagulation for non-rheumatic atrial fibrillation
    (e) Aspirin

3 The risk of stroke during the first few years following a non-disabling cerebrovascular ischaemic event:
   (a) Is approximately 20% per annum
   (b) Is higher in patients with ocular ischaemic events than cerebral events
   (c) Is only related to the degree of carotid stenosis in patients with 'lacunar' events
   (d) Decreases with time since the last ischaemic event
   (e) Is approximately double the risk of fatal stroke over the same period

4 With reference to applying the general overall result of a clinical trial to individual patients:
   (a) The absolute benefit derived from treatment will depend on the relative risk reduction with treatment
   (b) The absolute benefit derived from treatment will depend on the absolute risk of a poor outcome without treatment
   (c) The overall relative treatment effect is likely to be least generally applicable for treatments associated with a significant risk of serious harm
   (d) The overall relative odds reduction will decrease as the absolute risk of a poor outcome in the control group increases
   (e) Basing treatment decisions only on the overall trial result is, on balance, likely to do more good than harm

5 With reference to the incidence of ischaemic stroke in the population as a whole:
   (a) Optimal use of carotid endarterectomy for patients presenting with recently symptomatic >70% carotid stenosis could potentially reduce stroke incidence by 30–40%
   (b) Mean systolic blood pressure in the elderly population would have to be reduced by at least 15 mmHg before there would be a detectable decrease in stroke incidence
   (c) The population prevention strategy is only applicable for interventions with a significant risk of harm
   (d) Approximately 20% of first strokes are disabling
   (e) The high-risk prevention strategy traditionally requires screening of asymptomatic populations

ANSWERS

1a False	2a False	3a False	4a True	5a False
b False	b True	b False	b True	b False
c True	c False	c False	c True	c False
d False	d True	d True	d False	d False
e True	e True	e False	e True	e False

Disease modifying treatments in multiple sclerosis

Alastair Compston

☐ MULTIPLE SCLEROSIS: THE PROBLEM

Multiple sclerosis is the most common potentially disabling disorder of the central nervous system (CNS) affecting young adults in the western world. The symptoms and signs arise from patchy inflammation within the brain and spinal cord. Disability occurs as a direct consequence of this inflammatory process and its failure to repair. The cause is unknown, present treatment is unsatisfactory, and the disease represents an enormous burden for affected individuals, their families and for society. Clinically, multiple sclerosis can be considered as having three phases – relapse with full recovery, relapse with persistent disability, and slow progression. These usually follow in sequence, the evolution taking many years, but not all patients move through each stage and 20% follow a progressive course from onset.

After the initial clinical assessments have been made, the challenges are to achieve temporary improvement at times of recent symptomatic deterioration, to mask individual symptoms, to improve the quality of everyday life in the face of significant disability, and to modify the long-term course of the disease. The evidence that immunological mechanisms are involved has prompted the use of immunological therapies, and partial success has sustained these efforts. However, since a significant proportion of affected individuals remain free from disability despite having intermittent symptoms over several decades, physicians have been cautious when considering the use of immunosuppressive drugs, even when these are of proven value in other forms of inflammatory or autoimmune disease.

☐ MULTIPLE SCLEROSIS: THE PATHOGENESIS

The disease process is established early in life and preferentially selects certain individuals within high-risk ethnic groups. Genetic susceptibility is determined by a combination of alleles encoded at linked and unlinked loci on several chromosomes [1]. Exogenous factors are thought to be involved in initiating the disease process, but these remain to be identified. The interplay of genetic and environmental factors culminates in an inflammatory process that is confined to the CNS, but begins with the migration of activated lymphocytes across brain and spinal endothelial barriers. Cells that recognize antigen remain within the brain, release cytokines and establish a local inflammatory response. Lack of antigen recognition leads to lymphocyte removal by apoptosis. Cytokines appear to have a direct effect on electrical performance in myelinated nerves and symptom recovery is mainly due to reversible conduction block, without demyelination necessarily having occurred. Cytokines (especially interferon-gamma; IFN-γ) also activate microglia, which function both as antigen presenting cells and phagocytes in the CNS. If myelin or oligodendrocytes are opsonized with the ligands for receptors on activated microglia, cell–cell interaction and lethal injury occurs, mediated by high concentrations of cell surface bound tumour necrosis factor alpha (TNFα). Demyelinated axons have a reduced safety factor for nerve transmission and this is the basis for persistent symptoms. The failure of remyelination is associated with axon degeneration, which is thought to account for the chronic progressive phase of the disease. Reactive astrocytes eventually replace areas of persistent demyelination to form the glial scar that inhibits the migration of oligodendrocytes, or their precursors, into the plaque and so limits attempts at remyelination (Fig. 1); for review of the pathogenesis see Scolding et al. [2].

☐ MULTIPLE SCLEROSIS: LIMITING THE DAMAGE

A *cure* for multiple sclerosis would be any treatment given early in the clinical course that prevents the establishment of persistent disabilities and onset of the progressive phase, and a *useful* treatment is one that slows the rate at which persistent disabilities accumulate or the disease progresses; by comparison, reduction in relapse rate represents only a modest effect on the course of the disease.

Although the use of drugs that inhibit the primary vascular lesion is logical, until recently immunotherapy inflicted prolonged punishment on the whole immune system for the misdemeanours of a small proportion of its lymphocytes, and most available drugs had many undesirable side effects. Ideally, treatment should focus on those lymphocytes that are sensitized to the target antigens, leaving innocent clones free to patrol the nervous system; but since these antigen-specific cells have yet to be identified (if they exist) an alternative strategy is to interfere with the release of soluble mediators on which these cells depend for activation and/or effector mechanisms.

A list of drugs shown to reduce the duration or frequency of relapse, those that are of symptomatic use, and reagents currently (or recently) under assessment for disease modifying effects in multiple sclerosis is shown in Tables 1 and 2. Formerly, a review of the last group would have dealt only with non-specific immunosuppressants such as azathioprine, cyclosporin-A, cyclophosphamide, mitazanthrone and methotrexate, and with procedures such as plasmapheresis or total lymphoid irradiation. These may (or may not) modestly influence the course of the disease but they have significant adverse effects and, for the moment, attention is mainly directed at anti-inflammatory cytokines, monoclonal antibodies and synthetic or natural fragments of myelin proteins, which may be involved in the pathogenesis of multiple sclerosis.

Interferons

Interferons were first used in multiple sclerosis because of their antiviral properties. At first, no great distinction was placed on the type of interferon and each was assessed after administration either by the systemic or intrathecal route. A series of

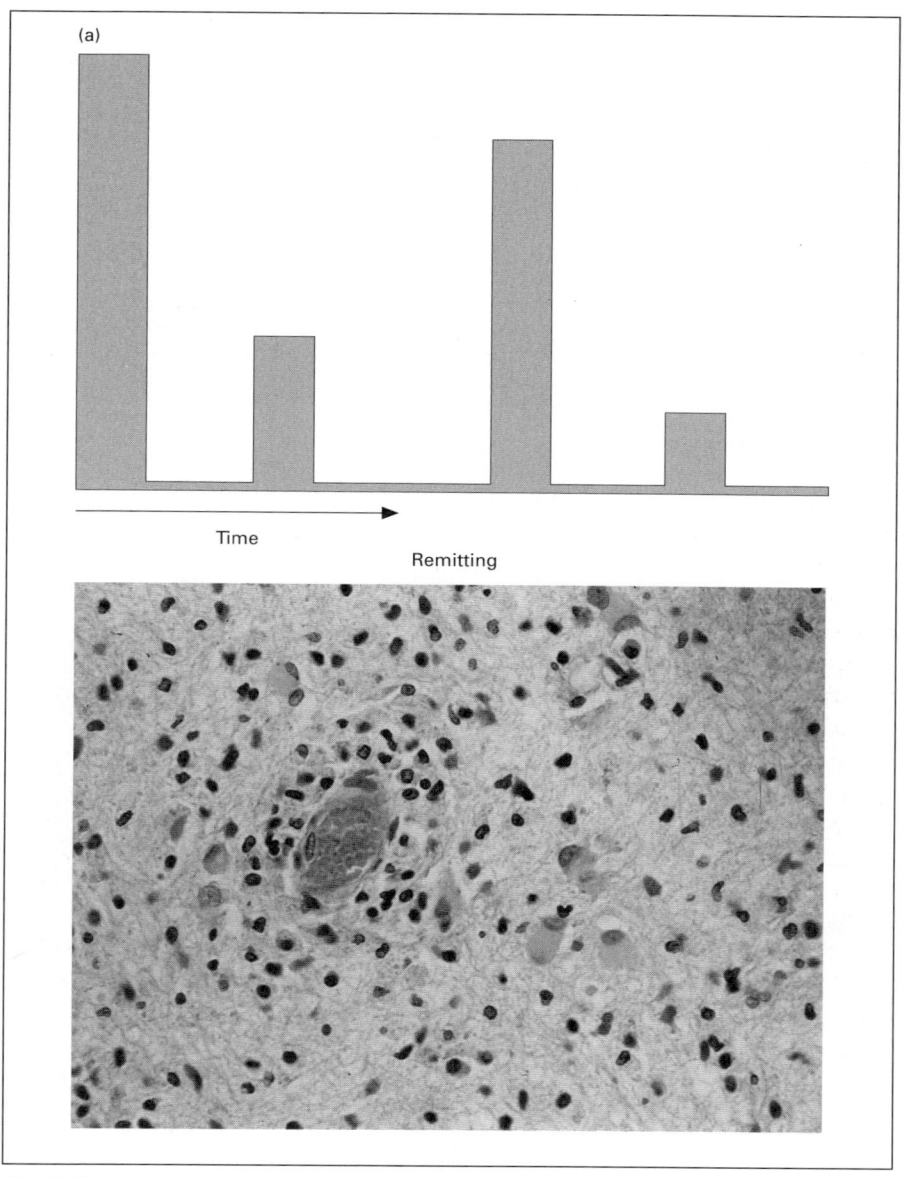

Fig. 1 Three stages in the clinical course of multiple sclerosis: (a) remitting episodes associated with perivascular cuffs of infiltrating lymphocytes; (b) persistent symptoms due to demyelination with minimal inflammation and limited repair; (c) disease progression – inflammation and active myelin breakdown are no longer apparent, the demyelination is associated with astrocytosis and there is axonal pathology leading to axon degeneration.

pilot studies, often uncontrolled and involving small numbers of patients, performed in the 1980s involved interferon-alpha (IFN-α), interferon-beta (IFN-β; given systemically or by the intrathecal route) and IFN-γ. The recognition that the immunological effects and physiological situations that characterize release of the naturally occurring interferons differ for IFN-α/IFN-β (type 1) and IFN-γ (type 2), and the results of further clinical trials, later led to the conclusion that IFN-γ makes multiple sclerosis worse [3] and that IFN-α is not obviously effective [4], although its use has not altogether been abandoned [5]. By contrast, the use of IFN-β has attracted increasing attention, due to the accumulation of modest evidence for efficacy and to vigorous marketing.

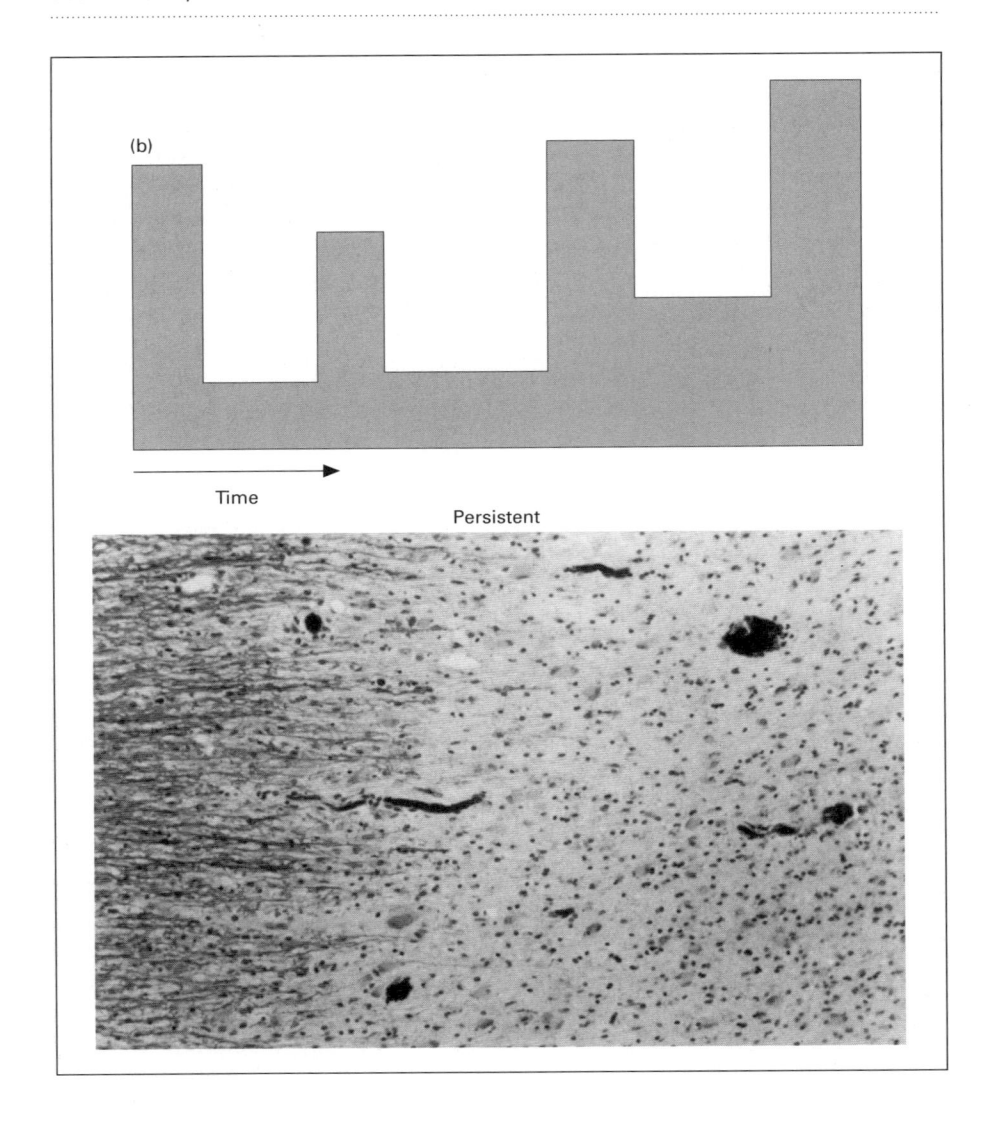

The definitive trial of IFN-β1b (marketed as Betaferon in the UK; given as alternate day subcutaneous injections) involved 372 patients, each having two relapses in the previous 2 years and with pre-entry scores on the Kurtzke expanded disability status scale (EDSS) of <5.5 [6]. Those who did not complete the trial (19%) were considered to have remained stable from the point of drop-out; the study was not

(c)

Time

Progressive

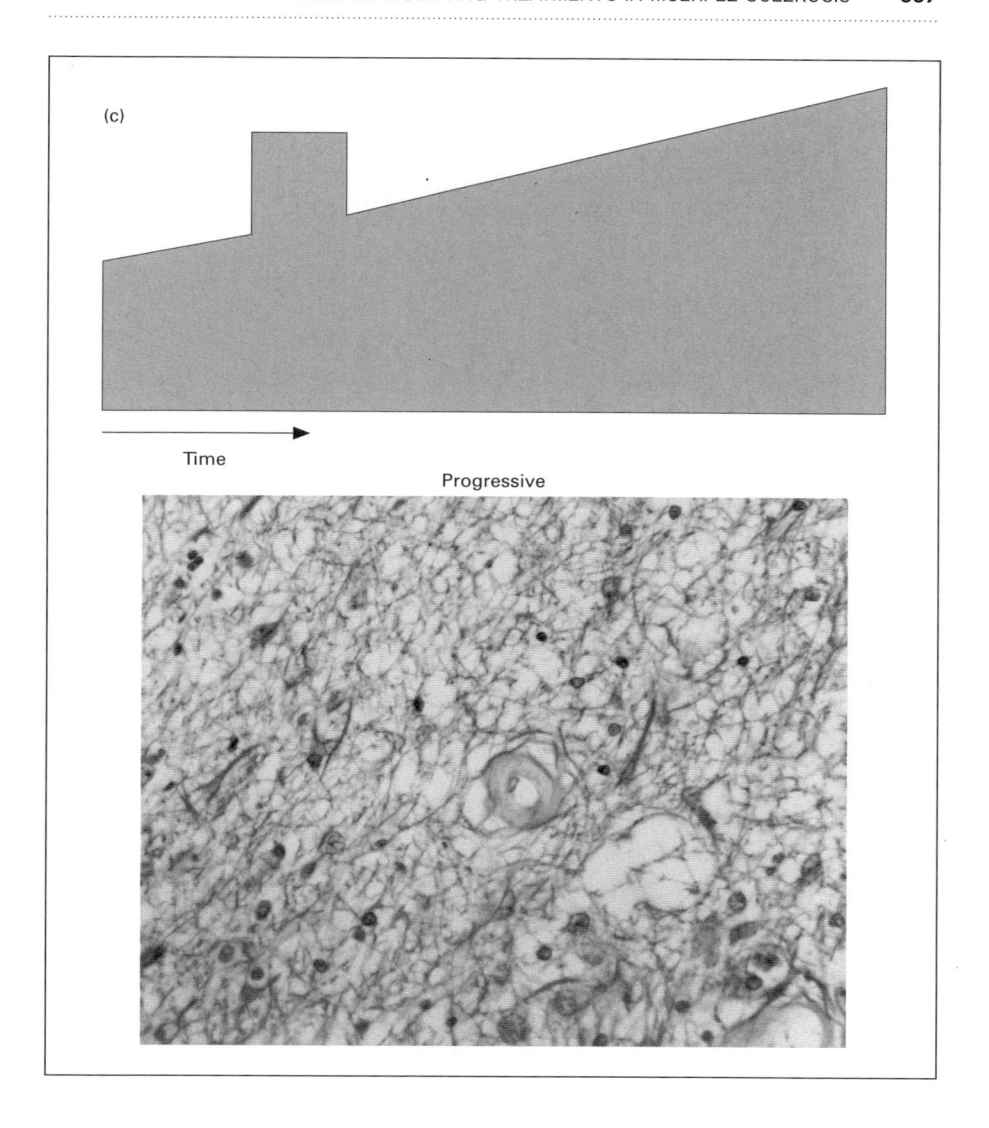

therefore strictly analysed on an intention-to-treat basis. The results of the initial and final reports, showing effects on relapse rate and magnetic resonance lesions but not disability, are summarized in Table 3. The overall tone of the follow-up report [7] is more moderate than the initial paper and accompanying editorials. At follow-up, participants had remained in the study for a median time of just under 4 years. Taking this entire period, the reduction in relapse rate associated with the use of IFN-β1b, reported in 1993, was maintained into the fifth year; however, the main effect was achieved in the first year, since when the reduction in relapse rate, which characterizes the natural history of multiple sclerosis, was actually greater in the placebo (−0.63 between years 2 and 5) than the treated group (−0.39). Much was made of the reduction in magnetic resonance activity seen in the IFN-β1b study and the extent to which this provides evidence for a disease modifying effect [8].

Table 1 Symptomatic treatments used in multiple sclerosis.

Symptom	Early persistent symptoms	Late persistent symptoms
Spasticity	☐ baclofen ☐ threonine ☐ tizanidine	☐ botulinum ☐ phenol ☐ tendon surgery
Tremor	☐ beta blockers ☐ glutethamide ☐ clonazepam ☐ isoniazid	☐ stereotactic thalamotomy
Bladder	☐ oxybutinin ☐ anticholinergics ☐ alpha blockers ☐ self-catheterization ☐ desmopressin	☐ bladder neck surgery ☐ artificial sphincters ☐ permanent catheterization
Bowel	☐ bulk laxatives ☐ *mini* enemas	☐ faecal containment
Sexual	☐ papaverine	☐ mechanical devices
Paroxysmal symptoms	☐ carbamazepine	
Pain	☐ anticonvulsants ☐ antidepressants	☐ nerve section
Fatigue	☐ amantidine ☐ pemoline ☐ fluoxetine	
Strength		☐ 4-aminopyridine ☐ 3,4-diaminopyridine ☐ electrical stimulation

The results of the trial using IFN-β1a (Avonex; given as 6 million units intramuscularly on a weekly basis) are summarized in Table 4 [9]. Three hundred and one patients with clinically definite multiple sclerosis in the relapsing phase (some with persistent symptoms and signs), and with disabilities <3.5 on the Kurtzke scale, were included; each had two or more (physician) documented relapses in the preceding 3 years, but none in the previous 2 months, and the pre-treatment exacerbation rate was >0.67 a year. Fewer treated patients had three or more exacerbations during the study than controls; annual exacerbation rates were reduced, as was the proportion free from any relapse at 2 years. This study differed from the trial of IFN-β1b in also showing a modest effect on disability and the probability of sustained progression. Conversely, the IFN-β1a study did not confirm the reduction in magnetic resonance lesion load claimed for IFN-β1b, even though the number of lesions was fewer in treated patients and there was a reduction in the number of active lesions.

The main adverse effects of IFN-β1b and IFN-β1a are local reactions at the

Table 2 Trials and claims for disease modifying treatments in multiple sclerosis.

Duration of relapse	☐ corticotrophin
	☐ pulsed i.v. methylprednisolone
	☐ oral prednisolone
Frequency of relapse	☐ interferon (IFN) β1a and β1b
	☐ IFN-α
	☐ copolymer 1
	☐ oral myelin
	☐ i.v. immunoglobulin
	☐ mitozanthrone
Rate of progression	☐ azathioprine
	☐ IFN-β1a
	☐ cladribine
	☐ total lymphoid irradiation
	☐ methotrexate
	☐ cyclophosphamide
	☐ plasma exchange
	☐ cyclosporin-A
	☐ mitozanthrone
Not effective	☐ isoprinosine
	☐ IFN-γ
Under investigation	☐ deoxyspergualin
	☐ FK806
	☐ linomide
	☐ pentoxifilline
	☐ mabs anti CD2/3/4/6/52/T-cell receptor (TCR)-β/VLA-α
	☐ TCR peptide blockers
	☐ T-cell vaccination
	☐ tumour necrosis factor-α (TNFα) antibodies/soluble receptor
	☐ cytokines, eg tumour growth factor-β (TGFβ)

injection site, flu-like symptoms and hyperthermia, but there is no evidence for significant drug hypersensitivity; based on the evidence available from the clinical trials and post-marketing experience, contraindications include the use of IFN-β in pregnant women, in patients with epilepsy, and in those with depression. The long-term adverse effects are still not known. It has now been revealed that up to 45% of patients on high doses (8 MIU) of IFN-β1b develop neutralizing activity, usually in the first year (34/124; 7/124 in year 2, and 2/124 in year 3). In the trial of IFN-β1a, persistent neutralizing anti-interferon activity was seen in 14% of treated individuals by 1 year and 23% at 2 years compared with 4% of the placebo-treated patients (in whom antibody activity disappeared on repeat testing). There is now much uncertainty on the extent to which these findings indicate that IFN-β would be even more effective, were it not for the development of neutralizing antibody; or conversely, that IFN-β is doomed to short-term efficacy by immunogenicity. In

Table 3 Interferon-β1b (Betaferon).

	Treatment		
	placebo	1.5 MIU	8 MIU
Number enrolled	123	125	124
Number entering year 5	56	52	58
Exacerbation rates			
Overall exacerbation rate	1.12*	0.96	0.78*
(baseline – year 5)	(1.02–1.23)	(0.87–1.06)	(0.70–0.88)
Year 1	1.44	1.22	0.96
Year 2	1.18	1.04	0.85
Year 3	0.92	0.80	0.66
Year 4	0.88	0.68	0.67
Year 5	0.81	0.66	0.57
Reduction in exacerbation rate			
Baseline to year 1	–0.36	–0.48	–0.74
Years 2 to 5	–0.63	–0.56	–0.39
Disability			
Number with EDSS >1 point	56/122 (46%)	59/125 (47%)	43/122 (35%)†
Baseline EDSS <3	26/58 (45%)	30/59 (51%)	20/55 (36%)
Baseline EDSS >3	30/64 (47%)	29/66 (44%)	23/67 (34%)
Median time to progression	4.18 years	3.49 years	4.79 years‡
Magnetic resonance imaging: lesion load (% change)			
Number enrolled	73	66	78
Number entering year 5	72	61	75
Completing year 1	+6.7	+5.7	–4.9
Completing year 4	+30.2§	+10.6	+3.6§
Increase in year 2–5	+23.5	+4.9	+8.7

*$p = 0.0001$; †$p = 0.096$; ‡$p = 0.087$; §$p = 0.00$

support of the first interpretation is the conclusion that patients who do not develop neutralizing activity have an even lower relapse rate than has been reported for all IFN-β1b treated patients (Table 5). It follows that the development of neutralizing activity is associated with a relapse rate that is higher than the reported rate for other treated patients.

The logic for using IFN-β in multiple sclerosis has, in the main, been assembled retrospectively and rests on the argument that IFN-β inhibits the actions of IFN-γ. Information gathered from a variety of sources shows that IFN-β has both pro- and anti-inflammatory effects; in summary, it inhibits the antigen presenting properties of microglia by restricting the expression of class 2 major histocompatibility antigens while increasing their cytotoxic properties [10].

These two studies [6,7,9] have generated more discussion, public debate and manoeuvring for position among those who organize the provision and funding of medical services than all other treatments that have previously been proposed for

Table 4 Interferon-β1a (Avonex).

	Treatment	
	placebo	IFN-β1a
Number enrolled	143	158
Number completing year 2	87	85
Disability		
Sustained progression at year 1	22%	13%
Sustained progression at year 2	33%	21%
Change in EDSS at 2 years by −<1 point	12%	19%
Change in EDSS at 2 years by +<1 point	37%	24%*
Relapse frequency		
Relapse frequency (<2) at 2 years	56%	68%
Relapse frequency (>2) at 2 years	44%	32%
Change in relapse rate at 2 years	−0.30	−0.59†
Magnetic resonance imaging		
Number of Gd+ lesions at baseline	>174	>196
Mean number of Gd+ lesions at baseline	2.32	3.17
Number of Gd+ lesions at year 2	>78	>49
Mean number of Gd+ lesions at year 2	1.65	0.80‡
Change in T2 lesion volume at year 2	−7%	−13%

*$p = 0.02$; †$p = 0.0002$; ‡$p = 0.05$

multiple sclerosis. Sandwiched between the primary publications has been a deluge of professional commentaries, much manipulation of public opinion by the pharmaceutical companies who stand to gain (and lose) from the marketing of these products, and the jottings of some seriously ill-informed journalists. The consequence has been that from late 1993 neurologists have frequently been asked to

Table 5 Interferon-β1b (Betaferon).

	Treatment		
	placebo	1.5 MIU	8 MIU
Enrolled	123	125	124
Number completing year 4	56	52	58
Exacerbation rates			
Before treatment	1.8	1.7	1.7
After year 1	1.44	1.22	0.96
Antibody positive	1.06*	–	1.08
Antibody negative	–	–	0.56

* A cohort studied between 1 and 3 years

prescribe IFN-β, and they have had to develop unsavoury tactics for deferring these decisions on the basis of uncertain efficacy and cost. This dilemma has led to the production of restrictive guidelines for rationing the use of IFN-β which seek to limit its use to a minority of patients. Debate has continued on the managed entry of Betaferon in the UK, with jockeying for position on who should take the decision to prescribe, who pays, and from what pot. In Europe, where a product licence was granted late in 1995, the take-up of prescriptions has been slow and in many countries this results from delay in establishing guidelines for clinical use, closely linked to funding decisions. Once these issues are resolved it is likely that at least 15% of patients will qualify for a prescription and this number will increase with the availability of Avonex (IFN-β1a); resources available from most health commissions or trusts are likely to fund prescriptions for fewer than 5% of affected individuals – a gap that will cause distress and debate among patients, practitioners, providers and purchasers (see Fig. 2).

Monoclonal antibodies

The use of non-specific agents proved the concept that immunosuppression is a valid approach to treatment in multiple sclerosis even if the magnitude of the effect often failed to establish a role for any one drug, given alone or in combination. With developments in therapeutic immunology came the opportunity to design small molecules and monoclonal antibodies which selectively target the immune system; humanization reduces the immunogenicity of therapeutic antibodies and (in theory) allows repeated treatment. Experimentally, pulsed treatment with a combination of depleting and blocking monoclonals targeted at lymphocyte antigens can induce prolonged alterations in immunological behaviour [11].

Using a non-humanized murine antibody that recognizes an antigen present on most (post-thymic) T lymphocytes (T12) together with corticosteroids, Hafler *et al.* [12] reported clinical stabilization in 6/12 patients with secondary progressive multiple sclerosis at 6 months, which was maintained for a further 3 months in 3/12; most patients developed human anti-mouse antibodies. Weinshenker *et al.* [13] treated 16 patients, selected on the basis of rapid deterioration or a high relapse rate, with anti-CD3 (OKT3). Despite receiving corticosteroids and non-steroidal anti-inflammatory drugs, a variety of systemic symptoms occurred in each of these patients; the systemic manifestations of OKT3 administration correlate with sequential release of circulating TNFα and IFN-γ followed by interleukin 6 (IL-6), which can be suppressed by methylprednisolone. There were no obvious clinical benefits from the use of OKT3, and two patients died from the disease. Serial magnetic resonance imaging (MRI) failed to show an effect on lesion load. Rapid but transient reductions were seen in circulating lymphocytes and their subpopulations and all patients developed high titres of human anti-mouse antibodies. While not promoting the continued use of murine monoclonals in multiple sclerosis, Weinshenker *et al.* [13] advocated the development of more specific and less toxic reagents, manipulated to restrict their immunogenicity.

The first reported study using murine anti-CD4 monoclonal antibody therapy in multiple sclerosis [14] included 21 patients with disease progression or frequent

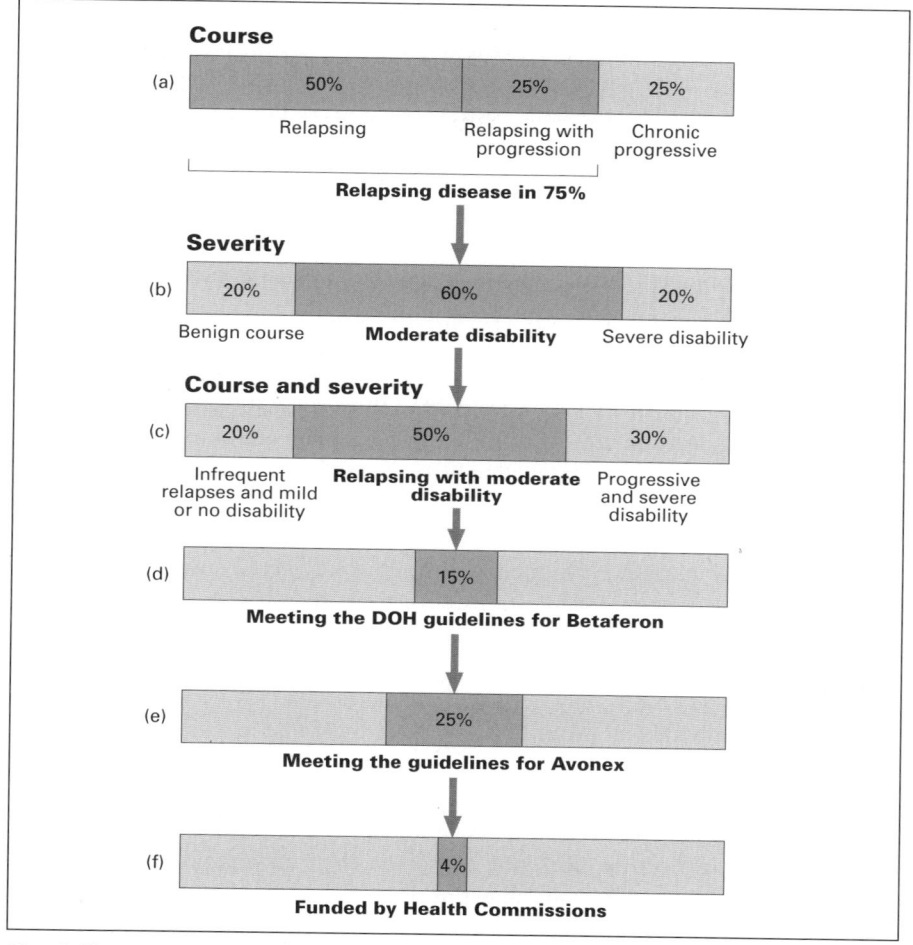

Fig. 2 The course and severity of multiple sclerosis showing the proportion of patients in a population based sample likely to meet guidelines and seek a prescription for IFN-β. (a) The proportion with relapsing disease (with or without progression). (b) The proportion with mild, moderate and severe disabilities. (c) The proportion who are relapsing and neither trivially nor severely disabled. (d) The proportion likely to meet the Department of Health guidelines (two or more disabling attacks in the previous 2 years, age >18 years, not pregnant, and without epilepsy or depression) for the use of Betaferon. (e) The proportion likely to meet guidelines for the use of Avonex. (f) The estimated proportion likely to receive health commission funding for a prescription.

relapse; there were no acute effects (good or bad) and clinical stabilization was reported by 8/20 at 6 months; no new relapses were recorded. The phenotypic immunological effects had returned to normal by 3 months. A transient elevation was observed in circulating TNFα, soluble TNF receptor and IL-6 but not IFN-γ, IL-1 or soluble CD8 and CD4 antigen; unlike most other investigators, Racadot et al. [14] reported a rise in cerebrospinal fluid TNFα levels from detectable pre-treatment levels.

Lindsey et al. [15] treated 29 patients in an open uncontrolled study, using a chimaeric anti-CD4 antibody in doses ranging from 10 to 200 mg given as a single infusion or over 3 days. The partial reduction in total circulating lymphocytes recovered within 6 months; the same pattern was observed for CD4 cells but without complete return to the normal range. Five patients developed antimurine antibodies. Modest improvements were noted in 3/26 patients, whereas 16 were unchanged and seven deteriorated. Fourteen of 25 patients in whom serial scans were obtained had enhancing lesions on baseline MRI; 100 enhancing lesions were seen on 91 scans obtained during follow-up, and 17/25 patients showed an increase in T_2-weighted lesions. The patients reported minor systemic symptoms, and there was an increase in infections requiring treatment. Most of these patients were considered for re-treatment if the CD4 count returned to >300 cells per mm^3 [16]. Twenty one of the original cohort received up to three re-treatments (a total of 36), responding with a decrease in CD4 count on each occasion and sometimes showing prolonged lymphopenia. There seemed to be no increase in the development of anti-idiotype antibodies with re-treatment. One patient improved, three worsened, 16 remained unchanged and one was lost to follow-up. Magnetic resonance activity was present in 10/16 scans before treatment and 12/26 scans (performed in 16 patients) at follow-up. Other than minor infections, sometimes requiring treatment, and one episode of herpes zoster, there were few complications of re-treatment. On the basis of these preliminary results, a double-blind placebo controlled study of anti-CD4 monoclonal antibody has been completed but the results [17] do not suggest that this particular antibody will prove to have a long-term role in the management of patients with multiple sclerosis.

Lymphopenia is rapid and prolonged after administration of CAMPATH-1H since the target antigen (CD52) is expressed in high density on the lymphocyte cell membrane. A single course does not appear to elicit an antiglobulin response. Moreau et al. [18] treated patients shown to have one or more active (gadolinium diethylenetriamine penta-acetic acid enhanced) magnetic resonance abnormalities with a cumulative dose of 120 mg in a single course over two weeks. Lymphopenia was rapid, profound and prolonged with CD4 counts remaining below the normal range for >2 years. On 61 MRI carried out either during pre-treatment assessments or follow-up in the seven patients, there were 68 T_2-weighted magnetic resonance abnormalities which were known to be both new and active (28 areas of enhancement detected on the initial pre-treatment scans and 44 areas of enhancement which appeared on more than one scan were not counted as new lesions). Fifty one out of 68 lesions were seen on the 18 MRI scans carried out before treatment. In the first 3 months after treatment, 15 new lesions were seen on 20 MRI scans whereas only two more were seen on 23 subsequent investigations carried out during follow-up for between 6 and 28 months; this indicates a 90% reduction in disease activity (Table 6).

In an extension of this series the release of cytokine coinciding with the first infusion of CAMPATH-1H and the induction of lymphopenia was shown to be associated with transient symptomatic *deterioration* and altered conduction through previously affected CNS pathways – findings that are informative with respect to the production of neurological symptoms in multiple sclerosis [19]. Patients

Table 6 Disease activity in patients with multiple sclerosis at monthly intervals before and after treatment with CAMPATH-1H. The number of enhancing lesions seen on the initial pretreatment scan ($n = 28$), and new enhancing ($n = 63$), new but non-enhancing ($n = 4$), and old enlarging but non-enhancing ($n = 1$) lesions is shown prior to treatment and during follow-up. Lesions that continued to enhance from a previous examination ($n = 44$) are not included. The Kurtzke expanded disability status scale score (EDSS) is shown for each patient at entry and on completion of the study.

Case		(EDSS)	Number of lesions (scans)			
			First scan	-4/12 to C-1H	C-1H to +3/12	>3/12
1	F	(6.0–4.5)	22 (1)	24 (2)	2 (2)	0 (3)
2	M	(6.0–6.0)	3 (1)	4 (2)	2 (3)	1 (5)
3	F	(5.5–5.0)	1 (1)	1 (2)	0 (3)	0 (3)
4	F	(6.0–6.0)	2 (1)	5 (3)	3 (3)	0 (3)
5	F	(4.5–4.5)	0 (1)	9 (3)	2 (3)	0 (3)
6	M	(6.0–5.5)	0 (1)	2 (3)	1 (3)	0 (3)
7	F	(6.0–6.0)	0 (1)	6 (3)	5 (3)	1 (3)
Total			28 (7)	51 (18)	15 (20)	2 (23)

experienced a worsening of persistent symptoms or a recurrence of clinical manifestations that had characterized previous episodes of demyelination; these changes occurred 2–4 h after starting the first infusion and usually recovered within 12 h. The neurological symptoms always manifested as reactivation of pre-existing symptoms and were associated with transient conduction block; they were prevented by the use of corticosteroids. Although most patients developed headache, rigors and pyrexia, the symptomatic deteriorations were not directly a result of elevated temperature. With the exception of those patients who received corticosteroids, there was a substantial increase in the serum concentrations of TNFα, IL-6 and IFN-γ during CAMPATH-1H infusion. The time course of cytokine release and symptomatic deterioration, and the suppression of both responses following corticosteroid treatment, is one line of evidence providing circumstantial evidence that cytokines, directly or indirectly, increase pre-existing symptoms in patients with multiple sclerosis through an effect on conduction in partially demyelinated pathways.

Immunological tolerance

In view of the conditional benefits of immune suppression in the treatment of patients with multiple sclerosis, attention has turned to alternative means of interfering with the sequence of events that lead to tissue injury.

One approach has been to eliminate antigen-specific autoreactive T cells by vaccination with X-irradiated cells primed against myelin basic protein. In a small pilot study involving eight patients, five showed a reduction in relapses from 16 to three in the 2 years before and after treatment compared with a change from 12 to

10 in controls; this was accompanied by a difference in magnetic resonance lesion size of +8% and +39.5%, respectively. Lesion size and clinical relapses worsened in three patients in whom autoreactive T cells (showing antigenic drift) reappeared after vaccination [20].

The elimination of antigen-specific autoreactivity has also been approached by the use of peptides that block antigen recognition. Bornstein et al. [21] first reported in detail on the therapeutic use in 16 patients with multiple sclerosis of a synthetic peptide composed of L-alanine, L-glutamic acid, L-lysine and L-tyrosine (Copolymer 1: Cop-1); designed to mimic the structure of myelin basic protein, Cop-1 was shown to be neither encephalitogenic nor toxic and it suppressed experimental allergic encephalomyelitis (EAE) perhaps by inducing antigen-specific suppressor cells.

In a subsequent blinded and placebo-controlled study [22], 50 patients with at least two relapses in the previous 2 years and Kurtzke EDSS scores of <6 at entry were randomized and self-injected subcutaneously with Cop-1 or placebo for up to 2 years. Taking absence of relapse during the trial as the primary end-point, a greater proportion of individuals in matched pairs receiving Cop-1 were relapse-free on completion (10/22, compared with 2/22 in whom the placebo partner but not the Cop-1 treated individual was free from relapse, and 10/22 in whom the course was concordant within pairs; $p = 0.04$). There were 62 exacerbations in 23 placebo-treated patients compared with 16 amongst 25 Cop-1 treated individuals; although the placebo group showed a reduction in relapse rate during the trial (as part of the natural history or regression to the mean), the relapse rate was ×4.9 in placebo cases during the first year and ×3.3 in the second year. Overall, 14/25 treated patients were free from relapse compared with 6/23 in the placebo group, and placebo patients tended to have more relapses ($p < 0.001$). An apparent difference in the rate at which Cop-1 and placebo-treated patients deteriorated (5/25 Cop-1 and 11/23 placebo), which was especially marked in individuals with low EDSS scores at entry, was not statistically significant. There was, however, a delay in the time to progression by 1 EDSS point amongst Cop-1 treated patients. Local injection site reactions seriously undermined blinding in this study and 29/40 participants (in whom information was available) correctly guessed treatment assignments (the authors suggest that unblinding was also influenced by the response to treatment).

On the basis of this evidence, a phase III trial was carried out involving 251 patients randomized to Cop-1 (20 mg by daily subcutaneous injection for 2 years; $n = 125$) or placebo ($n = 126$ [23]). The relapse rate over 2 years in treated patients was 1.19 ± 0.13 compared with 1.68 ± 0.13 in controls (a 29% reduction giving annual rates of 0.59 and 0.84, respectively; $p < 0.007$). There were more Cop-1 treated patients who were free from relapse and treatment also favoured a delay in relapse. The proportion of patients who were unchanged, improved or worsened (by 1 EDSS point) did not differ between groups.

An alternative approach to the induction of immunological tolerance, and one that has received preliminary clinical application [24], is to desensitize myelin protein reactivity with oral antigen. Thirty patients, having at least two relapses in the previous 2 years, ingested 30 mg of bovine myelin for 1 year; 6/15 treated individuals had *major* attacks compared with 12/15 in the placebo group. A rather contrived subgroup analysis claimed an effect on disability in DR2(15) negative males. These clinical observations could not be correlated with changes in the proportion or specificity of T cell clones reactive to myelin basic protein, or its encephalitogenic peptides. In other contexts, oral feeding of antigen has been shown to favour the induction of T cells which secrete IL-4, TGF-B and IL-10 at low doses and to delete Th1 and Th2 cells at higher doses [25].

☐ MULTIPLE SCLEROSIS: GLIAL REPAIR

A major challenge for research in multiple sclerosis is to overcome the failure of repair that characterizes the chronic plaque. Here, the questions that need to be answered are whether the failure of significant remyelination reflects the relative absence of oligodendrocyte lineage precursor cells (needed to remyelinate damaged axons) in the adult brain and spinal cord, or failure of these cells to enter sites of demyelination, through lack of appropriate signals and/or glial scar formation. Quite probably, each of these is a problem and remyelination may require restoration of signals provided by growth factors that are present during development and organize the growing brain, improved migration through the postinflammatory glial scar, and (perhaps) implantation of autologous or donor glial cells. Repairing the areas of brain inflammation makes little sense if the disease process has not already been checked; conversely, limiting the damage will in itself do little for affected individuals who are already disabled unless remyelination is also achieved.

Spontaneous attempts at remyelination are seen in a high proportion of active lesions in multiple sclerosis and in experimental demyelinating disease. Although it has been argued that the fully differentiated oligodendrocyte (a postmitotic cell) can re-enter the cell cycle, the consensus would be that remyelination requires the juxtaposition of glial progenitor cells (which have the ability to proliferate, migrate and differentiate) with naked axons. The obvious growth factor candidates for attracting cells into demyelinated areas are basic fibroblast growth factor (bFGF), platelet derived growth factor (PDGF) and neurotrophin-3 (NT-3) perhaps also with sequential use of survival factors (insulin-like growth factor: IGF-1), once differentiation and myelination are proceeding. After glial progenitor cell implantation, donor derived astrocytes, oligodendrocytes and myelin can each be detected in experimental demyelinated lesions [26]. The potential for remyelination by glia derived from *adult* nervous system has also been studied using both rodent and human cells. A mixed population of progenitor and fully differentiated adult rat cells transplanted into the rat spinal cord, demyelinated by ethidium bromide and X-irradiated to prevent host remyelination, shows expansion of the donor oligodendrocyte pool by proliferation of progenitors which differentiate into oligodendrocytes and achieve extensive remyelination; transplantation of human glia using cell cultures that include a proportion of progenitor cells shows that oligodendrocyte lineage cells survive in clumps within the lesion and extend processes that wrap around and separate rat axons but these do not compact and often end in loops where the processes abut onto naked axons [27]. An important question not resolved by these histologically orientated studies is whether remyelination will restore function and, if so, what proportion of demyelinated fibres need to be repaired. Conduction velocity is reduced by 75% in rats that are myelin deficient due to the absence of proteolipid protein (PLP), but myelination can be achieved in these animals after transplantation of cells from healthy litter mates and this is sufficient to overcome conduction block and improve the velocity of conducting fibres 3-fold [28].

REFERENCES

1. Compston DAS, Sawcer S, Kellar-Wood H, Wood NJ. The genetic epidemiology of multiple sclerosis. *Acta Neurol Scand* 1995; **Suppl 161**: 43–51.
2. Scolding NJ, Wood N, Zajicek JP, Compston DAS. Mechanisms of demyelination. *Prog Neurobiol* 1994; **43**: 143–73.
3. Panitch HS, Hirsch RL, Haley AS, Johnson KP. Exacerbations of multiple sclerosis in patients treated with gamma interferon. *Lancet* 1987; **i**: 893–5.
4. Knobler RL, Panitch HS, Braheny JC, Sipe JC, *et al.* Systemic alpha interferon therapy of multiple sclerosis. *Neurology* 1984; **34**: 1273–9.
5. Durelli L, Bongiopanni MR, Cavallo R, Ferrero B, *et al.* Chronic systemic high-dose recombinant interferon alfa-2a reduces exacerbation rate, MRI signs of disease activity, and lymphocyte interferon gamma production in relapsing-remitting multiple sclerosis. *Neurology* 1994; **44**: 406–13.
6. The IFNB Multiple Sclerosis Study Group. Interferon beta-1b is effective in relapsing-remitting multiple sclerosis. 1. Clinical results of a multicenter, randomized, double-blind, placebo-controlled trial. *Neurology* 1993; **43**: 655–61.
7. The IFNB Multiple Sclerosis Study Group and the University of British Columbia MS/MRI Analysis Group. Interferon beta-1b in the treatment of multiple sclerosis: final outcome of the randomised controlled trial. *Neurology* 1995; **45**: 1277–85.
8. Paty DW, Li DKB, The IFNB Multiple Sclerosis Study Group. Interferon beta-1b is effective in relapsing-remitting multiple sclerosis: MRI results of a multicenter, randomized, double-blind, placebo-controlled trial. *Neurology* 1993; **43**: 662–7.
9. Jacobs LD, Cookfair Dl, Rudick RA, *et al.* Intramuscular interferon beta-1a for disease progression in relapsing multiple sclerosis. *Ann Neurol* 1996; **39**: 285–94.
10. Hall G, Compston DAS, Scolding NJ. Beta-interferon and multiple sclerosis. *Trends Neurosci* 1997; **20**: 63–7.
11. Qin S, Cobbold SP, Pope H, Elliott J, Kioussis D, Davies J, Waldmann H. 'Infectious' transplantation tolerance. *Science* 1993; **259**: 974–7.
12. Hafler DA, Ritz F, Schlossman SF, Weiner HL. Anti-CD4 and anti-CD2 monoclonal antibody infusions in subjects with multiple sclerosis: immunosuppressive effect and human anti-mouse responses. *J Immunol* 1988; **141**: 131–8.
13. Weinshenker BG, Bass B, Karlik S, Ebers GC, Rice GPA. An open trial of OKT3 in patients with multiple sclerosis. *Neurology* 1991; **41**: 1047–52.
14. Racadot E, Rumbach L, Bataillard M, Galmiche J, *et al.* Treatment of multiple sclerosis with anti-CD4 monoclonal antibody. *Autoimmunity* 1993; **6**: 771–86.
15. Lindsey JW, Hodgkinson S, Mehta R, Siegel RC, Mitchell DJ, *et al.* Phase 1 clinical trial of chimeric monoclonal anti-CD4 antibody in multiple sclerosis. *Neurology* 1994; **44**: 413–9.
16. Lindsey JW, Hodgkinson S, Mehta R, Mitchell DJ, *et al.* Repeated treatment with chimeric anti-CD4 antibody in multiple sclerosis. *Ann Neurol* 1994; **36**: 183–9.
17. van Oosten EW, Lai M, Hodgkinson S, Barkhof F, *et al.* Treatment of multiple sclerosis with the monoclonal anti-CD4 antibody cM-T412: results of a randomized, double-blind placebo-controlled, MR monitored phase II trial. *Neurology* (in press).

18 Moreau T, Thorpe J, Miller D, Moseley I, Hale G, Waldmann H, Wing M, Scolding N, Compston DAS. Reduction in new lesion formation in multiple sclerosis following lymphocyte depletion with CAMPATH-IH. *Lancet* 1994; **344**: 298–301.
19 Moreau T, Hale G, Waldmann H, Isaacs J, Wing M, Compston DAS. Cytokine release increases conduction block in partially demyelinated pathways due to multiple sclerosis. *Brain* 1996; 119: 225–37.
20 Medaer R, Stinissen P, Truyen L, Raus J, Zhang J. Depletion of myelin basic protein autoreactive T cells by T-cell vaccination: pilot trial in multiple sclerosis. *Lancet* 1995; **346**: 807–8.
21 Bornstein MB, Miller A, Teitelbaum D, Arnon R, Sela M. Multiple sclerosis: trial of a synthetic polypeptide. *Ann Neurol* 1982; 11: 317–9.
22 Bornstein MB, Miller A, Slagle S, Weitzman M, *et al.* A pilot trial of Cop-1 in exacerbating-remitting multiple sclerosis. *New Engl J Med* 1987; 317: 408–14.
23 Johnson KP, Brooks BR, Cohen JA, Ford CC, *et al.* Copolymer 1 reduces relapse rate and improves disability in relapsing-remitting multiple sclerosis: results of a phase III multicenter, double-blind placebo-controlled trial. *Neurology* 1995; 45: 1268–76.
24 Weiner HL, Mackin GA, Matsui M, Orav EJ, Khoury SJ, Dawson DM, Hafler DA. Double-blind pilot trial of oral tolerisation with myelion antigens in multiple sclerosis. *Science* 1993; 259: 1321–4.
25 Chen Y, Inobe J, Marks R, Gonnella P, Kuchroo VK, Weiner HL. Peripheral depletion of antigen-reactive T cells in oral tolerance. *Nature* 1995; 376: 177–80.
26 Franklin RJM, Blakemore WF. Glial-cell transplantation and plasticity in the O-2A lineage – implications for CNS repair. *Trends Neurosci* 1995; 18: 151–6.
27 Targett M, Sussman J, Scolding NJ, O'Leary MT, Compston DAS, Blakemore WF. Failure to remyelinate rat axons following transplantation of glial cells obtained from the adult human brain. *Neuropath Appl Neurobiol* 1996; 22: 199–206.
28 Utzschneider DA, Archer DR, Kocsis JD, Waxman SG, Duncan ID. Transplantation of glial cells enhances action potential conduction of amyelinated spinal cord axons in the myelin deficient rat. *Proc Natl Acad Sci USA* 1994; 91: 53–7.

☐ MULTIPLE CHOICE QUESTIONS

1 One of your patients with multiple sclerosis has not attended for 3 years but presents with recent severe difficulty in using her right hand. You would:
   (a) Indicate that this is a common manifestation of multiple sclerosis and arrange to see her again in two months
   (b) Refer routinely to the neurology clinic
   (c) Request admission to the regional neurology unit for a course of intravenous methylprednisolone
   (d) Prescribe a six-week course of intramuscular ACTH
   (e) Refer her to the community physiotherapist

2 A 33-year-old unmarried shop assistant with mild multiple sclerosis is embarrassed about her long-standing bladder urgency with occasional incontinence. You would:
   (a) Prescribe oxybutinin
   (b) Advise the use of an indwelling catheter
   (c) Refer for education in self intermittent catheterization
   (d) Refer for gynaecological assessment of stress incontinence
   (e) Prescribe long-term prophylactic antibiotics

3 Your patient, aged 45, has secondary progressive multiple sclerosis and uses a wheelchair for visits outside her home. She has read in the newspaper about a breakthrough in treatment and wants a prescription for interferon-beta. You would:
   (a) Provide a trial course for 6 months
   (b) Indicate that there is no evidence for efficacy of interferon-beta in multiple sclerosis
   (c) Advise that interferon-beta is not indicated in secondary progressive multiple sclerosis
   (d) Indicate that all decisions on prescribing interferon-beta are devolved to neurologists and refer to the regional neurology centre for a decision
   (e) Suggest that she seeks involvement in a clinical trial

4 Multiple sclerosis:
   (a) Has a recurrence risk of 5% in the siblings of affected individuals
   (b) Causes severe disability requiring the use of a wheelchair in 80% of affected individuals
   (c) Is due to an autoimmune response to measles virus
   (d) Has a population prevalence in the UK of $120/10^5$
   (e) Is primarily a disorder of astrocytes

5 Placebo-controlled trials in multiple sclerosis have shown that:
   (a) Anti-CD4 monoclonal antibodies reduce relapse rate
   (b) Copolymer 1 prevents onset of the progressive phase
   (c) Interferon-beta reduces lesion load on magnetic resonance imaging
   (d) Cyclophosphamide is indicated in the treatment of secondary progressive disease
   (e) Pulsed methylprednisolone does not influence the course of the disease

ANSWERS

1a False	2a True	3a False	4a True	5a False
b False	b False	b False	b False	b False
c True	c True	c True	c False	c True
d False	d False	d False	d True	d False
e False	e False	e False	e False	e True

Management of status epilepticus

D W Chadwick

☐ INTRODUCTION

Status epilepticus in its many different forms and with its many different causes is a relatively rare medical emergency but one that presents great challenges and pitfalls. It can claim to be possibly the most frequently mismanaged of medical emergencies.

There is no commonly agreed definition of status epilepticus. Most authors accept it as a state in which epileptic activity persists continuously or intermittently for at least 30 minutes. This is a practical definition that recognizes that acute medical interventions will be justified in most circumstances after such a period of time has elapsed. This article will only consider the management of status epilepticus in adults, but it is important to recognize that it is much more common in children and that the clinical phenomena it can cause in children are much more varied than in adults [1].

A number of different classifications of status epilepticus have been proposed and none are wholly adequate [1]. A simple approach is to accept that any form of seizure can become continuous and exhibit status, so one classification would simply be an extension of the classification of seizures [2]. The classification contained in Table 1 is very much a pragmatic one, recognizing the differences between convulsive and non-convulsive status. While the major part of this article will concentrate on the management of tonic-clonic status, it is important at this point to discuss other forms of status epilepticus.

☐ DIFFERENT FORMS OF STATUS EPILEPTICUS

Myoclonic status in coma

This can be seen in any acute or chronic, severe encephalopathy but is most commonly seen after acute hypoxic brain damage following cardiopulmonary resuscitation. It usually develops 1 or 2 days into the coma and can last for hours or days. The jerks comprise irregular asynchronous myoclonic jerks of different parts of the body that are commonly provoked by any disturbance or movement. This phenomenon often carries a very adverse prognosis for recovery from coma, but

Table 1 Classification of status epilepticus.

Convulsive status	Non-convulsive status
Tonic–clonic	Absence
Myoclonic status in coma	Complex partial
Epilepsia partialis continua	

where recovery does occur patients may be left with posthypoxic action myoclonus. Burst suppression is commonly seen in the electroencephalogram (EEG) [3]. It is doubtful whether this phenomenon deserves aggressive antiepileptic drug treatment as the prognosis is relatively poor and treatment is of doubtful benefit until such time as the patient is recovering, when persisting myoclonus may become a major functional problem.

Epilepsia partialis continua

This consists of spontaneous regular or irregular clonic jerks confined to one part of the body and continuing for hours, days or weeks. This may occur as part of either an acute [4] or chronic encephalitis [5], or as part of a more obvious structural pathology (tumour, stroke or trauma). The phenomenon tends to be highly resistant to antiepileptic drugs and in acute cases seizures will usually stop spontaneously. Treatment is indicated to prevent any secondary generalization, but often only drug-induced coma can stop the continuous motor seizure. Treatment for chronic encephalitis has included steroids or γ-globulins with the alternative of resective neurosurgery [6].

Non-convulsive status

While absence status can occasionally be seen in adults, it is much more common for this to be due to complex partial status. This is an important differential diagnosis for acute confusion in an epileptic or elderly population. It tends to be very varied in its symptomatology. It commonly comprises a twilight state of varying awareness, often associated with stereotyped automatisms typical of complex partial seizures. On occasions, however, it may simply be characterized by withdrawal and apparent drowsiness, or by other apparent psychiatric symptoms. The EEG is, of course, of considerable importance in the diagnosis of non-convulsive status, where it will usually show continuous slow wave or spike wave abnormalities that may be localized or varyingly generalized. This form of status is relatively common in patients with temporal lobe epilepsy where up to 10% or 15% of patients may exhibit periods of partial status. The status can usually be treated with acute benzodiazepines given under EEG control as part of a diagnostic procedure. This will always have to be followed, however, by the administration of appropriate long-acting antiepileptic drugs (see below).

☐ FREQUENCY AND CAUSES OF STATUS EPILEPTICUS

Rowan and Scott [7] suggested that status epilepticus accounted for 0.01% of all admissions to a general hospital. Most hospital-based series suggest that approximately half of such admissions will be due to status complicating an acute cerebral lesion and about half will be due to the development of status in people with a prior epilepsy. Table 2 provides an illustration of the causes of status epilepticus in these two different groups of patients [8]. About 3% of adults with a history of epilepsy have episodes of status compared with 10–15% of children with

Table 2 Causes of status epilepticus in 98 patients.

	Preceding seizure disorder	No previous seizures
Non-compliance	27	–
Alcohol	11	4
Drug overdose	0	10
Stroke	4	11
Metabolic	3	5
Hypoxia	0	4
Tumour	0	4
Trauma	1	2
Infection	0	4
Unknown	11	4

Totals are greater because more than one factor might be present in an individual patient; alcohol abuse occurred with non-compliance in five cases [8].

epilepsy [1]. The pathophysiology and consequences of tonic-clonic status epilepticus are determined by both continuing cerebral discharge and the motor activity that it provokes, which results in a wide variety of central nervous system (CNS) and systemic changes. This has been well documented in primate studies [9]. There is initially a massive increase in cerebral blood flow and metabolism with catecholamine release resulting in hyperglycaemia and lactic acidosis. Blood pressure and cardiac output rise, associated with tachycardia and the rapid development of hyperpyrexia. As convulsive status continues, cerebral autoregulation fails and intracranial pressure may rise rapidly with the development of cerebral oedema. Systemically later changes include the development of hypoglycaemia with metabolic and respiratory acidosis. Reflex pulmonary oedema may occur. A consumptive coagulopathy may develop with hepatorenal failure, rhabdomyolysis and myoglobinuria. Blood pressure falls with a falling cardiac output and temperature continues to rise. This latter is an important management issue as there is good evidence that hyperpyrexia predisposes cerebral neurons to hypoxic ischaemic necrosis. However, even when the systemic disturbances are controlled by the institution of neuromuscular paralysis and ventilation, neuronal cell loss may still occur as long as seizure discharge continues. For this reason some form of continuous EEG or monitoring of cerebral function should be undertaken in patients with established status. For all these reasons, tonic-clonic status is a condition that demands intensive monitoring and therapy in an environment that can only be provided by an intensive treatment unit (ITU).

However, before advocating a protocol for the management of status epilepticus it is important to recognize that a differential diagnosis of this condition exists and that pseudoseizures or non-epileptic attacks can mimic status [10]. This represents an extreme form of abnormal illness behaviour that in some circumstances may represent a Münchhausen syndrome. The condition is not uncommon, and in tertiary referral units, such as regional neurological centres, it may be more common than true status epilepticus. Pseudoseizures are usually convulsive in nature, though they may not be very convincing to the experienced observer. However, in some cases even experienced observers may have the greatest difficulty in differentiating pseudoseizures from some forms of frontal seizures. The key to the diagnosis is often in the background. Pseudoseizures usually develop no earlier than mid-to-late adolescence and most commonly occur in patients with no previous severe cerebral disease. The attacks are highly resistant to antiepileptic drug therapy in contradistinction to tonic-clonic seizures in true epilepsy developing at this age. There are many other positive pointers towards a diagnosis of pseudoseizures and pseudostatus. Episodes of pseudostatus tend to be repetitive and result in multiple hospital admissions. In spite of this, all investigations are resolutely normal. While a normal EEG cannot completely exclude a diagnosis of epilepsy, a normal interictal EEG probably does exclude an epilepsy severe enough to be characterized by recurrent episodes of convulsive status! It is an almost exclusively female form of behaviour and pseudostatus is usually preceded by a history of self-injury or self-poisoning, psychiatric disorder and other unexplained physical symptoms [10]. Failure to recognize pseudostatus can result in inappropriate treatment with powerful sedative drugs leading to respiratory arrest and septicaemia related to instrumentation. While the author has no direct evidence, it is possible that people have died of this condition through overenthusiastic medical intervention!

☐ MANAGEMENT OF STATUS EPILEPTICUS

Figure 1 includes a flow diagram for a suggested protocol for the management of tonic-clonic status. The main elements of this comprise the administration of appropriate antiepileptic drugs, the institution of supportive care, the diagnosis and identification of a cause for status, and, where necessary, the treatment of any underlying condition and the institution of longer-term maintenance antiepileptic drug treatment.

A wide variety of antiepileptic drugs are available, but relatively few can be given parenterally. Conventionally, benzodiazepines have been widely used because of their rapid onset of activity. However, diazepam has a relatively short period of activity and longer-acting benzodiazepines such as lorazepam should now be preferred. Most commonly, this should be administered with a bolus of phenytoin into a rapidly running drip so as to give a loading dose of approximately 18 mg/kg, which should be sufficient to obtain therapeutic brain levels within 30–40 minutes. This cocktail should be administered as soon as status has been established for 20–30 minutes. Some would advocate the administration of a bolus of glucose at this time to exclude hypoglycaemia. If the status continues, it is important to consider the background and whether this could be pseudostatus. If there are concerns in this area, transfer to a regional neurological centre with facilities for EEG monitoring would be essential. If there is no doubt that this is true status and the seizures are continuing, then an infusion of a rapidly acting antiepileptic drug should be undertaken. Chlormethiazole is useful for this, with dosage titrated to response at 0.5–5 ml

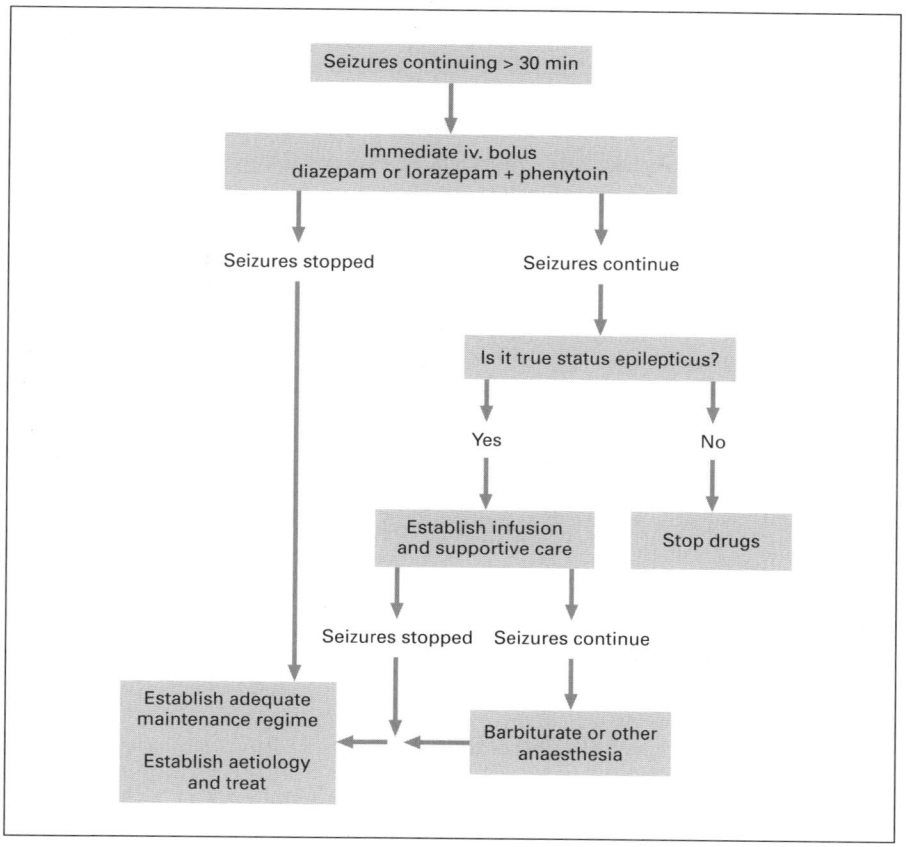

Fig. 1 Flow diagram of the management of status epilepticus.

per minute. At this stage, transfer to an ITU setting with full cardiorespiratory support should occur. The parenteral anticonvulsant should then be increased up to a dose that stops the seizures, with supportive ventilation being provided where respiration is compromised. (One common fault in management is the use of subtherapeutic doses of a succession of different parenteral drugs.) If this fails to control the seizures, then full anaesthesia with respiratory support should be undertaken. In the past this has usually taken the form of treatment with thiopentone, but shorter-acting agents such as midazolam and propofol may now be used. These drugs have advantages in being of shorter duration of activity and therefore more rapidly reversible than thiopentone. These stages can usually be accomplished within 2–3 h of an acute admission if status is ongoing. It will then become possible to undertake any necessary further investigations, including imaging and EEG monitoring. It may also be important to establish and continue longer-acting antiepileptic medication. From the point of view of continuity, this is often best done by administering conventional drugs by a nasogastric tube once it is certain that patients are absorbing via the oral route.

☐ OUTCOME OF STATUS EPILEPTICUS

The outcome of status epilepticus is varied and different hospital-based series over recent years give widely different results [1]. Mortality rates of between 15% and 60% are quoted in some recent series. This is largely dependent on the cause of status. Some studies include large numbers of patients following cardiorespiratory arrest in whom the outcome is likely to be very poor. Certainly, it is universally the case that presentation in status carries a worse prognosis than status in patients with previous epilepsy. There is no doubt that the longer that status is established before the institution of adequate treatment, the worse the outcome both in terms of mortality and morbidity, which in most series runs at about 10% for significant neurological sequelae.

Status epilepticus tends to present to casualty departments and the initial management is often directed by junior hospital doctors who may have little experience of managing this challenging condition. It is important that all acute district general hospitals have a protocol for the management of status epilepticus that is readily available and easily understood by their staff.

REFERENCES

1. Shorvon S. *Status Epilepticus*. Cambridge University Press, 1994.
2. Commission on Classification and Terminology of the International League Against Epilepsy. Proposal for revised clinical and electroencephalographic classification of epileptic seizures. *Epilepsia* 1981; **22**: 489–501.
3. Lowenstein DH, Aminoff MJ. Clinical and EEG features of status epilepticus in comatose patients. *Neurology* 1992; **42**: 100–4.
4. Kojewnikof AY. A particular type of cortical epilepsy; tranl. DM Asher. In: Andermann F, ed. *Chronic Encephalitis and Epilepsy: Rasmussen's Syndrome*. London: Butterworth-Heinemann, 1991: 245–62.
5. Ogouni H, Andermann F, Rasmussen TB. The natural history of chronic encephalitis and epilepsy: a study of the MNI series of forty-eight cases. In: Andermann F, ed. *Chronic Encephalitis and Epilepsy: Rasmussen's Syndrome*. Boston, MA: Butterworth-Heinemann, 1991: 7–36.
6. Dulac O. Rasmussen's syndrome. *Cur Opinion Neurol* 1996; **9** (issue 2).
7. Rowan AJ, Scott DF. Major status epilepticus: a series of 42 patients. *Acta Neurol Scand* 1970; **46**: 573–84.
8. Aminoff MJ, Simon RP. Status epilepticus: causes, clinical features and consequences in 98 patients. *Am J Med* 1980; **69**: 657–66.
9. Meldrum BS, Horton RW. Physiology of status epilepticus in primates. *Arch Neurol* 1973; **28**: 1–9.
10. Howell SJL, Owen L, Chadwick DW. Pseudostatus epilepticus. *Q J Med* 1989; **71**: 507–19.

☐ MULTIPLE CHOICE QUESTIONS

1. Convulsive status epilepticus:
   (a) Is a common occurrence in people with epilepsy
   (b) Is more common in adults than children
   (c) Is commonly associated with increasing pyrexia
   (d) May be complicated by hepatorenal failure

(e) Is responsive to intramuscular diazepam

2 Non-convulsive status:
(a) May cause confusional states in the elderly
(b) Is usually due to absence in adults
(c) Is never a presentation of epilepsy
(d) Does not require treatment with parenteral antiepileptic drugs
(e) Can readily be diagnosed by EEG recording

3 Pseudoseizures:
(a) Are more common in males than females
(b) Are often associated with a previous episode of self-injury and poisoning
(c) Are common in childhood
(d) Are most commonly seen in patients who also have epilepsy
(e) Are easily confused with front lobe seizures

ANSWERS

1a	False	2a	True	3a	False
b	False	b	False	b	True
c	True	c	False	c	False
d	True	d	False	d	False
e	False	e	True	e	True

Management of medical coma

D Bates

☐ INTRODUCTION

When asked to see an unconscious patient in the intensive care unit, the physician must remember that the patient may be suffering delayed effects of trauma, such as subdural haematoma or meningitis arising from a basal skull fracture. In addition, the possibility of raised intracranial pressure following a parenchymal haematoma, the decompensation of a cerebral tumour or the presence of a collection of pus means that all possible causes of loss of consciousness must be considered. It is therefore imperative that, when examining the individual patient, the possibility of trauma be considered and excluded before the decision is taken that the patient is in a coma of non-traumatic aetiology.

Few problems are more difficult to manage than the unconscious patient because the potential causes of loss of consciousness are considerable, and because the time for diagnosis and effective intervention is relatively short. Coma is a potentially life-threatening emergency until vital functions are stabilized, the underlying cause of the coma is diagnosed and reversible causes are corrected. Delay in instituting treatment for a patient with raised intracranial pressure may have obvious consequences in terms of pressure conning, but similarly the unnecessary investigation of patients in metabolic coma with imaging techniques may delay the initiation of appropriate therapy. It is therefore essential for the physician to adopt a systematic approach to ensure resuscitation and to direct tests towards producing the most rapid diagnosis and most appropriate therapy.

☐ ASSESSMENT AND TREATMENT OF COMA

Causes of coma

Consciousness depends on an intact ascending reticular activating substance (ARAS) in the dorsal brain stem and functioning cerebral cortex of both hemispheres [1]. Disruption of the ARAS will occur with focal lesions in the brain stem, mass lesions in the posterior fossa and chemical depressants, most commonly ingested drugs. The cerebral cortex provides the content of consciousness, which is an amalgam of all cognitive function. Coma arising from disruption of cortical activity requires a diffuse pathology, such as generalized anoxia or ischaemia, either systemic following cardiac arrest or anaesthetic accidents, or cerebral due to cortical vasospasm in infective meningitis or subarachnoid haemorrhage.

The physician diagnosing the cause of coma must therefore consider the following factors:

(i) *Supra- or infra-tentorial mass lesions:* there will usually be evidence of raised intracranial pressure and focal signs are common.

(ii) *Subtentorial destructive lesions or the local effect of a toxin:* these pathologies will directly damage the ascending reticular activating substance.

(iii) *Diffuse damage to the cerebral cortex:* this is most commonly seen in hypoxia and ischaemia, but is also found in meningitis, subarachnoid haemorrhage, hypoglycaemia, keto-acidosis and electrolyte abnormalities.

Resuscitation

Resuscitation is usually established before medical consultation, but the physician should recognize the importance of protecting the patient's airway, supporting respiration and circulation, and providing an adequate supply of glucose to stabilize the patient.

Once oxygenation and circulation are ensured and monitored, blood can be withdrawn to determine blood glucose, for biochemical estimations and toxicology, and then a bolus of 25–50 g of dextrose can be given.

History

Once the patient is stable, it is important to obtain information from those people who accompanied the patient to hospital or who saw the onset of coma. Coma is likely to present in one of three ways: (i) as the predictable progression of underlying illness; (ii) as an unpredictable event in a patient with previously known disease; or (iii) as a totally unexpected event. It is obvious that a history of a sudden collapse in the midst of a busy street or office indicates the need for different investigations from those required for the patient who is discovered at home in bed surrounded by bottles emptied of sedative tablets.

Examination and monitoring

A rapid but careful systematic examination may help to identify possible causes of the coma and it is important that the temperature, heart rate, blood pressure and respiration be monitored and the integument examined to identify anaemia, jaundice, cyanosis or the cherry-red colour of carbon monoxide poisoning. Bruising or bleeding from orifices must be identified and any exanthem, or hyperpigmentation, be noted. It is imperative that examination for neck stiffness, Kernig's and Brudzinski's signs be undertaken to identify the presence of meningeal irritation. Fundal examination is vital to identify the presence of papilloedema, fundal haemorrhages, emboli, hypertensive or diabetic retinopathy and the rare finding of subhyaloid haemorrhages.

☐ NEUROLOGICAL EXAMINATION

Formal neurological examination consists of eliciting various reflex responses. The most important aspects of the examination are those that define the level of consciousness, identify the activity of the brain stem and demonstrate evidence of lateralization.

Level of consciousness

The Glasgow Coma Scale is the most useful hierarchical assessment of the level of consciousness (Table 1) [2].

Eye opening is relatively easy to assess; the fixed and unresponsive opening of the eyes sometimes seen in deep coma should not be confused with volitional or reflex opening of the eyes from a closed position in response to stimuli. All four limbs are tested for movement and the best response is recorded, though asymmetry may be an important finding. A grimace response to painful stimulation indicates intact corticobulbar function, but patients in coma, particularly after hypoxic ischaemic insult, may show grimace in response to minor peripheral stimulation yet have no associated peripheral motor response. This finding always raises the question of a ventral pontine lesion (the locked-in syndrome) or of a cervical cord injury. However, it is more commonly seen in patients who will evolve into a vegetative state and is, generally, a poor prognostic sign. The level of coma should be documented serially and is one of the most important indicators of the need for further investigations.

Brain stem function

The brain stem reflexes are particularly important in identifying those lesions that may affect the reticular activating substance, explaining the reason for coma, and help in identifying the viability of the patient.

Pupillary reaction

The size, equality and reaction of the pupils to light is recorded. Unilateral dilatation of the pupil with loss of the light response suggests uncal herniation or a posterior

Table 1 The Glasgow coma scale.

Eyes	Open	Spontaneously	4
		To verbal command	3
		To pain	2
		No response	1
Best motor response	To verbal command	Obeys	6
	To painful stimulus	Localizes pain	5
		Withdrawal	4
		Flexion	3
		Extension	2
		No response	1
Best verbal response		Orientated	5
		Disorientated	4
		Inappropriate words	3
		Incomprehensible sounds	2
		No response	1

communicating artery aneurysm. Mid-brain lesions typically cause loss of the light reflex with mid-position pupils; pontine lesions cause miosis but a retained light response. Fixed dilatation of the pupils is an indication of a central diencephalic herniation.

Hepatic or renal failure and other forms of metabolic coma may make the pupillary reflexes appear unduly brisk and the pupils therefore relatively small. Most drug intoxications tend to cause small but sluggish pupil reaction and a pontine haemorrhage will cause pinpoint pupils owing to parasympathetic stimulation.

Corneal responses

The corneal responses are usually retained until coma is very deep but may be lost in association with corneal oedema after prolonged coma. If absent in a patient who is in otherwise light coma, then the possibility of drug-induced coma or of local causes of anaesthesia to the cornea should be considered. The loss of a corneal response when drug overdose or corneal oedema is excluded is a poor prognostic sign [3].

Spontaneous eye movement

The resting position of the eyes and the presence of spontaneous eye movements should be noted. Conjugate deviation of the eyes suggests an ipsilateral hemisphere or contralateral brain stem lesion. Depression of the eyes below the meridian may be seen with damage at the level of the mid-brain tectum and in states of metabolic coma. The eyes will be dysconjugate if there is damage to the oculomotor or abducens nerves within the brain stem or along their paths.

Roving eye movements seen in light coma are similar to those of sleep. They cannot be mimicked and their presence excludes psychogenic unresponsiveness. Ocular bobbing, an intermittent jerking downward eye movement, is seen with destructive lesions in the low pons and with cerebellar haematoma or hydrocephalus.

Reflex eye movements

These are tested by the oculocephalic and oculovestibular responses. The oculocephalic or doll's head response is tested by rotating the patient's head from side to side and observing the position of the eyes. In coma with an intact brain stem, the eyes will move conjugately and in a direction opposite to the head movement. In a conscious patient, such a response can be imitated by deliberate fixation of the eyes, but is not common. In patients with pontine depression the oculocephalic response is lost and the eyes remain in the mid position when the head is turned.

The oculovestibular response is more accurate and more useful. It is elicited by instilling between 50 and 200 ml of ice-cold water into one external auditory meatus. The normal response is the development of nystagmus with the quick phase away from the side of stimulation. A tonic response with conjugate movement of the eyes towards the stimulated side indicates an intact pons and suggests a supratentorial cause for the coma. A dysconjugate response or no response at all indicates brain stem damage or depression. Each ear should be stimulated separately, and if unilateral irrigation causes vertical eye movements the possibility of drug overdose arises because many drugs affect lateral eye movements.

Respiration

Modern techniques of assisted respiration, and the need to examine patients in intensive care units where their respiration is controlled, complicate the assessment of normal respiratory function. If the patient is seen before respiration is controlled then the presence of long-cycle periodic respiration suggests a relatively high brain stem lesion, central neurogenic hyperventilation implies a lesion at the level of the upper pons and short-cycle periodic respiration, which carries a poor prognosis, is seen with lesions lower in the brain stem. In general, the presence of rapid regular respiration correlates with pulmonary complications and a poor prognosis rather than with the site of neurological disease.

Motor function

The finding of lateralization implies a focal cause for the coma. The observation of the involuntary movements affecting the face or limbs and asymmetry of the reflexes will help to support this possibility. Focal seizures are an important indicator of a focal cause for coma and the observation of more generalized seizures or of multi-focal myoclonus raises the possibility of metabolic or ischaemic-anoxic cause for the coma with diffuse cortical irritation and carries a poor prognosis.

☐ INVESTIGATIONS OF THE PATIENT IN COMA

On clinical grounds patients can be allocated to one of three patterns of response.

Coma with focal signs

Except in those patients in whom an underlying and irreversible terminal disease is known, a computerized tomography (CT) scan or magnetic resonance imaging (MRI) scan should be undertaken to identify the cause of coma. This will define whether or not a structural abnormality is present and in many instances give a clue to the underlying pathology. If the CT scan is normal, then the possibility of a non-structural focal abnormality antedating the onset of the coma or being part of the coma, as occasionally happens with hypoglycaemia or hepatic encephalopathy, should be considered. If there is no focal structural abnormality with imaging then other investigations, including metabolic and cerebrospinal fluid examinations should be carried out.

Coma with meningeal irritation but without focal signs

Such patients will usually be suffering from subarachnoid haemorrhage, acute bacterial meningitis or viral meningo-encephalitis. The distinction between infective and non-infective causes can usually be made on the basis of fever, and a lumbar puncture will be expected to reveal the cause. As a counsel of perfection, a CT scan should be undertaken before lumbar puncture to identify the possibility of a collection of pus or the site of a subarachnoid haemorrhage.

Presence of coma without focal signs or meningismus

This represents the most common finding in patients in coma who are likely to have a metabolic or anoxic cause for their condition. It is important to withdraw blood for toxicology to exclude the possibility of drug overdose and to seek evidence of hepatic failure, renal failure, hyperglycaemia, hypoglycaemia or disturbances of electrolytes or acidosis.

☐ PREDICTION OF OUTCOME IN COMA

In non-traumatic coma, other than that which is drug induced, the factors that determine outcome include the cause of coma, the depth of coma, the duration of coma and certain clinical signs, among the most important of which are brain stem reflexes.

Overall, only 15% of patients in non-traumatic coma for more than 6 h will make a good or moderate recovery; the other 85% will die, remain vegetative, or reach a state of severe disability in which they remain dependent [4]. Patients whose coma is due to metabolic causes, including infection, organ failure and biochemical disturbances, have a better prognosis, and 35% of them will achieve moderate or good recovery; of those whose coma follows hypoxic ischaemic insult, only 11% will make such a recovery; of those in coma due to cerebrovascular disease only 7% can be expected to make such a recovery. About 20% of patients who are in coma following hypoxic ischaemic injury will enter the vegetative state because of the likelihood of hypoxic ischaemic injury resulting in bihemispheric damage with relative sparing of the brain stem (Table 2).

The depth of coma is prognostic, with those patients showing no eye opening after 6 h of coma having only a 10% chance of making a good or moderate recovery, whereas those whose eyes open in response to painful stimuli have a 20% chance of

Table 2 Outcome of coma.

	No recovery	Vegetative state	Severe disability	Moderate disability	Good recovery	Total
Hypoxia ischaemia	121 (58%)	43 (20%)	23 (11%)	7 (3%)	16 (8%)	210
Cerebrovascular	134 (74%)	12 (7%)	21 (12%)	8 (4%)	6 (3%)	181
Hepatic	25 (49%)	1 (2%)	8 (16%)	5 (10%)	12 (24%)	51
Other	26 (45%)	6 (10%)	8 (14%)	3 (5%)	15 (26%)	58
Total	306 (61%)	62 (10%)	60 (12%)	23 (5%)	49 (10%)	500

making such a recovery. The longer the coma persists the less likely the patient is to recover; 15% of patients in coma for 6 h make a good or moderate recovery compared with only 3% who remain unconscious at 1 week. Of individual clinical signs, the most significant are: (i) the loss of corneal reflexes early in coma, which indicates poor prognosis; (ii) the loss of pupillary reflex after 24 h in coma, which is similarly indicative of a poor prognosis; and (iii) the absence of volitional motor responses by 3 days or the absence of roving eye movements by 7 days, which indicate a poor outcome [5].

The presence of roving eye movements within 6 h of coma identifies a group of patients of whom 25% will achieve a moderate or good recovery, and the use of combinations of clinical signs improves the accuracy of these predictors.

The most accurate prediction of outcome in patients in medical coma remains that identified by the use of clinical signs. Little is added by more sophisticated tests other than to identify the cause of the coma.

☐ CONTINUATION OF CARE

The long-term care of patients in coma may be undertaken in an intensive care unit, on a specialist ward or later in a long-stay hospital. It is important that those patients in whom prognosis is hopeless should not be permanently exposed to the rigours of intensive care medicine, but should continue to receive basic care within routine hospital wards. So long as patients are considered to have a realistic potential for recovery, they should be looked after on intensive care units or on specialist wards [6,7]. Their respiration, skin, circulation and bladder and bowel function need attention, seizures should be controlled and the level of consciousness monitored. It is important that mobility of joints and circulation to pressure areas be maintained during the long-term care of the patient, and the possibility of aspiration pneumonia, peptic ulceration and other complications of long-term intensive care be avoided. Techniques such as elective ventilation and the use of steroid therapy should not be used routinely in the management of the comatose patient as they do not improve prognosis and may compromise recovery.

REFERENCES

1. Plum F, Posner JB. *Diagnosis of Stupor and Coma*, 3rd edn. Philadelphia: Davis, 1980.
2. Teasdale G, Jennett B. Assessment of coma and impaired consciousness: a practical scale. *Lancet* 1974; 2: 81–4.
3. Jorgensen EO, Malchow-Moloer A. A natural history of global and critical brain ischaemia. *Resuscitation* 1981; 9: 133–91.
4. Levy DE, Bates D, Caronna JJ, *et al.* Prognosis of non-traumatic coma. *Ann Intern Med* 1981; 94: 293–301.
5. Bates D. The management of medical coma. *J Neurol Neurosurg Psychiat* 1993; 56: 589–98.
6. Sazbon L, Zagbreba F, Ronen J, Solzi P, Costeff H. Course and outcome of patients in vegetative state of nontraumatic aetiology. *J Neurol Neurosurg Psychiat* 1993; 56: 407–9.
7. The Multi-Society Task Force on PVS. Medical aspects of the persistent vegetative state. *New Engl J Med* 1994; 330: 1499–508; 1572–9.

MULTIPLE CHOICE QUESTIONS

1. The management of a patient in coma with focal signs should include:
   (a) Brain imaging
   (b) Lumbar puncture
   (c) Measurement of blood glucose
   (d) Electroencephalography
   (e) Measurement of blood metabolites in blood

2. The presence of a vegetative state:
   (a) Always indicates a hopeless prognosis
   (b) May be a transient phase in recovery from coma
   (c) Is most commonly seen as the result of cerebrovascular disease
   (d) Indicates damage to the brain stem but preserved cortical function
   (e) Can be regarded as 'permanent' after 1 week

3. Of patients in coma following non-traumatic and non-drug-related injury for more than 6 h:
   (a) Almost 50% will make a full recovery
   (b) The vegetative state is most commonly seen following hypoxic ischaemic injury
   (c) The cause of the coma is not related to outcome
   (d) An electroencephalogram is an essential investigation to identify prognosis
   (e) Imaging techniques are important only in helping to achieve the diagnosis

4. In patients who are unconscious following a cardiopulmonary arrest the following signs indicate a good prognosis:
   (a) Absent pupillary responses after 24 h
   (b) Spontaneous conjugate eye movements at 24 h
   (c) Localization of painful stimuli by 24 h
   (d) Nystagmus seen on oculovestibular testing
   (e) Multifocal myoclonus

5. The following statements about coma are true:
   (a) Coma occurring after sedative drug overdose characteristically results in active brain stem but depressed cortex
   (b) Hypoxic ischaemic coma is most likely to result in cortical damage with preserved brain stem function
   (c) The absence of a corneal response 24 h after a cardiac arrest indicates a poor prognosis
   (d) The patient in a persistent vegetative state will have lost all deep tendon reflexes
   (e) Hypoglycaemia may cause coma with focal neurological signs

ANSWERS

1a	True	2a	False	3a	False	4a	False	5a	False
b	False	b	True	b	True	b	True	b	True
c	True	c	False	c	False	c	True	c	True
d	False	d	False	d	False	d	True	d	False
e	False	e	False	e	True	e	False	e	True

Headaches: how good are we at early management?

David L Stevens

☐ INTRODUCTION

This chapter is primarily about headaches and it describes a study of headache management by family doctors. Because of the way the study was done, it is more than a review of how to diagnose and manage certain headache disorders, for we also gain an insight into doctors' behaviour. This simple study started as a teaching aid on how to manage headaches and ended up as an exploration of how clinical data are interpreted and why doctors behave in certain ways. We end up with more questions than answers.

☐ PATIENTS WITH HEADACHES

Headache is a common symptom. Waters [1] estimates that approximately 80% of adults (females more than males) have a significant headache each year and 16% (13% of males and 20% of females) consult their family doctors about the problem. Some are then referred on for specialist advice. It has been estimated that 1–2% of patients present with headache when consulting general practitioners (GPs) in the UK [2] and the USA [3,4] and that 14–17% of new patients consulting neurologists [5–7] have headache as their primary problem. It is clear that we are dealing with large numbers here, so this is a condition that family doctors and neurologists should be good at managing.

Before proceeding further, it is legitimate to consider the expectations of patients when they present to a doctor with headache and, at the same time, to ask what GPs expect when they refer such patient for specialist advice. I think it is reasonable to conclude that both patients and GPs are asking the same questions:

- ☐ Is the headache due to something nasty?
- ☐ If it is, then can anything be done to help?
- ☐ If it isn't, then can it be treated?

The study described below looks at certain aspects of how doctors address these questions.

☐ HOW WAS THE STUDY DONE AND WHAT EMERGED?

What follows is a description of a simple technique to look at how doctors interpret data on headache and what they do with patients with this problem. The device used involves fictitious patients. The doctors were presented with three histories describing headache problems, given as if by real patients and containing enough detail to allow certain questions to be asked about the doctor's ideas on diagnosis, investigation and management. These case histories are given below. Each case history was accompanied by a questionnaire, which first requests a diagnosis and then poses a series of 'What would you do next?' questions:

- ☐ Would you do blood tests?
- ☐ Would you do X-rays?
- ☐ Would you do anything else?
- ☐ How would you treat? (Cases A and B only)
- ☐ Would you refer to a specialist?

The case histories and questionnaires were given to a total of 100 GPs who were attending three different residential postgraduate meetings. These doctors were away from home and therefore they did not have access to text-books or journals. The same documents were later given to ten consultant neurologists, who were asked to give their perception of perfect GP answers in the hope of establishing a sort of gold standard for diagnosis and management. A summary of the answers concerning each of these fictitious patients is given following the relevant case history.

Patient A

Miss A is a single lady of 38. She is a solicitor and she is on the local council. She lives on her own. She doesn't come to see you very often; she says she never has the time, but things are getting on top of her and she hopes that you can do something about the headaches. They are getting worse.

'Yes, I've had them for years. I can remember them when I was at school, but I would only have a bad one about once a year. Now I'm getting two or three a month and they knock me for six for three days. My work is suffering, so I hope you can help.'

'I can tell when one is coming, because I feel a niggle here', she puts her hand to her temple, 'and after about ten minutes it starts to pound. Then I feel sick and if I'm not careful, I'm actually sick.' She indicates one half of the head: 'It spreads all over, so that I have to take something. If I can, I lie down, but if I'm at work, I have to try and carry on. When I get home, I go to bed and just stay there until it goes.'

'It's messing up my life. If I just had them at weekends, like I did when I was young, I could cope, but now I get them at any time.'

[This one is easy.]

Patient A – response to questions

    Characteristics of the condition:
    Common   YES
    Classic text-book description   YES

Question	Response	100 GPs	10 Consultant neurologists
What is the diagnosis?	Migraine	85%	40%
	Common migraine	4%	60%
	Classic migraine	8%	
	Migrainous neuralgia	1%	
	Cranial arteritis	2%	
Do you do blood tests?	Yes	21%	0%
	Haematology	8%	
	ESR or viscosity	14%	
	Chemistry	6%	
	Hormone studies	2%	
Do you do X-rays?	Yes	2%	0%
	CT or MRI	2%	
How do you treat?			
For attacks	Analgesics	51%	30%
	Ergotamine	7%	
	Sumatriptan	33%	70%
	'Migraine treatments'	9%	
Preventive	Beta blockers	31%	30%
	Pizotifen	54%	40%
	Clonidine	1%	
	Prednisolone	2%	
	Antidepressants	1%	
	Dietary advice	8%	
	Counselling	8%	
Specialist referral	Yes	4%	40%

Patient B

Mr B is an ex-soldier and saw 30 years of service. He is a fitness fanatic and prides himself on being healthy. He describes himself to his friends as a hard man. He likes to give the impression that he can take anything. But not this time.

'It started 10 days ago and I've been getting it every night. It starts at two in the morning and wakes me up. It is behind my eye and all round here' (he puts the heel of his hand over his right eye) 'and it hurts like hell. I get up and walk about, I've even banged my head on the wall, but it doesn't make it go away. I've been a leader of men and it seems pathetic that I, of all people, should cry with pain, but I tell you doctor, it makes me crack up. It goes on for ages, at least two hours, then I can get back to sleep. Sometimes it wakes me up again, but usually it's only once a night.'

'Yes, I do get a runny eye with it, and yes, it does look a bit red, but I thought that was because I keep rubbing it.'

'The nose does feel blocked, you are quite right, I'd noticed that. I wondered if it was my sinuses. What do you think?'

[This one is easy if you know what it is, but difficult if you do not recognize it.]

Patient B – response to questions

Characteristics of the condition:
Common   NO
Classic text-book description   YES

Question	Response		100 GPs	10 Consultant neurologists
What is the diagnosis?	**Migrainous neuralgia**		**44%**	**100%**
(some gave more than	Migraine		3%	
one answer)	Orgasmic migraine		1%	
	Trigeminal neuralgia		7%	
	Temporal arteritis		8%	
	Optic neuritis		1%	
	Glaucoma		10%	
	Sinusitis		14%	
	Raised intracranial pressure		8%	
	Unknown		14%	
Do you do blood tests?	**Yes**		**41%**	**20%**
	Haematology		20%	10%
	ESR or viscosity		34%	20%
	Chemistry		9%	
	Other		7%	
Do you do X-rays?	**Yes**		**40%**	**20%**
	CT or MRI		11%	20%
	Skull X-ray		19%	
	Sinus X-ray		27%	
	Chest X-ray		7%	
Specialist referral?	**Yes**		**44%**	**0%**

Patient C

Mr C is 56 and you have known him for years. He is, and always has been, a worrier. He sees you a lot for all sorts of symptoms. The year before last it was the bowels and the wind, last year it was a mysterious tightness in the chest that defied analysis, and now it is headache. He has complained of headache on and off over the years and you have notes written by yourself and by your predecessor describing his chronic headache problem.

'They started two months ago. I know I've talked to you about headaches before, but these are different and they're getting worse. I have it every day doctor. I wake up with it and it's awful. It's a tightness and a pressure all over the head. Sometimes it's throbbing as well and if I exert myself, even a little bit, then the throbbing gets worse. I only have a bit of peace in the afternoons; it can settle down at lunchtime. Then I have a few hours of peace and it comes back and stays until bed time. Pills are no good; I've taken hundreds. I don't know why they never work. I know I've told you about headaches before, but these are different; they're much worse than they've ever been. You ask my wife, she'll tell you how much I suffer . . . I can't do my job, I can't concentrate and my memory is awful . . . I haven't got any energy. You've got to do something. One of my friends at work thinks I should see a specialist. What do you think?'

[This one is potentially difficult.]

Patient C – response to questions

Characteristics of the condition:
Common   YES
Classic text-book description   NO

Question	Response	100 GPs	10 Consultant neurologists
What is the diagnosis?	**Tension headache**	**48%**	**60%**
	Anxiety/depression	20%	10%
	Migraine	1%	
	Vascular disease	2%	
	Raised intracranial pressure	11%	10%
	Cerebral tumour	18%	20%
Do you do blood tests?	**Yes**	**74%**	**50%**
	Haematology	50%	30%
	ESR or viscosity	50%	40%
	Chemistry	56%	10%
Do you do X-rays?	**Yes**	**62%**	**50%**
	CT or MRI	47%	50%
	Skull X-ray	29%	
	Chest X-ray	25%	10%
	Cervical spine X-ray	5%	
	Arteriogram	2%	
Do you do anything else?	**Full examination**	**32%**	**70%**
	Fundus examination	28%	
	Blood pressure	28%	
Specialist referral?	**Yes**	**64%**	**80%**

☐ HOW DO WE EVALUATE CLINICAL DATA?

A lot of what we doctors do is pattern recognition. When we try to recognize the pattern or patterns presented by a patient with a particular problem, we draw upon a body of information that we have tucked away in our heads which relates to that problem. Because we have all been educated differently, and we have different personalities and different attitudes, it is inevitable that within any group of doctors there will be a variety of ways of approaching the same clinical problem. The present study reveals that doctors do indeed vary in their approaches.

Before going any further, it must be acknowledged that it is obvious that what we are discussing here is not real life. The fictitious histories have been constructed to be realistic, but it is obvious that they and the questionnaires are artificial devices. However, they do have the one advantage of allowing a large number of doctors to be faced with exactly the same problem and the same set of questions. Here the clinical data are the same for everybody. Real life is not like that.

When a patient consults us about a particular symptom, we analyse it by using the relevant knowledge that we have in our heads, so when the opening phrase is 'Doctor, it's about these headaches . . .', we call up what can be thought of as the headache files in our memories. These files contain the accumulated knowledge that we have tucked away which relates to headache. We have information we were given as students, facts we have been taught since, things we have learned from colleagues, and other pieces of information we have gathered from books, journals, television programmes, drug company advertising and many other sources. All of these facts are mixed with additional information that we have learned as we have practised: the accumulated experience gathered from seeing hundreds, if not thousands, of previous patients with headaches. All of this constitutes our knowledge data base. When we react to a patient by using this data base, we also add our own distinctive approach to their problem, which is coloured by who we are and how we react generally to things. We reveal in our approach to clinical problems a lot about ourselves: whether we tend to worry or whether we are always supremely confident, whether our attitudes are rigid or fluid and whether, to us, clinical problems are black, white or some shade of grey.

Because no two of us are alike, and because we have all had different experiences over the years, it is inevitable that our data bases are different as well. Some of us have very compartmentalized ways of storing facts. We all know physicians who, if asked about a particular problem, seem to click on to the lists they have in their heads, and out come catalogues of clinical and other features, differential diagnoses, treatment statistics, survival figures, and so on. They seem to be able to open up files in their minds, which contain well organized, but rather rigid, sets of facts that relate to the problem under discussion. Others seem to store their knowledge differently. They define things less rigidly, they emphasize the blurred edges of definitions, they discuss things in general terms and they are often not so good with the lengthy lists of clinical features, complications and other statistics. In reality, I think we all do a bit of both.

Another variable concerns how much we know, for it is inevitable that some of us know more than others. We all have colleagues who seem to have heard of everything, so that we wonder how it is that we don't know what they know. Their lists are longer than ours and they seem to know more answers than we do. All of these considerations must be relevant when we try to analyse why a large group of doctors, when faced with exactly the same problem, come up with such varied solutions.

The patient with migraine

Our doctors, the GPs and the neurologists, when offered some fictitious patients with headache syndromes, reveal this varied approach. They were, with very few exceptions, spot-on when diagnosing the migraine suffered by Miss A, the solicitor. They all recognized this case because she has a common problem with classic textbook features. They varied in terms of what they did next, for some did tests and others did not, but in general they were all conventional in their approach to the investigation and management of the problem. So, all of them, GPs and neurologists, have similar templates in their heads concerning migraine.

Why the GPs did so many blood tests is not clear. I suspect that this is a cultural phenomenon. There are many possible explanations, but it seems likely that this is a piece of ritualized behaviour. Some doctors may do blood tests on patients as a way of saying 'I am taking you seriously and these blood tests are the symbolic evidence of this'. Over the years, they have got into the habit of encouraging their patients to believe that the doctor is only being serious when he or she enacts this blood test ritual. It is doubtful if any of them could call upon solid evidence to justify such testing. While it is likely that the explanation for this is as given already, it has to be acknowledged that some of the doctors may have felt that if they were asked in a questionnaire: 'Would you do blood tests?' they had better answer 'Yes', just to be on the safe side, whereas in real life they would act differently.

The patient with migrainous neuralgia

The ex-soldier with migrainous neuralgia illustrates some further facets of doctors' behaviour. This is an uncommon disorder, but with classic text-book features. The neurologists all recognized the case, but the GPs, on the other hand, were rather varied. If they did not recognize it, they proposed a wide variety of other diagnoses, which suggests that some of them are unclear about the classic features of many different disorders, not just the one illustrated here. Clearly, it is unreasonable to expect the average GP to know everything about such diverse conditions as migrainous neuralgia, trigeminal neuralgia, temporal arteritis, glaucoma and optic neuritis (all suggested as an explanation for Mr B's symptoms), but it could be argued that further education is necessary to help them to sort out the features of these relatively unusual, but important, disorders. However, other specialists, in different disciplines, could make similar lists of relatively obscure disorders that they feel GPs should learn about and it is obvious that there is a limit as to how expert we can reasonably expect GPs to be across the whole of medicine. There is no easy answer, but we should at least try to acknowledge all of this when we educate undergraduates or offer postgraduate education to GPs. We should ask 'What is going to be important to them in their practice and what isn't?' I do not think we have achieved the right balance yet and the eccentricities of the curriculum for undergraduate education in some UK universities is proof of this. From a neurological perspective, the education of the undergraduates that come to the hospitals where I work is extremely varied in quality and quantity. It can range from quite exceptional in some instances, to frankly awful in others. It seems that the amount of time allocated to neurology at some universities takes no account of the fact that 20% of acute medical admissions are neurological [8] and that each year almost 10% of the population consult their GPs about a neurological problem [9].

The patient with chronic headache

The third patient, poor Mr C with his chronic headache problem, illustrates some further issues. He has a disorder that is diffuse and somewhat ill-defined. No clear-cut text-book description here, and it shows. From exactly the same data, the family doctors and the neurologists were split 2:1 on whether he had a banal problem or something serious. This makes no sense and it is not easy to explain.

I think some of this reflects the cautious approach – 'He *could* have something serious, so we had better make sure'. This is likely to be part of the explanation, because both groups of doctors scanned him with enthusiasm, and approximately 20% did this even though they had previously diagnosed him as having a tension headache or an anxiety/depression syndrome. They were being careful. But why? There are many possible explanations, including the 'nasty surprise' syndrome ('I saw one of these before and he turned out to have a tumour, so I scan all of them now . . .'), fear of litigation should something be missed or a belief that patients want scans (which many do).

Some of this behaviour suggests a general lack of confidence in their own ability to make a robust clinical diagnosis, which is clearly understandable if the story given by the patient does not conform to a simple classic pattern and the clues that reveal the true nature of the problem are not obvious. The problem, however, is that some thought like this and some did not. That is the real puzzle. I would find all of this so much easier to understand if everybody agreed that his headaches were benign or if they all agreed that he could have something serious but, as the figures show, opinion is divided. How do such disparate approaches come about? Why don't we all share the same view? I do not think we know, but it might be useful to find out.

Some general comments

The question 'Would you do anything else?' was almost a trick question. If this one had been worded 'Would you perform a physical examination?' then it is likely that everyone would have answered 'Yes', but physical examination was not always mentioned in the answers given and the data on the man with the chronic headache illustrate this. I think that this result resembles what happens in real life, for many patients referred to my neurology clinics express surprise when told that a physical examination will be performed, and some admit that they have not previously been examined. Clearly GPs need further education on this point, for we cannot really condone the omission of such a valuable part of the assessment.

Much of what has been discussed so far can be looked at from an economic point of view. Blood tests and scans cost money, so it is reasonable for us to ask whether our doctors should have been more conservative in their investigations. There are no robust data on how useful blood tests are likely to be in the three headache disorders discussed here, but one's instinctive feeling is that in the majority of such patients they are likely to be unhelpful. There are data, however, on the value of scans, for the American Academy of Neurology [10] has looked at this and the figures are instructive. In patients with migraine who have had no recent change in the pattern of the disorder and who do not have focal signs or a history of seizures, the yield from scanning is 0.4%. We do not have data on migrainous neuralgia, but in patients with chronic headache and no physical signs the yield is 2.4%. So the scans requested by our doctors are likely to be negative. An expensive exercise.

Referral to a specialist is also expensive. Our data on that topic are completely bizarre. The GPs were good at migraine and only 4% felt referral was likely to be useful, but 40% of the neurologists thought that the lady with migraine should be referred. It would seem that neurologists want to see more migraine. With migrainous neuralgia, 44% of the GPs felt that referral would be a good plan, but the neurologists were not interested: all of them said that no referral was needed. And with the patient with chronic headache, 64% of the GPs and 80% of the neurologists felt that referral might be best. What does one make of this? It is not clear but, if we think about waiting lists, pressures on hospital services, the wish of the government that more care should be given by primary physicians and, most important of all, that referrals cost a lot of money, then we really should be trying to find out.

One very obvious message emerges from this study. If a disorder is classic and common, then we all recognize it; if it is classic, but rare, then experts recognize it, but non-experts do not, and if it is not classic, even though it may be common, then there is much disagreement, even among experts. All of this is important for we are living in an era when much enthusiasm is being put into designing guidelines and protocols. If we take our very simple examples, then we could design wonderful protocols for migraine, but we do not need them because everybody is good at recognizing this condition. We could design migrainous neuralgia protocols, but because the condition is unusual they would never be used. And what about chronic headache? The data presented here suggest that we would have great difficulty in getting ten neurologists to agree on a set of guidelines, so when we really need them it looks as if we cannot create them.

☐ CONCLUSION

This simple study on the management of headache has revealed much about how different doctors behave when presented with the same data, and it has highlighted some curious facets of doctors' behaviour. There are lessons to be learned about the way we should teach both undergraduates and postgraduates about headaches, and it is likely that, if this technique were applied to other common conditions, similar results would be obtained.

REFERENCES

1. Waters WE. *Headache*. London: Croom Helm, 1986.
2. Logan WPD, Cushion AA. Morbidity statistics from general practice. *Studies on Medical and Population Subjects*. Number 14. London: HMSO, 1958.
3. Leviton A. Epidemiology of headache. In: Schoenberg BS, ed., *Neurological Epidemiology: Principles and Clinical Applications*. New York: Raven Press, 1978.
4. National Center for Health Statistics, 1979.
5. Stevens DL. Neurology in Gloucestershire: the clinical workload of an English neurologist. *J Neurol Neurosurg Psychiat* 1989; **52**: 439–46.
6. Hopkins A, Menken M, DeFriese G. A record of patient encounters in neurological practice in the United Kingdom. *J Neurol Neurosurg Psychiat* 1989; **52**: 436–8.
7. Association of British Neurologists. *United Kingdom Audit of the Care of Common Neurological Disorders*. 1991.

8 Morrow JI, Patterson VH. The neurological practice of a district general hospital. *J Neurol Neurosurg Psychiat* 1987; **50**: 1397–401.
9 Hopkins A. Lessons for neurologists from the United Kingdom Third National Morbidity Survey. *J Neurol Neurosurg Psychiat* 1989; **52**: 430–3.
10 American Academy of Neurology. Quality standards committee, 1994.

Imported infections

G Pasvol

☐ INTRODUCTION

There was a time when travel by sea was sufficiently prolonged for imported infections to reveal themselves, and often resolve by natural cure or death, long before arrival on home shores. Today jet aircraft can bring strange diseases to our doorstep in a short space of time. While insect vectors may carry the agents of many infections acquired abroad, the jet aircraft is now the 'vector' of often unfamiliar disease on a scale requiring all practising physicians to possess some knowledge of imported diseases. Moreover, the age of infections, as was once thought, is by no means over. Emerging and re-emerging infections are graphically described in a recent compelling, highly recommended (and referenced) book by Laurie Garrett, perhaps prophetically entitled *The Coming Plague* [1]. Climatologists have, moreover, predicted an unprecedented rise in global temperature of about 2°C by the year 2100 which might well affect the incidence of infectious diseases especially of mosquito-borne disease such as malaria, dengue fever and viral encephalitides [2].

The number of international travellers has escalated dramatically [3]. Each year over a billion and a half journeys are embarked on worldwide, of which about 500 million are for tourism. Over 30 million are for travel to developing countries and over a million of these are from the UK. Moreover, the adventurous traveller is seeking out more exotic destinations and activities than ever before. Up to 50% of those going abroad become ill in some way, mainly due to diarrhoeal disease or a respiratory tract infection. Superimposed on these maladies are illnesses related to excess alcohol, sunshine and overindulgent eating, as well as coincidental illnesses not necessarily of an infectious nature. Young people may find the 'culture shock' especially on return, sometimes after recreational drug experience, sufficient to lead to a psychological breakdown, while older returning expatriates may experience stress reactions after prolonged periods abroad. Travellers may put themselves at risk from sexually transmitted diseases. Travel has undoubtedly played a role in the increase in prevalence of human immunodeficiency virus (HIV).

The concept that imported diseases are necessarily exotic is erroneous, well reflected by the range of diagnoses made in patients presenting to the Lister Unit at Northwick Park Hospital in 1994 (Table 1). Of the tropical imported infections, malaria is by far the most important, not only numerically but because of its lethal potential. Enteric fever, dengue fever and hepatitis are next in importance, whereas the more exotic such as tick typhus, amoebiasis, leishmaniasis, trypanosomiasis, onchocerciasis and cysticercosis are infrequent (Table 2). A number of imported illnesses such as schistosomiasis, giardiasis and cutaneous larva migrans seldom require hospital admission, explaining their underrepresentation in Table 1. Whilst the scientific basis of many of these infections has expanded relatively rapidly in

Table 1 Primary diagnosis in 360 cases of imported disease admitted to the Infection and Tropical Medicine (Lister) Unit, Northwick Park Hospital. January–December, 1994.

Total inpatient episodes	**1212**
Total imported episodes	**360**
	Cases
Malaria (12 *Plasmodium vivax*, rest *P. falciparum*)	79
Enteric fever (*Salmonella typhi* and *S. paratyphoid*)	12
Dengue fever	10
Hepatitis (A 7; B 1; E 1; EBV 1)	10
Tuberculosis: mainly in asylum seekers (suspected 30, pulmonary 37, extrapulmonary 4)	71
Gastroenteritis (organism not identified)	45
Gastroenteritis (Shigella 8, Giardia 6, Salmonella 2, enterohaemorrhagic *E. coli* 1)	17
Respiratory tract infections (upper 18, lower 20)	38
Urinary and genital tract infections	7
Soft tissue infection (cellulitis and infected insect bites)	7
Febrile undiagnosed, presumed viral illnesses	43
Other viral illness (meningitis 1, chicken-pox 1, influenza 1)	3
HIV, first presentation (Cryptosporidium, pelvic TB, lymphoma)	4
Amoebic liver abscess	2
Leishmaniasis	1
Schistosomiasis	2
Leptospirosis	1
Miscellaneous (one each of meningococcal septicaemia, meningococcal meningitis, neutropenia following dapsone, confusion following mefloquine, Addison's disease, Ciguatera fish poisoning, cardiac failure)	7

recent years, there are suprisingly few advances in practical management. We still, for example, do not have an effective malarial vaccine. The major problem with imported infections remains that of diagnosis and treatment.

☐ CLINICAL APPROACH TO THE PATIENT WITH AN IMPORTED INFECTION

History

It is critical in a patient with an imported infection to take a detailed history. The destination, conditions and duration of travel often provide clues to the diagnosis, especially in the case of the more common tropical diseases (Table 2). On our unit at Northwick Park Hospital, for example, up to 70% of cases with falciparum malaria have visited one of four countries, namely Ghana, Nigeria, Kenya or India. Most of our cases of enteric fever are from the Indian subcontinent, schistosomiasis from swimming in the lakes of central or southern Africa, whereas dengue fever is most frequently diagnosed in travellers from south-east Asia, the Indian subcontinent and the Caribbean. Giardiasis is common in those who have been to Nepal and Russia, whereas filariasis is diagnosed in those who have been to the Cameroons and other West African countries. These observations might, of course,

Table 2 Most common imported tropical diseases.

Disease	Distribution	Suggestive findings
Malaria	Endemic areas	Fever, jaundice, diarrhoea
Tick typhus (Rickettsia conori)	Game parks of Africa	Eschar of tick bite, maculo-papular rash, lymphadenopathy
Giardiasis	Worldwide, especially Indian subcontinent	Diarrhoea, wind, malaise
Amoebiasis	Worldwide, especially Indian subcontinent	Dysentery, point tenderness over liver, neutrophilia, raised alkaline phosphatase and erythrocyte sedimentation rate (ESR) ultrasound/computerized tomography (CT)
Trypanosomiasis (usually T. brucei rhodesiense)	East and southern African game parks	Tsetse fly bite (painful), chancre, rash, lymphadenopathy
Schistosomiasis	Lakes and rivers of Africa, South America	Swimmer's itch; Katayama fever; haematuria/diarrhoea/myelopathy
Cysticercosis	Worldwide, especially India and Mexico	Neurological signs; subcutaneous nodules

merely reflect the most common destinations among our sample of travellers. Many unusual imported infections are not necessarily acquired in the tropics (Table 3), and gastroenteritis and tuberculosis have even been acquired on aircraft. It is important to establish which travel vaccinations and which antimalarials were used, as this information might well modify the likelihood of a particular infection such as hepatitis A. Many of the vaccines in use are not a hundred percent effective, and severe malaria, for example, may occur despite compliant chemoprophylaxis.

The estimated incubation period may give a clue to the diagnosis. There are infections with a short incubation of under a week (eg dengue and most infectious diarrhoeas), those with an intermediate incubation period of 2–3 weeks (which include the majority of falciparum malaria cases) and those with a long incubation, which may present weeks or months after return (eg giardia, schistosomiasis and filariasis).

Specific symptoms often provide clues to the nature of the illness. The most common are fever, diarrhoea, rash, jaundice, sexually transmitted disease or impairment of consciousness (Table 4). It is also important to know if the patient has any underlying medical condition that predisposes to a particular diagnosis or might require adjustment of drug therapy. For example, patients on histamine H_2-antagonists are at greater risk from enteric fevers. A sexual history may be appropriate.

Table 3 Imported infections not necessarily tropical.

Disease	Distribution	Suggestive findings
Central European encephalitis (CEE)	Alpine regions of Europe, eastern Europe	Seasonal, encephalopathy
Russian spring summer encephalitis (RSSE)	Russia	
Lyme disease (Borrelia burgdorferi)	Forested areas of Europe and North America	Tick bite, rash, arthralgia neurological signs
Ehrlichiosis	North America	Tick bite, fever
Leishmaniasis	Warm climates including the Mediterranean	Cutaneous: non-healing lesion/ulcer Visceral: fever, anaemia, splenomegaly, hyper-immunoglobulin G (IgG)
Leptospirosis	Worldwide	Recreational water contact

Table 4 Common presentations of disease in the returning traveller.

Fever	Malaria Viral infections especially dengue fever Enteric fevers (typhoid and paratyphoid) Pneumonia (including legionnaire's disease) Early hepatitis (mild fever) Rickettsial illnesses, eg tick typhus Amoebic liver abscess Brucellosis Relapsing fever (Borrelia recurrentis)
Diarrhoea	Malaria See causes of traveller's diarrhoea (Table 6)
Jaundice	Malaria Hepatitis A, B and E Enteric fevers Cytomegalovirus (CMV), Epstein-Barr virus (EBV) and toxoplasmosis
Sexually transmitted disease	Gonorrhoea Chlamydia Chancroid (Haemophilus ducreyi) Hepatitis B Syphilis HIV infection
Impairment of consciousness	Cerebral malaria Typhoid Encephalitis, eg herpes simplex, Japanese B Drug addiction: intoxication or withdrawal

The examination

A thorough physical examination is important. Although the pattern of a fever is often not as helpful as is classically taught, a dramatically high peak of fever with classic rigors may suggest malaria, pneumonia or septicaemia rather than viral hepatitis, where the fever may only be moderate. A relative bradycardia may point to enteric fever but may also be present in brucellosis and other conditions. Careful examination is necessary to detect skin rashes [eg petechial and/or blanching in dengue (see Plate 13), the rose spots of typhoid or the eschar of tick typhus], hepato- or spleno-megaly (suprisingly uncommon in acute malaria, but present in leishmaniasis), or point tenderness over the liver in amoebic liver abscess. Often there may be very few clues apart from a fever. In this case, the approach needs to be one of considering those most frequent in the first instance.

Investigations

Investigations should include a full blood count (with a malaria film; Plate 14), blood culture, liver function tests and stool microscopy, where relevant. Anaemia may suggest malaria or leishmaniasis. A normal or low white blood cell count supports a diagnosis of uncomplicated malaria, typhoid or dengue, whereas a raised neutrophil count is more in favour of a respiratory or urinary tract infection or an amoebic liver abscess. The most common causes of an eosinophilia in travellers are schistosomiasis, filarial infection (eg onchocerciasis presenting with itching) or strongyloidiasis. Acute schistosomiasis may have an incubation period of 3–8 weeks, whereas filariasis or chronic schistosomiasis may take years to declare themselves. Protozoal infections do not generally cause eosinophilia. A thrombocytopenia (<150 000 platelets/µl) is present in the majority of cases of acute malaria caused by any of the four species. Thrombocytopenia also suggests dengue fever. Serological diagnosis of many of the exotic infections is necessary since non-immune individuals may carry only a small parasite burden (Table 5). Diagnosis of enteric fever requires blood, stool and sometimes bone marrow culture.

☐ MAJOR CLINICAL SYNDROMES

Fever

Malaria

The most important diagnosis to exclude is malaria, and it is often necessary to obtain at least three daily blood films to exclude the diagnosis, especially when patients have been on prophylaxis. It is more helpful to repeat the blood film whether the patient is febrile or not rather than to examine the same film a second

Table 5 The more common serological tests helpful in the diagnosis of imported disease.

Amoebiasis	Hydatid disease	Strongyloidiasis
Cysticercosis	Leishmaniasis	Trichinella infection
Filariasis	Schistosomiasis	Trypanosomiasis

time. A novel antigen capture diagnostic test for *P. falciparum*, the *Para*Sight™-F test, requires no expertise, is sensitive and is very promising [4]. Diarrhoea and jaundice, both symptoms of malaria, can be misleading. Fever may be the only physical sign present. In acute malaria, splenomegaly or clinical pallor are unusual unless the patient has been ill for a prolonged period, eg over a week. Quinine is currently the drug of choice for the treatment of falciparum malaria but always requires a second drug such as Fansidar™ (pyrimethamine and sulphadoxine) or a tetracycline to prevent recrudescence [5]. Primaquine is only needed for the eradication of the exoerythrocytic forms of *P. vivax* and *P. ovale* thus preventing relapse.

Qinghaosu (artemisinin) derivatives, especially artemether, arteether and artesunate (all converted into a commonly biologically active metabolite, dihydroartemisinin) are showing promise as relatively non-toxic, rapidly acting drugs against *P. falciparum*, including chloroquine-resistant strains [5]. The major problem using these drugs is the high incidence of recrudescence. We still await an effective vaccine – the Patarroyo SPf66 vaccine has met with only limited success [6].

Enteric fever

After malaria, the next most important diagnosis to consider in the event of a high fever, is that of typhoid and paratyphoid. Enteric fever in travellers may not be severe and at the onset the fever may be mild and the constitutional symptoms unimpressive. Clues to the diagnosis are the findings of slight confusion or inattentiveness, coughing, sometimes constipation, relative bradycardia compared to the temperature and infrequent, but tell-tale, rose spots. The diagnosis is confirmed by positive blood, stool or bone marrow culture.

Dengue and other arboviral infections

In our experience the next most common febrile illness in the returning traveller is dengue fever, an arboviral infection. This disease is now on the increase worldwide possibly due to urbanization and climatic change. Dengue presents as a non-specific febrile illness and, in common with malaria, demonstrates thrombocytopenia. There may also be a blanching macular and/or a non-blanching petechial rash (see Plate 13). Postural hypotension and bleeding of the gums on brushing the teeth are clues. Defervescence coincides with a recovery in platelet count and disappearance of the virus as detected by polymerase chain reaction (PCR) [8].

It is important to note, where patients have come from certain high-risk areas for Lassa fever (ie the high plateaux of Nigeria and Sierra Leone, particularly where travellers have been in contact with patients in a hospital setting) and Ebola virus infection from the appropriate endemic area in central Africa, that the recently revised national guidelines are applied in management [9].

Other febrile illnesses

Other diseases presenting with a high fever include leptospirosis, rickettsial disease (eg tick typhus), trypanosomiasis, leishmaniasis and amoebiasis (see Tables 2 and 3).

Each of these conditions has its own specific characteristics, but they need only to be considered when the other more important common infections have been excluded.

There have been some advances in our understanding and management of these diseases. Difluoromethyl ornithine (DFMO) is effective in *Trypanosoma brucei gambiense* (but not *rhodesiense*) infections. Liposomal amphotericin, although expensive, has heralded a major advance over the pentavalent antimonials sodium stibogluconate and meglumine antimonate in the treatment of visceral leishmaniasis (see Plate 15) [10]. Two distinct species of *Entamoebae*, namely *E. histolytica* and *E. dispar* have recently been identified. *Entamoeba dispar*, the more prevalent, is asymptomatic whereas *E. histolytica* is the pathogenic species [11]. They can be distinguished by patterns of isoenzymes on gels (zymodemes) or by means of PCR. This discovery explains the finding of asymptomatic infection in individuals who to all intents and purposes were previously thought to have *E. histolytica* infection.

Diarrhoea

Diarrhoea in the returning traveller is a subject on its own. Diarrhoea as a group of illnesses is one of the most common presentations in patients returning from abroad and two recent newcomers to the growing list of identifiable causes must include *Cryptosporidium* and *Cyclospora* [12]. Both of these require highly trained microscopists to make a diagnosis on faecal concentrates. *Cyclospora* responds to cotrimoxazole; there is no treatment for *Cryptosporidium* at present. Stool culture and where necessary a rectal scrape with immediate microscopy looking for amoebae is essential (see Plate 16). The principal identifiable causes of imported diarrhoea are given in Table 6.

Jaundice

Patients returning from abroad with jaundice present an extremely wide differential diagnosis. Once again the important diagnosis to exclude is malaria. Enteric fever may also present as jaundice The viral hepatitides present clinically with a low grade

Table 6 Principal identifiable causes of imported diarrhoea.

Bacteria	Protozoa
Enterotoxigenic *E. coli* (ETEC)	*Giardia lamblia*
Shigella spp.	*Entamoeba histolytica*
Salmonella spp.	*Cryptosporidium parvum*
Campylobacter jejuni	*Cyclospora cayetanensis*
Vibrio cholera	*Microsporidium* spp. (rare in non-HIV-infected subjects)
Non-cholera vibrios, eg *V. parahaemolyticus*	
Viruses	
Rotavirus	
Small round viruses, eg Norwalk agent	

fever, and hepatitis A, B and E must first be excluded. Hepatitis C serology may only become positive many weeks after acute infection. Other hepatitides presenting in travellers include EBV, CMV and toxoplasma infection. No doubt further, as yet unidentified, causes of hepatitis will be identified in travellers.

Rashes

Some of the most common causes of rashes, particularly papules, are insect bites, often infected and each with its own distinctive clinical appearance. Another common infection is cutaneous larva migrans, due to the migration of animal hookworm larvae under the skin usually causing severe itching and a serpiginous track. The urticarial lesions of Katayama fever, an early manifestation of schistosomiasis, are characteristic (see Plate 17), as are the fleeting linear wheals of larva currens due to strongyloidiasis. Other dermatological conditions include ulcers due to cutaneous leishmaniasis, sinuses caused by various maggots (myiasis such as *Dermatobia hominis* and *Cordylobia anthropophaga*), itching due to onchocerciasis, and subcutaneous nodules of onchocerciasis or cysticercosis.

Sexually transmitted diseases

Travellers who are at risk from sexually transmitted disease may present with genital ulcers or urethral discharge. Genital ulcers might suggest syphilis, chancroid or herpes simplex virus (HSV). A discharge suggests gonorrhoea or a non-specific urethritis due to *Chlamydia*. HIV infection is an important diagnosis to exclude in two situations: an acute glandular fever-like illness with a rash as part of a seroconversion illness, or in long-term travellers with risk factors who return from abroad severely ill. The process of diagnosis and management of HIV positive cases is quite different, and a negative HIV test may be a useful starting point in any prolonged undiagnosed infection.

The management of imported infections can be summarized into five main practice points (Table 7). Recent scientific advances are given in Table 8.

Table 7 Summary of practice points in relation to management of imported infections.

All patients require a careful travel history including the places visited, the duration of their visit, the risk factors to which they have been exposed and the immunizations and prophylaxis taken.

Malaria must be excluded by blood film in any ill patient who has travelled to an endemic area regardless of whether they have taken antimalarials compliantly or not. In order to exclude especially falciparum malaria in a febrile patient, at least three daily films are required.

A thrombocytopenia in a returning traveller suggests, among other infections, malaria and dengue fever.

The majority of patients with falciparum malaria can no longer be treated with chloroquine but require quinine and a second drug to avoid recrudescence.

Helminthic rather than protozoal infections produce an eosinophilia.

Table 8 Scientific advances in the treatment of imported infections.

Artemisinin (Qinghaosu) derivatives have shown promising results in the treatment of mild and severe chloroquine-resistant falciparum malaria [5].

The ParaSight™-F test, an antigen capture test using a monoclonal antibody to the histidine rich protein II (HRP II), is showing promise in the specific diagnosis of falciparum malaria [4].

The SPf 66 antimalarial vaccine appears to be only marginally effective [5,6].

Isolation of the *var* (variable) genes coding for the erythrocyte membrane protein 1 of *P. falciparum* (Pf EMP-1) has heralded a major step forward in the identification of a parasite protein expressed on the surface of the infected red cell, which may be of relevance in the design of a subunit malarial vaccine [7].

Salmonella typhi has shown plasmid-mediated resistance to chloramphenicol and amoxycillin and non-plasmid related to the quinolones (eg ciprofloxacin). The organism has retained sensitivity at the current time to the third generation cephalosporins, eg cefotaxime, ceftriaxone and cefoperazone.

Liposomal amphotericin is a major advance in the treatment of visceral leishmaniasis [10].

Albendazole, a rediscovered anthelminthic, is showing increasing promise in the treatment of cutaneous larva migrans, hydatid diseases, cysticercosis etc.

☐ PATIENTS WITH ALTERATION IN CONSCIOUSNESS

Malaria must always be excluded in patients with any alteration in consciousness level before any other diagnosis is considered in travellers returning from an endemic area (Table 4). Mefloquine, and very occasionally chloroquine, may rarely cause ataxia, dizziness or confusion. A range of viral encephalitides needs to be considered once malaria has been excluded.

☐ CONCLUSION

Diagnosing disease in returning travellers presents an exciting challenge to the physician. More often than not the diagnosis is neither exotic nor obscure. Every now and then problems arise in which the diagnostic possibilities are wide and pose some of the greatest challenges to the diagnostician. At times the problem turns out not to be an infection. Patients often relate the acquisition of symptoms to travel which may purely be coincident. We have seen cases where subarachnoid haemorrhage has been confused with meningitis, simple hepatic cysts confused with hydatid cysts, primary lymphoedema with elephantiasis and inflammatory bowel disease, phaeochromocytoma and hyperthyroidism with an infectious diarrhoea. The physician attending the traveller may need to extend the differential diagnosis well into the realms of general medicine.

It may be appropriate to end with a quote from Laurie Garrett's book *The Coming Plague* mentioned in the introductory paragraph [1]. 'The planet (earth) is nothing but a crazy quilt of micro (biological) soups scattered all over its 196 936 800-square-mile surface. Rapid globalization of human niches requires that human beings everywhere on the planet go beyond viewing their neighbourhoods, provinces, counties or hemispheres as the sum total of their personal ecospheres. Microbes and their vectors recognize none of the artificial boundaries recognized by human beings. Theirs is the world of natural limitations: temperature, pH, ultraviolet light, the presence of vulnerable hosts and mobile vectors.' With the emergence of new infections and the re-emergence of old ones, the physician now and in the future will need to have an increased awareness of the more important infections related to travel.

REFERENCES

1. Garrett L. *The Coming Plague: Newly Emerging Infections in a World Out of Balance.* New York; Penguin, 1994.
2. Patz JA, Epstein PR, Burke TA, Balbus JM. Global climate change and emerging infectious diseases. *J Am Med Assoc* 1996; **275**: 217–23.
3. Cook GC, ed. *Travel-associated Disease.* London: Royal College of Physicians of London, 1995.
4. Shiff CJ, Premji Z, Minjas JN. The rapid manual ParaSight™-F test: a new diagnostic tool for *Plasmodium falciparum* infection. *Trans Roy Soc Trop Med Hyg* 1993; **87**: 646–8.
5. Pasvol G, ed. *Malaria.* London: Bailliere Tindall, 1995.
6. Tanner M, Teuscher T, Alonso PL. SPf66-the first malaria vaccine. *Parasitol Today* 1995; **11**: 10–13.
7. Borst P, Bitter W, McCulloch R, van Leeuwen F, Rudenko G. Antigenic variation in malaria. (Minireview). *Cell* 1995; **82**: 1–4. (A further three original papers on the same subject are to be found in the same volume of *Cell*.)
8. Brown JL, Wilkinson R, Davidson RN, Wall RA, Pasvol G. Rapid diagnosis and duration of viraemia in dengue fever using reverse transcriptase polymerase chain reaction. *Trans Roy Soc Trop Med Hyg* 1996; **90**: 140–3.
9. Advisory Committee on Dangerous Pathogens. *Management and Control of Viral Haemorrhagic Fevers.* London: HMSO, 1996.
10. Davidson RN, Di Martino L, Gradoni L, *et al.* Liposomal amphotericin B (Ambisome™) in Mediterranean visceral leishmaniasis: a multicentre trial. *Quart J Med* 1994; **87**: 75–81.
11. Ravdin JI. Amebiasis. *Clin Inf Dis* 1995; **20**: 1453–66.
12. Bendall RP, Lucas S, Moody A, Tovey G, Chiodini PL. Diarrhoea associated with cyanobacterium-like bodies: a new coccidian enteritis of man. *Lancet* 1993; **341**: 590–2.

☐ MULTIPLE CHOICE QUESTIONS

1. The presence of thrombocytopenia in a returning traveller should raise the suspicion of:
    (a) Amoebiasis
    (b) Dengue fever
    (c) Leishmaniasis
    (d) Malaria
    (e) Typhoid

2. A case of falciparum malaria in a non-immune traveller from Kenya:
    (a) Can be treated with chloroquine
    (b) Needs primaquine to eradicate the liver forms
    (c) Should be treated with quinine alone

(d) Usually has splenomegaly
(e) Can present with diarrhoea

3 An incubation period of under a week is incompatible with the diagnosis of:
(a) Malaria
(b) Dengue fever
(c) Lassa fever
(d) Schistosomiasis
(e) Shigella dysentery

4 In the returning traveller:
(a) Cerebral malaria can occur despite chemoprophylaxis
(b) Serology is usually positive in an amoebic liver abscess
(c) Giardia can produce an eosinophilia
(d) Typhoid should be treated with chloramphenicol
(e) Cysticercosis is caused by the beef tapeworm

5 Rare conditions that may be acquired abroad include:
(a) Trypanosomiasis transmitted by ticks
(b) Tick typhus in the game parks of Africa caused by *Rickettsia conori*
(c) Cutaneous larva migrans is caused by a filarial worm
(d) Visceral leishmaniasis presenting with anaemia and hypergammaglobulinaemia, chiefly IgG
(e) Onchocerciasis transmitted by the black biting fly *Simulium*

ANSWERS

1a False	2a False	3a True	4a True	5a False
b True	b False	b False	b True	b True
c False	c False	c True	c False	c False
d True	d False	d True	d False	d True
e False	e True	e False	e False	e True

Prevention and treatment of hospital acquired infection

J Cohen

☐ INTRODUCTION

Hospital acquired, so-called nosocomial, infection is in many respects a hidden epidemic, one that has been ignored by most people other than hospital infection specialists and microbiologists. Yet the clinical and financial impact of this problem is not so easily ignored. A number of studies have shown that something like 10% of all patients acquire an infection while they are in hospital, and this figure is rising. More importantly, patients with a nosocomial infection stay in hospital longer, and have a higher in-hospital mortality. Not surprisingly, they attract a very considerable marginal cost, as shown by Wenzl [1]. Estimates of the additional health care expenditure associated with nosocomial infection are staggering, and amount to millions of pounds per year.

The most common nosocomial infections are those associated with surgical wounds and intravascular lines, urinary tract infections and pneumonia, but there are others, less apparent, that also need to be considered (Table 1). In this chapter, I will focus on one group in which infection has a particularly large impact on the clinical course – infection on the intensive care unit (ICU).

Table 1 Common nosocomial infections.

Urinary tract infections (catheter related)
Indwelling vascular lines
Wound infections
Pneumonia
Bacteraemia/fungaemia
Associated with blood/blood products
Complicating orthopaedic (and other) implants
Acquired from health care worker
In immunocompromised patients

A recent large investigation, the European Prevalence of Infection in Intensive Care (EPIC) study, provided very valuable epidemiological data on the scale of the problem. A point prevalence study carried out in 1417 ICUs in 17 European countries showed that approximately 20% of patients had an infection acquired on the ICU [2]. The most common infection was pneumonia, but it is interesting that 12% of the infections were bacteraemia or fungaemia (Table 2). The organisms causing these infections were largely those one would have predicted: Gram-negative

Table 2 Epidemiology of infection seen in the EPIC study [2]. Prevalence of ICU-acquired nosocomial infection in 2064/10038 (20.6%) ICU patients.

Infection	Patients infected (%)
Pneumonia	49.6
Lower respiratory tract	17.8
Urinary tract	17.6
Bloodstream (bacteraemia or fungaemia)	12.0

enteric bacteria, *Pseudomonas aeruginosa*, and staphylococci (Table 3). Several of these merit closer discussion.

☐ FUNGAL INFECTIONS

Epidemiology

One of the most surprising statistics to emerge from the EPIC study was that fungi accounted for more than 15% of the documented bloodstream infections. In fact, almost all of these were yeast infections due to *Candida* spp, and indeed there is a growing awareness that disseminated Candida infections are a rapidly emerging problem on ICUs. Risk factors for the development of fungal infection include prolonged use of broad-spectrum antibiotics, recent major surgery, and heavy skin colonization with Candida.

Diagnosis

Unfortunately, the diagnosis of disseminated candidiasis can be very difficult. There are few pathognomonic clinical signs. In the ICU setting, the typical presentation will simply be the development of fever in a 'high risk' patient who is currently receiving antibiotics, or who has not responded to an empirical change in antibiotic therapy. In some cases, evanescent, rose-pink maculopapular skin lesions may

Table 3 Microbiology of nosocomial infection recorded in the EPIC study [2]. Microbiological documentation from 1754/2064 (85%) patients with ICU-acquired infections.

Cause of infection	Percentage of total isolates*
Enterobacteriaceae *E. coli*, Klebsiella, Enterobacter	34.4
Staphylococcus aureus	30.1
Ps. aeruginosa	28.7
Coagulase-negative staphylococci	19.1
Fungi	17.1

*55% of ICU-acquired infections were polymicrobial

appear, but in my experience they are rare. In contrast, a much underappreciated and extremely valuable physical sign is the development of endophthalmitis (see Plate 18). In one recent study, as many as 15% of patients with candidaemia had eye lesions, and regular ophthalmoscopy is to be encouraged.

Diagnostic microbiology is also not entirely satisfactory. Candida will grow in blood cultures, and if found should never be ignored or dismissed as a contaminant. However, it is well recognized that blood cultures may remain sterile despite a subsequent confirmed diagnosis of disseminated candidiasis. Conversely, the isolation of *Candida* spp from a non-sterile site does not imply deep infection; the most important example is Candida in sputum or tracheal washings, which does not of itself make a diagnosis of Candida pneumonia, in fact a rather rare condition. There are a number of serological tests that are designed to detect Candida antigen in blood; in the correct clinical setting a positive test should prompt antifungal therapy, but they cannot be used to confidently exclude the diagnosis.

Treatment

The treatment of disseminated candidiasis has become considerably easier with the availability of imidazole drugs such as fluconazole. Rex *et al.* [3] carried out a comparative study of fluconazole and amphotericin B in 206 ICU patients with documented infection. They compared a regimen of fluconazole (400 mg a day) with amphotericin B (0.5–0.6 mg per kg a day) for 14 days. The two regimens were of equal efficacy, but the fluconazole group had significantly less toxicity. It is therefore reasonable to recommend fluconazole as first-line therapy in this condition, but it is important to be aware of the limitations of this approach. First, fluconazole is not active against all fungi, notably *Aspergillus* spp, so it cannot be used empirically unless the diagnosis has been microbiologically confirmed. Furthermore, some *Candida* species are intrinsically insensitive (notably *Candida krusei*), and even some isolates of *Candida albicans* can develop resistance to fluconazole, although this is uncommon.

In cases in which non-albicans species are isolated, or where antifungal therapy must be started empirically, then amphotericin B must be used. The usual dose is 0.3–0.6 mg per kg a day. Much of the toxicity of amphotericin B can be lessened by the concomitant use of hydrocortisone, chlorpheniramine and/or pethidine, but despite these devices some renal impairment is almost inevitable. In response to these difficulties, a number of lipid-based formulations of amphotericin B have lately become available, which claim to reduce the toxicity of the agent. These new drugs include liposomal amphotericin B (Ambisome®), amphotericin B lipid complex (Abelcet®), and amphotericin B colloidal dispersion; in addition, there have been several reports suggesting that conventional amphotericin B mixed with Intralipid® can be used as a cheaper alternative. There is no doubt that these lipid formulations are less toxic, but at present there are few data comparing their efficacy with native drug in this population of patients. For the time being they should be used cautiously, if at all. The management of deep fungal infections in patients on the ICU has recently been reviewed [4] (Table 4).

Table 4 Principles of treating Candida infections on the ICU. Full details are given in the report of the British Society for Antimicrobial Chemotherapy Working Party [4].

Management of deep Candida infection in surgical and ICU patients
Isolation of Candida from any sterile site is always significant
In an at-risk patient, heavy colonization is a strong indication for treatment
Removal of devices and catheters is essential
Precise mycological diagnosis is important
Sensitivity testing is valuable, antifungal drug levels are not
Serological diagnosis is unreliable

☐ NOSOCOMIAL PNEUMONIA

Pneumonia is one of the most common infections encountered in ICUs, but its true incidence is unknown because of the lack of consensus about diagnostic criteria. A working definition is that it is a condition characterized by new infiltrates on the chest radiograph, raised white blood cell count (>11 000/mm^3), pyrexia of 37.5°C or higher, and the production of purulent secretions; it has a crude mortality rate ranging between 33% and 71%, but infections associated with Gram-negative bacilli have a higher mortality rate than Gram-positive infections [5].

Diagnosis of ventilator associated pneumonia

The microbiology differs from unit to unit and depends on the type of patient involved. Gram-negative bacilli predominate, but common respiratory pathogens such as *Haemophilus influenzae* and *Streptococcus pneumoniae* cannot be excluded. *Staph. aureus* is an uncommon cause of pneumonia, even though it is not infrequently isolated from sputum. On occasion, less common Gram-negative bacteria such as *Stenotrophomonas (Xanthomonas) maltophilia*, *Pseudomonas aeruginosa*, *Pseudomonas* spp and *Acinetobacter* spp are isolated.

Unfortunately, microbiological diagnosis is difficult. A wide variety of techniques have been evaluated including endotracheal aspirates and the use of protective specimen brush, bronchoalveolar lavage and transbronchoscopic balloon-tipped catheters, but none is ideal. Furthermore, these invasive techniques are not without complications, such as hypoxaemia, bleeding and arrhythmias.

Treatment

It is generally necessary to start treatment without the benefit of a microbiological diagnosis; indeed care must be taken not to put undue emphasis on the results of sputum culture since this can be misleading. A cephalosporin such as cefotaxime is a reasonable first-line agent; alternatives are a quinolone or imipenem. If *Ps. aeruginosa* is isolated, I add an aminoglycoside. If aspiration is a possibility, then co-amoxiclav or imipenem will have an appropriate spectrum of activity. When the patient fails to respond to the initial therapy, consideration should be given to unusual pathogens such as tuberculosis, fungi, the 'atypical' group (*Legionella* spp etc), or viruses, and also to non-infective conditions that can mimic pneumonia, such as pulmonary oedema or haemorrhage.

Prevention

Despite intensive investigation, no entirely satisfactory strategy has yet been evolved which will reduce the mortality associated with this condition. Two approaches have been used, both of which aim to reduce the likelihood of colonization of the respiratory tract with potentially pathogenic micro-organisms.

Selective decontamination

This procedure is based on a large body of work, originally conducted by Dutch investigators who showed that in mice the gastrointestinal tract was normally covered with a 'wallpaper' of anaerobic organisms that prevented attachment (and subsequent invasion) of enteric organisms such as *E. coli* and Klebsiella. By choosing antibiotics that tended to preserve this 'wallpaper', the risk of systemic Gram-negative infection was lessened. This approach was then extended to the respiratory tract, and the method adopted was a combination of short-course treatment with a systemic antibiotic followed by topical therapy with agents such as polymyxin B and gentamicin, applied as a paste to the oral cavity, usually together with oral amphotericin B. A very large number of studies have been done, but there has been much criticism of the methods used and considerable debate as to how they should be interpreted. The general conclusion [6] is that while there is some suggestion that the rate of Gram-negative pneumonia may be reduced there is no corresponding reduction in mortality. Furthermore, the cost of the treatment, and the potential for encouraging the emergence of resistant Gram-negative bacteria, means that this method has not found widespread acceptance.

Reducing gastric pH

The alternative means of reducing gastric colonization is with anti-stress-ulcer prophylaxis regimens such as antacid, ranitidine or sucralfate. A study by Prod'hom *et al.* [7] concluded that sucralfate was the most effective of the three regimens in reducing late-onset pneumonia, but once again there was no clear effect on mortality. This approach has the advantage that it has little effect on the resistance patterns of the prevailing bacteria in the ICU, but it is still clearly not ideal.

☐ ANTIMICROBIAL RESISTANCE

Antibiotic-resistant organisms have caused nosocomial infections and hospital outbreaks ever since the introduction of penicillin. However, in recent years the list of clinically relevant organisms that have developed resistance to commonly used antimicrobial agents has grown alarmingly (Table 5). On the ICU, the most pressing problem at the moment is vancomycin-resistant enterococcus.

Table 5 Current clinical problems associated with emerging antimicrobial resistance.

Antibiotic-resistant organism	Antibiotic
Strep. pneumoniae	Penicillin
Staph. aureus	Methicillin
Salmonella typhi	Chloramphenicol (and many others)
H. influenzae	Ampicillin
Enterococcus faecium	Vancomycin
Mycobacterium tuberculosis	Multiple
Falciparum malaria	Multiple

Vancomycin-resistant enterococci

Enterococci, a common cause of nosocomial infection, are intrinsically resistant to most antimicrobials and readily acquire additional resistance. Vancomycin-resistant enterococci (VRE) have caused clusters of nosocomial infections since 1988, but lately they have swept through ICUs in the USA and they are now appearing with increased frequency in the UK. Most VREs are in fact isolates of *Enterococcus faecium*. There are two principal phenotypes: *van A* are the most resistant, and have diminished susceptibility to ampicillin, quinolones, vancomycin and teichoplanin. *van B* isolates are slightly more susceptible, but still pose a significant problem [8].

Prevention and treatment

With so few therapeutic options, prevention assumes even greater importance than usual. The Hospital Infection Control Committee of the Centers for Disease Control in the USA have recently published a series of guidelines [9] (Table 6), and these should be considered very carefully by all clinicians and infection control teams in the UK.

If prevention fails, treatment is very difficult. There are small and anecdotal studies suggesting that in some patients chloramphenicol may be used, and several investigational agents are being evaluated. We have used a streptogramin antibiotic, quinupristin/dalfopristin, with some success in a small number of patients, but much more clinical experience is needed before any clear recommendations can be made.

Table 6 Measures to prevent the spread of vancomycin resistance.

Prudent vancomycin use
   guidelines for use and restrictions
Continuing education programmes
Microbiological surveillance and testing
Isolate vancomycin-resistant enterococcus infected/colonized patients
Identify infected/colonized patients who need readmission or transfer to/from elsewhere
Focus infection control on high-risk areas

☐ CONCLUSIONS

Hospital acquired infections cover a huge and rapidly evolving field that has an enormous impact on health care. At the institutional level, epidemiologists, microbiologists and the infection control team need to be proactive in attempting to influence prescribing and implementing measures to control the spread of resistant organisms. At the level of the individual patient, physicians should not hesitate to seek advice from colleagues specializing in infectious diseases in dealing with some of the more difficult aspects of diagnosis and treatment.

REFERENCES

1. Wenzl RP The economics of nosocomial infections. *J Hosp Infect* 1995; **31**: 79–87.
2. Vincent J, Bihari D, Suter P, et al. The prevalence of nosocomial infection in intensive care units in Europe. Results of the European Prevalence of Infection in Intensive Care (EPIC) Study. EPIC International Advisory Committee. *J Am Med Assoc* 1995; **274**: 639–44.
3. Rex JH, Bennett JE, Sugar AM, et al. A randomized trial comparing fluconazole with amphotericin B for the treatment of candidemia in patients without neutropenia. *New Engl J Med* 1994; **331**: 1325–30.
4. British Society for Antimicrobial Chemotherapy Working Party. Management of deep Candida infection in surgical and intensive care unit patients. *Intensive Care Med* 1994; **20**:522–8.
5. Mehtar S. Ventilator-associated pneumonia. *Curr Opn Infect Dis* 1995; **8**: 283–6.
6. Kollef MH. The role of selective digestive tract decontamination on mortality and respiratory tract infections: meta-analysis. *Chest* 1994; **105**: 1101–8.
7. Prod'hom G, Leuenberger P, Koerfer J, et al. Nosocomial pneumonia in mechanically ventilated patients receiving antacid, ranitidine, or sucralfate as prophylaxis for stress ulcer: randomized controlled trial. *Ann Intern Med* 1994; **120**: 653–62.
8. Nicoletti G, Stefani S. Enterococci: susceptibility patterns and therapeutic options. *Eur J Clin Microbiol Infect Dis* 1995; **14** Suppl 1: S33-7.
9. Hospital Infection Control Practices Advisory Committee. Recommendations for preventing the spread of vancomycin resistance. *MMWR Morb Mortal Wkly Rep* 1995; **44**: 1–13.

☐ MULTIPLE CHOICE QUESTIONS

1. The prevalence of nosocomial (hospital acquired) infection is approximately:
   (a) 1%
   (b) 2.5%
   (c) 5%
   (d) 7.5%
   (e) 10%

2. The single most common site for infection in patients on an ICU is:
   (a) Intra-abdominal
   (b) Lower respiratory tract
   (c) Urinary tract
   (d) Bloodstream
   (e) Skin/soft tissue

3. Vancomycin resistance:
   (a) Is common in *Streptococcus (Enterococcus) faecalis*
   (b) Is common in *Staphylococcus epidermidis* (coagulase negative staphylococci)
   (c) Is an indication for strict infection-control procedures
   (d) Is usually associated with the *vanA* genotype
   (e) Has now been reported in *Staph. aureus*

4. In patients on ICUs:
   (a) The isolation of Candida from any sterile site is an absolute indication for treatment
   (b) Device-associated fungal infections can usually be managed without the need to remove the device
   (c) A positive test for Candida antigenaemia is a reliable indicator of deep infection
   (d) Amphotericin B drug levels are a useful adjunct to management
   (e) Heavy yeast colonization is a risk factor for deep infection

5. Fluconazole:
   (a) Is suitable empirical therapy for presumed deep fungal infection
   (b) Is active against *Aspergillus* spp
   (c) Is active against *Candida krusei*
   (d) Drugs levels should be measured routinely
   (e) Is appropriate first-line therapy for deep infections due to *Candida albicans*

ANSWERS

1a False	2a False	3a False	4a True	5a False
b False	b True	b False	b False	b False
c False	c False	c True	c False	c False
d False	d False	d True	d False	d False
e True	e False	e False	e True	e True

Progress in the diagnosis and treatment of human virus infections

J G P Sissons

☐ INTRODUCTION

Virus infections account for a considerable burden of human disease and are recognized as causes of chronic disease and of certain tumours. This chapter discusses recent advances in their diagnosis and treatment; space prevents a comprehensive discussion of these areas, but principles are illustrated by selected examples of important human virus infections.

☐ IMPACT OF MOLECULAR VIROLOGY ON THE DIAGNOSIS AND TREATMENT OF VIRUS INFECTIONS

Advances in molecular virology now have a major influence on both diagnosis and treatment. Until recently the large viral DNA genomes (such as cytomegalovirus, or vaccinia virus) remained the largest contiguous pieces of DNA of any sort to have been sequenced. The techniques for rapid DNA sequencing were developed on the large DNA viruses and are now being applied to the sequencing of prokaryotic and eukaryotic chromosomes. Whereas 15 years ago the protein structure of a new virus would be identified by a classic biochemical approach, now a prime goal of research on any new virus is to obtain its genomic sequence. Much information can be derived: genetic homology to other viruses can be recognized and facilitates classification, identification of homologues of other viral genes and of cellular genes enables function of the protein products to be predicted, genetic variation or mutation can be identified and related to pathogenesis, and analysis of the genome by deletion and mutation becomes possible. This is well exemplified in the case of herpes viruses. These viruses are conventionally divided into three major subfamilies – α (HSV1 and VZV), β (CMV) and γ (EBV) herpes viruses – based on their tissue tropism and pattern of latency/replication. The gene organization and complete DNA sequence of members of the individual subfamilies are known, and each has a characteristic orientation of blocks of homologous genes. Three new members of the herpes viruses have been identified in the last 6 years – human herpes virus 6 (HHV6), 7 and 8; before the biology of HHV6 could be defined, it was clear that by sequence homology and gene orientation this virus would be a member of the β-herpes virus subfamily.

Other advances include the identification of the cellular receptors for some viruses, human immunodeficiency virus (HIV), rhinoviruses, Epstein-Barr virus (EBV), and the solution of the fine structure of viral proteins by X-ray crystallography. All this knowledge aids identification of virus-specific targets for chemotherapy, and the availability of chemotherapy in turn creates a stimulus to rapid and precise diagnosis.

☐ PROGRESS IN VIRUS DIAGNOSIS

The introduction of techniques based on the polymerase chain reaction (PCR) is discussed as an example of the impact of new methods on virus diagnosis (Table 1).

Table 1 Application of polymerase chain reaction (PCR) to viral diagnosis.

Detection of virus *presence* in patient (usually in blood):
  HIV, HCV
Detection of virus in *abnormal site*:
  cerebrospinal fluid (HSV, enteroviruses)
  plasma (CMV)
Detection of *virus load* by quantitative PCR:
  HIV RNA (assessing response to therapy)
Detection of virus *subtypes or mutants*:
  HCV genotypes
  drug resistance mutations (HIV RT215 Thr → Tyr)
Identification of *novel agents*

HCV, hepatitis C virus; HSV, herpes simplex virus; CMV, cytomegalovirus

Use of polymerase chain reaction in virus diagnosis

The principle of the PCR is well known. A known target DNA sequence can be amplified by adding synthetic oligonucleotide primers and a thermostable DNA polymerase enzyme. In repeated cycles of heating and re-annealing the primers bind to their complementary sequence in the target DNA, and the polymerase then extends the DNA strand from the primer, copying the target sequence. Very small amounts of initial target DNA are thus exponentially amplified. Target *RNA* can also be amplified if it is first transcribed to complementary DNA by reverse transcriptase enzyme (so-called 'RT-PCR'). PCR is potentially able to detect single copies of viral DNA or RNA genomes in samples, but because of this sensitivity it is prone to contamination and artefact, and rigorous controls are essential. The technique is potentially particularly useful where significance attaches to: (i) finding virus in an individual at all, as in the case of hepatitis C virus (HCV) or HIV, or (ii) finding virus in a site where it is not normally present (although it may normally be present elsewhere in the individual); examples would include the detection of herpes simplex virus (HSV) in cerebrospinal fluid (CSF) in HSV encephalitis, or of human cytomegalovirus (HCMV) in plasma in CMV disease [1,2].

PCR is routinely used to detect HIV RNA in infants born to infected mothers, as the presence of maternal antibody makes serological tests on the infant difficult to interpret. Quantitative PCR techniques are also being applied to measure the virus load in the plasma of patients with HIV or HCMV disease, an increasingly important surrogate endpoint in clinical trials.

Diagnostic kits are now available for detecting HCV RNA, but the use of PCR in other situations is still semi-experimental: one laboratory has developed a PCR system to detect multiple causes of virus encephalitis on a single sample [3]. PCR-based tests available through the virology laboratory may include those for HSV and other viruses in CSF, but until these newer tests are fully standardized, validated and subjected to quality control, results have to be interpreted in a clinical context and with caution. However, this situation is likely to change rapidly as tests improve and become commercialized (as for HCV RNA).

Use of PCR-based techniques for identifying novel infectious agents

PCR-based techniques have also been used to detect novel infectious agents instead of the more traditional methods of isolation by culture. In the case of bacteria, Falkow and colleagues used PCR (with common primers based on bacterial 16S ribosomal sequences) with striking success to identify the hitherto undescribed agents of bacillary angiomatosis and cat scratch disease (*Bartonella hensellae*) and Whipple's disease (*Tropheryma whippelii*) [4]. Within the past 2 years, Chang and Moore [5] have reported the application of a PCR-based method (representational difference analysis), which allows selective amplification of small amounts of foreign DNA present in diseased but not normal tissue, to Kaposi's sarcoma tissue. Foreign DNA sequences were identified which showed homology to known γ-herpes viruses (such as Epstein-Barr virus and herpes virus saimirii – an oncogenic monkey virus), indicating the presence of a novel human herpes virus provisionally called KS-associated herpes virus (KSHV) or human herpes virus 8 (HHV8). Further studies with *in situ* DNA hybridization showed the presence of KSHV sequences in every cell of Kaposi's sarcoma lesions, and detection of virus in blood is predictive of the later development of Kaposi's sarcoma [6] – all strengthening the case for an association of this new virus with Kaposi's sarcoma, although much more work will be required to establish causality. The epidemiology of Kaposi's sarcoma, which is seen in epidemic form in homosexual men with AIDS, has long suggested a viral aetiology. However, previous attempts to detect a virus had failed, indicating the power of the PCR based approach. We now know the sequence of this virus before having any serological tests for it; it remains to be seen whether, like other herpes viruses, it is widely distributed in the normal population.

☐ VIRUS INFECTIONS FOR WHICH THE USE OF CHEMOTHERAPY IS ESTABLISHED

An increasing number of antiviral drugs are now becoming available; the advent of HIV has been a major factor promoting increased research on antivirals by pharmaceutical companies. Table 2 lists those human virus infections for which antiviral chemotherapy is currently used. Therapy for acute (non-persistent) virus infections is not discussed here, although there have been some significant advances. The use of ribavarin for severe respiratory syncitial virus (RSV) infection in young children is relatively established. Ribavarin is also used for the treatment of viral haemorrhagic fevers caused by arenaviruses, although there are no prospective controlled trials. In this country, amantadine is rarely used for influenza A infection,

Table 2 Human virus infections for which there is effective chemotherapy.

Persistent		Acute	
Infection	Treatment	Infection	Treatment
Herpes simplex	Aciclovir	Respiratory syncitial virus	Ribavarin (by nebuliser)
Varicella zoster	Valaciclovir Famciclovir	Haemorrhagic fevers: arenaviruses (Lassa) hantaviruses (HFRS)	Ribavarin (intravenous)
Cytomegalovirus	Ganciclovir Foscarnet	Influenza	Amantadine Rimantadine
HIV	Reverse transcriptase inhibitors Protease inhibitors Others		
Hepatitis B	Interferon-α Reverse transcriptase inhibitors		
Hepatitis C	Interferon-α		

because of its CNS side effects and the difficulty in obtaining early confirmation of the diagnosis in clinical practice. There are a number of compounds directed against rhinoviruses in development, based on detailed structural knowledge of the interaction between the virus and its receptor, but none has yet obtained a licence. In this review I will focus on therapy of persistent viruses, those that stay on in the host after acute primary infection, using two contrasting viruses to illustrate how knowledge of the virus life-cycle and pathogenesis determines the approach to therapy (the important area of therapy for hepatitis B and C is covered in the chapter by Ahmed and Elias).

Background

Herpes viruses

Herpes viruses – HSV, varicella zoster virus (VZV), EBV, CMV, HHV 6 and 7 – are DNA viruses that infect most normal adults, establishing latent infection at limited tissue sites (sensory ganglia, B cells or monocytes) with no virus being produced for much of the time. These DNA viruses have a very low mutation rate. Maintenance of the virus in the latent state only requires very limited expression of viral genes but periodically reactivation occurs with full virus production; reactivation in normal patients may be accompanied by symptomatic disease (such as oro-labial or genital lesions with HSV, or zoster with VZV), or simply be reflected by asymptomatic virus shedding. However, in immunosuppressed patients, reactivation may lead to uncontrolled replication and disseminated infection with organ disease.

Lentiretroviruses

Lentiretroviruses (such as HIV), in contrast, do not show classic latency but replicate continuously in the infected host. They reverse-transcribe their RNA genome into proviral DNA, which then integrates into the cell chromosomal DNA. Reverse transcription is error prone and retroviruses have a high mutation rate, which in the case of HIV, coupled with its high rate of replication, results in the infected individual rapidly acquiring many related but differing variant viruses, creating a 'moving target' for the immune system.

These contrasting features, one group of viruses latent with periodic reactivation and the other producing a continuous high load of rapidly mutating virus, require very different therapeutic approaches, illustrated by the following two specific examples.

Human cytomegalovirus (HCMV)

Antiviral therapy

Aciclovir is well established as the first safe targeted antiviral active against HSV and VZV; it is a nucleoside analogue preferentially phosphorylated in virus-infected cells by virus-specified thymidine kinase, and then incorporated into the viral DNA where it blocks the virus DNA polymerase. Newer analogues licensed for the treatment of zoster include penciclovir (Famvir) and the prodrug of aciclovir, valaciclovir (Valtrex), with less frequent oral daily dosage; none of these is active against HCMV, which has no thymidine kinase. However, two other antiviral drugs are currently licensed for the treatment of HCMV disease: ganciclovir (GCV) is also a nucleoside analogue, which is specifically phosphorylated by a HCMV encoded enzyme and inhibits the HCMV DNA polymerase, and foscarnet (Foscavir), which is a non-nucleoside DNA polymerase inhibitor. Both have to be given by intravenous injection. GCV frequently causes neutropoenia and foscarnet can cause hypocalcaemia; both have been shown in trials to be effective treatment for CMV retinitis and enterocolitis using two weeks of induction therapy. In patients with severe continuing immunosuppression, who have retinitis, as in acquired immune deficiency syndrome (AIDS), maintenance intravenous (i.v.) therapy is necessary to prevent progression and loss of sight. This emphasizes the fact that none of these drugs can ever eradicate latent virus, and that some immune response is needed to control reactivation. Oral GCV has recently become available but is less effective than i.v. GCV in limiting HCMV replication; in patients with advanced AIDS *primary* prophylaxis with oral GCV significantly reduces the risk of HCMV disease, and it may also have a role in *secondary* prophylaxis of HCMV retinitis where retinitis is not sight-threatening and i.v. administration is not feasible [7,8]. Intravenous GCV has also been used for *primary* prophylaxis of HCMV disease in bone marrow transplant recipients, instituted when surveillance cultures show HCMV viraemia, although recent work suggests its use may just postpone the onset of HCMV disease in bone marrow transplant recipients. Resistance to both GCV and foscarnet can occur, but usually only after prolonged administration of the drugs, as in maintenance therapy for retinitis. Several newer antiviral drugs directed against HCMV are in development. Cidofovir is the most advanced in trials.

Immunotherapy

The currently unsatisfactory state of chemotherapy for HCMV is illustrated by the continuing interest in adjunctive immunological approaches to therapy. GCV alone is not effective for therapy of HCMV pneumonitis which tends to be a particular problem in bone marrow transplant recipients; however, its use in combination with anti-CMV immunoglobulin results in substantial reduction in mortality in this serious disease. In a novel approach to prophylaxis of HCMV disease, a group in Seattle have generated HCMV-specific cytotoxic T lymphocytes *in vitro* from donors and infused them into bone marrow transplant recipients (analogous to 'adoptive transfer' in mouse experiments); the transferred cytotoxic T lymphocytes survive and restore recipient cytotoxic T lymphocyte responses, but it has yet to be formally shown that this reduces the incidence of HCMV disease [9]. A similar adoptive transfer approach using EBV-specific cytotoxic T lymphocytes has also been reported for the *treatment* of B cell lymphomas in bone marrow transplant recipients. Although these are extremely interesting clinical experiments, in view of its complexity it seems doubtful whether adoptive transfer will become a widely applicable therapy.

Post-infective immunization refers to the use of vaccines in subjects already infected with a virus, to enhance or alter their immunity. There is as yet no unequivocal evidence for its efficacy in any human infectious disease (*post-exposure* immunization for rabies is a different situation), but there are current trials of post-infective immunization with a recombinant HSV vaccine in patients with recurrent genital herpes simplex.

Human immunodeficiency virus

Recent work has shown that, although there are peaks of viral replication during primary infection and in late infection, high levels of HIV RNA are present in plasma throughout infection, including the long clinically asymptomatic period (Fig. 1). Estimates are that 10^9 HIV virions are produced every day and half the plasma virus load is turned over every 2 days [10]. This rate of replication, coupled with the high mutation rate of HIV, means that drug-resistant viruses have a rapid selective advantage. The major currently available antivirals against HIV are listed in Table 3. Evidence for their clinical efficacy can only derive from clinical trials, of which many are in progress; trials with *clinical* endpoints are generally more informative than those with *surrogate* endpoints such as changes in CD4 cell count or virus load, but the former become more difficult to design as the number of drugs entering trials increases.

Reverse transcriptase inhibitors

Zidovudine (AZT) was the first drug of this class and has been shown to retard progression from AIDS to death. However, the recent Concorde trial of zidovudine monotherapy started in patients with CD4 cell counts of 200–500 showed no benefit on either survival or progression from asymptomatic infection to AIDS [11]. This result contradicted an earlier NIH trial (ACTG 019), which was stopped early after

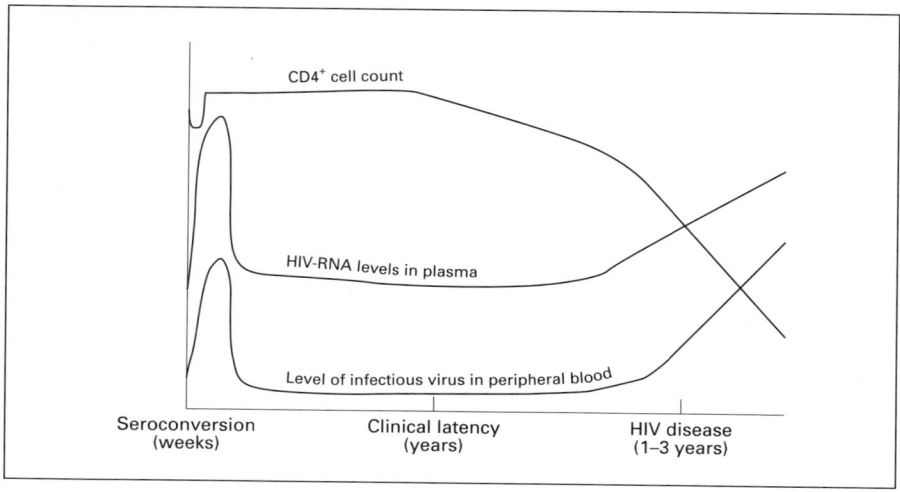

Fig. 1 Schematic course of HIV infection.

Table 3 Antivirals currently available for chemotherapy of HIV.

Nucleoside reverse transcriptase inhibitors
  Zidovudine (AZT)
  Zalcitabine (ddC)
  Didanosine (ddI)
  Lamivudine (3TC)
  Stavudine
	Protease inhibitors
	  Ritonavir
	  Saquinavir
	  Indinavir

Non-nucleoside reverse transcriptase inhibitors
  Nevirapine
  Delavirdine
  Loviride	

zidovudine appeared to slow clinical progression, and emphasizes the advantage of clinical endpoints [12]. Resistant virus rapidly emerges with such monotherapy, and most interest now focuses on combination chemotherapy. The recent Delta trial [13] of zidovudine combined with either didanosine (ddI) or zalcitabine (ddC) in patients with CD4 counts <350/µl showed a relative reduction in mortality of 42% for AZT/ddI and of 32% for AZT/ddC, compared to AZT alone. The effects were less in the treatment groups who had received AZT monotherapy prior to the trial (Table 4). The molecular background to combination therapy is that the acquisition of a mutation conferring resistance to ddI in a virus already resistant to AZT results in reversion to sensitivity to AZT. The combination of zidovudine and lamivudine (another reverse transcriptase inhibitor) has recently been shown to result in greater improvement in CD4 counts and plasma HIV RNA than either agent alone, and newer non-nucleoside reverse transcriptase inhibitors such as nevirapine lower plasma viraemia by 1–1.5 logs, compared to 0.7 for the above drugs. Toxicity of these nucleoside reverse transcriptase inhibitors is partly attributable to their effect on mitochondrial DNA [14].

Table 4 Summary of results from Delta trial of combination chemotherapy.

	Delta 1 (AZT naive)		Delta 2 (AZT >3/12)	
	AZT/ddI	AZT/ddC	AZT/ddI	AZT/ddC
Reduction in mortality*	42%	32%	23%	NS
Reduction in risk of progression to AIDS or death	36%	17% (NS)	NS	NS

*Figures are relative reductions in mortality or risk of developing AIDS or dying, compared to patients taking AZT alone
NS, no significant difference from patients taking AZT alone

Protease inhibitors

Another class of antiretroviral drugs acts by inhibiting the HIV protease. Indinavir, saquinavir and ritonavir reduce plasma viraemia by about 2 logs, although resistant virus rapidly emerges when they are used as monotherapy. Trials are currently in progress using combinations of these newer drugs with reverse transcriptase inhibitors.

Who and how to treat?

In summary, there is good evidence to support the use of combination reverse transcriptase inhibitor chemotherapy in patients with HIV who have CD4 counts <350/µl (see Table 5). There is no proven case for the use of monotherapy, and it may make subsequent combination therapy less effective. An exception is the use of antepartum and intrapartum zidovudine, followed by 6 weeks administration to the neonate, to lower transmission of HIV from mother to child (trials show reduction

Table 5 Trial proven treatment for HIV.

Clinical stage	Trial proven therapy
Primary infection	AZT monotherapy improves CD4 count over 15 months
Asymptomatic:	
CD4 count >350	No benefit from AZT monotherapy
CD4 count <350	Benefit from reverse transcriptase inhibitor combination therapy (Delta, ACTG 175)
Symptomatic infection	Benefit from reverse transcriptase inhibitor combination therapy
	Lesser benefit from AZT monotherapy
Prior nucleoside monotherapy	Reverse transcriptase inhibitor combinations reduce viral load (Delta)
Pregnancy transmission	AZT monotherapy reduces transmission
CNS disease	AZT monotherapy

in risk from 25% to 8% [15]). There are persuasive theoretical arguments for attempting to reduce the load of HIV early in primary infection (where this is clinically recognized). HIV is more homogeneous at this stage and selection for resistant virus may take longer. The subsequent plasma virus load may then remain lower for a substantial period [10], and recent evidence suggests that a lower plasma virus load correlates with a better prognosis. The optimum therapy for asymptomatic HIV carriers with CD4 counts >350/µl is not yet clear from trials.

At the time of writing, initial reports of trials of two reverse transcriptase inhibitors (such as AZT and lamivudine) with a protease inhibitor are arousing great interest. Virus levels in blood are reduced below the level of detection by PCR in many treated subjects for periods up to a year of follow-up. Such results suggest the possibility of major improvements in the therapy of HIV if they translate into equivalent survival benefit.

☐ CONCLUSION

An increasing range of antiviral drugs is becoming available, particularly in response to the need to treat the major persistent pathogenic virus infections such as HIV, CMV and hepatitis B and C (see chapter by Ahmed and Elias). Their rational use depends on understanding the virus life-cycle and (at least in the trial setting) on the ability to obtain quantitative measures of viral load and resistant virus using PCR techniques. The availability of effective therapies is an incentive to accurate and rapid diagnosis using similar techniques.

REFERENCES

1. Whitley RJ, Lakeman F. Herpes simplex virus infections of the central nervous system: therapeutic and diagnostic considerations. *Clin Infect Dis* 1995; **20**: 414–20.
2. Lakeman F, Whitley RJ. Diagnosis of herpes simplex encephalitis: application of polymerase chain reaction to CSF from brain biopsied patients and correlation with disease. *J Infect Dis* 1995; **171**: 857–63.
3. Jeffery K, Reed SJ, Peto T, *et al.* PCR diagnosis of CNS infections. *Lancet* 1997; **349**: 313–7.
4. Relman DA, Schmidt TM, MacDermott RP, Falkow S. Identification of the uncultured bacillus of Whipple's disease. *New Engl J Med* 1992; **327**: 293–301.
5. Moore PS, Chang Y. Detection of herpesvirus-like DNA sequences in Kaposi's sarcoma in patients with and those without HIV infection. *New Engl J Med* 1995; **18**: 1181–5.
6. Whitby D, Howard MR, Tenant-Flowers M, *et al.* Detection of Kaposi sarcoma associated herpesvirus in peripheral blood of HIV-infected individuals and progression to Kaposi's sarcoma. *Lancet* 1995; **346**: 799–802.
7. Drew WL, Ives D, Lalezari JP, *et al.* Oral ganciclovir as maintenance treatment for cytomegalovirus retinitis in patients with AIDS. *New Engl J Med* 1995; **333**: 615–20.
8. Spector SA, *et al.* Oral ganciclovir for the prevention of cytomegalovirus disease in persons with AIDS. *New Engl J Med* 1996; **334**: 1491–7.
9. Walter EA, Greenberg PD, Gilbert MJ, *et al.* Reconstitution of cellular immunity against cytomegalovirus in recipients of allogeneic bone marrow by transfer of T-cell clones from the donor. *New Engl J Med* 1995; **333**: 1038–44.
10. Ho DD. Time to hit HIV, early and hard. *New Engl J Med* 1995; **333**: 450.
11. Concorde Coordinating Committee. Concorde: MRC/CNRS randomised double-blind

controlled trial of immediate and deferred zidovudine in symptom-free HIV infection. *Lancet* 1994; **343**: 871–81.
12. Volberding PA, Lagakos SW, Grimes JM, et al. A comparison of immediate with deferred zidovudine therapy for asymptomatic HIV-infected adults with CD4 cell counts of 500 or more per cubic millimeter. *New Engl J Med* 1995; **333**: 401–7.
13. Delta Coordinating Committee. Delta: a randomised double-blind controlled trial comparing combinations of zidovudine plus didanosine or zalcitabine with zidovudine alone in HIV-infected individuals. *Lancet* 1996; **348**: 283–91.
14. Swartz MN. Mitochondrial toxicity – new adverse drug effects. *New Engl J Med* 1995; **333**: 1146–8.
15. Peckham C, Gibb D. Mother-to-child transmission of the human immunodeficiency virus. *New Engl J Med* 1995; **333**: 298–302.

☐ MULTIPLE CHOICE QUESTIONS

1. In Kaposi's sarcoma:
   (a) The epidemiology is that of a virus-associated tumour
   (b) Sequences of a novel γ-herpes virus are detectable in blood and tumour
   (c) This virus is most closely related to herpes simplex virus
   (d) These sequences are present in every cell in the tumour

2. Regarding herpes simplex virus:
   (a) The virus is normally latent in sensory ganglia
   (b) The virus thymidine kinase phosphorylates acyclovir in infected cells
   (c) Acyclovir eradicates latent virus
   (d) Virus may be detected by PCR in cerebrospinal fluid in HSV encephalitis with high specificity

3. In treating human cytomegalovirus (CMV) infection:
   (a) Ganciclovir and foscarnet are equally effective on current evidence
   (b) Maintenance therapy is essential in patients with AIDS and CMV retinitis
   (c) Ganciclovir alone is effective in treating CMV pneumonitis in bone marrow transplant recipients
   (d) Oral ganciclovir is the first choice for the treatment of CMV retinitis

4. The following are true of HIV infection:
   (a) HIV in plasma in primary infection is relatively homogeneous
   (b) Virus disappears from plasma during asymptomatic infection
   (c) The quantity of viral RNA in plasma is a predictor of prognosis
   (d) Reverse transcription of HIV RNA is associated with a low rate of mutation

5. In treating HIV infection
   (a) Patients with CD4 lymphocyte counts above 350 should be given zidovudine monotherapy
   (b) Combinations of reverse transcriptase inhibitor drugs prolong survival in patients with AIDS
   (c) Zidovudine monotherapy reduces the risk of mother-to-child transmission of HIV in pregnancy

(d) Resistance rapidly occurs due to mutations in reverse transcriptase in patients given monotherapy

ANSWERS

1a	True	2a	True	3a	True	4a	True	5a	False
b	True	b	True	b	True	b	False	b	True
c	False	c	False	c	False	c	True	c	True
d	True	d	True	d	False	d	False	d	True

Infections in the immunocompromised host

W A Lynn

☐ INTRODUCTION

Modern medicine has seen great progress in the ability to treat previously incurable conditions with a vast array of new techniques. Great strides have been made in our ability to manipulate the immune system with immunosuppressive drugs, treat cancers with cytotoxic chemotherapy, and organ transplantation has now become almost routine practice. However, the price for this is an increasing population of patients whose immune system is impaired, placing them at risk of developing life-threatening infectious complications. Furthermore, improvements in our ability to sustain critically ill patients, increased use of invasive monitoring and the rising prevalence of drug-resistant pathogens further increase the exposure of vulnerable patients to infectious agents.

☐ DEFINITIONS AND EPIDEMIOLOGY

Immunocompromised host

There is no standard definition of 'immunocompromised'. In the widest sense, one interpretation could be any individual who has a less than optimal host response to infection. Used in this broad context, almost all chronically ill patients would be considered immunocompromised. Such a definition clearly has limited applicability, and a more pragmatic approach is to consider as immuno-compromised any individual with a specific defect in host defence, such that they are at significantly increased risk of unusual or opportunistic infections. This is a heterogeneous group of patients with a wide spectrum from patients with severe life-threatening immunodeficiency to those with more subtle problems that only become apparent under specific circumstances [1].

Incidence and prevalence

As well as the lack of a precise definition of 'immunocompromise', there are also few data available to estimate the numbers of patients at risk in the UK. However, where figures are available, it is clear that the numbers are considerable and rising. For example, in 1993 there were 2500 solid organ transplants in England and Wales with 3000 in 1995. By the end of 1995, there were an estimated 15 000 patients in England and Wales with a functioning renal transplant. The prevalence of some immuno-suppressive conditions in the general population is known, for example systemic lupus erythematosus at 1:2000 and systemic vasculitis at 1:10 000 (K. Davies, personal communication). To the end of January 1996, 25 635 patients had been reported as human immunodeficiency virus (HIV) positive with 8201 acquired immune deficiency syndrome (AIDS) related deaths. The Public Health Laboratory Service (PHLS) has estimated that there will be 3–4000 patients with AIDS alive each year into the next century [2]. The potential impact of chronic medical conditions is much greater, with 10 000 patients currently on haemodialysis (G. Gaskin, personal communication) and an estimated 500 000 diabetics (H. Mather, personal communication). If we add the patients receiving immunosuppressive drugs, including corticosteroids, all patients with cancer or on chemotherapy, and patients with other chronic medical conditions, it can be appreciated that the total number of people with serious immunosuppression is very significant and that medical practitioners in all fields need to be familiar with such patients.

Opportunistic infection

An opportunistic infection is an infection caused by a pathogen that does not, or rarely, infect an immunocompetent host. Thus the particular pathogen lacks the necessary virulence factors to cause disease in the presence of a normal immune system; good examples would be *Pneumocystis carinii* pneumonia, invasive aspergillosis or bacteraemia due to 'normal' skin flora in patients with indwelling central venous catheters.

☐ PRINCIPLES IN THE PRESENTATION AND MANAGEMENT OF INFECTION IN IMMUNOCOMPROMISED PATIENTS

The type of infection, and response to therapy, seen in the immunocompromised patient is determined by host and environmental factors (Fig. 1). Thus, it is important to take all of these factors into account in each individual case to guide the diagnostic process and arrive at the correct therapy.

Nature of immune dysfunction

Broadly speaking, immunodeficiency may be due to congenital defects in host response systems or acquired as a result of immunosuppressive diseases [1] and therapeutic insults as described in Table 1. Patients may be faced with a permanent but stable problem such as splenectomy, a progressive deterioration in immune function in conditions such as AIDS, or there may be severe but transient immunosuppression, for example during cancer chemotherapy. Thus the type of immune dysfunction, the severity of the defect and the duration/prognosis of the underlying disease are all important host factors that combine to determine what infections occur and what the overall outcome will be in individual patients.

The type of immune defect can be extremely helpful in predicting the specific infections that the individual is most at risk from, as outlined in Table 2. For example, patients without a functional spleen have a problem clearing encapsulated bacteria from the circulation and are, therefore, at increased risk from pneumococcal infection. However, in practice many patients have multiple factors impairing different aspects

INFECTIONS IN THE IMMUNOCOMPROMISED HOST

Immunosuppression
- Nature of defect
- Duration
- Degree

Therapeutic interventions
- Immunosuppressive drugs
- Radiotherapy
- Surgery
- Prosthetic material

Environmental exposure
- Hospitalization
- Nosocomial outbreaks of resistant infections
- Ethnic origin/previous places of residence
- Past history of infections
- Blood transfusions and blood products
- Recent disease exposures

Co-morbidities
- Progressive underlying disease
- Indwelling vascular lines
- Poor nutrition
- Diabetes
- Renal or hepatic failure
- Breakdown in mucosal barriers

Outcome
- Resolution?
- Progression?

Antimicrobial therapy
- Antibiotic selection pressures
- Effective therapy available

Host ↔ **Pathogen**

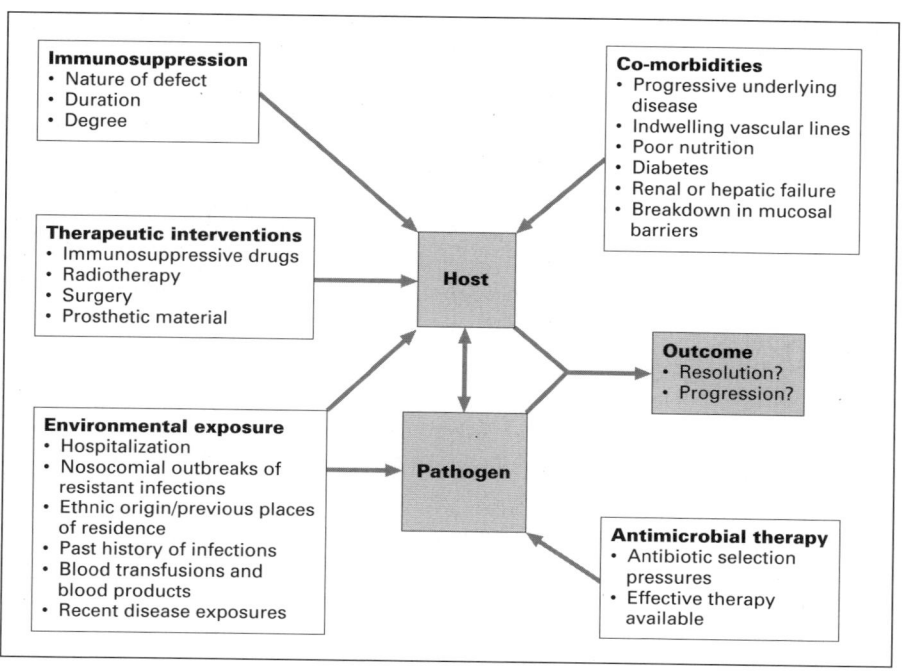

Fig. 1 Schematic relation between the various host, pathogen and environmental factors that interact to determine outcome from infectious diseases in immunocompromised patients.

of the immune system and, apart from specific situations such as splenectomy or congenital defects, it is uncommon to see pure immunodeficiencies. A good example of this is the patient undergoing heterologous bone marrow transplantation for leukaemia. Pre-transplantation, the patient is immunosuppressed by the leukaemia itself plus any initial chemotherapy. Conditioning for transplantation involves bone marrow ablative chemotherapy and total body irradiation. The early post-transplant phase is dominated by bacterial infections due to breakdown in mucous membranes plus neutropenia. As the period of neutropenia is prolonged beyond 2 weeks, there is the onset of fungal infections associated with neutropenia, namely candidiasis and aspergillosis. Once the new marrow engrafts, neutrophils return and the importance of bacterial infections recedes. The picture is then dominated by impaired cell-mediated immunity from the immunosuppressive drugs used to control graft-versus-host disease. The pattern of bacterial infections shifts towards atypical or intracellular pathogens, such as mycobacteria; aspergillus remains a problem but other fungi emerge including cryptococcosis. Herpetic infections become more important, particularly cytomegalovirus (CMV), and more unusual opportunistic pathogens appear including *Pneumocystis carinii* pneumonia (PCP) and intestinal cryptosporidiosis. Late post-transplantation, the degree of immunosuppression correlates with the level of graft-versus-host disease, but in addition patients have a long-lasting defect in humoral responses and splenic function as a result of the total body irradiation. During this period, they remain at risk from overwhelming

Table 1 Types of immunodeficiency.

Immune defect	Congenital causes	Acquired causes

Humoral	Hypogammaglobulinaemia
	   X-linked agammaglobulinaemia
	IgA deficiency
	Common variable
	   immunodeficiency
		Myeloma, some leukaemias/
		   lymphomas, AIDS
		Impaired humoral response to
		   vaccination in diabetes, renal
		   failure and many chronic medical
		   conditions

Impaired opsonization of bacteria	Complement deficiencies
	   Classic pathway
	   Alternative pathway
	   Mannose-binding protein deficiency
		Systemic lupus erythematosus
		   (SLE) nephrotic syndrome

Splenic dysfunction	Congenital absence of spleen	Splenectomy Sickle cell disease Splenic leukaemia/lymphoma Irradiation

Neutrophil dysfunction	Cyclic neutropenia
	Chronic granulomatous disease
	Leucocyte adhesion deficiency
	Neutrophil granule deficiency
		Neutropenia
		   Disease-related, drug-induced
		Neutrophil dysfunction
		   Diabetes, renal or hepatic failure

Cell-mediated immune dysfunction	Severe combined immuno-
	   deficiency (SCID)
	Adenosine deaminase deficiency
	Defective MHC molecule
	   expression
	IL-2 deficiency
	Digeorge syndrome
	Ataxia telangiectasia
	Wiskott-Aldrich syndrome
		Infections, eg HIV/AIDS,
		   leprosy, tuberculosis, measles
		Immunosuppressive drugs
		   Cyclosporin, corticosteroids etc.
		Immunosuppressive diseases
		   Lymphoreticular malignancy,
		   systemic lupus erythematosus
		   (SLE), sarcoidosis

Failure of non-specific defence mechanisms	Kartagener's syndrome
	   (immotile cilia)
		Mucositis, indwelling venous
		   lines/catheters, foreign bodies,
		   malnutrition

pneumococcal infection, are particularly vulnerable to primary varicella or measles infection, and experience an increased incidence of second malignancies.

Underlying disease

It is important to remember that the outcome from infections will often depend as much on the underlying disease process as on the recognition and treatment of the infecting organism. Thus, survival from invasive aspergillosis in neutropenic patients requires recovery from neutropenia. Therefore, when managing immunocompromised patients, as much therapeutic effort should be directed towards the underlying illness as to the infection. Diabetes, renal and hepatic failure should be corrected, nutritional support addressed and immunosuppressive illnesses treated. This may lead to the paradoxical situation of giving immunosuppressive therapy, ie chemotherapy for lymphoma, to an infected patient but, on occasion, this may be the only viable option.

Table 2 Infections typically associated with specific immune deficits.

Immune defect	Infections typically encountered
Humoral	*Bacteria* Recurrent infection, soft-tissue, respiratory tract, sinusitis and bronchiectasis
Complement deficiency/splenic dysfunction	*Bacteria* Encapsulated bacteria, eg Pneumococcus and Haemophilus. Recurrent Neisseria and Salmonella infections *Protozoa* Overwhelming malaria or babesiosis
Neutrophil dysfunction	*Bacteria* Recurrent severe bacterial infections, *Staphylococcus* spp., viridans streptococci, enteric Gram-negative bacilli and *Pseudomonas* spp. are most common isolates *Viruses* Recurrent mucocutaneous herpes simplex *Fungi* Invasive candidiasis (candidaemia, endophthalmitis, hepatosplenic candidiasis) Invasive aspergillosis, invasive dermatophyte infection
Cell-mediated immune dysfunction	*Bacteria* Mycobacteria (TB and atypical mycobacteria), *Salmonella* spp., listeriosis, legionellosis, melioidosis (*Burkholderia pseudomallei*), bacillary angiomatosis (*Bartonella hensulae*) *Viruses* Herpes viruses: HSV 1 and 2, VZV, CMV Respiratory viruses: adenovirus, respiratory syncytial virus, parainfluenza and influenza Polyoma viruses (JC/BK): PML, haemorrhagic cystitis *Fungi* Mucocutaneous candidiasis, invasive aspergillosis, cryptococcosis, histoplasmosis *Parasites* PCP, scabies, leishmaniasis, cryptosporidiosis, microsporidiosis, strongyloidiasis *Infection-related malignancy* B-cell lymphoma (EBV), Kaposi sarcoma (HHV8), cervical carcinoma (papilloma virus), squamous carcinoma of the skin (papilloma virus)

HSV, herpes simplex virus; VZV, varicella zoster virus; CMV, cytomegalovirus; PML, progressive multifocal leucoencephalopathy; EBV, Epstein-Barr virus; HHV8, human herpes virus-8

Environmental factors

Environmental factors also influence the precise pathogens seen in individual cases. For example, if the particular hospital where a patient has been treated is undergoing building work increasing exposure to aspergillus spores may occur, or if a transplant unit has an outbreak of antibiotic-resistant bacteria, then the diagnostic and therapeutic process must be adjusted accordingly. Furthermore, the patients' ethnic origin and travel history are very important. Immunocompromised patients may reactivate latent pathogens acquired many years earlier and therefore may present with infections that are not endemic in the UK, for example histoplasmosis, strongyloidiasis or leishmaniasis. This was most dramatically illustrated by veterans from the Far East campaign of the Second World War, some of whom developed strongyloides hyperinfection syndrome when given corticosteroids more than 30 years after returning to the UK.

Invading pathogens

As mentioned above, when considering the immunocompromised host we typically consider unusual opportunistic pathogens. It is important, however, to remember that immunocompromised patients are also at increased risk of 'conventional' infections and we must not overlook the obvious, for example a dental abscess, when evaluating these patients. Immunocompromised patients also break many of the 'rules' of standard infectious diseases. We generally think of infections being due to an acute invasion of the body by a single pathogen. In the immunocompromised host it is common to have multiple infections, either simultaneously or sequentially. Furthermore, some pathogens may be impossible to eradicate and require suppressive therapy for as long as the patient is immunocompromised, for example invasive CMV infection in AIDS. In this context, many infections are not acute but are actually re-activation of old disease, for example toxoplasmosis in AIDS or CMV infection post-transplantation, and so it is not possible to protect patients from these infections by isolation or infection control.

Clinical features of disease presentation

The manifestations of any infection are due to a combination of host and pathogen factors. After invasion of a normally sterile body site, there is a brisk host inflammatory response that leads to the symptoms and signs of that infection, for example fever, cough, pleurisy and purulent sputum in pneumococcal pneumonia. In a successful host response the infection is localized and the patient survives. In the immunocompromised host the balance is shifted and disease presentation and course may be altered.

The reduced constraining effect of the immune system means that there may be increased organism numbers or dissemination within the host. Thus patients with early HIV infection tend to present with typical pulmonary tuberculosis, but when there is severe immune dysfunction in AIDS there is an increase in extrapulmonary sites of tuberculosis. The potential for massive replication of infecting pathogens and unusual disease presentations is graphically shown in Plates 19 and 20.

Conversely, the abnormal host response means that physical signs may be reduced or even absent. For example, fever may not be present during bacteraemia and, in the neutropenic patient with pneumonia, pulmonary infiltrates may not be seen due to the lack of neutrophil migration into the lung. Thus, a high index of suspicion is required and all symptoms should be taken seriously, as often the only clue may be that the patient is non-specifically unwell. Meticulous assessment may then reveal the underlying cause. Plate 21 shows an asymptomatic patch of CMV on the retina of an AIDS patient whose presenting complaint was that he felt unusually tired; prompt recognition and therapy saved the sight in that eye.

☐ NEW TRENDS IN INFECTIONS IN THE IMMUNOCOMPROMISED HOST

Investigations

A detailed discussion of the merits of different investigations is beyond the scope of this chapter, but several points are worthy of comment. The application of new technology is revolutionizing the diagnosis of unusual infections. One of the major difficulties is the lack of signs localizing infection and diagnostic radiology has much to offer in detecting and then guiding invasive procedures to establish a diagnosis; Fig. 2 shows one such case. Furthermore, new microbiological diagnostic techniques will enable us to detect, and hopefully treat, infections at a much earlier stage. The use of the polymerase chain reaction (PCR) in routine diagnostics is still at an early stage but the potential power of this technique is shown in Fig. 3 where varicella

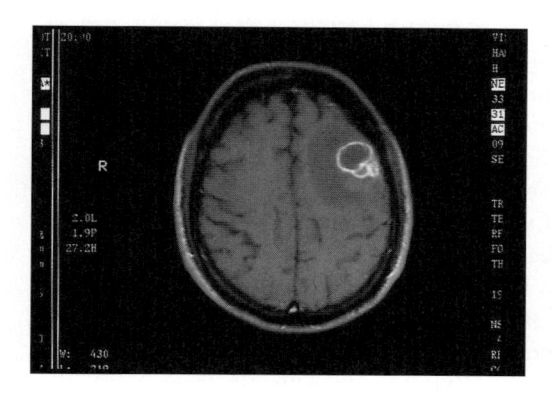

Fig. 2 Magnetic resonance imaging (MRI) scan of the brain in a severely immunocompromised patient with headache and fever. MRI revealed a complex abscess in the left frontal lobe subsequently confirmed histologically as being due to *Mycobacterium tuberculosis*. (By courtesy of Dr Sunil Shaunak.)

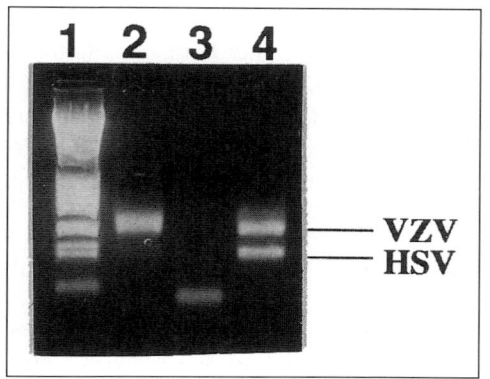

Fig. 3 A 28-year-old patient with advanced AIDS presented with a fever and mild paraparesis. MRI of the spinal cord was normal and the cerebrospinal fluid revealed a lymphocytic pleiocytosis. The patient was taking oral acyclovir and culture of cerebrospinal fluid was negative, but PCR revealed the presence of varicella zoster virus DNA consistent with varicella zoster virus transverse myelitis. Lane 1, DNA standard ladder; lane 2, patient's CSF sample; lane 3, negative control; lane 4, VZV and HSV DNA positive control. (By courtesy of Dr C Bangham.)

zoster virus was detected in the cerebrospinal fluid from a febrile patient with an evolving paraplegia within 48 hours of the lumbar puncture. By detecting antimicrobial resistance genes, PCR also has the ability to identify resistance in organisms where this is difficult to measure rapidly by conventional methods, and this is already being applied to tuberculosis and HIV isolates. PCR has also been pivotal in the discovery of novel infectious agents and has been used to find human herpes virus type 8 (HHV8) in Kaposi sarcoma [3].

Emerging pathogens

Three main themes emerge when examining the changing epidemiology of infections in the immunocompromised patient.

First is the recognition of new organisms. I have already mentioned HHV8 as the probable cause of Kaposi sarcoma; another herpes virus HHV6 (the causative agent of roseola infantum) has been implicated in interstitial pneumonitis following bone-marrow transplantation. Hepatitis C is the major cause of parenterally acquired non-A non-B hepatitis and is increasingly recognized as a cause of chronic hepatitis after organ transplantation [4]. *Bartonella hensulae* and *B. quintana* are Gram-negative bacteria that have been identified by PCR from specimens from patients with bacillary angiomatosis [5]. This condition is seen in patients with severe cell-mediated immunodeficiency and consists of multiple skin lesions resembling Kaposi sarcomata. The disease spectrum associated with these organisms is still being defined, but includes cat-scratch disease in normal hosts and endocarditis, peliosis hepatitis and pyrexia of unknown origin in the immunocompromised patient. Of various parasites, the two organisms that merit particular attention are cryptosporidiosis and microsporidiosis [6]. Cryptosporidiosis has emerged as a major cause of essentially untreatable chronic diarrhoea in AIDS and is increasingly recognized in other immunocompromised patient groups. Microsporidia can be detected by electron microscopy of small bowel biopsies or with special stains of faecal preparations. In addition to diarrhoea microsporidia may widely disseminate, including to the brain, kidneys and liver [6]. Microsporidiosis is probably under-diagnosed, which is important as it often responds to therapy with albendazole.

Second, the range of organisms, previously thought to be non-pathogenic, isolated as opportunistic pathogens continues to expand. In particular there is an ever increasing list of fungi that may cause invasive disease including dermatophytes [7]. Finally, there are the problems associated with drug resistance both in commonly encountered organisms such as pneumococcus and in true opportunists [8] (Table 3). This will have major implications in patient management not only relating to the efficacy of therapy but also in infection control. Furthermore, when the infection is also a pathogen for immunocompetent hosts, the possibility of disease spread in the community exists, as has been highlighted for drug-resistant tuberculosis [9].

Antimicrobial therapy

It is beyond the scope of this chapter to discuss all of the therapeutic developments in the treatment of opportunistic pathogens. In general, prevention is always better

Table 3 Emerging problems with antimicrobial resistance.

Pathogen	Nature of clinical problem
Bacteria	
MRSA	Major problem in some centres, central-line infections
Methicillin-resistant *S. epidermidis*	Most hospital isolates are resistant, most common cause of central-line infections
VRE	Outbreaks in some renal units and some transplant centres
Resistant Gram-negative bacilli	Sporadic outbreaks in most hospitals, rely on local surveillance/sensitivity
Mycobacteria	
Mycobacterium tuberculosis	Increasing outbreaks of MDR-TB; homelessness, drug/alcohol use, HIV infection major risk factors, nosocomial outbreaks described
Atypical mycobacteria	Responds poorly to standard anti-TB therapy and resistance may develop on treatment or during prophylaxis
Fungi	
Candida albicans	Increasing azole resistance particularly in HIV, encouraged by low-dose antifungal prophylaxis
Non-albicans *Candida* spp.	Prevalence of non-albicans yeast isolation increasing, azole resistance high particularly with *C. krusii* and use amphotericin for initial therapy
Viruses	
Herpes simplex	Acyclovir resistance well described in HIV and transplantation, foscarnet second-line choice
Varicella zoster	Acyclovir resistance described in varicella zoster infections in AIDS
Cytomegalovirus	Increasing problem with ganciclovir and/or foscarnet-resistant CMV, particularly in AIDS

MRSA, methicillin-resistant *Staphylococcus aureus*; VRE, vancomycin-resistant enterococcus; MDR-TB, multiply resistant *Mycobacterium tuberculosis*

than cure, and one of the most important advances has been the recognition that 'high-risk' patients can be targeted with health advice, vaccinations and selected prophylactic antibiotics to reduce the morbidity and mortality of infectious diseases [10]. Some of these strategies are described in Table 4, but it should be stressed that this is a rapidly changing area and specific advice will often depend on trends in local antimicrobial resistance patterns.

Adjunctive immunotherapy

For certain pathogens, for example *Cryptosporidium parvum*, we do not have suitable antimicrobial therapy, and for many other infections cure rates are very low, even in the face of effective antimicrobial therapy. This reflects the fact that for many infections an effective immune response is required to clear the organism and antimicrobial agents simply tilt the balance in favour of the host. Therefore, much attention has focused on ways of manipulating the immune response to try to

Table 4 Commonly used antimicrobial prophylaxis in the immunocompromised host.

Clinical situation	Antimicrobial prophylaxis
Splenic failure	*Pneumococcus* 　Penicillin or ampicillin daily. Erythromycin in allergic patients. 　Pneumococcal vaccination (?Haemophilus and meningococcal vaccines)
Neutropenia	*Bacterial infections* 　Unless neutropenia likely to be transient consider quinolone prophylaxis
Bone marrow transplantation	*Bacterial infections* 　Quinolone prophylaxis during neutropenic phase, life-long penicillin prophylaxis for pneumococcus *Fungal infections* 　Topical antifungals when mucositis present, oral fluconazole reduces invasive candida but may increase resistance, systemic amphotericin B does reduce aspergillus infection but is toxic *Viral infections* 　Acyclovir reduces HSV and may reduce CMV infection rates, consider ganciclovir for patients at high risk of CMV infection *Pneumocystis* 　Prophylaxis for one year with co-trimoxazole
AIDS	*Pneumocystis* 　Primary prophylaxis if CD4 <200, secondary prophylaxis in all cases of PCP 　Preferred drug co-trimoxazole 960 mg 3 times a week *Toxoplasmosis* 　Should be covered by co-trimoxazole, secondary prophylaxis with sulphadiazine/pyrimethamine *Fungal infections* 　Candida: primary prophylaxis not recommended due to increasing azole resistance 　Cryptococcus: life-long maintenance therapy required after infection, azole or amphotericin B *Viral infections* 　Acyclovir may be needed if frequent HSV or VZV infections 　After CMV life-long maintenance required (ganciclovir and/or foscarnet), role of oral ganciclovir unclear *Mycobacterial infections* 　Consider isoniazid for patients at high risk of tuberculosis (controversial) 　Consider rifabutin or clarithromycin if CD4 <100 for atypical mycobacteria such as MAI

redress the balance [11]. Some of the more promising of these are highlighted in Table 5. In many chronic infections, such a leishmaniasis or tuberculosis, persistence of the organism is associated with a Th2 lymphocyte response and successful clearance of the infection with a Th1 cytotoxic T-cell response. Therefore, there is much interest in trying to push the response from Th2 to Th1, for example with interferon-γ or interleukin-12 [12]. In most other cases, the application of immunomodulating therapy is experimental, except for the colony stimulating factors, G-CSF or GM-CSF, for patients with neutropenia. These cytokines induce

Table 5 Cytokines of potential benefit in infection.

Cytokine	Activity
TNF-α	Enhances intracellular killing of bacteria and fungi; low-dose may protect against bacterial sepsis
IL-1	Enhances antibody responses as vaccine adjuvant; low-dose may protect against bacterial sepsis
IL-2	Stimulates T-cell proliferation, cytotoxicity and NK cell activity, vaccine adjuvant effects
IL-12	Induces Th1 response, stimulates NK cells and has vaccine adjuvant effects
Interferon-γ	Induces Th1 response, enhances intracellular killing of bacteria, mycobacteria, fungi and parasites
G-CSF	Shortens duration of neutropenia, enhances neutrophil function
GM-CSF	Shortens duration of neutropenia, enhances neutrophil function, activates macrophages and enhances intracellular killing of bacteria and fungi, vaccine adjuvant effects

TNF, tumour necrosis factor; IL, interleukin; NK, natural killer; G-CSF, granulocyte colony stimulating factor; GM-CSF, granulocyte/macrophage colony stimulating factor.

the accelerated maturation and release of neutrophils from the bone marrow and thus shorten the duration of neutropenia following chemotherapy. A number of studies have now shown that this has a significant impact on infective episodes, although which patients will benefit the most, and what the best regimen is, still needs to be elucidated.

☐ CONCLUSION

The population of patients with significant defects in immune function is likely to continue to expand. This, coupled with the threat of emerging drug-resistant pathogens, means that the prevention, recognition and therapy of infections in this group will be of increasing importance. In the future, it may be possible to improve immune function and resolve some of these difficulties, but until then the problem of infection in the immunocompromised host is one of which all medical practitioners need to be aware.

REFERENCES

1 Buckley RH. Immunodeficiency diseases. *J Am Med Assoc* 1992; **268**: 2797–806.
2 Public Health Laboratory Service. The incidence and prevalence of AIDS and prevalence of other severe HIV disease in England and Wales for 1995 to 1999: projections using data to the end of 1994. *CDR Review* 1996; **6**: R1–R24.
3 Whitby D, Howard MR, Tenant-Flowers M, Brink NS, *et al*. Detection of Kaposi sarcoma associated herpesvirus in peripheral blood of HIV-infected individuals and progression to Kaposi's sarcoma. *Lancet* 1995; **346**: 799–802.
4 Garcia G, Terrault N, Wright TL. Hepatitis C virus infection in the immunocompromised patient. *Semin Gastrointest Dis* 1995; **6**: 35–45.

5   Webster GF, Cockerell CJ, Friedman-Kien AE. The clinical spectrum of bacillary angiomatosis. *Brit J Dermatol* 1992; **126**: 535–41.
6   Gunnarsson G, Hurlbut D, DeGirolami PC, Federman M, Wanke C. Multiorgan microsporidiosis: report of five cases and review. *Clin Infect Dis* 1995; **21**: 37–44.
7   Perfect J, Schell W A. The new fungal opportunists are coming. *Clin Infect Dis* 1996; **22**: S112–S117.
8   Shlaes DM, Binczewski, Rice LB. Emerging antimicrobial resistance in the immunocompromised host. *Clin Infect Dis* 1993; **17**: S527–S536.
9   Salomon N, Perlman DC, Friedmann P, Buchstein S, Kreiswirth BN, Mildvan D. Predictors and outcome of multidrug-resistant tuberculosis. *Clin Infect Dis* 1995; **21**: 1245–52.
10 Avery RK. Infections and immunizations in organ transplant recipients: a preventive approach. *Cleve Clin J Med* 1994; **61**: 386–92.
11 Murray HW. Cytokines as antimicrobial therapy for the T-cell-deficient patient: prospects for treatment of nonviral opportunistic infections. *Clin Infect Dis* 1993; **17**: S407–S413.
12 Brunda MJ. Interleukin-12. *J Leukoc Biol* 1994; **55**: 280–8.

☐ MULTIPLE CHOICE QUESTIONS

1   Following bone marrow transplantation:
    (a) Aspergillosis is a frequent problem in the first 2 weeks
    (b) Life-long penicillin prophylaxis is required
    (c) Gram-positive organisms are the most common cause of bacteraemia
    (d) Patients with graft-versus-host disease suffer from less infectious complications
    (e) Acyclovir-resistant CMV infection is an increasing problem

2   The following vaccines can safely be administered to a patient with cell-mediated immunodeficiency:
    (a) Hepatitis B
    (b) Pneumovax
    (c) Oral polio
    (d) Influenza
    (e) Oral typhoid

3   The following conditions display the immune deficits shown:
    (a) Sickle cell disease: hyposplenism
    (b) Cyclosporin A: neutrophil dysfunction
    (c) Systemic lupus erythematosus: complement deficiency
    (d) Diabetes: impaired neutrophil function
    (e) Sarcoidosis: impaired cell-mediated immunity

4   The following cytokines enhance host responses to infection:
    (a) Interleukin 10
    (b) Transforming growth factor beta
    (c) Interleukin 12
    (d) Interferon-γ
    (e) GM-CSF

5   Regarding patients with AIDS:
   (a) The number of cases of AIDS is rapidly declining in the UK
   (b) Infection with CMV can be eradicated by ganciclovir therapy
   (c) Humoral immune responses are impaired early in HIV infection
   (d) Microsporidiosis is an increasingly recognized complication
   (e) Candidaemia is a frequent complication

ANSWERS

1a False	2a True	3a True	4a False	5a False
b True	b True	b False	b False	b False
c True	c False	c True	c True	c True
d False	d True	d True	d True	d True
e False	e False	e True	e True	e False

Modern management of acute tubular necrosis: prevention of oliguria

M G A Palazzo and J Cordingley

☐ INTRODUCTION

Acute renal failure may be defined as the inability of urine output to maintain normal plasma urea, creatinine, hydrogen ion balance and volume status. In normal 70 kg adults a sustained urine output of less than 0.5 ml/kg/h will usually result in a gradual rise in plasma creatinine and urea concentrations. However, some patients may develop or be converted into a non-oliguric form of acute renal failure where high urine volumes (100–200 ml/h) are associated with a high creatinine level.

Acute renal failure (ARF) is a common development among patients with an acute systemic illness. Its incidence may be as high as 30% in the intensive care population. The most common cause is a hypovolaemic/ischaemic incident, particularly in patients with an underlying predisposing condition such as reno-vascular disease, hypertension or diabetes, or the administration of drugs such as non-steroidal anti-inflammatory drugs (NSAIDs) and aminoglycosides. Table 1 shows the most common conditions associated with ARF. Hypovolaemia accounts for up to 90% of all hospital cases of acute renal failure.

ARF is classified anatomically as prerenal, renal and postrenal. In practice, prerenal and renal (intrinsic) are frequently a continuum of the same pathological

Table 1 The most common conditions related to development of acute renal failure.

Hypovolaemia or ineffective circulating volume	Haemorrhage
	Sepsis
	Cardiac arrest
	Post major surgery
	Burns
Toxins (more likely if there is chronic impairment or associated hypovolaemia)	NSAIDs
	Radiocontrast
	Aminoglycosides
	Amphotericin B
	Cyclosporin
	Antineoplastic agents
Hypertension	
Diabetes	
Renal artery stenosis	
Renal artery thrombosis	
Renal vein thrombosis	

process, since hypovolaemia is responsible for virtually all prerenal and the majority of intrinsic renal failure. The extent of the damage ranges from mild tubular to severe cortical necrosis and is inversely related to the chances of recovery. Restoration of function occurs in about 95% of patients following ARF. The development of acute renal failure during acute illness is closely related to hospital outcome. For example, patients with acute respiratory failure who develop ARF show increased hospital mortality from 30% to 70–80% in spite of renal support. Table 2 outlines the mortality among intensive care patients with ARF.

A number of factors may account for the poor outcome. The most important determinant is the severity of the precipitating condition. However, renal support is also not without problems the most serious of which are gastrointestinal and cerebral haemorrhage. Furthermore there is some evidence that during haemofiltration there may be continuing renal tubular damage which prolongs the need for haemofiltration. Finally, haemofilters might alter the balance of pro- and anti-inflammatory cytokines.

The unimpressive performance of sick patients on renal support has prompted a re-evaluation of the management of impending ARF with efforts directed toward preventive therapy. There have been a number of approaches, mostly of the 'magic bullet' type in animal models. Similar human studies have been unsatisfactory because of small numbers, short duration or failure to use appropriate clinical end points (Table 3). Few studies have been strictly controlled with respect to blood pressure and volume status. Dopamine, used in nearly every intensive care unit, has yet to undergo a prospective randomized controlled trial in patients in which the need for renal support is used as the end point. Some authors have suggested that, unless evidence is forthcoming, dopamine should be abandoned altogether [20].

☐ STRATEGIES IN THE PREVENTION OF ACUTE RENAL FAILURE

Low-dose dopamine

Endogenous dopamine is produced by the kidney and its action promotes sodium

Table 2 Outcomes associated with patients with ARF in intensive care units.

Author	Year	Technique	Mortality
Kramer [1]	1980	CAVH	64
Klehr [2]	1985	CAVH	78
Weiss [3]	1987	CAVH	55
Stevens [4]	1988	CAVHD	69
Wendon [5]	1989	CVVH	46
Storck [6]	1990	CVVH	87
Macias [7]	1991	CVVH	84

CAVH, continuous arteriovenous haemofiltration;
CAVHD, continuous arteriovenous haemodialysis;
CVVH, continuous veno-veno haemofiltration

Table 3 The effect of various prophylactic agents on the need to provide renal support.

Agent	Pathology	Effect on need for support	Reference
Dopamine	Cardiac surgery	None	PCR–Myles 1993 [8]
	Critically ill	None	PCR–Duke 1994 [9]
	Liver transplant	None	PCR–Swygert 1991 [10]
Verapamil	Post-transplant	None	PCR–Duggan 1985 [11]
Diltiazam	Post-transplant	Benefit	PCR–Wagner 1987 [12]
Atrial natriuretic Peptide	Post-transplant	None	Sands 1991 [13]
	Mixed	Benefit	PCR–Rahman 1994 [14]
Mannitol	Post-transplant	Benefit	PCR–Tiggeler 1984 [15]
	Post-transplant	Benefit	PCR–Weimar 1983 [16]
Frusemide	Ischaemic, toxic	Variable	PCR–Solomon 1994 [17]
	Ischaemic, toxic	None	PCR–Kleiknecht 1976 [18]
	Ischaemic, toxic	None	PCR–Brown 1981 [19]

PCR: prospective, controlled, randomized trial

excretion through dopamine receptors in the renal vasculature, glomeruli and proximal tubules.

Low-dose dopamine results in renal vasodilatation, reduces the need for Na^+/K^+ adenosine triphosphatase (ATPase) in the proximal tubule and can significantly increase cardiac output. The sum of these effects is increased renal blood flow, increased glomerular filtration rate (GFR) and natriuresis.

The evidence for dopamine's prophylactic effectiveness is derived from perioperative studies in which urine volumes and creatinine clearance have been measured. Unfortunately, most of these studies were uncontrolled and in some frusemide was also administered [21,22]. Although there is evidence that dopamine increases urine output there are no definitive data that low-dose dopamine in addition to the restoration of normal haemodynamics, prevents the need for renal support in oliguric patients.

Diuretics

Traditionally when urine output is consistently below 0.5 ml/kg/h high doses of frusemide and occasionally mannitol are given to 'kick start' the kidneys. In a prospective randomized controlled study of 58 patients with established ARF, Brown et al. [23] found that frusemide (3 g daily) increased urine output but had no effect on the number of dialyses, time course of renal failure or mortality.

Mannitol was initially investigated as a possible renal protective agent in the early 1960s. Apart from its osmotic diuretic effect, suggested mechanisms for potential benefits include reduction in cell swelling following renal ischaemia, a rise in tubular flow preventing obstruction by casts, free-radical scavenging, increased renal prostaglandin (PGE_2) concentrations and mitochondrial protection after ischaemia and reperfusion.

Mannitol was popularized by Dawson in 1965, who in a non-randomized controlled study found that mannitol substantially reduced the postoperative fall in urine output and creatinine clearance in jaundiced surgical patients. A recent randomized prospective controlled trial reported that perioperative mannitol resulted in a significantly worse creatinine clearance on the second postoperative day [24]. In another randomized controlled study of 27 patients undergoing infrarenal aortic clamping, in which intravascular fluid loading was guided by pulmonary artery wedge pressure (PAWP), no significant differences in creatinine clearance were found between patients who received perioperative saline alone or saline combined with mannitol and dopamine [25]. Again, although there is no clinical doubt that mannitol increases urine output, there is little evidence to suggest that it prevents the need for haemofiltration.

Calcium antagonists

It has been known for some time that arteriolar vasoconstriction is mediated by cytosolic calcium. Dihydropyridine calcium antagonists preferentially vasodilate afferent arterioles by inhibiting calcium influx and might be expected to increase renal blood flow (RBF) and GFR and possibly protect autoregulation. Calcium antagonists are also thought to limit calcium accumulation in tubular cells following ischaemic damage. They have been shown to improve creatinine clearance and reduce the incidence of acute tubular necrosis (ATN) after renal transplantation.

Natriuretic peptides

Atrial natriuretic peptide (ANP), its analogues and urodilatin are being investigated as possible therapeutic agents in the prevention and treatment of ATN. ANP increases GFR by dilation of the afferent arteriole and constriction of the efferent arteriole resulting in a rise in filtration pressure. In addition, ANP increases glomerular permeability and promotes tubular sodium and water loss.

In a prospective randomized controlled trial, Rahman *et al.* investigated the effects of ANP in patients with established ARF [26]. In a complicated protocol, 53 patients were randomized to receive ANP. Significantly fewer of the patients who received ANP required dialysis (23% *vs* 52%). This study is difficult to interpret because of changing randomization procedures, the influence of diuretics and paucity of data on severity of illness. Urodilatin, which unlike ANP does not cause hypotension, has produced some encouraging results in postoperative cardiac transplant patients but unfortunately these were compared to historical controls [27].

Nitric oxide and endothelin antagonists

Nitric oxide production by the inducible type of nitric oxide synthase is thought to play an important role in producing the cardiovascular hyperdynamic response to sepsis. Nitric oxide is involved in many physiological roles within the kidney, including cortical and medullary haemodynamics, tubuloglomerular feedback and mesangial cell and tubular function. Nitric oxide protects against medullary ischaemia and glomerular thrombosis after endotoxin administration. However, in a recent animal study of hyperdynamic septic shock, N-nitro-L-arginine methyl ester (L-NAME) returned systemic haemodynamics to the pre-septic state, and increased urine output and GFR. The authors suggested that nitric oxide synthase inhibition in sepsis may improve glomerular filtration pressure by preferentially increasing efferent vascular tone.

Endothelins (ETs) are potent vasoconstrictor peptides secreted by many types of cells. So far, two receptors have been identified, ETa and ETb. In the kidney ET-1 produces dose-dependent vasoconstriction. Low doses affect the afferent and efferent arterioles equally, leaving glomerular filtration pressure unchanged. At higher doses, afferent arteriolar constriction dominates, reducing GFR. ET also causes dose-dependent effects on sodium excretion and mesangial cell contraction. Hypoxia stimulates the release and enhances the effects of ET. Elevated concentrations of ET-1 have been found in patients with acute renal failure and these return to normal as function is restored. Studies in which ET action has been reduced by receptor antagonists or ET antibodies have shown an amelioration of some of the results of hypoxic renal injury.

Adenosine antagonist

Locally produced adenosine is released during renal ischaemia and is thought to alter tubuloglomerular feedback. It also causes a redistribution of blood flow favouring the renal medulla. Antagonists such as theophylline may restore glomerular arteriolar haemodynamics but in so doing worsen the precarious medullary perfusion (see below). The doses of theophylline to provide competitive receptor antagonism are considerably smaller than those needed for phosphodiesterase inhibition. In animal models these agents have provided both protection and restoration of renal function; however, controlled randomized clinical studies demonstrating a reduced need for haemofiltration in high-risk groups are not available.

☐ RENAL RESCUE – A STRUCTURED APPROACH TO PREVENTING DETERIORATION OF RENAL FUNCTION

The findings of animal-based studies for many of the agents mentioned have mostly been encouraging, only to find that their application in the complex clinical environment has failed to make an impression. The disappointing response to these therapies and high mortality on haemofiltration has led us to consider a more rigorous approach, which aims to provide the best conditions for facilitating urine production and reducing the need for haemofiltration. We have developed a protocol, currently under evaluation, which is directed at rapidly achieving the seemingly simple aims of normovolaemia, normotension and an improvement in renal medullary oxygen balance (Table 4).

Table 4 Charing Cross renal rescue protocol.

1 **Precondition – normovolaemia:**
   GTN 2 mg/h maintained throughout protocol
   Warm colloid challenge
   CVP/PAOP increased against stroke volume and clinical end points
   Warm feet, warm dry torso, falling heart rate
2 **Precondition – patient related normotension:**
   Noradrenaline to achieve normal systolic blood pressure
   (as soon as clinically normovolaemic)
3 **Offload work of the mTAL:**
   Once preconditions 1 and 2 achieved
   Frusemide 10 mg bolus, followed by 1–4 mg/h

Aim to achieve urine output 100–200 ml/h
Replace magnesium, potassium and phosphate as required

Identification of the 'at risk' patient

In most cases, it is easy to identify patients who have sustained overt renal insults. These include episodes of hypotension in patients exposed to NSAIDs, contrast media or nephrotoxic antibiotics. It is more difficult to recognize the patient with unrevealed renal impairment, ie those with apparently normal function but in whom a small insult results in significant renal impairment. It is well known that serum creatinine remains normal until there has been a large reduction in GFR (Fig. 1). A small change in GFR at a reduced performance level (B–C) results in a

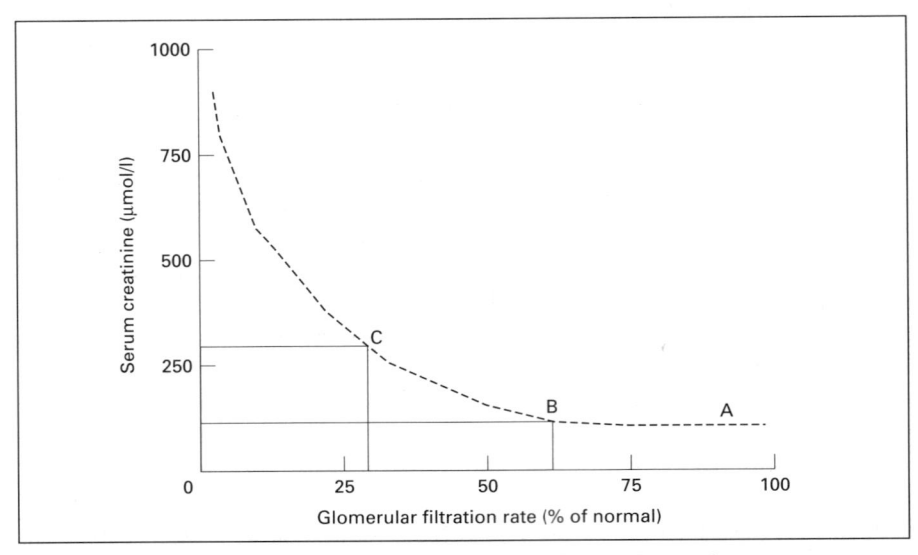

Fig. 1 The relationship between serum creatinine and GFR. For details, see the text.

larger rise in creatinine than a similar change in GFR at normal performance levels (A–B). Consequently, serum creatinine concentration at the upper end of normal, particularly among small patients, hypertensives, diabetics and those on angiotensin-converting enzyme (ACE) inhibitors, is a warning that they might be at the limit of compensation.

Normovolaemia

The first precondition of the 'renal rescue protocol' is achievement of optimum intravascular volume. Fluid loading has the immediate effect of reducing release of aldosterone and anti-diuretic hormone (ADH) and stimulates ANP production. Ramamoorthy et al. demonstrated that aggressive fluid loading reversed the fall in urine output, sodium excretion and ANP levels caused by positive-pressure ventilation [28]. The seemingly simple task of achieving normovolaemia is complicated by the absence of any reliable measurement that confirms normovolaemia for an individual patient. Common guides to volume status are based on dynamic measurements of right atrial and pulmonary artery occlusion pressures (PAOP). The derivation of volume from pressure is complicated by differences in myocardial compliance, venous tone and use of vasoconstrictors. However, even in a normal heart, right atrial pressure measurements in hypovolaemia can be misleading. Techniques for absolute measures of blood volume, eg double indicators or carbon monoxide haemoglobin labelling, are cumbersome for routine use and in the absence of reference to clinical signs still do not make judgement of normovolaemia any easier.

Far greater emphasis should be placed on clinical end points in individual patients during volume loading, such as warm dry torso, warmth of feet and decreasing heart rate, rather than on absolute central venous pressure (CVP). The filling pressures to achieve these clinical end points, in our experience, have not been predictable and are not the same for every patient. Many hypovolaemic patients develop high venous tone which may conceal their low volume state. When these patients are resuscitated it is not uncommon to see a rapid rise in PAOP or CVP which may be interpreted as overtransfusion when they are plainly still hypovolaemic (cold, tachycardic). The concomitant use of inotropes during fluid resuscitation can also be misleading by providing patients with 'perfect' filling pressures and blood pressures but with poorly perfused peripheries. Inotropes should be withheld until signs of clinical normovolaemia have been achieved and is accompanied by a reduction in base deficit.

In the protocol, rapid warm fluid loading is commenced *simultaneously* with a low-dose infusion of glyceryl trinitrate (GTN, 2 mg/h). The rationale of GTN infusion is to reduce venous tone and so reveal hypovolaemia. This approach may lead to the use of a substantial quantity of fluid to achieve a warm well-perfused periphery. GTN also provides nitric oxide to offset the effects of intrarenal ET in response to hypoxia. An alternative approach to chemical vasodilation is use of an external warming blanket (Bair Hugger). Patients with a poor myocardium may warm very slowly, particularly if fluid loading is cautious. Although either crystalloid or colloid solutions can be used, it is generally agreed that colloids are more effective, ie smaller volumes are needed initially to achieve the same clinical result.

Patient-related normotension

The second precondition is achievement of the patient's normal premorbid systolic blood pressure. Although RBF and GFR are autoregulated, urine production increases with blood pressure. This is a normal phenomenon known as pressure diuresis or natriuresis (Fig. 2). In addition, there is animal evidence from ischaemic ATN and sepsis models that autoregulation is impaired or absent, which implies that renal blood flow in these conditions may also be directly related to blood pressure. Sadly, the practice to allow septic patients to remain at pressures considered 'acceptable', often no more than 100 mmHg regardless of their premorbid blood pressure, is widespread and may worsen renal injury.

In the protocol, once normovolaemia is achieved, normal blood pressure is restored by titration with noradrenaline as quickly as possible (<5 min), to promote urine output. Care is taken to maintain warm peripheral temperature and a normal base deficit with GTN and fluids. In elderly hypertensive patients this can mean increasing systolic blood pressure to 180 mmHg or more. The advantages of noradrenaline over adrenaline, dopamine and dobutamine in a normovolaemic patient are lower heart rates, higher diastolic pressures (coronary perfusion) and fewer dysrhythmias. Noradrenaline should not be used without Swan Ganz guidance or outside an intensive care unit. When noradrenaline is titrated with a full circulation, normal blood pressure will be reached at normal systemic vascular

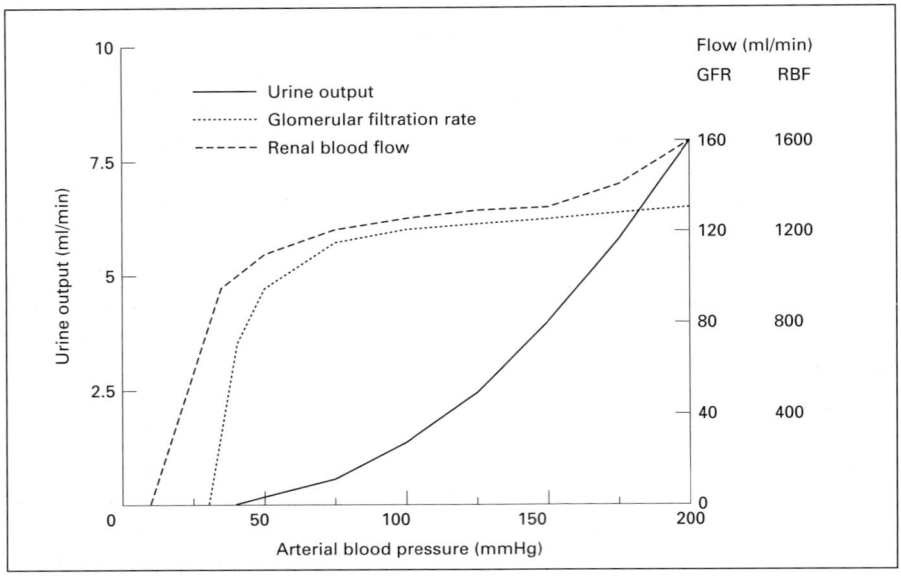

Fig. 2 The relationship between mean arterial blood pressure and renal blood flow (RBF), GFR and urine output.

resistance values for an individual patient. The dangers of increased afterload occur when the circulation is poorly repleted. Some patients with very poor myocardial performance (cardiac index <2.5 l/m²) may be unable to sustain both a normal arterial pressure and good peripheral perfusion. In these circumstances, careful use of a β-agonist such as dobutamine may be useful. Introduction of dobutamine should be as much guided by clinical signs as by numbers. A cardiac index of 2.5 l/m² may be acceptable in a well-perfused 80-year-old, but clearly not in a peripherally cold, fit young adult.

There have been many reports of the beneficial effect of noradrenaline on renal function including urine output, creatinine and free water clearance [29]. Indeed, Martin *et al.* in a prospective randomized double-blind trial comparing noradrenaline and dopamine for management of septic shock found that noradrenaline produced a significantly greater increase in urine output than dopamine [30].

The possible reasons for noradrenaline's effectiveness are diverse. It has been shown in man that afferent and efferent arteriolar resistances increase but efferent constriction dominates and accounts for the rise in filtration fraction. Noradrenaline also stimulates ANP release. The relative effects of ANP and direct noradrenaline action have not been separated.

Improving renal medullary oxygen tension

Once normovolaemia and normotension have been achieved, attention is directed towards improving renal medullary oxygen balance. Renal oxygen extraction ratio is low and suggests that oxygen delivery is more than adequate to meet consumption needs. However, in the outer medulla, pO_2 is low and oxygen supply is only just sufficient to meet demand. The low pO_2 is due to high oxygen utilization by Na⁺K⁺-ATPase in the thick ascending limb of the loop of Henle (mTAL) and a pO_2 counter-current mechanism similar to that for solutes. In this region the oxygen extraction ratio is as high as 79% compared with 8% for the kidney as a whole. Consequently oxygen availability and consumption in mTAL is highly susceptible to a reduction in oxygen delivery. Brezis *et al.* [31] demonstrated in an isolated perfused kidney preparation that inhibition of Na⁺K⁺-ATPase by ouabain reduced development of mTAL necrosis and increased medullary oxygen tension.

Frusemide reduces the activity of Na⁺K⁺2Cl⁻ co-transporter which reduces the need for Na⁺/K⁺-ATPase. Frusemide also increases renal PGE_2 concentrations, which results in peritubular capillary vasodilatation and inhibits mTAL metabolic activity. The sum of these effects is an improvement in medullary oxygen tension.

In the protocol, 10 mg frusemide is given as a bolus and continued as an infusion at 1–4 mg/h to promote better tubular oxygen balance. Failure to produce volumes of urine above 80 ml/h indicates that haemofiltration is likely to be required. Patients with a sustained urine response >150 ml/h for 4–5 days leads to a plateau in creatinine concentrations followed by a decrease. With urine outputs of this magnitude, losses of K⁺, Mg²⁺ and phosphate are high and need aggressive replacement. It is common for these electrolyte losses to precipitate atrial dysrhythmias: 4–8 g of magnesium and 200–300 mmol of potassium may be needed daily.

Anecdotal evidence in our institution has been sufficiently promising to explore the protocol in a randomized prospective controlled study currently in progress. Retrospective data for 1993 have shown that of 90 patients with creatinine >150 µmol/l, 49 patients went on to fulfil standard criteria for acute renal failure and need for haemofiltration (creatinine >360 µmol/l, urea >36 mmol/l, urine volume <480 ml/24 h). All were treated with the protocol; 32 patients did not require haemofiltration at any stage in their illness. Of the 17 that did, five were patients with diuretic supported chronic renal disease, one had gross aortic regurgitation and two were severely oliguric (<30 ml/day) for more than 24 h.

☐ CONCLUSION

The management of impending renal failure and techniques to provide protection of renal function, particularly in sepsis or after major surgery, have been disappointing. We have outlined a renal rescue protocol based on bedside clinical signs and physiological principles, which for many patients provides sufficient urine output to avoid the need for haemofiltration and its attendant risks and costs. The protocol includes achievement of two preconditions, patient-related normovolaemia and normotension and the use of a low-dose frusemide infusion to improve oxygen balance in the renal medulla. Failure to respond with this approach will require renal support; this is most likely in the more severely ill patients in whom there is often little one can do until the precipitating condition is cured.

REFERENCES

1. Kramer P, Kaufhold G, Grone H. Management of anuric intensive care patients with arteriovenous hemofiltration. *Int J Artif Organs* 1980; **3**: 225–30.
2. Klehr H, Kaschell H, Kuckenbecker C, *et al.* Clinical result of continuous arteriovenous hemofiltration. In: Sieberth H, Mann H, eds. *Continuous Hemofiltration.* Basel: Karger, 1985: 159–65.
3. Weiss L, Danielson B, Wikstrom B, *et al.* Continuous arteriovenous haemofiltration in the treatment of 100 critically ill patients with acute renal failure: report on clinical outcome and nutritional aspects. *Clin Nephrol* 1987; **31**: 184–9.
4. Stevens P, Davies S, Brown E, *et al.* Continuous arteriovenous haemodialysis in critically ill patients. *Lancet* 1988; **ii**: 150–2.
5. Wendon J, Smithies M, Sheppard M, *et al.* Continuous high volume veno-venous hemofiltration in acute renal failure. *Intensive Care Med* 1989; **15**: 358–63.
6. Storck M, Hartl W, Zimmerer E, *et al.* Comparison of pump-driven and spontaneous continuous haemofiltration in postoperative acute renal failure. *Lancet* 1990; **337**: 452–5.
7. Macias W, Mueller B, Scarim S, *et al.* Continuous venovenous hemofiltration: an alternative to continuous arteriovenous hemofiltration and hemodiafiltration in acute renal failure. *Am J Kidney Dis* 1991; **18**: 451–8.
8. Myles P, Buckland M, Schenk N, *et al.* Effect of 'renal dose' dopamine on renal function following cardiac surgery. *Anaesth Intensive Care* 1993; **21**: 56–61.
9. Duke G, Briedis J, Weaver R. Renal support in critically ill patients: low-dose dopamine or low-dose dobutamine? *Crit Care Med* 1994; **22**: 1919–25.
10. Swygert T, Roberts L, Valek T, Brajtbord D, Brown M, Gunning T, Paulsen A, Ramsay M. Effect of intraoperative low-dose dopamine on renal function in liver transplant recipients. *Anesthesiology* 1991; **75**: 571–6.

11 Duggan K, Macdonald G, Charlesworth J, et al. Verapamil prevents post-transplant oliguric renal failure. *Clin Nephrol* 1985; 7: 287–91.

12 Wagner K, Albrecht S, Neumayer H-H. Prevention of post-transplant acute tubular necrosis by the calcium antagonist diltiazem: a prospective randomised study. *Am J Nephrol* 1987; 7: 287–91.

13 Sands J, Neylan J, Olson R, O'Brien D, Whelchel J, Mitch W. Atrial natriuretic factor does not improve the outcome of cadaveric renal transplantation. *J Am Soc Nephrol* 1991; 1: 1081–6.

14 Rahman SN, Kim GE, Mathew AS, Goldberg CA, Allgren R, Schrier RW, Conger JD. Effects of atrial natriuretic peptide in clinical acute renal failure. *Kidney Int* 1994; 45: 1731–8.

15 Tiggeler R, Berden J, Hoitsma A, Koene R. Prevention of acute tubular necrosis in cadaveric kidney transplantation by the combined use of mannitol and moderate hydration. *Ann Surg* 1984; 201: 246–51.

16 Weimar W, Geerlings W, Bijnen A, et al. A controlled study on the effect of mannitol on immediate renal function after cadaveric donor kidney transplantation. *Transplantation* 1983; 35: 99–101.

17 Solomon R, Werner C, Mann D, D'Elia J, Silva P. Effects of saline, mannitol and furosemide to prevent acute decreases in renal function induced by radiocontrast agents. *New Engl J Med* 1994; 331: 1416–20.

18 Kleinknecht D, Ganeval D, Gonzalez-Duque L, et al. Furosemide in acute oliguric renal failure: a controlled trial. *Nephron* 1976; 17: 51–8.

19 Brown C, Ogg C, Cameron J. High dose frusemide in acute renal failure: a controlled trial. *Clin Nephrol* 1981; 15: 90–6.

20 Vincent J. Renal effects of dopamine: can our dream ever come true? (editorial). *Crit Care Med* 1994; 22: 5–6.

21 Henderson I, Beattie T, Kennedy A. Dopamine hydrochloride in oliguric states. *Lancet* 1980; ii: 827–8.

22 Lindner A. Synergism of dopamine and furosemide in diuretic resistant oliguric acute renal failure. *Nephron* 1983; 33: 121–6.

23 Brown C, Ogg C, Cameron J. High dose frusemide in acute renal failure: a controlled trial. *Clin Nephrol* 1981; 15: 90–6.

24 Gubern J, Sancho J, Simo J, Sitges-Serra A. A randomized trial on the effect of mannitol on postoperative renal function in patients with obstructive jaundice. *Surgery* 1988; 103: 39–44.

25 Paul M, Mazer C, Byrick R, Rose D, Goldstein M. Influence of mannitol and dopamine on renal function during elective infrarenal aortic clamping in man. *Am J Nephrol* 1986; 6: 427–34.

26 Rahman SN, Kim GE, Mathew AS, et al. Effects of atrial natriuretic peptide in clinical acute renal failure. *Kidney Int* 1994; 45: 1731–8.

27 Hummel M, Kuhn M, Bub A, et al. Urodilatin, a new therapy to prevent kidney failure after heart transplantation. *J Heart Lung Transpl* 1993; 12: 209–17.

28 Ramamoorthy C, Rooney M, Dries D, Mathru M. Aggressive hydration during continuous positive-pressure ventilation restores atrial transmural pressure, plasma atrial natriuretic peptide concentrations, and renal function. *Crit Care Med* 1992; 20: 1014–9.

29 Desjars P, Pinaud M, Bugnon D, Tasseau F. Norepinephrine therapy has no deleterious renal effects in human septic shock. *Crit Care Med* 1989; 17: 426–9.

30 Martin C, Papazian L, Perrin G, Saux P, Gouin F. Norepinephrine or dopamine for the treatment of hyperdynamic septic shock. *Chest* 1993; 103: 1826–31.

31 Brezis M, Agmon Y, Epstein F. Determinants of intrarenal oxygenation. I. Effects of diuretics. *Am J Physiol* 1994; 36: F1059–F1062.

☐ MULTIPLE CHOICE QUESTIONS

1 Dopamine:
  (a) Is a diuretic
  (b) Inhibits Na^+K^+-ATPase

(c) Is an endogenous product
(d) Has been shown to reduce the need for haemofiltration
(e) Causes release of renal PGE_2

2. Frusemide:
   (a) Causes release of renal PGE_2
   (b) Inhibits Na^+K^+-ATPase
   (c) Inhibits Na^+K^+ $2Cl^-$ co-transporter
   (d) Improves medullary thick ascending loop of Henle pO_2
   (e) In large doses prevents acute renal failure

3. Noradrenaline:
   (a) Is predominantly a beta-agonist
   (b) Is likely to cause more supraventricular tachyarrhythmias than dobutamine
   (c) Raises systolic and diastolic pressure
   (d) Always decreases cardiac output
   (e) Has been associated with increased glomerular filtration fraction

4. Haemofiltration:
   (a) Is associated with haemorrhage
   (b) May initially worsen acidosis
   (c) May result in a metabolic alkalosis
   (d) May remove cytokines
   (e) May generate cytokines

5. Acute renal failure:
   (a) The major cause in persistent hypovolaemia
   (b) Is infrequently caused by NSAIDs alone
   (c) Is associated with a 30% increase of hospital mortality in the critically ill
   (d) Is reversible in the vast majority of cases
   (e) Renal blood flow autoregulation remains unaltered

ANSWERS

1a True	2a True	3a False	4a True	5a True
b True	b False	b False	b True	b True
c True	c True	c True	c True	c True
d False	d True	d False	d True	d True
e False	e False	e True	e True	e False

Urinary tract infection

C R V Tomson

☐ INTRODUCTION

Urinary infection is a cause of significant morbidity and is a frequent cause of consultations in general practice. Asymptomatic bacteriuria is associated with increased mortality in elderly people, although whether this is cause or effect is unknown. Occasionally, urinary infection can cause life-threatening illnesses in previously healthy adults.

This review concentrates on selected aspects of the clinical management of urinary infection in adults. Information from existing reviews, eg [1,2], MedLine searches, and reference lists of original papers has been reviewed with an emphasis on interventions of proven value in the prevention or treatment of urinary infection.

☐ DIAGNOSIS

Urinary tract infection (UTI) is normally defined as the presence of bacteria in bladder urine. (The exception to this rule is localized upper tract infection, for instance a perirenal abscess.) The problem with making the diagnosis of UTI is that urine is frequently contaminated during micturition. Less than 2% of mid-stream urine samples taken from women are sterile. Culture of mid-stream urine therefore requires careful interpretation. Since the work of Kass in the 1950s, a colony count of $>10^5$ organisms per ml has been taken as 'significant' bacteriuria, anything less being considered as due to contamination. However, these criteria were validated in asymptomatic women, voiding without special precautions to avoid contamination. More recent work has shown that, in symptomatic women and in men, lower counts are often significant.

The accepted 'gold standard' for the detection of bladder bacteriuria is suprapubic aspiration of the bladder. Bladder urine may also be obtained by catheterization, although this procedure carries a 1–2% risk of introducing infection. Using a combination of these techniques in women with acute dysuria and frequency, Stamm *et al.* [3] showed a close correlation between the colony count in bladder urine and that in mid-stream urine specimens (Figs 1, 2) and suggested a diagnostic cut-off of 10^3 organisms per ml.

These findings should not detract from the importance of careful precautions to avoid contamination when mid-stream urine samples are obtained. In women these should include careful cleaning of the vulva and manual parting of the labia during passage of urine. In men, retraction of the foreskin may prevent contamination.

Although the absence of pyuria should cause suspicion that a pure growth of a uropathogen is due to contamination, suprapubic aspiration and catheter studies

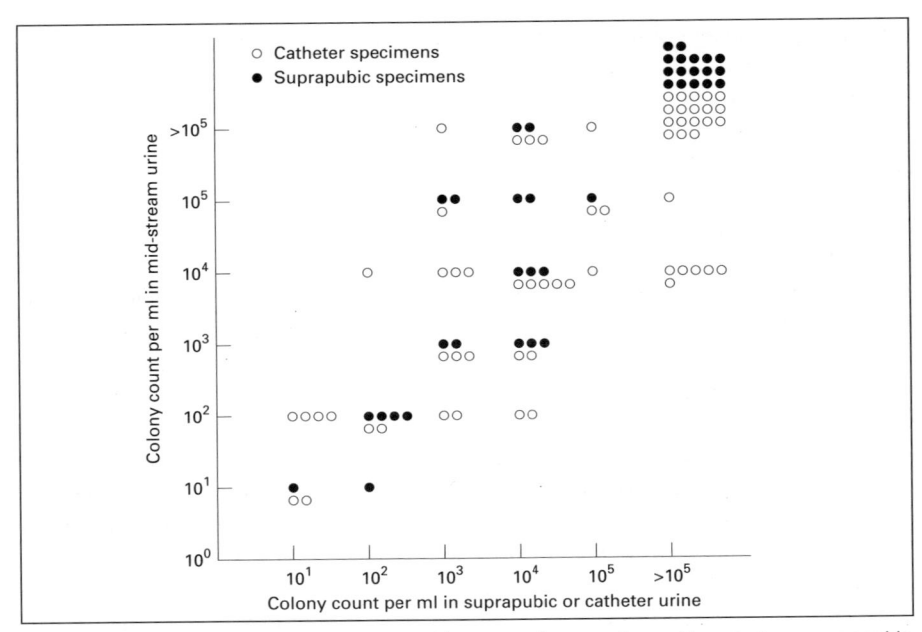

Fig. 1 Correlation between colony counts in mid-stream urine samples and in catheter or suprapubic aspiration samples in 98 women with acute frequency and dysuria. (From Stamm et al. [3].)

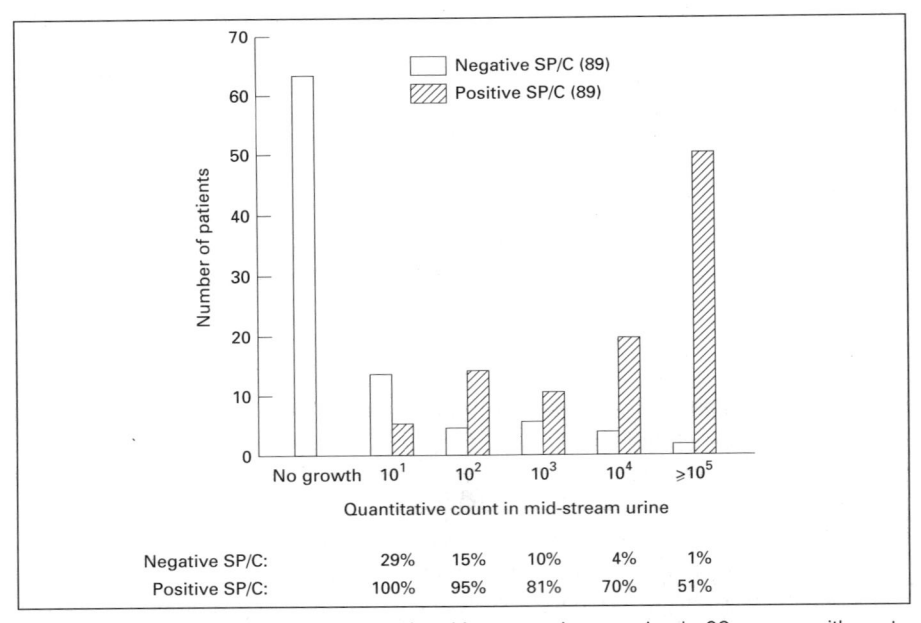

Fig. 2 Distribution of quantitative counts in mid-stream urine samples in 98 women with acute frequency and dysuria, split according to the presence or absence of true bladder bacteriuria as detected by suprapubic aspiration or catheterization (SP/C). Relying on a cut-off of 10^5 organisms per ml would falsely classify 51% of patients with bladder bacteriuria as non-infected. Figures below the graph indicate the cumulative percentages of patients included as the diagnostic standard is lowered from ≥105 to 101 organisms per ml of mid-stream urine. (From Stamm et al. [3].)

have shown bladder bacteriuria in some such cases in symptomatic women; this occurs either in the early stages of infection or because of laboratory errors in the detection of pyuria.

☐ LOCALIZATION OF URINARY TRACT INFECTIONS

Lower UTI (cystitis) is common and responds rapidly to treatment. In contrast, upper UTI may be difficult to eradicate and may be a pointer to anatomical abnormalities. Differentiation between upper and lower tract infection is therefore important. Clinical symptoms are unreliable in this regard: up to 50% of patients with confirmed lower UTI have flank pain and fever, symptoms that may be absent from patients with confirmed upper tract infection [4]. The 'gold standard' is selective ureteric catheterization, which requires cystoscopy and is rarely performed. Alternative diagnostic tests are available.

The Fairley test involves culture of bladder urine following catheterization, followed by a bladder washout with antiseptics and fibrinolytic enzymes, followed by further urine cultures during a water diuresis. Rapid re-appearance of organisms suggests upper UTI, but does not identify which side is infected.

Tests for antibody-coated bacteria are not routinely available and are of questionable validity.

Rising serum titres of antibodies to urinary pathogens or to Tamm–Horsfall glycoprotein are seen in upper tract infection but are of less use in recurrent upper tract infection.

The detection of white cell casts on phase-contrast microscopy is diagnostic of renal inflammation (Fig. 3).

The urethral syndrome

The term 'urethral syndrome' is generally used for the combination of frequency and dysuria with the absence of significant counts of a known urinary pathogen, ie 'culture-negative cystitis'. Situations in which this may occur include the following:

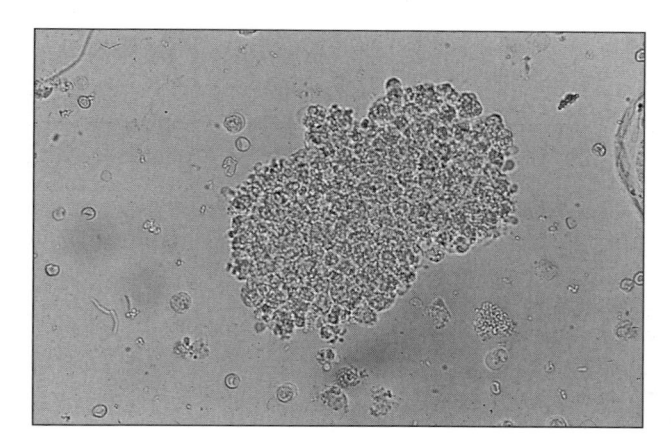

Fig. 3 White cell cast from a patient with acute pyelonephritis. Casts have straight edges, and must be distinguished from the white cell clumps that can occur in cystitis.

- ☐ the early stages of bacterial cystitis
- ☐ bacterial cystitis in a patient maintaining a high fluid intake
- ☐ urinary infection with an organism not usually recognized as a urinary pathogen or which does not grow on routine urine culture
- ☐ sexually acquired urethritis
- ☐ non-infective urethral inflammation

A role for paraurethral infection by lactobacilli has been suggested, but this remains controversial. A high proportion of women with urethral syndrome and pyuria have chlamydial urethritis and respond to appropriate antibiotics, eg doxycycline [5]. Sexual partners of patients suspected to have chlamydial infection should also be treated.

☐ RISK FACTORS FOR URINARY INFECTION

Numerous alterations in host defence can increase susceptibility to urinary infection.

Stasis

Stasis of urine permits bacterial replication in urine, which is an ideal culture medium for many bacteria. Stasis may result from scarring, eg reflux nephropathy, obstructive uropathy, or impaired bladder emptying, eg neurogenic bladder.

Foreign bodies

Foreign bodies in the urinary tract impair host defence – for instance urinary catheters, indwelling urinary tract stents, and urinary stones.

Blood group antigens

Susceptibility to coliform UTI depends on how well uropathogenic bacteria can adhere to cell-surface carbohydrate antigens. Increased susceptibility to urinary infections has been found in women with the Lewis non-secretor and recessive phenotypes. Acute pyelonephritis in children without reflux has been associated with the P1 blood group phenotype [6].

Sexual activity

Epidemiological studies show a close relationship between acute cystitis and sexual intercourse. Use of a diaphragm or condom and use of spermicidal gels have also been associated with increased risk (Fig. 4) [7]. Failure to empty the bladder after intercourse has also been associated with an increased risk of urinary infection.

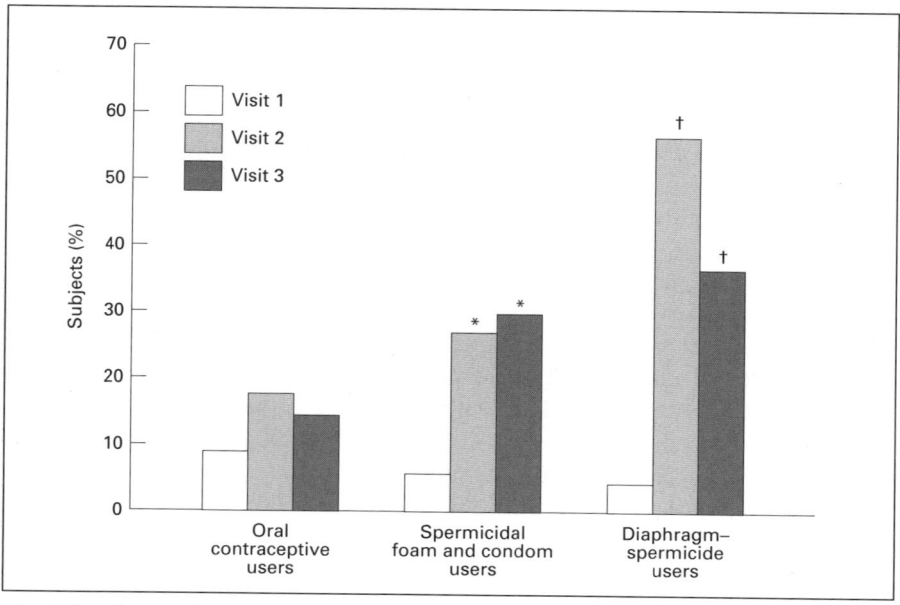

Fig. 4 Prevalence of *Escherichia coli* bacteriuria in 104 women before (visit 1), the morning after (visit 2), and 24 hours after sexual intercourse (visit 3), according to contraceptive method. *$p<0.01$ compared with prevalence at visit 1; †$p<0.001$. (From Hooton et al. [7].)

Periurethral colonization

Periurethral colonization by uropathogens is closely associated with subsequent cystitis. In healthy women, production of lactic acid by lactobacilli maintains a low vaginal pH, which inhibits such colonization. Oestrogen deficiency and inappropriate antibiotic treatment reduce growth of lactobacilli and thus may impair host defence.

☐ TREATMENT OF URINARY TRACT INFECTIONS

Uncomplicated UTIs (ie lower UTIs in women with normal bladder anatomy and emptying) may clear during symptomatic treatment alone. If treatment is required, a single high dose of antibiotic may be sufficient, although relapse rates are lower after a 3-day course. Symptoms persist for 2–3 days after eradication of bacterial infection. Laboratory confirmation of uncomplicated cystitis is not usually cost-effective, given that treatment will normally have been completed by the time the results are available. In this situation, the main role of the laboratory is to advise on the most appropriate antibiotic, taking into account local data on bacterial antibiotic resistance.

The ideal duration of treatment in acute pyelonephritis is uncertain. A 14-day course of an appropriate antibiotic is usually recommended, monitoring temperature and C-reactive protein to assess response.

In patients with prostatitis or with infection of 'protected' regions of the urinary tract, such as renal cysts, 6 weeks treatment with an antibiotic that is known to penetrate tissues well (eg ciprofloxacin) is often necessary.

Patients with indwelling urinary catheters have 'inevitable bacteriuria' and should not be treated unless symptomatic. The infecting organisms change frequently, so there is no point in performing regular urine cultures in asymptomatic patients so as to be able to choose an antibiotic when symptoms do develop. There is a high rate of acquired resistance if prolonged courses of antibiotics are used in this situation. Similarly, urine infection in patients with urinary tract stones is ineradicable unless the stones are cleared.

Treatment of asymptomatic infection is seldom justified apart from in pregnancy, when there is a greatly increased risk of ascending infection. Urine should be cultured when booking-in all pregnant women, asymptomatic infections treated, and clearance of infection confirmed by a post-treatment urine culture. Recurrent infection should be treated and followed by antibiotic prophylaxis. There is no evidence that the treatment of asymptomatic urinary infections in adults with reflux nephropathy or in patients with polycystic kidney disease alters the progression of chronic renal failure.

Long-term prophylaxis

Long-term low-dose antibiotic prophylaxis is widely used in women who experience frequent recurrences of cystitis despite a high fluid intake, careful attention to perineal hygiene, voiding after intercourse, and care in ensuring complete bladder emptying. Although numerous studies using historical control groups or patients as their own controls suggest that this form of treatment is highly effective, only a few randomized placebo-controlled trials have been reported. These have confirmed the efficacy of nightly or postcoital prophylaxis (Fig. 5) [8].

If treatment is discontinued after 6 months, the risk of recurrence appears to return to pre-treatment levels. However, for reasons that are unclear, prophylaxis for 9–12 months appears to be followed by a sustained reduction in recurrent cystitis [2].

The ideal prophylactic antibiotic would have the following properties:

- ☐ minimal toxicity
- ☐ cheapness
- ☐ activity against most common urinary pathogens
- ☐ low incidence of vaginal candidiasis
- ☐ adequate concentration in urine or periurethral fluid
- ☐ low rate of development of bacterial resistance

Nitrofurantoin

This antibiotic has been widely used in long-term prophylaxis. Because it is so well absorbed, very little reaches the colon, and development of resistance among faecal

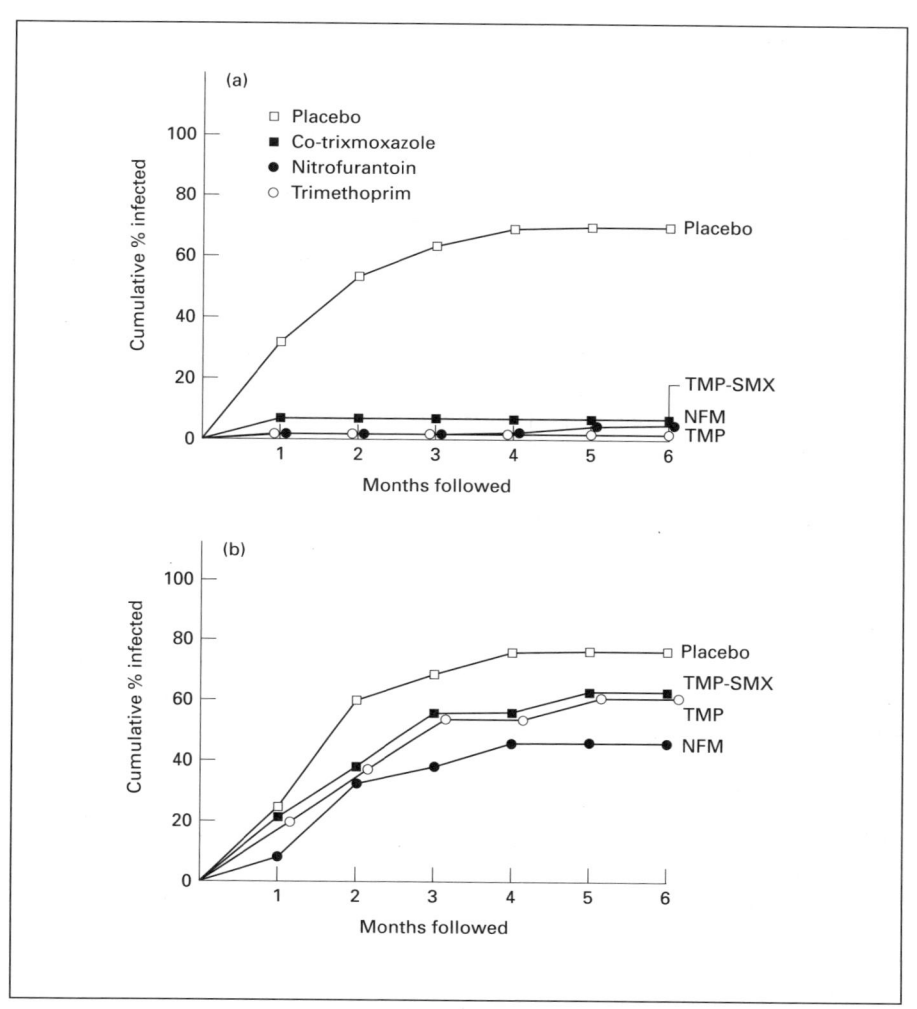

Fig. 5 Cumulative incidence of bacteriologically proven urinary tract infections in women with recurrent cystitis randomized to placebo (n = 15), co-trimoxazole (n = 15), macrocrystalline nitrofurantoin (n = 15) or trimethoprim (n = 15). (a) During treatment; (b) 6 months after drug treatment was stopped. (From Stamm et al. [8].)

flora is rare. However, the possibility of hepatic and pulmonary toxicity makes long-term treatment undesirable.

Trimethoprim

This antibiotic is secreted into vaginal fluid by ion trapping and thus achieves high local concentrations, resulting in eradication of periurethral colonization by coliforms. Toxicity is rare. Despite increasing resistance rates, breakthrough infection is relatively rare, and this is the drug of first choice.

Co-trimoxazole

This drug is no longer licensed for use in urinary infection owing to the toxicity of the sulphonamide component.

Quinolones

Quinolones such as ciprofloxacin achieve high tissue penetration and high urinary levels, but are expensive; development of resistant faecal flora is an increasing problem.

There is little experience with other antibiotics in long-term prophylaxis. There is no evidence that 'rotating' regimens are necessary; selection of resistant organisms is only a problem with long-term low-dose prophylaxis if there is persistent infection due to anatomical abnormalities, rather than recurrent re-infection.

Methenamine

Methenamine (mandelate or hippurate) releases formaldehyde in acid urine, thus delivering a potent antiseptic to the site of bacterial multiplication. Resistance to formaldehyde does not occur. One small double-blind trial has shown a reduction in recurrence of acute cystitis in women treated with methenamine hippurate, without formal attempts to ensure urine acidification. This agent has become unfashionable, but deserves further study.

☐ PREVENTION OF URINARY INFECTION

In patients with normal urinary tracts, host defence against infection may be enhanced by ensuring frequent and complete bladder emptying; a high fluid intake may help by increasing frequency of micturition. Voiding after sexual intercourse and avoidance of spermicidal gels are also justified.

Oestrogen replacement in postmenopausal women has been shown in several studies to decrease the rate of recurrent urinary infections, probably by restoring normal vaginal colonization by lactobacilli (Fig. 6) [9].

Cranberry juice has been a folk remedy for cystitis for years. Recent studies have suggested that a component of cranberry juice inhibits adherence of uropathogenic *Escherichia coli* to the bladder mucosa. Recently a randomized controlled trial showed that daily ingestion of 300 ml of commercially available cranberry juice significantly reduced the rate of urinary infection in elderly women, compared to ingestion of a placebo drink identical in taste, appearance and ascorbic acid content (Fig. 7) [10].

Infection stones

Stones made of magnesium ammonium phosphate, which may grow to occupy the whole renal pelvis ('staghorn' calculi) are one of the most serious complications of urine infection as they can cause renal failure by a combination of obstruction and

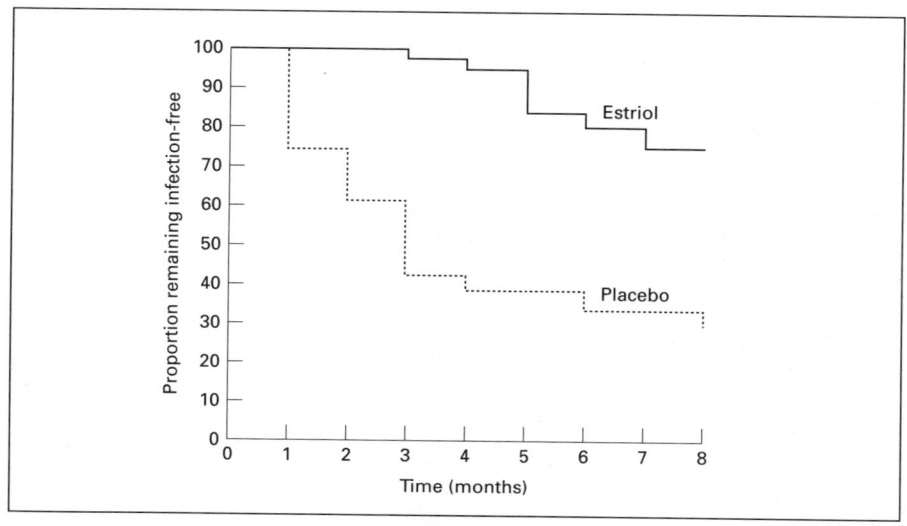

Fig. 6 Cumulative proportion of postmenopausal women with a history of recurrent UTI remaining free of infection during treatment with intravaginal estriol cream or placebo ($p<0.001$). (From Raz and Stamm [9].)

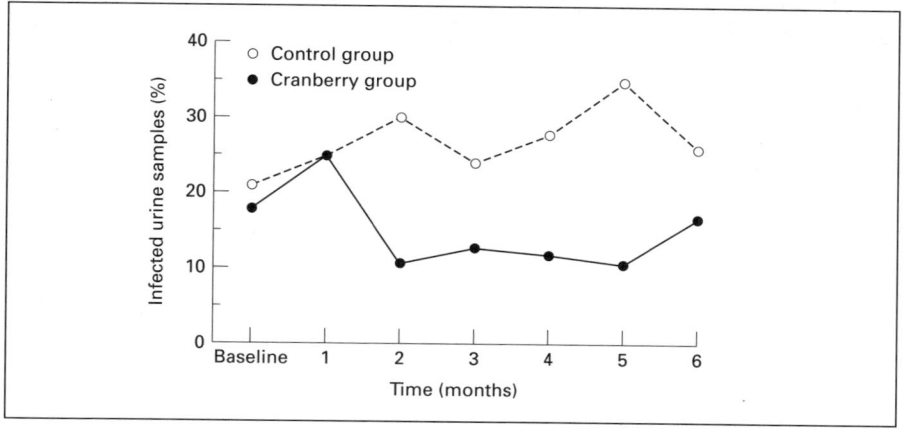

Fig. 7 Incidence of bacteriuria in mid-stream urine samples from 153 elderly women randomized to daily intake of 300 ml cranberry juice or to a placebo identical in taste, ascorbic acid content and appearance. The odds of subjects taking cranberry juice having bacteriuria with pyuria were 42% of those in the control group ($p = 0.004$) and those patients were also more likely to clear asymptomatic infection by the next month than the control group. (From Avorn et al. [10].)

infective scarring (Fig. 8). They are caused by persistent urine infection with urease-producing organisms such as *Proteus* spp, and commonly occur in patients predisposed to persistent urine infection by stasis within the urinary tract. Urease inhibitors (including hydroxyurea, acetohydroxamic acid and propionhydroxamic acid) reduce the formation and growth of infection stones, but all are considered too

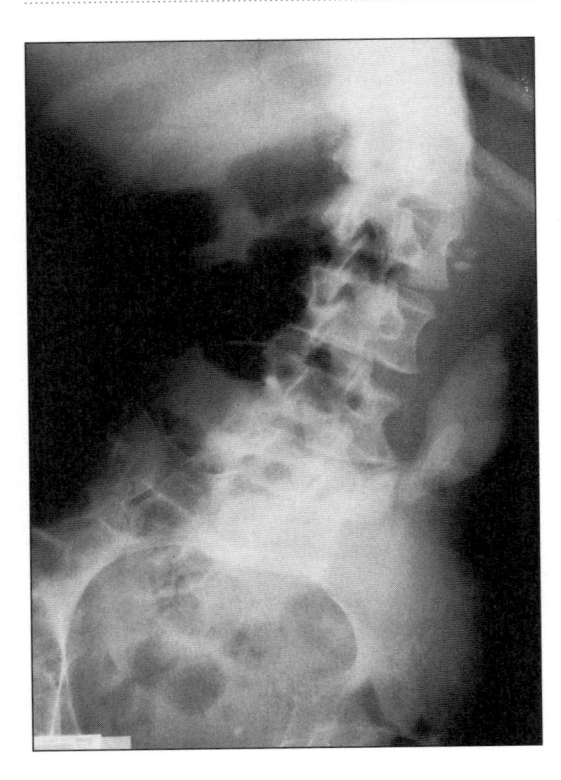

Fig. 8 Staghorn calculus in a patient with neurogenic bladder following spinal cord injury. The patient presented with septicaemic shock and severe renal impairment, and now has stable chronic renal impairment after stone clearance, having been taught intermittent self-catheterization.

toxic for routine use. Successful surgical treatment of staghorn calculi is necessary to eradicate infection, and should be covered by antibiotic prophylaxis and followed by a concerted attempt to prevent re-infection, including attempts to prevent stagnation of urine, and consideration of long-term antibiotic prophylaxis.

☐ URINE INFECTIONS IN PATIENTS WITH ABNORMAL BLADDERS

Impaired bladder emptying, for instance in spina bifida, after spinal cord injury, or complicating bladder reconstruction, is an important cause of urine infection and, occasionally, of progressive renal damage caused by obstruction and ascending infection. Management with long-term bladder catheterization is complicated by 'inevitable bacteriuria'. Long-term prophylactic antibiotics are ineffective, with a high rate of side effects and of acquired resistance. Asymptomatic infections should not be treated.

Clean intermittent self-catheterization has revolutionized the care of many patients with impaired bladder emptying. Most patients can be taught to catheterize themselves; re-usable catheters, which must be kept clean but do not have to be sterile, are available. In most patients this is preferable to construction of an ileal conduit.

Methenamine with ammonium chloride has been shown in one study to result in significantly reduced rates of infection over a relatively short period of follow-up (Fig. 9) [11]; long-term studies have not been performed.

Investigation of patients with recurrent UTI

In females with recurrent cystitis the yield from investigation with intravenous urography and cystoscopy is low. Recurrent re-infection should be differentiated from persistent or relapsing infection by typing organisms identified in pre- and post-treatment urine cultures. Investigation should be reserved for patients with atypical features [12], including the following:

- ☐ persistent infection (especially with *Proteus* spp)
- ☐ acute pyelonephritis
- ☐ persistent haematuria
- ☐ unusual organism or genuine mixed growth
- ☐ evidence of renal disease – hypertension, proteinuria, impaired renal function

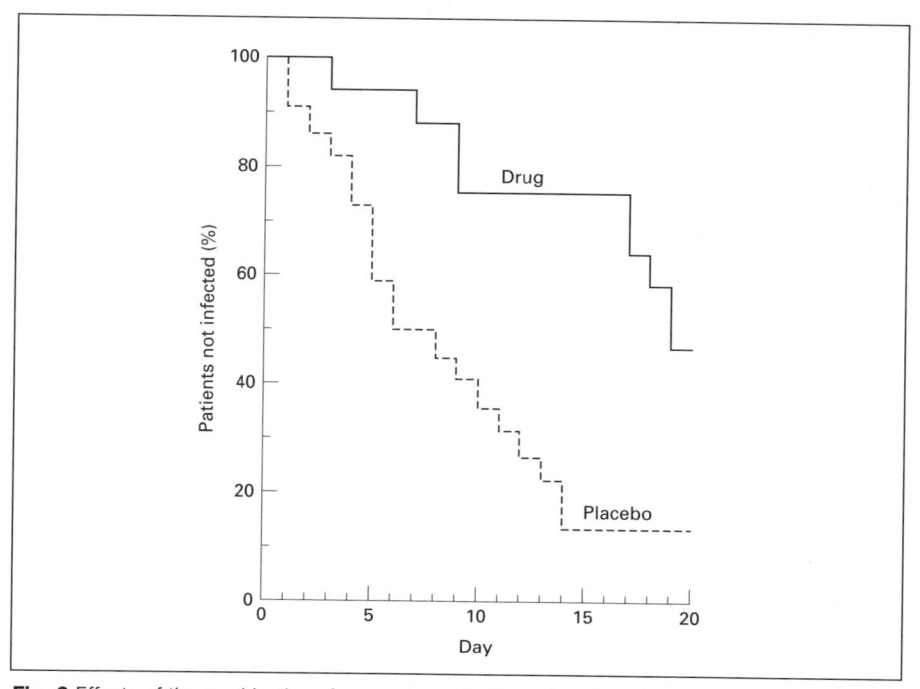

Fig. 9 Effects of the combination of ammonium chloride and methenamine mandelate compared to placebo in patients with neurogenic bladder during a period of bladder re-training and learning intermittent self-catheterization. Of those patients receiving the active drug, 53% developed infection during the 21-day period compared to 86% of those receiving placebo ($p<0.02$). (From Kevorkian et al. [11] © 1991–4 American Medical Association).

- history of childhood urinary infections
- family history of reflux nephropathy

It is conventional to recommend investigation for an underlying cause in all men with proven UTI. However, urological investigation is rarely rewarding in men under 50 who respond to treatment [1]. Chronic prostatitis should be considered in men with persistent frequency and dysuria, particularly in the presence of low counts of organisms on urine culture.

Impaired bladder emptying is an important treatable cause of recurrent urine infection, and is most reliably detected by ultrasound examination of the bladder after voiding. This simple test should be considered in any patient in whom urine infections recur despite advice on preventive measures.

Vesicoureteric reflux in adults allows persistence of residual urine in the bladder after micturition. Patients thought to have reflux (which may be intermittent) should be advised to void the bladder again 5 minutes or so after passing urine. The role of anti-reflux surgery in adults is unproven.

Renal damage resulting from urine infection

Renal scarring caused by the combination of urine infection and vesicoureteric reflux – so-called 'reflux nephropathy' or 'chronic pyelonephritis' – is very rare after the age of 5. In adults with established reflux nephropathy there is no evidence that treatment of asymptomatic urinary infections alters the risk or rate of progressive renal damage. However, urine infection can cause severe renal damage in the presence of obstruction (including that caused by stones), in diabetics, and in patients taking non-steroidal anti-inflammatory drugs [2]. Although defects in uptake of contrast media or isotope label can be demonstrated by computerized tomography (CT) or ^{99}Tc-labelled dimercaptosuccinic acid (DMSA) scanning in patients with acute pyelonephritis, in the absence of any of these complicating conditions, reports of significant loss of renal function as a result of adult acute pyelonephritis are very rare indeed.

REFERENCES

1. Stamm WE, Hooton TM. Management of UTIs in adults. *New Engl J Med* 1993; **329**: 1328–34.
2. Cattell WR, ed. *Urinary Tract Infection.* Oxford: Oxford University Press, 1996.
3. Stamm WE, Counts GW, Running KR, Finn S, Turck M, Holmes KK. Diagnosis of coliform infection in acutely dysuric women. *New Engl J Med* 1982; **307**: 463–8.
4. Busch R, Huland H. Correlation of symptoms and results of direct bacterial localization in patients with urinary tract infections. *J Urol* 1984; **132**: 282–5.
5. Stamm WE, Running K, McKevitt M, Counts GW, Turck M, Holmes KK. Treatment of the acute urethral syndrome. *New Engl J Med* 1981; **304**: 956–8.
6. Schoolnik GK. How *Escherichia coli* infects the urinary tract. *New Engl J Med* 1989; **320**: 804–5.
7. Hooton TM, Hillier S, Johnson C, Roberts PL, Stamm WE. *Escherichia coli* bacteriuria and contraceptive method. *J Am Med Assoc* 1991; **265**: 64–9.
8. Stamm WE, Counts GW, Wagner KF, *et al.* Antibiotic prophylaxis of recurrent urinary tract infections. *Ann Intern Med* 1980; **92**: 770–5.

9 Raz R, Stamm WE. A controlled trial of intravaginal estriol in postmenopausal women with recurrent urinary tract infections. *New Engl J Med* 1993; **329**: 753–6.
10 Avorn J, Gurwitz JH, Glynn RJ, Choodnovskiy I, Lipsitz LA. Reduction of bacteriuria and pyuria after ingestion of cranberry juice. *J Am Med Assoc* 1994; **271**: 751–4.
11 Kevorkian CG, Merritt JL, Ilstrup DM. Methenamine mandelate with acidification: an effective urinary antiseptic in patients with neurogenic bladder. *Mayo Clin Proc* 1984; **59**: 523–9.
12 Maskell R. Management of recurrent urinary tract infections in adults. *Prescribers J* 1995; **35**: 1–11.

☐ MULTIPLE CHOICE QUESTIONS

1 In a woman with recurrent cystitis:
   (a) Intravaginal oestrogen may reduce the rate at which infections recur if the patient is postmenopausal
   (b) Isolation of the same organism, with the same antibiotic sensitivities, on each attack should prompt further investigation
   (c) Long-term antibiotic prophylaxis with trimethoprim results in the frequent emergence of resistant strains and is ineffective at preventing recurrence
   (d) Changing contraceptive method from diaphragm plus spermicide to oral contraceptive pill may reduce the rate of infections
   (e) Renal damage from recurrent pyelonephritis is extremely rare in the absence of stones or obstruction

2 In a patient with spina bifida and a neurogenic bladder:
   (a) Persistent infections with *Proteus* spp may lead to staghorn stone formation
   (b) The risk of urinary infection can be reduced by regular intermittent self-catheterization with non-sterile re-usable catheters
   (c) Long-term antibiotic prophylaxis is effective at preventing infection
   (d) Hydroxyurea may inhibit the growth of infection stones
   (e) Severe renal failure may result from the combination of painless high-pressure retention of urine and urine infection

ANSWERS

1a	True	2a	True
b	True	b	True
c	False	c	False
d	True	d	True
e	True	e	True

Hypertension and the kidney: villains and victims

J D Firth

☐ INTRODUCTION

Advanced renal disease causes high blood pressure. The majority of patients with, or approaching, end-stage renal failure (from whatever cause) require treatment for hypertension. Patients presenting with hypertension often also have impaired renal function, and those found by chance to have abnormal renal function often have elevated blood pressure, if only marginally so. Does one cause the other? The situation is confused, leading Klahr in an editorial to describe the kidney in hypertension as being both 'villain and victim' [1]. In this chapter I will endeavour to tackle two important questions regarding the complex relationship between hypertension and the kidney. First, does hypertension cause renal failure? Second, does treating hypertension delay the progression of renal disease and, if so, are all antihypertensive agents equally effective? A limited number of recent high-quality studies will be discussed in detail.

☐ DOES HYPERTENSION CAUSE RENAL FAILURE?

Essential hypertension presenting in the malignant phase is frequently associated with impaired renal function, and those with substantial impairment at presentation are likely to progress. In one study of 24 patients with this condition, the mean serum creatinine at presentation of the seven people who went on to develop end-stage renal failure was 448 μmol/l, compared to 169 μmol/l in the 17 patients who did not [2]. Patients with malignant hypertension usually progress to end-stage renal failure when the serum creatinine is above 250–300 μmol/l at the time of diagnosis; those with a presenting serum creatinine below this level usually, but not always, escape this fate (Fig. 1).

If the answer to the question 'Does malignant hypertension cause renal failure?' has been clear for many years, the answer to the sequel 'Does non-malignant essential hypertension cause renal failure?' has not been so until very recently. Data from the USA and European renal registries might seem to provide a ready answer; figures from the mid-1980s suggest that hypertension was the cause of renal failure in about 5% of those entering renal replacement therapy programmes, with some estimates putting the figure much higher, but this information cannot be taken at face value. The proportion of patients classified as having renal failure caused by essential hypertension varies markedly between countries, and between different units within the same country. The situation reflects the fact that there are no generally accepted criteria for deciding whether a patient presenting to a renal clinic

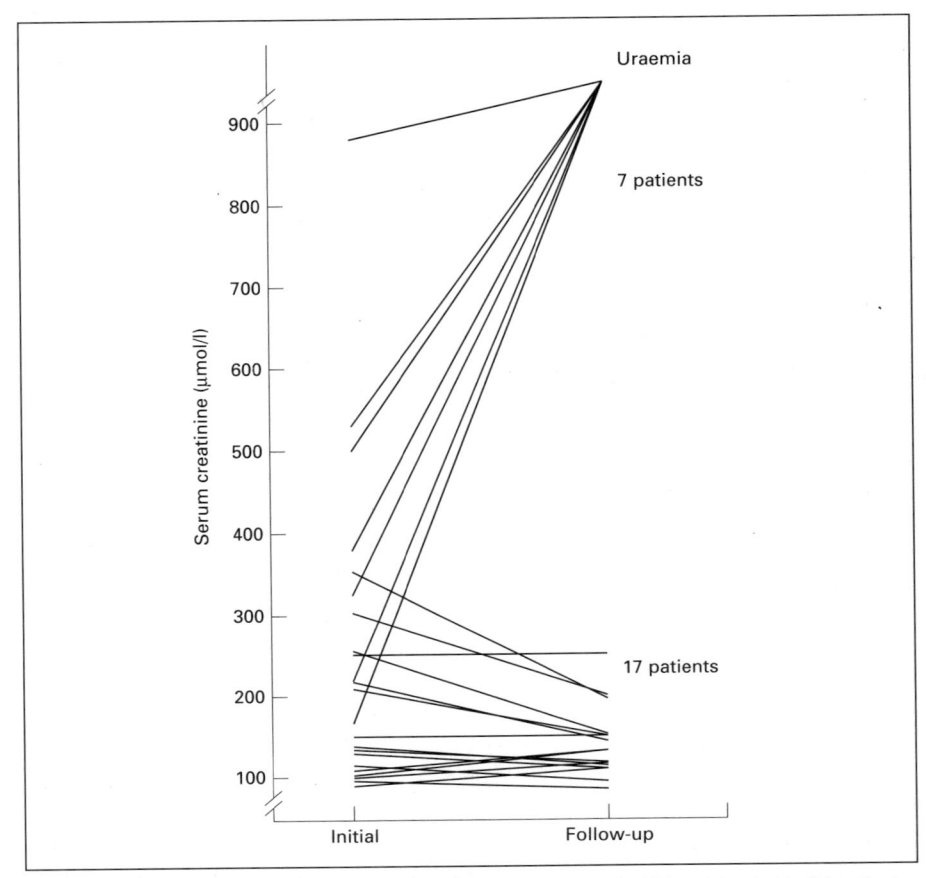

Fig. 1 Change in serum creatinine in the course of malignant essential hypertension in 24 patients. (From Herlitz *et al.* [2].)

with hypertension and significant renal impairment should be classified as having 'hypertensive renal failure' or 'renal failure, cause unknown' with hypertension as a complication.

It is well established from cross-sectional studies that, after maturity, glomerular filtration rate (GFR) declines with increasing age. The Baltimore Longitudinal Study on Aging was the first to track this decline systematically in a large cohort of individuals: between 1958 and 1981 five or more determinations of creatinine clearance rate were made in 446 participants. Multiple-regression analyses showed mean blood pressure to be an independent variable affecting the rate of decline of renal function. In the group as a whole, a significant correlation was found between it and the rate of decline of creatinine clearance over time: the higher the pressure, the faster the decline. Even when individuals with possible renal and/or urinary tract pathology and those treated with diuretic and/or antihypertensive agents were excluded, the relationship remained in the 254 'normal' subjects (Fig. 2) [3]. This study therefore demonstrates that the renal function of individuals with high blood

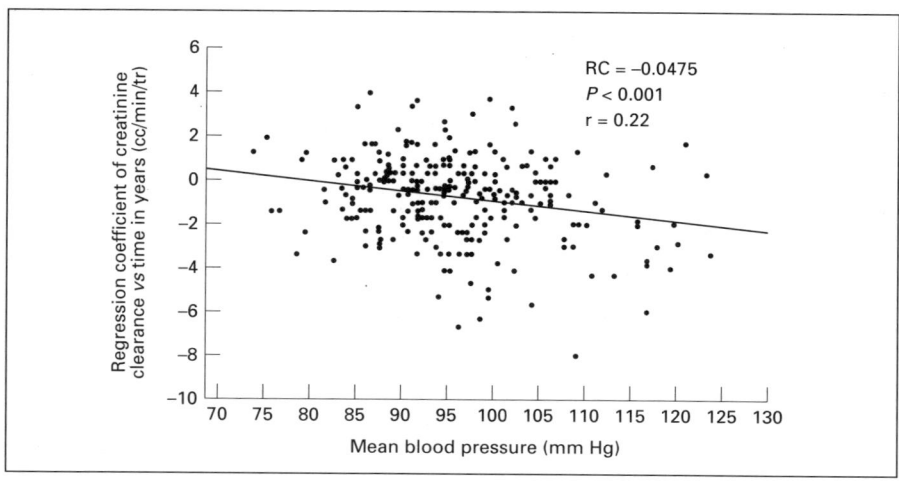

Fig. 2 Regression coefficient of creatinine clearance *vs* time in years plotted against mean blood pressure in 254 normal subjects. (From Lindeman et al. [3].)

pressure is likely to decline over the years at a faster rate than that of those with a lower blood pressure. It does not, however, demonstrate that the effect is a causal one.

The issue of causality was addressed, at least in part, by a prospective study of blood pressure and serum creatinine in 1399 individuals who had been fortuitously recruited into both the 'Clue' and ARIC (Atherosclerosis Risk in Communities) studies [4]. The 'Clue' study (from the slogan 'Give us a clue to cancer') was a cancer screening campaign conducted in 1974 in which individuals had their blood pressure measured. The ARIC study involved the measurement of blood pressure and serum creatinine level between 1986 and 1989. Both the serum creatinine level and the presence of hypercreatinaemia (arbitrarily defined as a serum creatinine level >115 µmol/l in men and >97 µmol/l in women) were better predicted by past rather than by current blood pressure. Creatinine values showed significant association with blood pressure recorded 12 to 15 years previously (the higher the blood pressure, the higher the creatinine), but not with blood pressure measured contemporaneously. This effect was observed across the range of 'normal' values of blood pressure and creatinine (Fig. 3), consistent with the hypothesis that elevated blood pressure, even within the normal range, might induce renal damage.

Strong evidence in support of this contention has come recently from a study of the development of end-stage renal disease in the 332 544 men screened between 1973 and 1975 for entry into the Multiple Risk Factor Intervention Trial (MRFIT) [5]. During an average of 16 years follow-up, 814 subjects either died of, or were treated for, end-stage renal disease. A strong, graded relation was observed between both systolic and diastolic pressure at screening, and the subsequent development of end-stage renal disease (Fig. 4). This relationship was not due to end-stage renal disease occurring soon after screening (Fig. 5); among those who survived for 10 years without developing end-stage renal disease the relative risk of developing

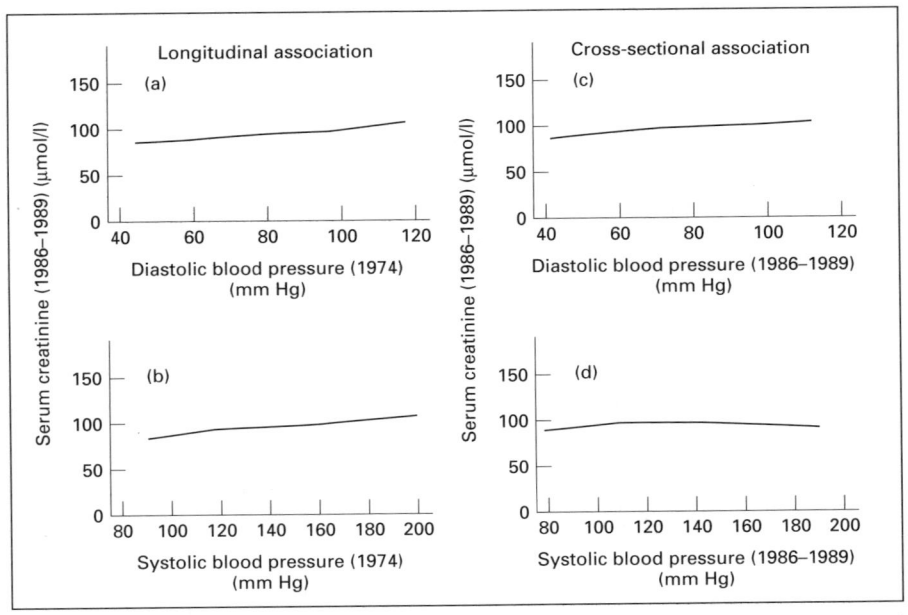

Fig. 3 From scatter plots of serum creatinine levels measured in 1986–1989 and diastolic and systolic blood pressure measured in 1974 (longitudinal association; a, b) and in 1986–1989 (cross-sectional association; c, d) in 1399 middle-aged residents of Washington County, Maryland, USA. Robust locally weighted regression lines are shown. Mean change in 1986–1989 adjusted serum creatinine for a 20 mmHg increment in BP (µmol/l [95% confidence limits]): 1974 systolic BP, 0.9 [−0.1, 1.9]; 1974 diastolic BP, 1.9 [0.4, 3.4]; 1986–1989 systolic BP, −0.7 [−1.7, −0.3]; 1986–1989 diastolic BP, 0.8 [−0.7, 2.4]. (From Perneger et al. [4].)

that condition was still markedly elevated in those with highest screening blood pressure (Table 1). Furthermore, in the 12 866 screened individuals who entered the MRFIT study, the relationship between blood pressure and risk of end-stage renal disease was not changed by taking into account the baseline serum creatinine concentration and urinary protein excretion, reasonable markers of established renal disease.

In summary, the finding in two well-conducted studies, one very large, of a graded relationship between blood pressure now and renal function in the future supports the hypothesis that 'benign' essential hypertension can cause renal failure in a small proportion of patients. The higher the blood pressure, the greater the chances of developing renal failure, even when all cases in which there is any other indication or suspicion of renal disease are excluded. This leads to the obvious question 'Why some and not others?'. The answer(s) is not known, and will be complex. Racial differences are certainly important: black patients are twice as likely as whites to have progressive renal insufficiency [6].

The key points can be summarized as follows:

- ☐ Patients with malignant hypertension usually, but not invariably, progress to end-stage renal failure if they present with a serum creatinine concentration above 250–300 µmol/l.

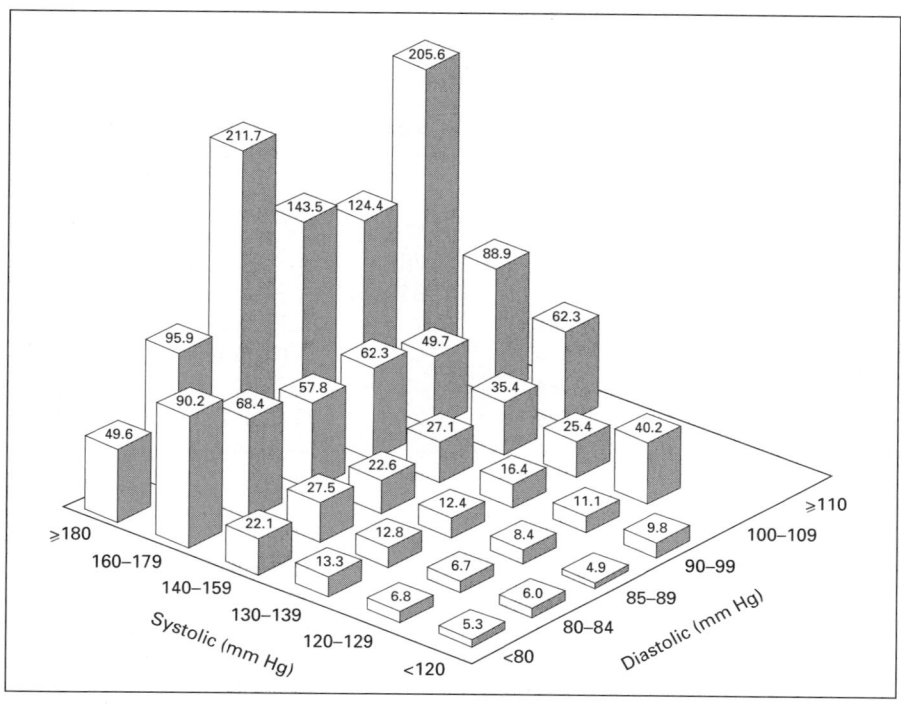

Fig. 4 Age-adjusted rate of end-stage renal disease, due to any cause, per 100 000 person-years, according to systolic and diastolic blood pressure in men screened for the Multiple Risk Factor Intervention Trial. (From Klag et al. [5]. Reprinted with permission. © Massachusetts Medical Society.)

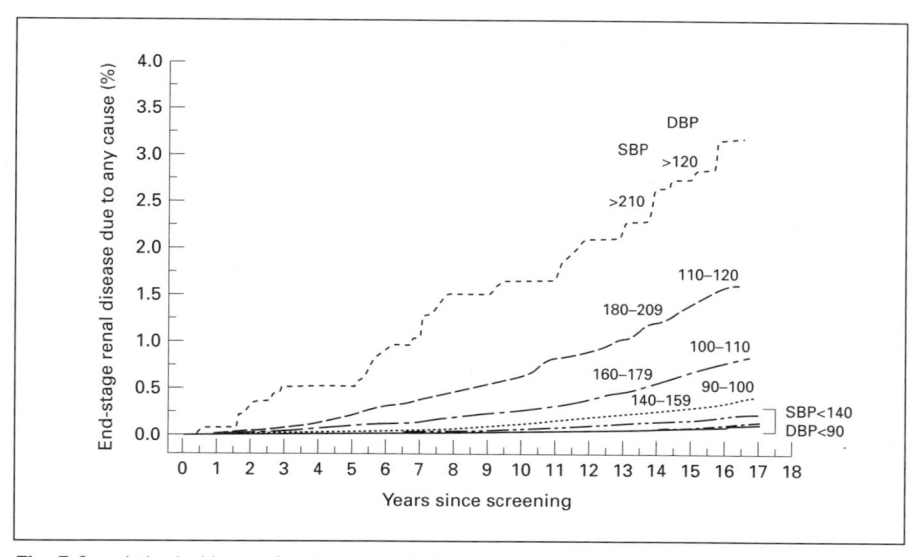

Fig. 5 Cumulative incidence of end-stage renal disease, due to any cause, according to blood pressure category in men screened for the Multiple Risk Factor Intervention Trial. SBP, systolic blood pressure; DBP, diastolic blood pressure. (From Klag et al. [5]. Reprinted with permission. © Massachusetts Medical Society.)

Table 1 Baseline blood pressure and incidence of end-stage renal disease (ESRD) in 332 544 men screened for the Multiple Risk Factor Intervention Trial. (Modified from Klag et al. [5].)

Blood pressure at screening (mmHg)		Number of men	Number developing ESRD	Adjusted relative risk (95% CI)	Adjusted relative risk in 10-year survivors
Systolic	Diastolic				
<120	<80	61 089	51	1.0	1.0
120–129	<84	81 621	86	1.2 (0.8–1.7)	
130–139	<90	73 798	134	1.9 (1.4–2.7)	
140–159	<100	85 684	275	3.1 (2.3–4.3)	2.8
160–179	<110	23 459	158	6.0 (4.3–8.4)	5.0
180–209	<120	5 464	73	11.2 (7.7–16.2)	8.4
>210	>120	1 429	37	22.1 (14.2–34.3)	12.4

☐ If a patient has benign essential hypertension, the higher the pressure the greater the chances of developing end-stage renal failure in the future. However, even those with grossly elevated pressure (systolic >210 mmHg, diastolic >120 mmHg) do not have a very high absolute level of risk (less than 3% over 16 years). It is not known why some are affected and not others.

☐ DOES TREATING HYPERTENSION DELAY THE PROGRESSION OF RENAL DISEASE?

Patients with high blood pressure should be treated, primarily to reduce their risk of cerebrovascular events. From an immediate non-nephrological clinical perspective it might therefore be thought that the answer to the question 'Does treating hypertension delay the progression of renal failure?' is not of great consequence since patients will be treated anyway. It would, however, be a mistake to think in this way. The majority of individuals with chronic renal impairment can expect to progress gradually to end-stage renal failure, and any treatment that slows down this process is of great benefit to them, as well as having considerable implications for health-care expenditure, given the high cost of renal replacement therapy. For these patients, those caring for them, and those concerned with finance, the debate about whether reducing blood pressure delays progression is far from sterile. Two matters need to be decided. First, 'What is the optimum target level for arterial pressure?'; there is no good reason to think that this is necessarily the same as that required, for example, for preventing strokes. Second, because it is known that equivalent reduction of arterial pressure with different antihypertensive agents can lead to different effects on end-organ damage, eg cardiac hypertrophy, it is of great interest to know whether one agent is better than another at protecting the kidney. On a theoretical level, finding out whether reducing blood pressure delays progression of renal disease, and whether there are class differences between antihypertensive agents in this respect, might also give useful insight into the confusing relationship that exists between hypertension and the kidney.

Patients with essential hypertension

A much quoted study followed 94 patients with essential hypertension and initially normal serum creatinine concentration (<133 µmol/l), treated with a range of antihypertensive agents [6]. After a mean period of 58 months, they were retrospectively divided into two groups on the basis of the level of their blood pressure during the follow-up period: one whose control had been good ($n = 61$, mean treated diastolic pressure of each individual <90 mmHg, mean treated diastolic pressure of group 84 mmHg) and one whose control had been poor ($n = 33$, mean treated diastolic pressure of each individual >90 mmHg, mean treated diastolic pressure of group 95 mmHg). A deterioration in renal function, defined as an increase in the serum creatinine concentration of >35 µmol/l, was seen in ten patients in the good control group (16%) and four of those in the poor control group (12%). The authors reasonably concluded that renal function could deteriorate in some patients despite good blood pressure control (by conventional standards).

A recent and much larger study measured serum creatinine levels annually for an average of 5.3 years in 2125 mild and moderately hypertensive men, identified through a screening programme and treated with a variety of drugs [7]. Multiple-regression analysis confirmed the correlations made in the Clue/ARIC and MRFIT studies [4,5] between initial diastolic pressure and subsequent renal function, in this study in the form of the final measure of serum creatinine concentration. However, no measure of blood pressure *during* treatment was independently associated with final serum creatinine levels. When the patients were stratified depending on the mean level of diastolic blood pressure achieved during treatment (less than or greater than 95 mmHg), the mean slopes of reciprocal serum creatinine plots were not significantly different in the two blood pressure groups. Changes in serum creatinine levels occurring over time appeared to reflect regression towards the mean (Fig. 6).

What can we deduce from these two observational studies in essential hypertension? [6,7] Despite the obvious limitations imposed by retrospective classification into high and low blood pressure groups, rather than prospective random allocation, a message for clinical practice comes across. Those patients with essential hypertension, whose diastolic pressure is reduced to below 90–95 mmHg by treatment, cannot expect to fare much better as regards change in renal function over a 5-year period than those whose diastolic pressure remains in the range 90/95 to 105 mmHg. This is not to say: (i) that benefit might not accrue over a longer timescale, and continued observation of these cohorts would be of great interest; or (ii) that benefit might not arise in some subgroup of patients yet to be identified, perhaps those treated with a particular type of antihypertensive agent.

Patients known to have chronic renal failure

While there is no doubt that treatment of those with grossly elevated blood pressure can prevent decline in renal function, the effect of treating more modestly elevated

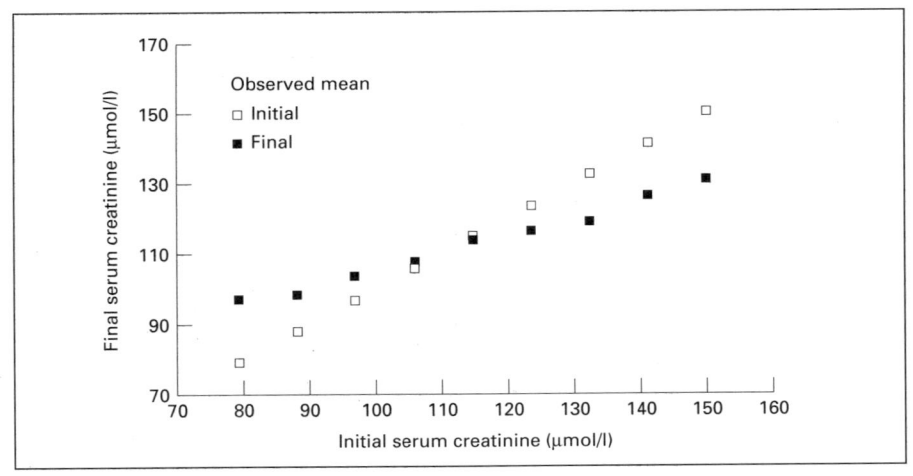

Fig. 6 Relation of initial to final serum creatinine, measured on average 5.3 years later, in 2125 mild and moderately hypertensive men. (From Madhavan et al. [7]. Reproduced by permission of The Lancet Ltd.)

pressure remains contentious. Klahr and colleagues used a 2 × 2 design to randomize 585 patients with moderate renal impairment (GFR 25–55 ml/min) and 255 with more severe renal failure (GFR 13–24 ml/min) between a 'usual' or 'low' protein diet, and between 'usual' (target <140–160/90 mmHg, depending on age) or 'low' (target <125–145/75 mmHg, depending on age) blood pressure groups [8]. The recommended first-line antihypertensive agent was an angiotensin converting enzyme inhibitor, but at least half of the patients received treatment with other agents in preference. Mean arterial pressure was the same in both groups at randomization but – despite the stated difference in targets – was only 4.7 mmHg lower in the low blood pressure group during an average of 2.2 years of follow-up. Glomerular filtration rate fell at the same rate in both groups (Fig. 7). It should be noted, however, that by the standards of most clinical practice in the UK, hypertension was treated very vigorously in the 'usual' blood pressure group, where the achievement of a mean blood pressure of about 97–98 mmHg implies an average sphygmomanometer recording of 145/75 mmHg.

Might one antihypertensive agent be better than another?

In animal models, angiotensin converting enzyme inhibitors can reduce glomerular capillary hypertension and glomerular hypertrophy, both of which are thought to be important factors in the progression of renal disease. Zucchelli and colleagues [9] therefore sought to determine whether an angiotensin converting enzyme inhibitor, captopril, would be better than a calcium antagonist, nifedipine, in preserving renal function in patients with gradually worsening renal failure. A group of 121 patients with established chronic renal failure and a serum creatinine level between 135 and 440 µmol/l were randomized to captopril or slow-release nifedipine for a 3-year study period. The dose of each was increased as required to obtain a supine diastolic

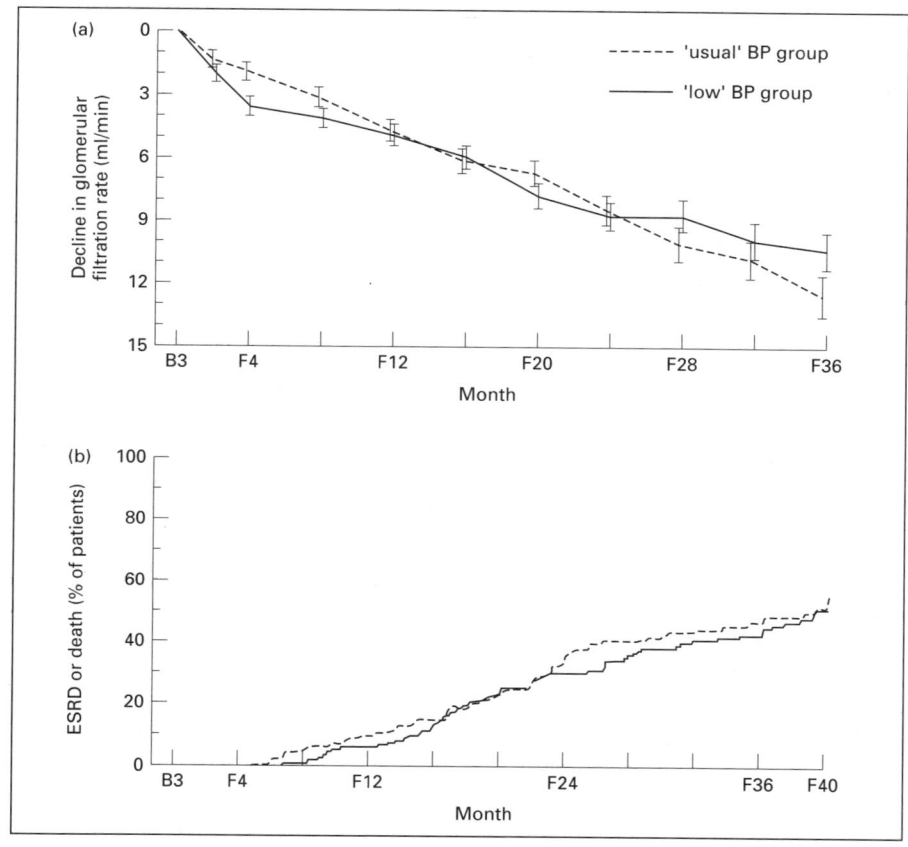

Fig. 7 (a) Decline in GFR from baseline (B) to selected follow-up times (F) in patients with an initial GFR of 25–55 ml/min. (b) The occurrence of end-stage renal disease (ESRD) or death during follow-up in patients with an initial GFR in the range 13–24 ml/min. (From Klahr et al. [8]. Reprinted with permission. © Massachusetts Medical Society.)

blood pressure of less than 95 mmHg, with the addition of frusemide and then clonidine if satisfactory control could not be achieved using monotherapy with the randomly allocated agent. The mean blood pressure values in the two groups were virtually the same throughout the study, and there was no difference between the groups in the rate of decline of renal function or in the number of patients requiring dialysis (Fig. 8).

Hannendouche et al. [10] performed a similar study, randomizing 100 patients with chronic renal failure and an initial serum creatinine level in the range 200–400 µmol/l to receive treatment with either the angiotensin converting enzyme inhibitor, enalapril, or a β-blocker (acebutalol or atenolol). The aim was to reduce diastolic pressure to below 90 mmHg. If this could not be achieved with monotherapy, then frusemide was added, followed if necessary by a calcium antagonist. Over 3 years there was no difference in the blood pressure levels achieved in the two groups, but renal function – as judged by the slope of reciprocal creatinine plots – deteriorated

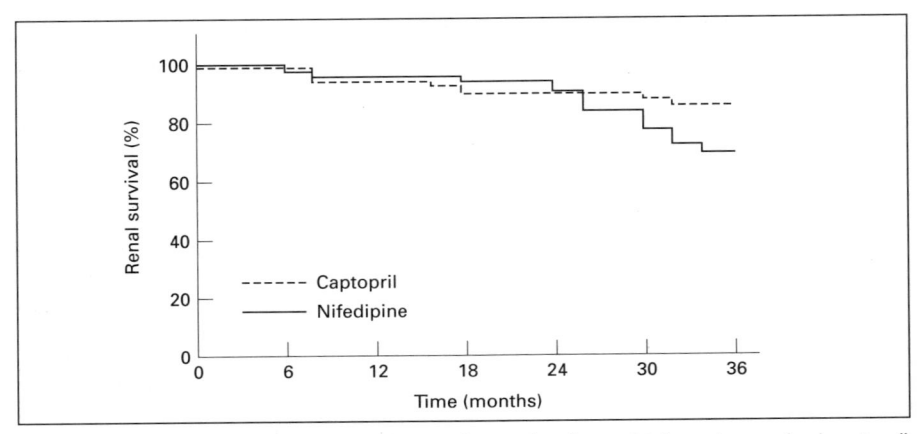

Fig. 8 Renal survival in patients with mild to moderate chronic renal failure who received captopril or nifedipine as initial antihypertensive agent. (From Zucchelli et al. [9].)

significantly less rapidly in those given enalapril, and 10 of 52, rather than 17 of 48, progressed to end-stage renal failure during the trial period (Fig. 9).

On the basis of these two well conducted studies it would seem better to initiate treatment of patients with renal impairment who are hypertensive using angiotensin converting enzyme inhibitors (keeping a close watch over the first week or so for a deterioration in function that could indicate the presence of renal artery stenosis) or calcium antagonists in preference to other agents.

The key points can be summarized as follows:

- In patients with chronic renal failure the control of gross hypertension reduces the rate of decline of renal function, but there is no firm evidence to suggest that the target level for reduction in blood pressure should be different from that usually advised.

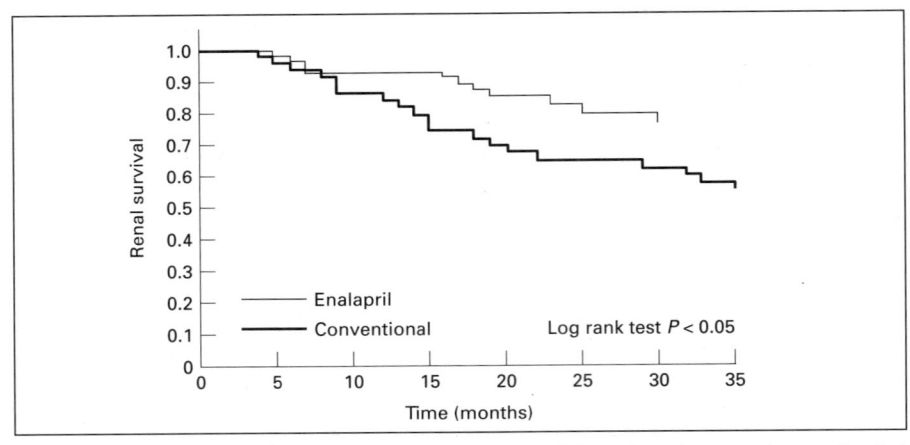

Fig. 9 Renal survival in patients with moderate chronic renal failure whose hypertension was treated initially with either enalapril or a β-blocker. (From Hannedouche et al. [10]. Reproduced by permission of BMJ Publishing Group.)

☐ Reduction of blood pressure using angiotensin converting enzyme inhibitors or calcium antagonists is better at preserving renal function than treatment using other agents.

REFERENCES

1. Klahr S. The kidney in hypertension – villain and victim. *New Engl J Med* 1989; **320**: 731–3.
2. Herlitz H, Gudbrandsson T, Hansson L. Renal function as an indicator of prognosis in malignant essential hypertension. *Scand J Urol Nephrol* 1982; **16**: 51–5.
3. Lindeman RD, Tobin JD, Shock NW. Association between blood pressure and the rate of decline in renal function with age. *Kidney Int* 1984; **26**: 861–8.
4. Perneger TV, Nieto FJ, Whelton PK, Klag MJ, Comstock GW, Szklo M. A prospective study of blood pressure and serum creatinine: results from the 'Clue' study and the ARIC study. *J Am Med Assoc* 1993; **269**: 488–93.
5. Klag MJ, Whelton PK, Randall BL, et al. Blood pressure and end-stage renal disease in men. *New Engl J Med* 1996; **334**: 13–8.
6. Rostand SG, Brown G, Kirk K, Rutsky EA, Dustan HP. Renal insufficiency in treated essential hypertension. *New Engl J Med* 1989; **320**: 684–8.
7. Madhavan S, Stockwell D, Cohen H, Alderman MH. Renal function during antihypertensive treatment. *Lancet* 1995; **345**: 749–51.
8. Klahr S, Levey AS, Beck GJ, et al. The effects of dietary protein restriction and blood-pressure control on the progression of chronic renal failure. *New Engl J Med* 1994; **330**: 877–84.
9. Zucchelli P, Zuccala A, Borghi M, et al. Long-term comparison between captopril and nifedipine in the progression of renal insufficiency. *Kidney Int* 1992; **42**: 452–8.
10. Hannedouche T, Landais P, Goldfarb B, et al. Randomised controlled trial of enalapril and β-blockers in non-diabetic chronic renal failure. *Brit Med J* 1994; **309**: 833–7.

☐ MULTIPLE CHOICE QUESTIONS

1. Regarding patients with hypertension:
   (a) Those presenting in the malignant phase almost invariably progress to end-stage renal failure
   (b) Benign essential hypertension is not associated with an increased risk of end-stage renal failure
   (c) Previous blood pressure level predicts renal function better than current blood pressure level
   (d) Above a pressure of 160/100 mmHg the risk of developing chronic renal failure increases dramatically
   (e) Black patients are more likely than whites to develop chronic renal failure

2. Regarding patients with chronic renal failure:
   (a) Treating blood pressure has little effect on the rate of progression
   (b) It is proven that the target level for blood pressure reduction should be lower than that usually advised for the prevention of strokes
   (c) Reducing diastolic blood pressure to below 90–95 mmHg has been shown to be critical for preserving renal function
   (d) Angiotensin converting enzyme inhibitors are better than β-blockers and other conventional agents at preventing progression of renal failure

(e) Calcium antagonists are as good as angiotensin converting enzyme inhibitors at preventing progression of renal failure

ANSWERS

1a	False	2a	False
b	False	b	False
c	True	c	False
d	False	d	True
e	True	e	True

Diabetic nephropathy: detection and intervention

R W Bilous

☐ INTRODUCTION

Diabetic nephropathy is a clinical diagnosis based on the finding of proteinuria using conventional urinalysis. Most patients will also have hypertension and retinopathy and will develop renal impairment. However, the diagnosis only depends upon the presence of proteinuria.

Routine urinalysis is now performed using dry chemistry dipsticks and these conventionally detect total protein (mainly albumin) concentrations of more than 300 mg/l. This roughly equates to a total protein excretion of approximately 500 mg/day. In 1963, the development of a sensitive radio-immunoassay for albumin made it possible to detect much lower concentrations in urine. At the same time, increased urinary albumin excretion (UAE) was discovered in newly diagnosed non-insulin-dependent diabetic (NIDDM) patients in Bedford. The significance of this finding was only realized much later when follow-up studies of patients revealed that those with increased UAE not only were more likely to develop nephropathy but also had an increased cardiovascular morbidity and mortality [1]. This phenomenon of increased UAE below the conventionally detected range was termed 'microalbuminuria' or 'incipient nephropathy', whereas those patients with proteinuria detected by conventional methods have 'overt' or 'clinical' nephropathy [1]. In this chapter the terms *microalbuminuria* and *clinical nephropathy* will be used.

Microalbuminuria is usually defined on the basis of an albumin excretion rate of 20–200 µg/min on a timed overnight collection or 30–300 mg/day on a 24 h sample (Table 1). Clinical nephropathy, on the other hand, is defined as a protein

Table 1 Definitions of microalbuminuria. (Adapted from Mogensen et al. [5].)

Excretion rate	20–200 µg/min or 30–300 mg/day (timed overnight or 24 h specimen)
Concentration	30–300 mg/l
Albumin : creatinine	2.5–25 mg/mmol (male) 3.5–25 mg/mmol (female)
False-positive results with:	biological variation posture/diurnal variation exercise urinary infection other renal disease/cardiovascular disease
False-negative results with:	dilute urine/diuresis

concentration of >300 mg/l or more than 0.5 g/day total protein (>300 mg/day albumin) excretion rate in a 24 h sample [1].

Finally, diabetic nephropathy is a clinical diagnosis and must be distinguished from glomerulopathy which is based on the finding of the characteristic pathological abnormalities in renal glomeruli. Glomerulopathy is invariably present in patients with clinical nephropathy and early changes are usually seen in those with microalbuminuria, but the term is not interchangeable with nephropathy.

☐ NATURAL HISTORY

This has mostly been described in insulin-dependent diabetes mellitus (IDDM) patients, but is likely to be similar in NIDDM. Cumulative incidence of clinical nephropathy is around 20% after 20 years diabetes duration in both IDDM and NIDDM, with a sharp rise between 12 and 20 years [2] (Fig. 1), and reaches a peak of 40% after 40 years diabetes in IDDM. Thus only a minority of diabetic patients ultimately develop the complication.

The incidence of clinical nephropathy in IDDM seems to be declining. Cohort studies from the Steno Hospital in Copenhagen and the Joslin Clinic in Boston have demonstrated a significant reduction of approximately 50% after 20 years diabetes duration, comparing patients diagnosed in the 1930s with those in the 1950s. In addition, a recent study from Sweden has shown no new cases of clinical nephropathy in 51 IDDM children diagnosed between 1976 and 1980 and followed for up to 15 years, compared with 10–30% in cohorts diagnosed in the 1960s and with a similar duration [3] (Fig. 2).

Nearly all patients with clinical nephropathy will have microalbuminuria beforehand, and in IDDM patients this period lasts on average 7 years [4]. The reported

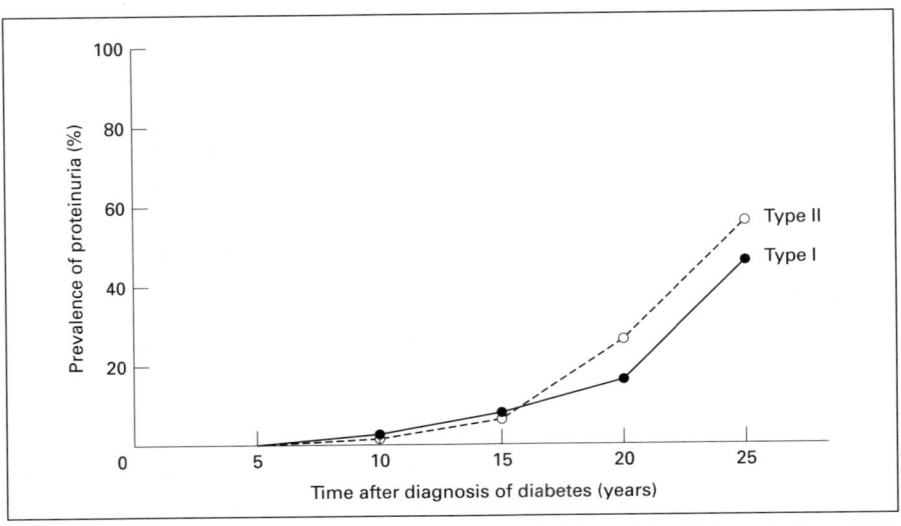

Fig. 1 Prevalence of proteinuria (clinical nephropathy) in 312 Type I (insulin-dependent) and 496 Type II (non-insulin-dependent) diabetic patients after 25 years duration of known diabetes. (From Hasslacher et al. [2].)

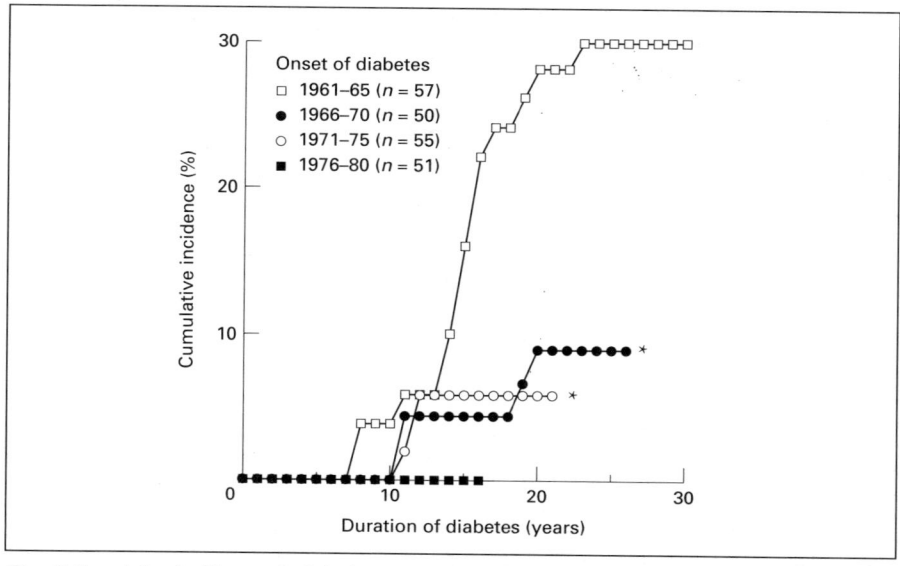

Fig. 2 Cumulative incidence of clinical nephropathy in insulin-dependent diabetic patients with age of onset < 15 years, minimum follow-up of 15 years and in whom diagnosis was made for 1961–5, 1966–70, 1971–5 and 1976–80. Asterisk denotes significant difference in incidence ($p = 0.01$) between the indicated cohort and patients diagnosed during 1961–5. (From Bojestig et al. [3].)

incidence of progression of normal UAE to microalbuminuria in IDDM is approximately 2% per year. There are few good incidence data in NIDDM.

Reported prevalence rates vary from 5% to 20% depending on the population under study and the duration and type of diabetes. In addition, for microalbuminuric patients, different definitions have been used based on various tests. Prevalence rates of 5–22% for IDDM and 10–42% for NIDDM have been reported (Table 2). Whereas most patients with microalbuminuria and IDDM will eventually progress to clinical nephropathy, the situation is less clear in NIDDM. In microalbuminuric IDDM the average rate of increase of UAE is approximately 20% per year [4].

Glomerular filtration rate (GFR) appears stable in patients with microalbuminuria, but declines steadily in those with clinical nephropathy (Fig. 3). This rate of decline has historically been reported in IDDM as a mean of 10 ml/min/year and tends to be linear in individuals, although there is considerable variation between patients. The average period of clinical nephropathy prior to end-stage renal failure is 6 years [1].

Systemic blood pressure rises in parallel with UAE although most patients with microalbuminuria will not have conventionally defined hypertension. Nonetheless, one of the features of those IDDM patients with normal UAE who progress to microalbuminuria is a rise in mean blood pressure [4] (Fig. 4). Consequently, newer definitions of hypertension have been developed for patients with microalbuminuria and clinical nephropathy of 130–140 systolic/85–90 mmHg diastolic [5], although

Table 2 Reported prevalence rates for microalbuminuria in IDDM and NIDDM patients.

Location	Population sample		Definition	Prevalence
IDDM				
Hospital clinics				
Denmark	102 children	7–18 years	>15 µg/min	20%
Denmark	982 adults	>18 years	>30 mg/day	22%
USA	627 adults	15–54 years	>20 µg/min	22%
Europe	3250 adults	15–60 years	>20 µg/min	21%
Newcastle	416 adults	14–87 years	>30 µg/min	6.7%
Population based				
Norway	351 adults	18–32 years	>15 µg/min	12.5%
USA	706 mixed	8–71 years	>30 mg/l	21.2%
UK (Poole)	121 mixed	?	>30 µg/min	5.0%
NIDDM				
Newly diagnosed				
UK (UKPDS)	585 mean	58±8 years	>50 mg/l	17%
Germany	68	56–66 years	>30 mg/l	19%
Denmark	1267 median	65.3 years	>2 mg/mmol (ACR)	33.6%
Hospital clinics				
Newcastle	524	19–86 years	>30 µg/min	9.7%
Belfast	216 mean	63.9 years	>25 mg/l	22%
Denmark	549	<76 years	>31 mg/day	27%
Japan	52	>35 years	>15 µg/min	35%
USA (Blacks)	116	29–88 years	>20 µg/min	31%
Population based				
Pacific Islanders	228	>20 years	>30 mg/l	42%
UK (Poole)	329	?	>30 µg/min	11.2%
Denmark	204	60–74 years	>15 µg/min	24.7%

ACR = albumin : creatinine ratio; UKPDS = UK Prospective Diabetes Study

there is some debate over the validity of these values for older NIDDM patients. More than 85% of patients with clinical nephropathy will develop hypertension defined as 160/90 mmHg, and nearly one-half of IDDM microalbuminuric patients will be on antihypertensive therapy within 4 years of diagnosis [4].

IDDM patients with clinical nephropathy have up to a 50-fold increased relative mortality compared to age and diabetes-duration matched non-proteinuric individuals (Fig. 5), although this mortality appears to be declining, with current 10-year rates recorded at one-fifth that of previously reported series (Fig. 6). In NIDDM, a 5-fold increase has been shown in the Pima Indians with clinical nephropathy, whereas Europid patients with microalbuminuria (>15 µg/ml) had an increased mortality over 10 years of approximately 50% compared to those with normal UAE at baseline [8].

In all series, the majority of deaths are recorded as due to cardiovascular disease (acute myocardial infarct, stroke, gangrene) and not renal failure. Many patients

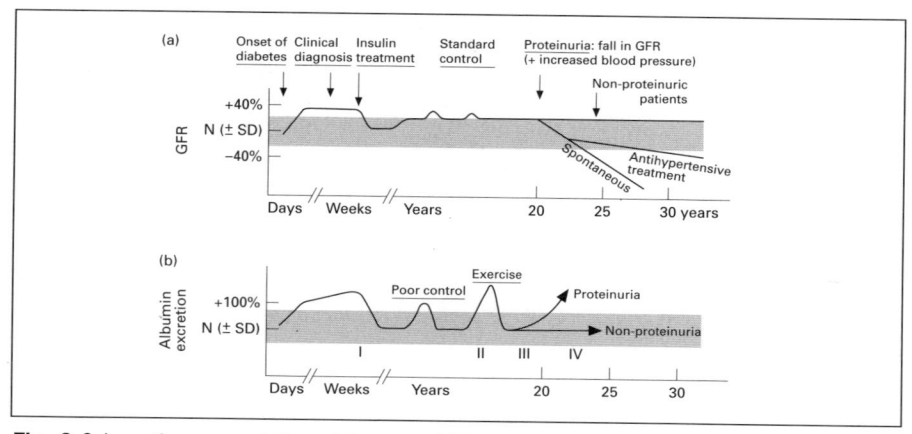

Fig. 3 Schematic representation of the natural history of GFR (a) and albuminuria changes (b) in insulin-dependent diabetes. The onset of proteinuria heralds a relentless decline in GFR. Roman numerals refer to stages of nephropathy: III, microalbuminuria; IV, clinical nephropathy. N, normal mean values. (From Mogensen et al. [1].)

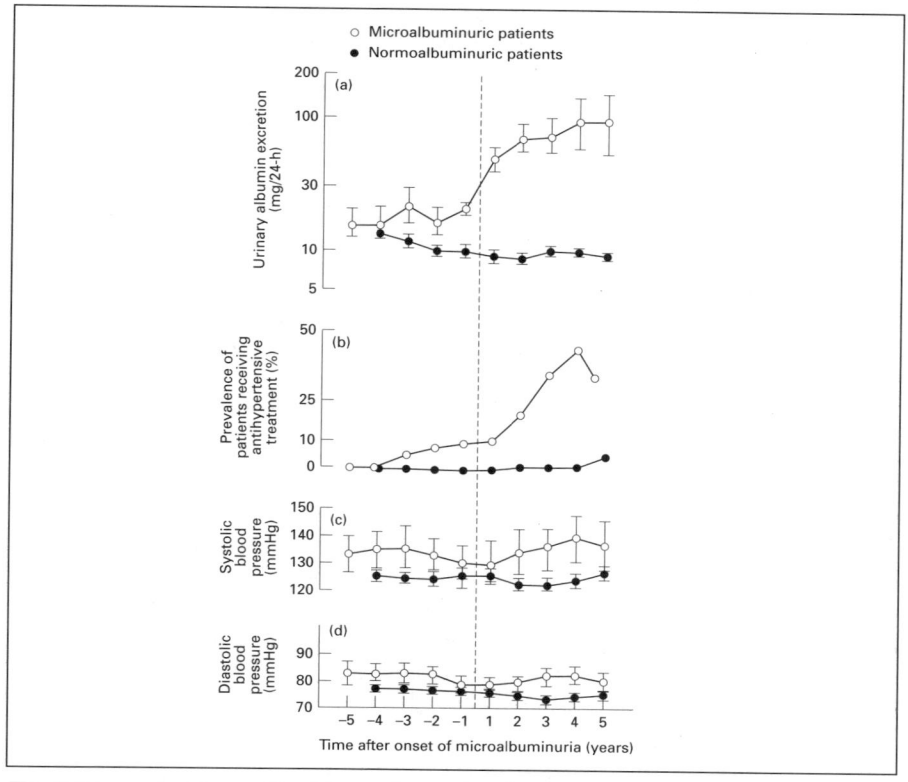

Fig. 4 Urinary albumin excretion (a), prevalence of antihypertensive treatment (b), and systolic (c) and diastolic (d) blood pressure in insulin-dependent patients who developed microalbuminuria ($n = 29$) and who remained normoalbuminuric ($n = 171$). Note: Albumin excretion and blood pressure are higher at baseline in patients who go on to develop microalbuminuria, and careful control of blood pressure cannot completely prevent its development. (From Mathiesen et al. [4].)

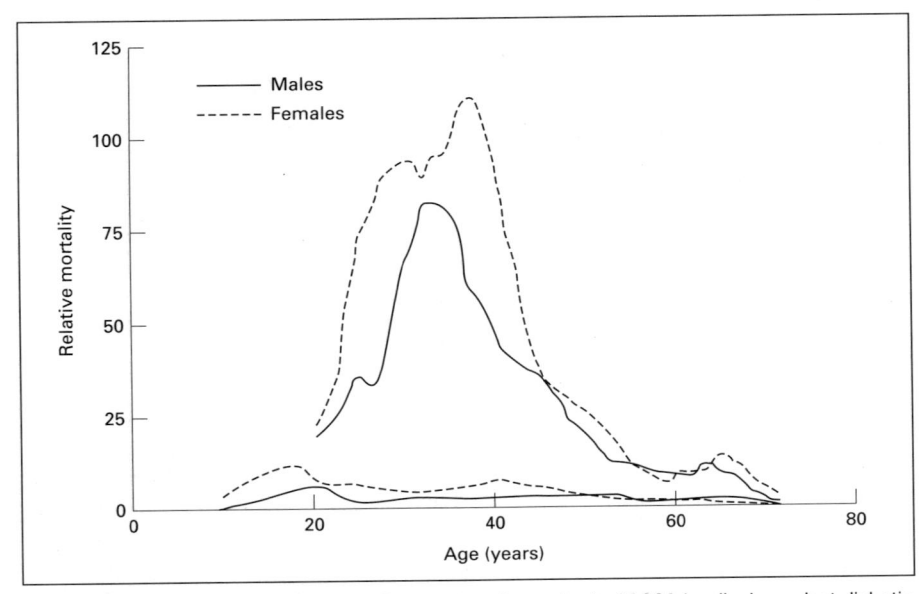

Fig. 5 Relative mortality as a function of current age in a cohort of 1001 insulin-dependent diabetic patients diagnosed in Denmark during 1933–52 and followed until 1982. The top two lines represent 406 patients with clinical nephropathy and the lower two 595 patients with urinary total protein excretion < 0.5 g/day. *Note:* 100-fold increase in mortality in proteinuric females aged 40 years. (From Borch-Johnsen et al. [6].)

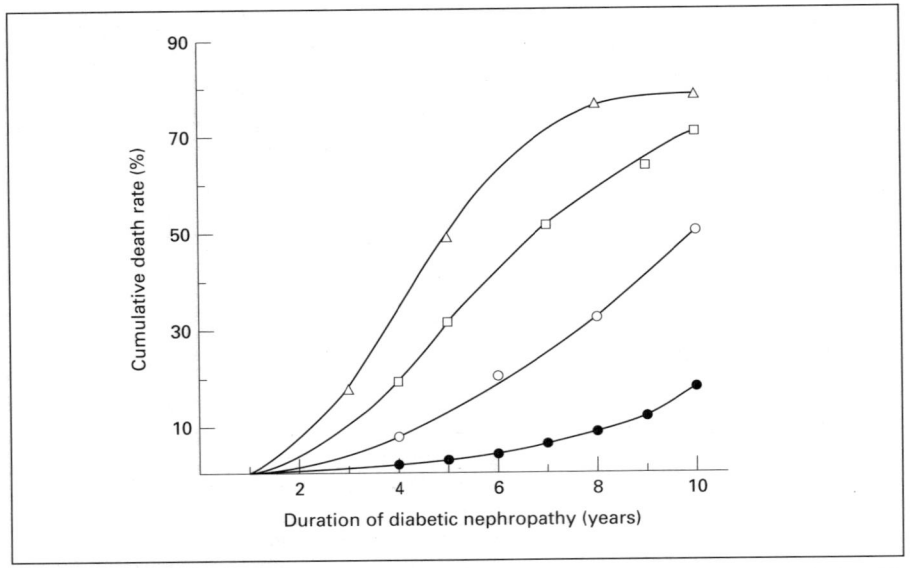

Fig. 6 Cumulative death rate in four historical series of insulin-dependent diabetic patients with clinical nephropathy derived from the following studies: △, Knowles, USA (1971), n = 45; □, Andersen, Denmark (1983), n = 360; ○, Krolewski, USA (1985), n = 67; and compared with ●, Parving, Denmark (1989), n = 45. Note that 5-year cumulative death rates have fallen by about 80% over the past 20 years. (From Parving et al. [7].)

with microalbuminuria and clinical nephropathy have so-called silent myocardial ischaemia with clinically unrecognized severe coronary artery disease. Those patients who enter renal replacement therapy retain this high risk of vascular disease and survival rates are approximately one-half those of non-diabetic patients [9]. Some centres are now performing routine coronary arteriography in diabetic patients before entering into renal replacement therapy, and have shown better survival rates in those undergoing coronary artery bypass grafting before dialysis or transplantation.

☐ DEFINITION AND DIAGNOSIS

For clinical nephropathy, detection and diagnosis is fairly straightforward. It depends upon the finding of conventional dipstick-positive proteinuria on three occasions at least 2–3 months apart, and/or a 24 h total protein excretion of 0.5 g. Microalbuminuria is defined on the basis of a timed excretion rate, and for all research or intervention studies either an overnight or 24 h urine collection should be used [5]. These samples are difficult to use in a routine clinical setting, however.

Recently, side-room tests for detection of low concentrations of albumin have been developed. These have acceptable specificity and sensitivity using a diagnostic cut-off of 20 mg/l, but tend to be expensive at approximately £1 per test. Because urinary albumin concentrations are subject to dilution error, and may increase after exercise or a protein meal, most authors suggest that early morning (first void) urine samples should be used. In addition, by relating the albumin and creatinine concentrations in a ratio (the albumin : creatinine ratio or ACR), an improvement in specificity and sensitivity over albumin concentrations alone is seen, up to 80–100% depending on the diagnostic cut-off [10]. The current guidelines of the St Vincent Declaration Expert Group use a diagnostic ACR of 2.5 mg/mmol for men and 3.5 mg/mmol for women, as urinary creatinine concentrations partly depend on muscle mass (Table 3). Patients with values less than these can have annual tests, those with results above should have confirmation by one or two further samples and, if possible, a timed collection [5].

Table 3 Currently recommended screening procedures. (From Mogensen *et al.* [5].)

Authority	Procedure and confirmation
St Vincent Declaration	First morning ACR >2.5 mg/mmol (men) or >3.5 mg/mmol (women). Repeated at least twice and preferably confirmed with overnight timed specimen. All NIDDM and IDDM >1 year duration.
World Health Organization	Annual test (not specified). Confirm with repeat test. All NIDDM <70 years; IDDM >5 years duration and >12 years old.
American Diabetes Association	Annual test ACR >30 mg/g. Confirm with timed collection. All NIDDM; IDDM >5 years duration and >14 years old.

☐ TREATMENT OF NEPHROPATHY

Blood glucose control

There are no data on the impact of improved glycaemic control in NIDDM patients with nephropathy. In IDDM patients, the Diabetes Control and Complications Trial (DCCT) conclusively demonstrated that improved blood glucose control using intensive insulin regimens could reduce the number of patients developing microalbuminuria by approximately 50% (ie primary prevention). For microalbuminuric patients the effect of improved glycaemic control is now less clear.

Two separate studies were carried out in Denmark in the early 1980s involving 70 patients in total, half of whom were treated with intensive insulin therapy: 16 patients in the first and 36 in the second had microalbuminuria in the range 30–300 mg/day. In the original analysis, intensive insulin therapy with an average reduction in HbA1c of 20 % appeared to stabilize UAE but in those patients on conventional therapy, in whom HbA1c did not change, UAE increased. A subsequent analysis of the patients 5–8 years later revealed that five times as many patients on conventional therapy, who had a baseline UAE >100 mg/day, had clinical nephropathy at follow-up [11].

However, these findings were not confirmed by the DCCT in the USA [12] or by the Microalbuminuria Collaborative Study Group in the UK. The DCCT patients had UAE measured at regular intervals and had a mean follow-up of 6.5 years. In 73 patients whose baseline UAE was 28–139 µg/min (40–200 mg/day) there was no significant reduction in the numbers progressing to clinical nephropathy.

In the UK study, 70 patients with UAE 30–199 µg/min (42–286 mg/day) were randomized to conventional and intensive insulin therapy and studied for a median of 5 years. Significant glycaemic separation (HbA1c reduction of approximately 14%), however, was only sustained for up to 3 years. No difference was seen in the number of patients in each treatment group who progressed to clinical nephropathy (Fig. 7).

Intensive insulin therapy carries with it significant risk of severe hypoglycaemia, and most patients gain weight appreciably. Current recommendations are to strive for the best possible glycaemic control in all our patients, but the evidence that such interventions can prevent progression from microalbuminuria to clinical nephropathy (secondary prevention) is now considerably weakened.

In clinical nephropathy a small study of six patients demonstrated no benefit of improved glycaemia on rate of decline of GFR (tertiary prevention). Although it is generally accepted that clinical nephropathy is too far advanced for metabolic improvement to have a positive impact, a recent study of pancreas transplantation in a small group of IDDM patients did show regression of glomerulopathy and reduction in UAE following normalization of glycaemia for 5 years [14].

Antihypertensive therapy

Several studies in IDDM patients with clinical nephropathy using conventional antihypertensive therapy (eg β-blockers, hydralazine, frusemide) have demonstrated a

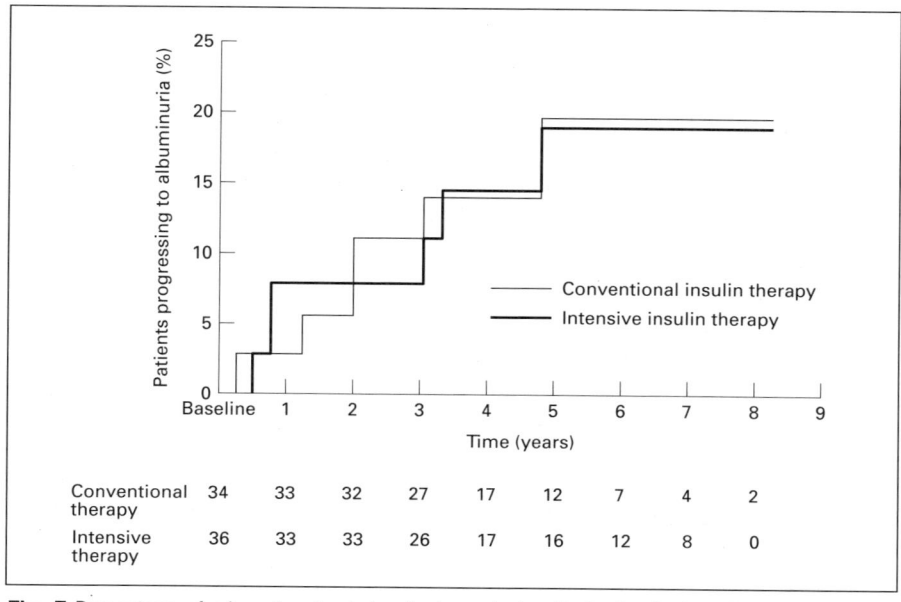

Fig. 7 Percentage of microalbuminuric insulin-dependent patients developing clinical nephropathy during intensive (n = 34) and conventional (n = 36) insulin therapy for up to 8 years. No impact of improved glycaemic control is apparent. (From Microalbuminuria Study Group [13].)

	Baseline	1	2	3	4	5	6	7	8
Conventional therapy	34	33	32	27	17	12	7	4	2
Intensive therapy	36	33	33	26	17	16	12	8	0

beneficial effect of lowering blood pressure to <160/90 mm Hg on the rate of decline of GFR (Fig. 8). There are fewer data in NIDDM, but these patients seem to show a similar benefit. Even intensive blood pressure management, however, cannot completely prevent IDDM patients with microalbuminuria from developing clinical nephropathy [4]. More recently, specific interest has focused on angiotensin converting enzyme inhibitor drugs (ACEI).

Angiotensin converting enzyme inhibitors

Animal work has suggested that a high intraglomerular capillary blood pressure is an important factor in initiating glomerular damage in experimental diabetes. ACEI drugs have been shown to reduce this pressure and subsequently prevent experimental glomerulosclerosis [16].

In man, there are many studies showing that ACEI drugs reduce UAE in both IDDM and NIDDM, hypertensive and normotensive patients with microalbuminuria. This reduction appears more marked with ACEI than other antihypertensive agents in most, but not all, studies. In IDDM, a recent combined analysis of a European and North American study of 2 years treatment with captopril *vs* placebo in 116 *vs* 119 normotensive patients respectively showed a 62.9% risk reduction (8 *vs* 25 patients) for the development of UAE >200 µg/min in the actively treated group ($p = 0.017$) (Fig. 9) [17]. In NIDDM, the use of enalapril *vs* placebo in two studies with a combined patient population of 76 *vs* 73 respectively for 4–5 years

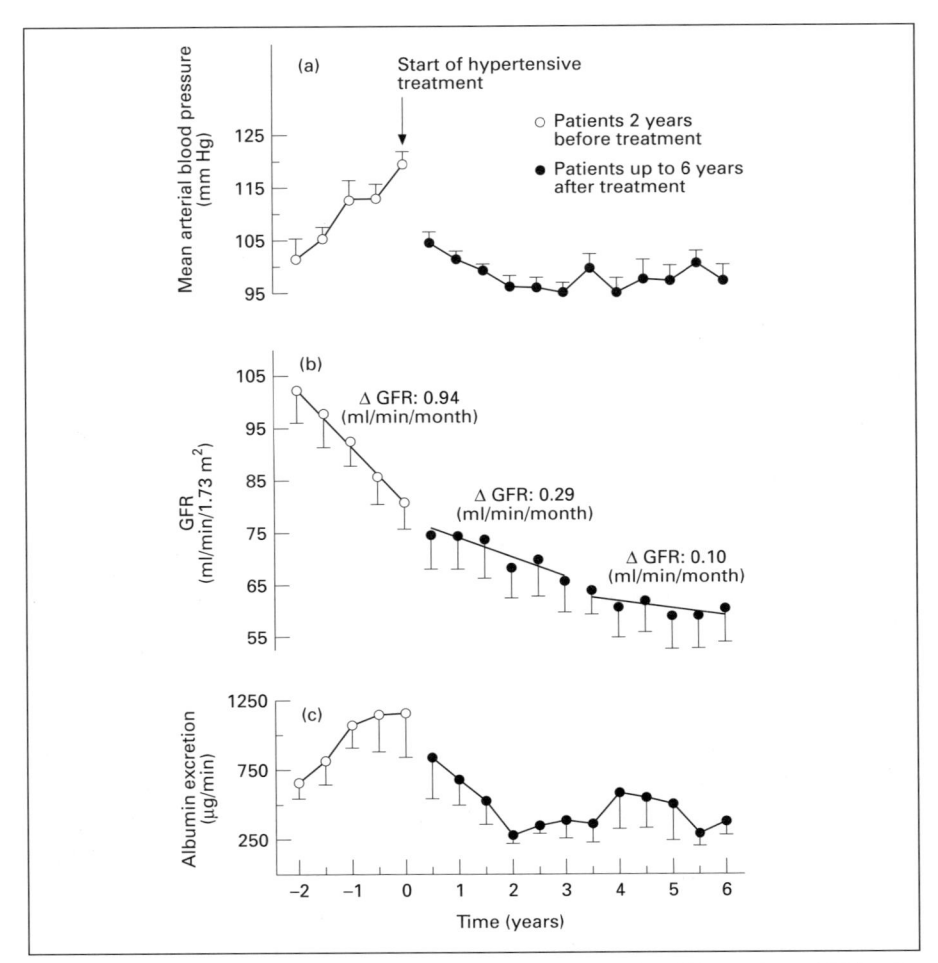

Fig. 8 Mean arterial blood pressure (a), GFR (b) and albumin excretion (c) in a cohort of 12 insulin-dependent patients with clinical nephropathy 2 years before and up to 6 years after receiving antihypertensive therapy with a treatment goal of < 160/90 mmHg. Note mean rate of loss of GFR of about 10 ml/min/year in the untreated state and the reduction of this by more than two-thirds following antihypertensive therapy. Treatment was β-blockers, hydralazine and frusemide. (From Parving et al. [15].)

showed a reduction or stabilization of UAE with 8 vs 25 developing levels >200 µg/min (a similar risk reduction to the IDDM studies). Encouragingly, less than 5% of patients had to discontinue therapy owing to side effects, and this number was not significantly different in those on placebo or active treatment.

Not all studies of ACEI in microalbuminuria have had such clear results, however, and the reasons for this discrepancy are uncertain. The balance of evidence is that such drugs at least slow down the rate of increase of UAE in microalbuminuric patients. It remains unproven that such a reduction in UAE translates to patient benefit in terms of harder clinical end-points such as loss of renal function (GFR), cardiovascular morbidity, end-stage renal failure (ESRF) and death.

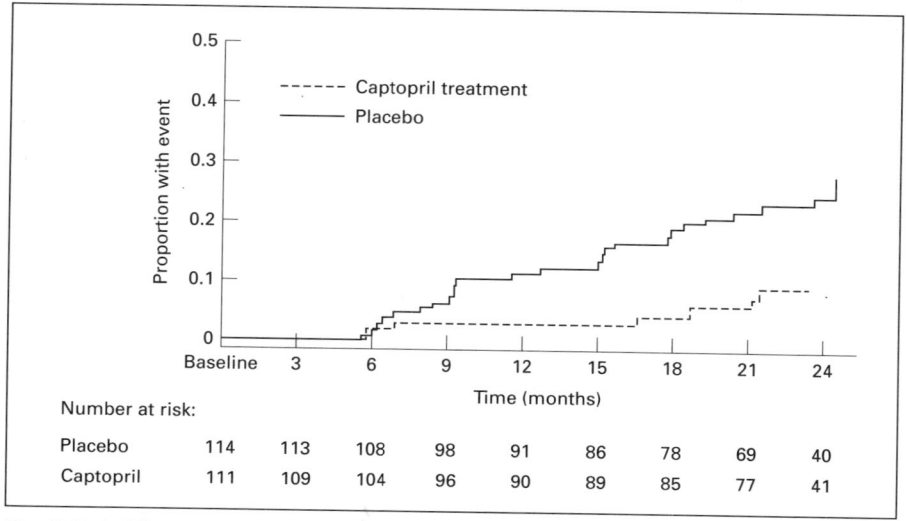

Fig. 9 Probability of progression to clinical nephropathy in 225 normotensive (< 145/90 in those under 35 years old; < 165/90 in those over 35 years) insulin-dependent patients with microalbuminuria who received captopril (50 mg twice daily) or placebo for two years. Risk reduction adjusted for blood pressure at baseline was 62.9% ($p = 0.017$). (From The Microalbuminuria Captopril Study Group [17].)

The only study to address these issues has been carried out using captopril in IDDM patients with clinical nephropathy when a 50% reduction in the combined end-point of death/ESRF was observed (Fig. 10) [16]. While it is tempting to extrapolate these findings to microalbuminuric patients, no confirming data yet exist in humans, largely because of the population size and length of time that such studies would require in order to have sufficient statistical power.

Dietary protein restriction

In experimental diabetes, protein restriction can prevent and delay renal functional loss and glomerulopathy. Studies in humans have not been so clear-cut.

Protein restriction reduces UAE in both microalbuminuria and clinical nephropathy, but evidence of a benefit on end-points such as loss of renal function is conflicting. Some patients dramatically slowed their rate of loss of GFR, whereas others did not. These studies used diets with approximately 50% of the usual protein content, compliance was difficult and the potential for protein malnutrition in heavily albuminuric patients is a real one. The large Modification of Diet in Renal Disease study in 804 non-diabetic, renal failure patients failed to show any impact on the rate of loss of GFR [16].

Other treatments

Because of the high prevalence of cardiovascular disease, the reduction of risk factors

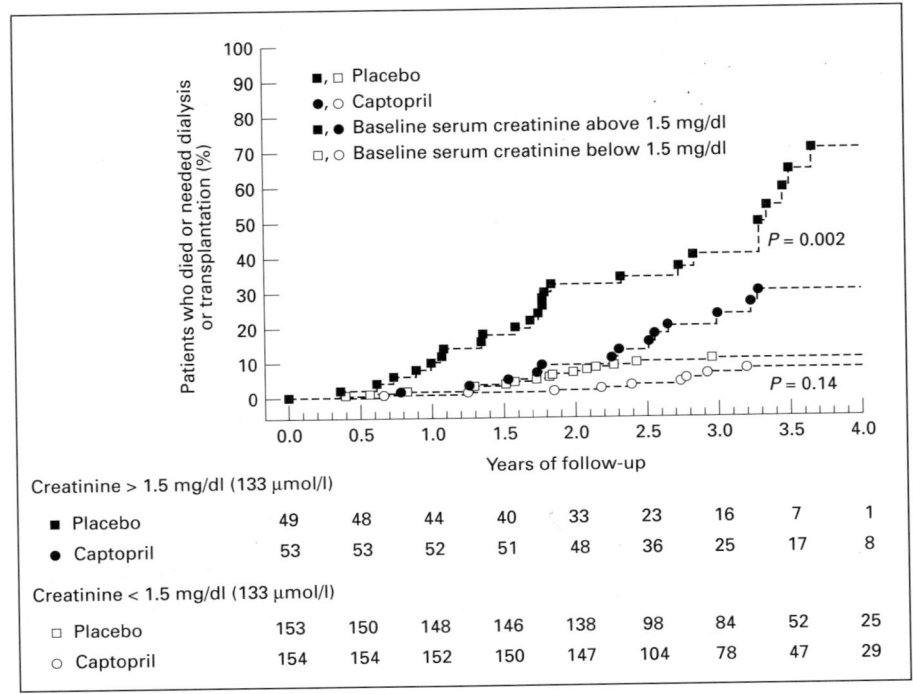

	0.0	0.5	1.0	1.5	2.0	2.5	3.0	3.5	4.0
Creatinine > 1.5 mg/dl (133 µmol/l)									
■ Placebo		49	48	44	40	33	23	16	7	1
● Captopril		53	53	52	51	48	36	25	17	8
Creatinine < 1.5 mg/dl (133 µmol/l)									
□ Placebo		153	150	148	146	138	98	84	52	25
○ Captopril		154	154	152	150	147	104	78	47	29

Fig. 10 Cumulative incidence of subjects dying, or requiring dialysis or transplantation in 409 insulin-dependent patients with clinical nephropathy and blood pressure < 140/90 mmHg who received placebo or captopril (25 mg three times daily) for up to 4 years. Patients are further subdivided into those with a baseline serum creatinine greater ($n = 102$) or less ($n = 307$) than 1.5 mg/dl (133 µmol/l). Note the 50% reduction in events in the captopril treated patients with the higher baseline serum creatinine. (From Lewis et al. [18].)

(such as hyperlipidaemia and smoking) and the routine use of aspirin have been proposed, but there are few conclusive supporting data.

Aldose reductase inhibitor drugs have shown benefit in experimental diabetic nephropathy but not in humans. These drugs reduce tissue levels of sorbitol, the accumulation of which is thought to lead to osmotically mediated tissue damage [16].

Another potential therapy has been the development of drugs that prevent aggregation of glycated tissue proteins into so-called advanced glycation end-products (AGE). It is thought that these modified structural proteins would be much more difficult to degrade and would thus accumulate and cause damage in sensitive tissue such as the renal glomerulus. Animal work using aminoguanidine has proved interesting, and long-term studies in humans are currently underway [16].

☐ SCREENING FOR MICROALBUMINURIA

The use of a laboratory test for screening for a disease or condition depends on satisfying six criteria.

- ☐ The condition must affect the quality or duration of life.
- ☐ Clinically (and cost) effective treatment must be available.
- ☐ Treatment in the asymptomatic phase reduces morbidity and/or mortality.
- ☐ The test should be cheap and easy to perform.
- ☐ The test should be highly sensitive.
- ☐ The disease prevalence must be sufficiently high so that the case finding cost is low.

Clinical diabetic nephropathy now satisfies all of these criteria but the case for microalbuminuria is not completely secure because of the third criterion: there are still no firm data on the impact of treatment on mortality and morbidity. However, if the proxy of progression to clinical nephropathy is used, then microalbuminuria qualifies.

Several papers have tried to prove cost effectiveness using a model of disease progression (Fig. 11) using assumptions of effectiveness from ACEI studies. Two studies differed in their estimate of quality adjusted life years (QALYs) obtained, ranging from 0.009 (US$ 75 000 per QALY) to 0.91 (US$ 10 000 per QALY) after 30 years treatment with ACEI. Another study estimated treatment efficacy as possibly increasing life expectancy by between 4 and 14 years, giving an overall saving per patient of US$ 800–7700 per lifetime [5]. Although all of these papers used similar models of disease progression, they incorporated differing evaluations of effectiveness (eg delaying onset of clinical proteinuria by 2 years or 24 years) and had

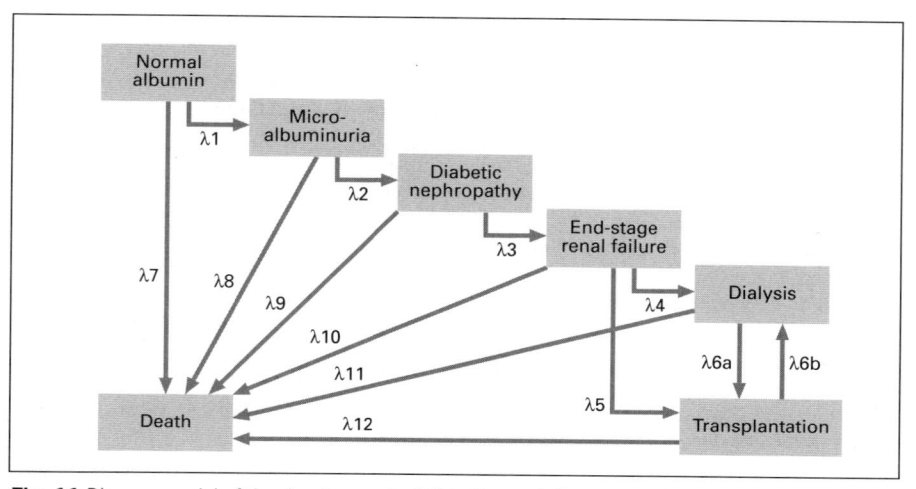

Fig. 11 Disease model of the development of diabetic renal disease used for the estimation of cost effectiveness of screening and intervention in insulin-dependent patients. Each lambda function (1–12) represents a transition probability specific for age, gender and duration of diabetes from one stage to the next. Derivation of these functions is highly dependent on individual basic assumptions of risk and probability. This partly explains the published differences in estimates despite using broadly similar models. (From Borch-Johnsen et al. [19].)

to use arbitrary evaluations of treatment outcomes by polling health-care professionals. Until more definitive long-term data are available on treatment efficacy, the critical question of cost effectiveness will remain unanswered. Nonetheless many national and international bodies recommend screening for microalbuminuria in diabetic patients (Table 3) [5].

REFERENCES

1. Mogensen CE, Christensen CK, Vittinghus E. The stages in diabetic renal disease with emphasis on the stage of incipient nephropathy. *Diabetes* 1983; **32**, Suppl. 2: 64–78.
2. Hasslacher C, Ritz E, Wahl P, Michael C. Similar risks of nephropathy in patients with type I or type II diabetes mellitus. *Nephrol Dial Transplant* 1989; **4**: 859–63.
3. Bojestig M, Arnqvist HJ, Hermansson G, Karlberg BE. Ludvigsson J. Declining incidence of nephropathy in insulin dependent diabetes mellitus. *New Engl J Med* 1994; **330**; 15–18.
4. Mathiesen ER, Ronn B, Storm B, Foght H, Deckert T. The natural course of microalbuminuria in insulin dependent diabetes: a 10-year prospective study. *Diabetic Med* 1995; **12**: 482–7.
5. Mogensen CE, Keane WF, Bennett PH, Jerums G, Parving H-H, Passa P, Steffes MW, Striker GE, Viberti GC. Prevention of diabetic renal disease with special reference to microalbuminuria. *Lancet* 1995; **346**: 1080–4.
6. Borch-Johnsen K, Andersen PK, Deckert T. The effect of proteinuria on relative mortality in type I (insulin-dependent) diabetes mellitus. *Diabetologia* 1985; **28**: 590–6.
7. Parving H-H, Hommel E. Prognosis in diabetic nephropathy. *Brit Med J* 1989; **299**: 230–3.
8. Schmitz A, Vaeth M. Microalbuminuria: a major risk factor in non-insulin dependent diabetes: a 10-year follow up study of 503 patients. *Diabetic Med* 1988; **5**: 126–34.
9. Raine AEG, Margreiter R, Brunner FP, et al. Report on management of renal failure in Europe XXII. *Nephrol Dial Transplant* 1992 ; **7**, Suppl 2: 7–35.
10. Marshall SM. Screening for microalbuminuria: which measurement? *Diabetic Med* 1991; **8**: 706–11.
11. Feldt-Rasmussen B, Mathiesen ER, Jensen T, Lauritzen T, Deckert T. Effect of improved metabolic control on loss of kidney function in type I (insulin-dependent) diabetic patients: an update of the Steno studies. *Diabetologia* 1991; **34**: 164–70.
12. The Diabetes Control and Complications Trial (DCCT) Research Group. Effect of intensive therapy on the development and progression of diabetic nephropathy in the DCCT. *Kidney Int* 1995; **47**: 1703–20.
13. The Microalbuminuria Study Group. Intensive therapy and progression to clinical albuminuria in patients with insulin-dependent diabetes mellitus and microalbuminuria. *Brit Med J* 1995; **311**: 973–7
14. Fioretto P, Mauer SM, Bilous RW, Goetz FC, Sutherland DER, Steffes MW. Effects of pancreas transplantation on glomerular structure in insulin-dependent diabetic patients with their own kidneys. *Lancet* 1993; **342**: 1193–6.
15. Parving H-H, Andersen AR, Smidt UM, Hommel E, Mathiesen ER, Svendsen PA. Effect of antihypertensive treatment on kidney function in diabetic nephropathy. *Brit Med J* 1987; **294**: 1443–7.
16. Breyer JA. Medical management of nephropathy in type 1 diabetes mellitus: current recommendations. *J Am Soc Nephrol* 1995; **6**: 1523–9.
17. The Microalbuminuria Captopril Study Group. Captopril reduces the risk of nephropathy in IDDM patients with microalbuminuria. *Diabetologia* 1996; **39**: 587–93.
18. Lewis EJ, Hunsicker LG, Bain RP, Rohde RD. The effect of angiotensin-converting enzyme inhibition on diabetic nephropathy. *New Engl J Med* 1993; **329**: 1456–62.
19. Borch-Johnsen K, Wenzel H, Viberti GC, Mogensen CE. Is screening and intervention for microalbuminuria worthwhile in patients with insulin-dependent diabetes? *Brit Med J* 1993; **306**: 1722–5.

MULTIPLE CHOICE QUESTIONS

1. Urinary albumin excretion can be increased by:
   (a) Exercise
   (b) Urinary infection
   (c) Low-protein diet
   (d) Posture
   (e) ACE inhibitors

2. Urinary albumin excretion can be reduced by:
   (a) Diuresis
   (b) Exercise
   (c) Low-protein diet
   (d) ACE inhibitors
   (e) Urinary infection

3. Improved glycaemic control with intensive insulin therapy:
   (a) Increases hypoglycaemia
   (b) Decreases weight
   (c) Prevents microalbuminuria developing
   (d) Slows the rate of decline in GFR
   (e) Usually prevents progression of albumin excretion from microalbuminuria to nephropathy

4. ACE inhibitors:
   (a) Reduce intraglomerular capillary pressure
   (b) Increase albumin excretion in NIDDM
   (c) Reduce cardiovascular mortality in nephropathy
   (d) Have higher rates of side effects in diabetes
   (e) Have no effect on albumin excretion in normotensive diabetic patients

5. Screening for microalbuminuria:
   (a) Satisfies all the criteria for an effective screening programme
   (b) Is of proven cost benefit
   (c) Is recommended by national bodies
   (d) Detects more cases in IDDM than NIDDM patients
   (e) Is best performed on a random daytime sample

6. Clinical diabetic nephropathy is defined as a urinary albumin excretion <300 mg/l.

7. Microalbuminuria in diabetic patients is defined as an albumin excretion of 30–300 mg/day.

8. Diabetic nephropathy is more common in insulin-dependent than non-insulin-dependent patients.

9   The incidence of diabetic nephropathy in IDDM is increasing.

10 The survival of diabetic patients on renal replacement therapy is the same as for non-diabetic patients.

11 Glomerular filtration rate is usually low in microalbuminuric diabetic patients.

12 Systemic hypertension (>160/90) is common in patients with microalbuminuria.

13 Relative mortality in NIDDM patients with nephropathy is at least five times that of patients with normal albuminuria.

14 Cardiovascular disease is a more common cause of death than renal failure in patients with nephropathy.

15 Coronary artery bypass grafting improves life expectancy in diabetic patients on renal replacement therapy.

ANSWERS

1a True	2a False	3a True	4a True	5a False
b True	b False	b False	b False	b False
c False	c True	c True	c True	c True
d True	d True	d False	d False	d False
e False	e False	e False	e False	e False
6 False	7 True	8 False	9 False	10 False
11 False	12 False	13 True	14 True	15 True

Assessment of prognosis in patients with angina and coronary artery disease

D S Dymond

☐ INTRODUCTION

It is now well accepted that angina that is refractory to medical therapy is an indication for revascularization either by angioplasty or by coronary bypass surgery. Given the potentially life-threatening nature of coronary disease, much attention has focused in recent years on the role of intervention for coronary disease for prognostic reasons, even when the symptoms may not be severe. Indeed, it is not uncommon for patients who are totally asymptomatic, but with severe coronary disease, to undergo revascularization.

Cardiologists have been searching for years for a systematic approach to the assessment of prognosis in order to try to pick out subgroups of patients with mild or no symptoms who will fare badly on medical therapy, and for whom revascularization might prolong life or reduce the risk of myocardial infarction. This is no easy task. Most physicians will have come across patients with sudden unheralded death and this still poses one of the greatest medical problems in the western world. Sudden death may be the first clinical manifestation of acute myocardial infarction in 20–25% of cases. Of more than 50 000 coronary deaths per year, as many as 60% may be unheralded. We know now that rupture of fairly small non-obstructing plaques, with subsequent clot formation inside the coronary artery, is often the substrate for acute coronary occlusion and sudden death in previously well patients. These minor plaques, which are often lipid rich, may be undetectable by coronary angiography or by the technology used to detect ischaemia.

In this chapter I will concentrate on a different group of patients, namely those with known coronary artery disease who are under the supervision of cardiologists; these, of course, represent a different cohort of patients from those who die suddenly having never seen a doctor.

☐ SEVERITY OF SYMPTOMS

Life would be easy if the severity of angina correlated with survival. Unfortunately, studies have shown no correlation with survival over a 7-year period when the severity of angina is measured by a scoring system on a questionnaire [1]. This is not surprising given the subjective nature of angina, the variability of symptoms in individual patients, and the fact that ischaemia may often be silent. This means that, even in patients who have angina, there are often episodes when the myocardium becomes ischaemic in the absence of symptoms. Patients with episodes of silent ischaemia have been shown to have a worse survival rate than those without [2]. On the basis of this, it is probably not adequate in the current era to rely on symptoms alone to decide which patients to investigate further.

☐ ANGIOGRAPHY

Over the past 20 years the availability of coronary angiography has increased enormously. Several studies have attempted to show a link between the number of diseased vessels (with disease variably defined as 50% or 70% luminal narrowing) and survival. As a rule, these studies showed that single vessel coronary disease has a good prognosis on medical treatment and that double vessel and triple vessel coronary disease have progressively worse survival rates, with left main stem stenosis having a generally poor prognosis without revascularization. An example of a left main stenosis is shown in Fig. 1. This information has little practical benefit unless one can do something about it; the Seattle Watch Heart Study [3] showed that surgery conferred no survival benefit in single vessel disease, but gave a definite improvement in survival in double and triple vessel disease. For a number of years angiography or 'tubular cardiology' was therefore used by many cardiologists to recommend conservative therapy or surgical revascularization. Clinical experience, however, shows that not all patients with single vessel disease run a benign course without revascularization and, conversely, many patients with multi-vessel disease do extremely well for many years without surgery. Single vessel disease involving the left anterior descending coronary artery, particularly if the lesion is proximal to the first septal branch, may have a mortality approaching 20% over a follow-up period of 3 months to 7 years, compared to 0% mortality in left anterior descending lesions distal to the diagonal branch [4]. Most cardiologists will have seen patients with single left anterior descending occlusions with extensive myocardial damage and syndromes of cardiogenic shock or left ventricular failure, who may even need cardiac transplantation. Although left main coronary disease remains an absolute indication for bypass surgery, it is clear that further refinement of the decision-making process is necessary to recommend revascularization for patients at high risk, and hence the search to identify and quantify inducible ischaemia.

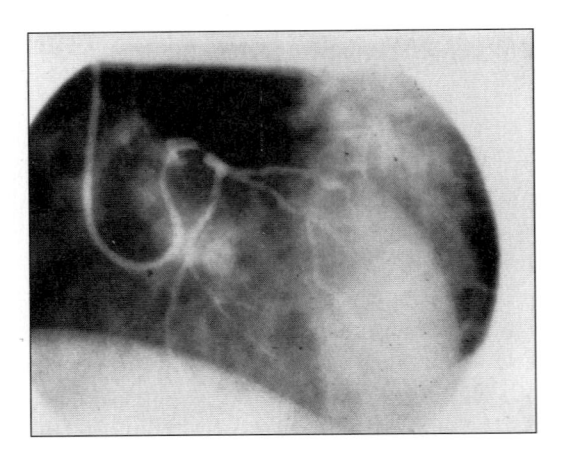

Fig. 1 Coronary arteriogram showing a significant left main stem stenosis.

☐ EXERCISE ELECTROCARDIOGRAM

The exercise electrocardiogram (ECG) is a widely available test, but fraught with difficulties in interpretation. Not every patient with abnormal ST segments on exercise has myocardial ischaemia. The relevance of the exercise test depends heavily on the population being studied. Asymptomatic patients with no cardiac risk factors who have abnormal ECG traces on exercise are likely to be false positive and of little diagnostic and prognostic value, but exercise testing in patients with proven coronary disease may be of prognostic value. The degree of ST segment depression, although visually striking, is less important than the stage of the exercise protocol at which depression of the ST segment appears. Five-year survival is significantly less in patients with both severe and mild angina who demonstrate ischaemia at stage 1 or stage 2 of the Bruce protocol compared to those who can get to stage 3 and beyond [5]. Weiner et al. [6] showed that, even in patients with triple vessel disease and normal left ventricular function, there was a statistically significant difference in the 4-year survival in patients who demonstrated ischaemia early in the exercise protocol from those with better exercise tolerance. In fact, patients with triple vessel disease who could exercise to stage 5 or beyond had a 100% 5-year survival [6].

As Table 1 shows, however, a large cohort of patients cannot have their risk identified by the exercise ECG. This may be due to other factors, such as electrolyte imbalance, left ventricular hypertrophy, conduction defects etc, which interfere with the interpretation of the trace. The exercise ECG remains an imperfect test.

☐ NUCLEAR CARDIOLOGY

Radioisotope scans are not subject to all the influences that can distort the exercise ECG and therefore may be accurate in assessing inducible ischaemia. The most commonly used radioisotope is thallium-201, a monovalent cation that behaves like potassium and distributes in the heart in relation to regional myocardial blood flow. Areas of underperfused myocardium on exercise or after pharmacologically induced increases in myocardial blood flow represent areas of underperfused myocardium which often, but not always, correlate with coronary stenosis. Areas of reversible ischaemia can be identified by comparing the images obtained under these stress circumstances with delayed images taken of the patient at rest. Plate 22 shows a normal thallium tomogram taken from a patient without significant coronary

Table 1 Identification of risk by the exercise ECG. (From Weiner et al. [6].)

Low-risk group (annual mortality less than 1%)	32%	Less than 1 mm of ST segment depression; exercise to stage 3 or beyond
High-risk group (annual mortality greater than 5%)	12%	More than 1 mm of ST segment depression; exercise to less than stage 1
?	56%	

artery disease; myocardial perfusion is normal and homogeneous at both stress and rest.

Early work with thallium always used the coronary angiogram as the gold standard, and a vast number of studies have been published producing results of sensitivity and specificity of the thallium images according to whether coronary disease was present or absent. The major flaw in this concept is to assume that every narrowing in a coronary artery will produce ischaemia, and many cardiologists who are dedicated angiographers have been sceptical about thallium scanning if the results fail to match the angiographic findings. Assuming that images are of high technical quality, it is perhaps more intellectually correct to accept the results of thallium scanning as independent evidence of the impact of a demonstrated coronary stenosis on myocardial perfusion. In other words, if an angiographically proven coronary stenosis fails to produce abnormalities of perfusion, that may be a good prognostic indicator on the benign nature of that stenosis rather than 'a false negative scan'. Proponents of nuclear cardiology have had some difficulty in having this concept accepted, although evidence is mounting that the thallium scan provides powerful prognostic evidence of a good or bad prognosis in patients with proven coronary artery disease. The thallium tomographic images lend themselves to segmental analysis and many workers have shown independently that the number of transient thallium defects (ie those that are present under stress but become normal at rest) predicts the risk of death or myocardial infarction. Adverse events after thrombolytic therapy may also be predicted [7].

Plate 23 shows thallium tomograms at stress and rest in the same format as Fig. 1. The early images demonstrate virtually absent myocardial perfusion under stress with marked improvement, but not normalization, on the resting images. Absent perfusion in multiple segments of the myocardium on all three sets of tomographic images might be expected to correlate with a stenosis of the left main stem. In fact, this patient had a subtotally occluded left anterior descending coronary artery with delayed filling and only partial collateralization from the right coronary artery. This particular left anterior descending artery was a large vessel that wrapped around the apex of the left ventricle and supplied part of the inferior wall. The impact of this stenosis on myocardial perfusion was hence global and this example shows how coronary disease which is defined as single vessel disease may produce a profound impact on myocardial flow. This patient was only mildly symptomatic, but on the basis of the thallium scan underwent left internal mammary grafting.

An alternative approach to myocardial perfusion scanning using radioisotopes is the assessment of left ventricular function by radionuclide angiography. Left ventricular ejection fraction (LVEF) can be measured accurately using the change in radioactive counts inside the left ventricle with each cardiac cycle. Segmental wall motion abnormalities can also be visualized. Patients with normal ventricular function at rest (see Plate 25) will exhibit a fall in ejection fraction if the ventricle becomes ischaemic on exercise and areas of ischaemia will become hypokinetic (Plate 25). The seminal work of Jones et al. [8] showed that exercise ejection fraction was a powerful predictor of prognosis in coronary disease and several other workers have examined the exercise ejection fraction response and have come to the same conclusion. Patients with triple vessel coronary artery disease who have a normal ejection fraction response to exercise have an excellent prognosis over a 4-year follow-up period, whereas those in whom the ejection fraction decreases have a much poorer outlook [9]. Many cardiac departments with an active nuclear cardiology laboratory use myocardial perfusion or left ventricular function studies as a prognostic guide to aid in the decision-making process for conservative therapy or for intervention.

Recent work from our own laboratory has examined the effect of treatment with anti-ischaemic medication on the ejection fraction response to exercise and whether an improved performance on medical therapy confers any prognostic benefit. Preliminary work indicates that the abolition of exercise-induced ischaemia confers a better short-term prognosis in medically treated coronary disease because patients in whom medical therapy did not lead to an improvement in exercise ejection fraction were the only ones who had adverse events in a 9-month follow-up period [10]. In patients who demonstrate an abnormal ejection fraction response to exercise off therapy, but who show a normalized response on therapy, the medication may be 'cardioprotective', whereas those patients who maintain an exercise induced fall in spite of anti-ischaemic medication would, by implication, have 'failure of cardioprotection'. These latter patients have a greater short-term risk of adverse outcome and need for revascularization [11]. Although these data on protective effects of medication are only preliminary, a large randomized trial is warranted to see if the exercise ejection fraction measured from radionuclide studies really can allow us to recommend revascularization in mildly symptomatic or asymptomatic patients on a more rational basis; this, of course, has implications for the best use of interventional sources.

Finally, patients with severely reduced left ventricular function may be turned down for coronary bypass surgery, particularly if they have clinical congestive cardiac failure. Recent work suggests that areas of myocardium that appear to be completely functionless may in fact be dormant or 'hibernating'. Radioisotopes can help identify areas of hibernating myocardium either by the use of resting thallium scans or, more elegantly, by the use of positron-emitting radioisotopes. These are not, unfortunately, widely available but in centres that have a cyclotron to produce these isotopes myocardial perfusion can be measured using ^{13}N-labelled ammonia and metabolism could be measured in the ischaemic myocardium using ^{18}F-labelled fluoro-deoxyglucose. Areas that demonstrate reduced or absent perfusion, but which continue to metabolize glucose, may be hibernating, and some work has demonstrated that these areas of 'perfusion/metabolism mismatch' may be those areas that can improve function after revascularization (see Plate 24) [12,13]. Again, this has major implications for the allocation of resources and allows the decision-making process to be based on science rather than whim.

☐ CONCLUSION

In summary, the complementary use of angiography and radioisotope imaging can aid prognostic assessment of patients with proven coronary disease. They can help guide the clinician towards recommending revascularization on prognostic grounds even in patients who may be minimally symptomatic, or those who are regarded as being, perhaps erroneously, beyond treatment.

REFERENCES

1. Holtgren HN, Peduzzi P. On behalf of VA Co-operative study. Relation of severity of symptoms of prognosis in stable angina pectoris. *Am J Cardiol* 1984; **54**, 988–93.
2. Weiner DA, Ryan TJ, McCabe CH, *et al.* Significance of silent myocardial ischaemia during exercise testing in patients with coronary artery disease. *Am J Cardiol* 1987; **59**: 725–9.
3. Rohen TA, Hammermeister HE, Dodge HT. *Circulation* 1981; **63**: 537–45.
4. Brooks N, Cattell M, Jennings K, Balcon R, Honey M, Layton C. Isolated disease of left anterior descending coronary artery; angiographic and clinical study of 218 patients. *Brit Heart J* 1982; **47**: 1189–96.
5. Dagenais GR, Rouleau JR, Christen A, Fabia J. Survival of patients with a strongly positive exercise electrocardiogram. *Circulation* 1982; **65**: 452–6.
6. Weiner DA, Ryan TJ, McCabe CH, *et al.* Value of exercise taking in determining the risk classification and the response to coronary artery bypass grafting in three-vessel coronary disease: a report from the Coronary Artery Surgery Study (CASS) registry. *Am J Cardiol* 1987; **60**: 262–6.
7. Basu S, Senior R, Dose C, Lahiri A. Value of thallium-201 imaging in detecting adverse events after myocardial infarction and thrombolysis: a follow up of 160 consecutive patients. *Brit Med J* 1996; **313**: 844–7.
8. Jones RH, Floyd RD, Austin EH, Sabiston DC, Jr, *et al.* The role of radioactive angiocardiography in the pre-operative prediction of pain relief and prolonged survival following coronary artery bypass grafting. *Ann Surg* 1983; **197**: 743–54.
9. Bonow RO, Kent LM, Rosing DR, *et al.* Exercise induced ischaemia in mildly symptomatic patients with coronary artery disease and preserved left ventricular function: identification of subgroups at risk during medical therapy. *New Engl J Med* 1984; **311**: 1339–45.
10. Lim R, Dyke L, Dymond DS. Effect on prognosis of abolition of exercise-induced painless myocardial ischaemia by medical therapy. *Am J Cardiol* 1992; **69**: 733–5.
11. Lim R, Dyke L, Dymond DS. Objective assessment of 'cardioprotective' efficacy as a prognostic guide to management of mildly symptomatic revascularisable disease. *J Am Coll Cardiol* 1995; **26**: 1140–5.
12. Bonow RO, Isizian V, Chocolo A, *et al.* Identification of viable myocardium in patients with chronic coronary artery disease and left ventricular dysfunction: comparison of thallium scintigraphy with reinjection and PET imaging with ^{18}F-fluorodeoxyglucose. *Circulation* 1991; **83**: 26–37.
13. Eitzman D, Al-Aouar Z, Kanter H, *et al.* Clinical outcome of patients with advanced coronary artery disease after viability studies with positron-emission tomography. *J Am Coll Cardiol* 1992; **20**: 559–63.

☐ MULTIPLE CHOICE QUESTIONS

1. The exercise electrocardiogram:
   (a) Is useful as a screening test in asymptomatic individuals
   (b) Is of prognostic value if ST segment depression >3 mm occurs
   (c) Predicts a poor prognosis if positive at stage 1
   (d) Is more reliable than radioisotope scans
   (e) Is often influenced by factors other than ischaemia

2. Coronary angiography:
   (a) Is valuable for predicting myocardial infarction

(b) Should be performed in a patient with limiting angina even if the exercise test is negative
(c) Has no prognostic value
(d) Always correlates with isotope scans
(e) Demonstrates plaques that are likely to rupture

3 Myocardial perfusion scanning under stress:
   (a) Is useful for predicting the number of diseased coronary arteries
   (b) Is a powerful predictor of prognosis independently of the number of diseased arteries
   (c) Can resolve the dilemmas caused by interpretation of exercise ECGs
   (d) Can measure absolute coronary blood flow
   (e) Is of no use after thrombolytic therapy as a prognostic tool

4 Radionuclide angiography under stress:
   (a) Cannot accurately assess left ventricular function
   (b) Always shows falls in ejection fraction in patients with coronary disease
   (c) May show normalization of an abnormal response with medical therapy
   (d) Is expensive and dangerous
   (e) Can be used to stratify risks in patients with angina, on and off therapy

5 In heart failure:
   (a) Coronary surgery is contraindicated in patients with poor left ventricular function and angina
   (b) Surgery may improve left ventricular function in some patients
   (c) Surgery may be indicated if akinetic areas are shown to be viable
   (d) Surgery can be justified if there is a match between disturbed flow and disturbed glucose metabolism
   (e) A resting thallium scan is of no value

ANSWERS

1a	False	2a	False	3a	False	4a	False	5a	False
b	False	b	True	b	True	b	False	b	True
c	True	c	False	c	True	c	True	c	True
d	False	d	False	d	False	d	False	d	False
e	True	e	False	e	False	e	True	e	False

Intervention in acute coronary syndrome: unstable angina and non-Q wave myocardial infarction

K A A Fox

☐ INTRODUCTION

The acute coronary syndrome comprises unstable angina, non-Q wave myocardial infarction (MI), Q wave myocardial infarction and sudden cardiac death. The common features in the syndrome are of disrupted atheromatous plaque with a variable contribution of intra-plaque and intra-luminal thrombosis (Table 1). The presence of occlusive thrombus and a large territory of myocardium supplied by the affected vessel will result in profound clinical manifestations of ischaemia (including the risks of arrhythmias and sudden death). Myocardial infarction results when the ischaemia is sufficiently profound and sustained to induce irreversible cell injury. This chapter will focus on interventions for unstable angina and non-Q wave MI.

The clinical diagnosis of unstable angina may be defined as new onset angina or angina that is worsening in its frequency or severity or duration, and it includes rest angina which occurs without provocation. Differentiation of unstable angina from

Table 1 Common features of acute coronary syndrome. (From Davies [1].)

Intimal lesions underlying major coronary thrombi		
Plaque fissure (deep intimal injury)*		74.7%
Mural thrombus	52%	
Occlusive thrombus	23%	
Endothelial damage (superficial injury)		25.3%
Mural thrombi	11%	
Occlusive thrombi	14.5%	

Mechanism of plaque fissuring
Reconstruction of 85 fissured plaques
    In 83%, tear entered extracellular lipid pool
    Most common site: plaque margin
    Predisposing factors
        Plaque cap: reduced collagen content
        Increased macrophage content
        Increased lipid content

*N = 166 lesions detected at postmortem angiography

non-Q wave MI can only be confirmed in retrospect, once the sequence of cardiac enzymes have been measured. However, this definition is not appropriate for interventions that need to be performed early in the course of the syndrome.

☐ OUTCOME IN UNSTABLE ANGINA

Early studies which employed a clinical definition of unstable angina, without electrocardiograph (ECG) change or other corroborating evidence, resulted in a heterogeneous population. Many of these patients may not have cardiac chest pain or true unstable angina. Thus, the overall event rate for this large group is relatively low (deaths approx. 2% in the first 7 days). The classification provided by Braunwald [2] has helped to differentiate unstable angina of primary origin from that due to non-cardiac causes or that following MI. It also separated recent onset from delayed and accelerating pattern angina (Table 2). However, the vast majority of patients who presented to hospital with unstable angina and ECG change fall into Braunwald classification IIIB. It is therefore necessary to devise a clinically relevant strategy to define a high-risk population (based on clinical and ECG criteria). On the basis of the ATACS study [3] (Table 3) and registry studies, it is possible to define a high-risk population (Table 4).

Recent trials of treatment strategies in unstable angina have employed similar inclusion criteria (excluding those with persistent ST segment elevation or other qualifications for thrombolysis) and have defined the risks of subsequent events.

By employing similar entry criteria, the risks of death from non-fatal MI are in

Table 2 Classification of unstable angina. (From Braunwald [2].)

Braunwald classification
I. New onset or accelerating angina
II. Angina at rest (not within 48 h)
III. Angina at rest (within 48 h)
Classification:
A   in the presence of extracardiac condition provoking angina
B   primary unstable angina
C   post-infarction (within 2 weeks)

Table 3 Results of the ATACS study which compared aspirin therapy and aspirin/heparin combination: 12-week follow-up of 358 patients with acute coronary syndrome. This study confirmed the high frequency of cardiovascular events in this study population (mainly recurrent angina). (From [3].)

	Recurrent angina	MI	Death	Total
Unstable angina	20%	4%	3%	27%
Non-Q MI	11%	11%	5%	27%

Table 4 Unstable angina in a high-risk population.

> Rest pain >10 min
> Repeated anginal episodes or crescendo pattern
> Associated ST/T wave changes on ECG
> Recent onset <24 h
> Elevated troponin-T
> Additional evidence of coronary artery disease

the range 3.8–5.1% within the first 7 days (ATACS and OASIS 1 studies [3,4]; see Table 5). In studies without the requirement for additional evidence of coronary artery disease the event rates are lower.

With more prolonged follow-up the event rates at 6–12 weeks range between 6.9% and 8.2% (ATACS study [3], HELVETICA study control arm [5], TIMI IIIb conservative arm [6]). By 12 months the frequency of death or MI is approximately 12% (TIMI IIIb study; $n = 733$, conservative arm [6]).

Risk of MI and death in unstable angina

Patients included in a randomized trial may not necessarily be representative of the population with unstable angina. Registry studies are useful in defining the overall risk rate in such a population. In a recent registry study involving 2800 patients in six countries, 6% of patients received a β-blocker, 90% aspirin, 60% calcium antagonist, 52% intravenous (i.v.) nitrate and 77% i.v. heparin. The mean hospital stay was 7 days. Overall, there was a 7% risk of death within the first 6 months (in-hospital plus follow-up) and a further 8.7% risk of MI. Thus, using simple clinical criteria *and* evidence of coronary artery disease, it is possible to define a high-risk population with a remarkable consistency of outcome findings in different

Table 5 The effect of aspirin or aspirin plus heparin on MI or death in unstable angina. Risk reduction is 0.44 (CI + 0.21 − 0.93) for heparin plus aspirin vs aspirin alone. (From the Theroux study [11], the RISC study [12], the OASIS study [4] and the ATACS study [3].)

		Patients suffering MI or death (%)	
Study	Follow-up treatment	Aspirin treatment	Aspirin plus heparin treatment
Theroux study ($n = 479$)	6 days	3.3	1.6
RISC study ($n = 796$)	5 days	3.7	1.4
ATACS study ($n = 214$)	5 days	8.3	3.8
OASIS study ($n = 253$)	7 days	—	5.1

countries. Based on an analysis of 21761 medically treated patients at Duke University Medical Center since 1985–1992, there were 9146 patients with an admission diagnosis of unstable angina. The highest risk of death was within the first 48 h and most of the remaining risk was within the first 4 weeks.

☐ PHARMACOLOGIC INTERVENTIONS IN UNSTABLE ANGINA

Based on the findings of the Veterans Association study [7] and the Canadian multi-centre trial [8] the evidence in favour of aspirin treatment following unstable angina is convincing. These trials resulted in a more than 50% reduction in the rates of death and non-fatal MI over a follow-up period of up to 2 years. Further evidence comes from the Antiplatelet Trialists' Collaboration [9,10] which involved 31 randomized trials in patients with a history of transient ischaemic attack, occlusive stroke, unstable angina or MI. A total of approximately 29 000 patients were studied and antiplatelet treatment resulted in a reduction in vascular mortality of 15% and a reduction in non-fatal vascular events (stroke or MI) of 30%. Overall, the total vascular events were reduced by about 25% (secondary prevention of vascular disease by prolonged antiplatelet treatment).

Role of heparin and aspirin

Based on the Theroux study [11], the RISC study [12] and the ATACS study [3], a total of 1489 patients have been randomized to heparin plus aspirin or aspirin alone and have revealed a risk reduction of approximately 56% with heparin (Table 5).

Recently, low-molecular-weight heparin has been shown to be better than placebo at reducing the risk of MI and refractory angina in patients who present with unstable angina and receive aspirin (FRISC study [13]). In a study with similar design, a comparison of heparin and low-molecular-weight heparin was undertaken with similar results (although this study was not powered to reveal small to medium differences in outcome FRIC study).

In the ESSENCE trial [14] a double-blind comparison was undertaken of a low-molecular-weight heparin (Enoxaparin) versus standard heparin treatment in unstable angina. Among 3171 patients there was a highly significant reduction in the combined frequency of death, myocardial infarction or recurrent angina (16.5% vs 19.8%; odds ratio 0.8 with 95% CI 0.49–0.95, $p = 0.19$). The results remained significant at 30 days and were accompanied by a lower rate of revascularization in the low-molecular-weight heparin group (27.7% vs 32.4%, $p = 0.01$). There was no difference in the instance of major bleeding complications.

Hirudin in unstable angina

The frequency of cardiac events in patients despite aspirin and heparin therapy has led to the search for more potent platelet-receptor antagonists and thrombin antagonists. In addition, recombinant hirudin has been used as an adjunctive treatment to thrombolytic therapy and aspirin in studies of acute MI. The latter include the GUSTO IIa study, the TIMI 9a study and the HIT study. Despite encouraging preliminary data, the combination of hirudin and thrombolytic agent resulted in an excess of major bleeds including cerebral haemorrhage and extracranial bleeds compared to heparin. These trials were stopped prematurely.

In contrast, studies of unstable angina in which hirudin was compared with heparin have been more encouraging and these do not involve concomitant thrombolytic therapy. The HELVETICA study [5] revealed a reduction in major cardiac events within the first 96 h of angioplasty in unstable angina with hirudin treatment. This difference did not persist in long-term follow-up. However, in the OASIS-1 pilot study [4] there was consistent evidence in favour of hirudin over heparin. The frequency of cardiovascular death, new MI, refractory or severe angina was 17% in heparin-treated patients, 15.4% low-dose hirudin and 8.7% with medium-dose hirudin (low-dose 0.2 mg/kg bolus and 0.1 mg/kg/h infusion and medium-dose 0.4 mg/kg bolus and 0.15 mg/kg/h). A total of 601 patients were randomized to these treatment strategies and the findings for cardiovascular death, new MI and refractory angina were similarly encouraging (heparin 6.3%, low-dose hirudin 4.6% and medium-dose hirudin 2.9%). There was no excess of major bleeds or strokes in this study. However, it does require confirmation in a larger scale investigation.

Platelet receptor antagonists

Platelet function is not completely inhibited by aspirin and experimental studies have shown that the effects are overcome with adrenaline-induced alpha-receptor modulation. The integrin glycoprotein IIb/IIIa occurs on the platelet surface and is the final common pathway for platelet aggregation. It binds circulating macromolecules like fibrinogen and von Willebrand factor and it cross-links platelets thus promoting aggregation (Fig. 1). Specific antagonists to the receptor may provide a potent way of inhibiting platelet-mediated thrombosis. The EPIC study [15] investigated 2099 patients in a double-blind prospective study of high-risk angioplasty/atherectomy. The end-points were death or non-fatal MI or unplanned coronary angioplasty with or without stent implantation or coronary artery bypass surgery (at 30 days). Bolus administration of the IIb/IIIa receptor antagonists (7EIII) reduced the combined end-point from 12.8% to 8.3% of cases (when administered as a bolus and infusion). However, this beneficial result was achieved at the expense of additional bleeding. Overall, there were four to five fewer cardiac events but at the cost of seven more major bleeds/100 patients treated.

☐ INVASIVE STRATEGIES

Intervention as opposed to conservative strategy in unstable angina and non-Q wave MI was studied in the TIMI IIIb trial [6]. The trial randomized 1473 patients with ischaemic rest pain or non-Q wave MI infarction to early invasive strategy (early angiography and revascularization when appropriate) or an early conservative strategy. The primary end-point was death, MI or an unsatisfactory symptom-limited exercise test. This end-point occurred in 18.1% of the patients consigned to

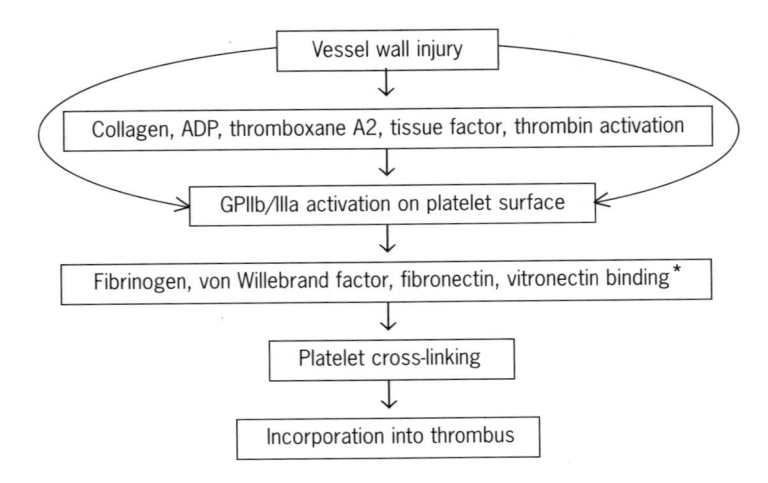

```
                    ┌─────────────────────┐
                    │  Vessel wall injury │
                    └─────────────────────┘
                               ↓
    ┌──────────────────────────────────────────────────────────────┐
    │ Collagen, ADP, thromboxane A2, tissue factor, thrombin activation │
    └──────────────────────────────────────────────────────────────┘
                               ↓
         ┌────────────────────────────────────────────┐
    →    │ GPIIb/IIIa activation on platelet surface  │   ←
         └────────────────────────────────────────────┘
                               ↓
    ┌───────────────────────────────────────────────────────────┐
    │ Fibrinogen, von Willebrand factor, fibronectin, vitronectin binding* │
    └───────────────────────────────────────────────────────────┘
                               ↓
              ┌──────────────────────────────┐
              │   Platelet cross-linking     │
              └──────────────────────────────┘
                               ↓
              ┌──────────────────────────────┐
              │  Incorporation into thrombus │
              └──────────────────────────────┘
```

* 50 000 fibrinogen receptors exposed per platelet
common amino acid sequence: arginine–glycine–aspartate

Fig. 1 The interaction between platelet activation and thrombin generation.

the conservative strategy and 16.2% for those assigned to the invasive strategy; the difference was not statistically significant.

The early invasive strategy reduced the average length of hospitalization and rehospitalization. After 1 year, death or MI occurred in 10.7% of patients assigned to early invasive strategy and 12.2% of patients consigned to the conservative strategy, which was not statistically significant. However, the relevance of the study was limited in view of the fact that 61% of the patients assigned to the invasive strategy underwent a revascularization procedure, whereas 49% of those assigned to the conservative strategy also underwent such a procedure. Thus, the differences in intervention rate were too small to reliably assess the impact of intervention. This question will be re-addressed in the larger RITA 3 study (3300 patients).

☐ CONCLUSION

Acute coronary syndromes include sudden death, Q-wave MI, non-Q wave MI and unstable angina. The last two conditions can be distinguished by the absence of a significant rise in cardiac enzymes in unstable angina. However, both of the last two conditions may involve release of other enzymes including troponin.

Unstable angina is a clinical syndrome with a heterogeneous outcome unless it is defined additionally by ECG criteria or other evidence of coronary artery disease. In doing so, a high-risk population can be identified. The hallmarks of standard treatment involve the use of aspirin and heparin and both have been shown to reduce the frequency of cardiac events. Although there is encouraging information on the use of more potent and specific platelet receptor antagonists and antithrombins, these data require confirmation in larger scale studies with mortality/MI end-points. The choice of conservative strategy or intervention strategy for unstable angina has not yet been resolved and requires formal testing.

REFERENCES

1. Davies MJ. A macro and micro view of coronary vascular insult in ischaemic heart disease. *Circulation* 1990; **82**: 38–46.
2. Braunwald E. Unstable angina: a classification. *Circulation* 1989; **80**: 410–4.
3. Cohen M, Parry G, Xiong J, *et al.* and the ATACS Research Group. Combination antithrombotic therapy in unstable rest angina and non-Q wave infarction in non-prior aspirin users: primary end points analysis from the ATACS trial. *Circulation* 1994; **89**: 81–8.
4. Organization to Assess Strategies for Ischemic Syndromes (OASIS) Investigators. Comparison of hirudin with heparin and warfarin with control for unstable angina and non Q wave MI in a randomized controlled trial. *Am Heart Assoc* 1995 (Abstract).
5. Serruys PW, Herrman J-PR, Simon R, *et al.* on behalf of the HELVETICA Investigators. A comparison of hirudin with heparin in the prevention of restenosis after coronary angioplasty. *New Engl J Med* 1995; **333**: 757–63.
6. The TIMI III Investigators. Effects of tissue plasminogen activator and a comparison of early invasive and conservative strategies in unstable angina and non-Q wave myocardial infarction: results of the TIMI III B trial. *Circulation* 1994; **89**: 1545–56.
7. Lewis HD Jr, Davis JW, Archibald DG, *et al.* Protective effects of aspirin against acute myocardial infarction and death in men with unstable angina. *New Engl J Med* 1983; **309**: 396–403.
8. Cairns JA, Gent M, Singer J, *et al.* Aspirin, sulfinpyrazone or both in unstable angina: results of a Canadian multicenter trial. *New Engl J Med* 1985; **313**: 1369–75.
9. Antiplatelet Trialists' Investigators. Secondary prevention of vascular disease by prolonged antiplatelet treatment. *Brit Med J* 1988; **296**: 320–31.
10. Antiplatelet Trialists' Investigators. Collaborative overview of randomised trials of antiplatelet therapy. 1. Prevention of death, MI and stroke by prolonged antiplatelet therapy in various categories of patients. *Brit Med J* 1994; **308**: 81–106.
11. Theroux P, Ouimet H, McCans J, *et al.* Aspirin, heparin or both to treat unstable angina. *New Engl J Med* 1988; **319**: 1105–11.
12. The RISC Group. Risk of myocardial infarction and death during treatment with low-dose aspirin and i.v. heparin in men with unstable coronary artery disease. *Lancet* 1990; **336**: 827–30.
13. Fragmin. Low-molecular-weight heparin during instability in coronary artery disease (FRISC) study group. *Lancet* 1996; **347**: 561–8.
14. Cohen M, Demers C, Gurfinkel E, Frommell G, Fox KAA *et al.* A double-blind comparison of Enoxaparin (a low-molecular-weight heparin) with standard heparin in the treatment of unstable coronary artery disease (the ESSENCE trial). (In press and presentation at the American Heart Association 1996 and British Cardiac Society 1997).
15. The EPIC Investigators. Use of a monclonal antibody directed against the platelet glycoprotein IIb/IIIa receptor in high-risk coronary angioplasty. *New Engl J Med* 1994; **330**: 956–61.

☐ MULTIPLE CHOICE QUESTIONS

1. Unstable angina: diagnosis and risk groups:
   (a) Unstable angina necessitates ECG change for the diagnosis
   (b) Elevated troponin T in unstable angina indicates increased risk of death and MI
   (c) Unstable angina can be distinguished from non-Q wave MI by clinical and ECG features

(d) Unstable angina carries a risk of subsequent MI or death of <5% in 6 months
(e) If associated with new and persistent left bundle branch block then the patient has sustained a myocardial infarction

2 Unstable angina: therapy:
(a) Aspirin treatment is associated with a 50% reduction in the frequency of death or non-fatal MI
(b) Heparin and aspirin treatment is associated with a 50% reduction in the frequency of death or non-fatal MI compared to aspirin alone
(c) Randomized trials have demonstrated a significant benefit for angioplasty in the first 48 h after presentation
(d) Platelet receptor antagonists (IIb/IIIa) reduce the frequency of cardiac events in conjunction with angioplasty
(e) Thrombolytic therapy reduces the frequency of death in unstable angina

3 Unstable angina:
(a) Oesophageal pain may mimic unstable angina including T-wave changes
(b) Hypertrophic cardiomyopathy can be distinguished from unstable angina by the absence of repolarization changes
(c) On coronary angiography, filling defects in relation to a stenosis, signify the presence of thrombus
(d) Complex angiographic lesions are associated with increased cardiac risk but no increase in the risk of intervention (angioplasty)
(e) In the presence of pre-existing stable angina, multivessel coronary artery disease is more likely than single vessel disease

ANSWERS

1a	False	2a	True	3a	True
b	True	b	True	b	False
c	False	c	False	c	True
d	False	d	True	d	False
e	True	e	False	e	True

Modern management of arrhythmias

R W F Campbell

☐ INTRODUCTION

The management of almost every cardiac disease has changed dramatically in the past 10 years. Nowhere is this more evident than in the management of cardiac arrhythmias. Following the inception of coronary care units with routine electrocardiogram (ECG) monitoring of infarct patients, cardiac arrhythmias were much feared and were energetically treated. Arrhythmia suppression was equated with benefit, but large-scale controlled trials in the 1980s showed that it was quite possible to suppress arrhythmias and to do harm [1]. While the results specifically addressed the arrhythmias that complicate myocardial infarction (MI), they prompted a reconsideration of the management of almost every cardiac arrhythmia. From the subsequent analyses, anti-arrhythmic drugs have emerged badly scarred. The efficacy of drug therapy to control arrhythmias is, in many situations, much less impressive than most would believe. Furthermore, in long-term management, unwanted side effects are being increasingly recognized. The height of disillusionment with drug therapy coincided with the remarkable advances in radio-frequency ablation and in the technical developments of implantable cardioverter defibrillators.

There are now so many treatment options available to practising clinicians who manage arrhythmias that selecting the optimal therapy has become extremely difficult. Arrhythmia management badly needs guidelines, but these are proving difficult to agree. Too few randomized controlled studies have been performed and, while it is easy to be critical of this situation, randomized controlled studies are difficult to perform when spontaneous events occur with a very low frequency and/or when events may be directly fatal.

The situation is not beyond hope. It is clear that there is no panacea for cardiac arrhythmias. Recent research has underscored the varied nature of the processes that create arrhythmias and it is to be expected that successful treatment will demand a range of different interventions. The key to successful management lies in detailed and accurate identification of the arrhythmia. Of the many new developments in modern arrhythmia management, three areas are worthy of special attention. All depend on arrhythmia diagnosis with differing degrees of sophistication.

☐ ACUTE MANAGEMENT OF TACHYCARDIAS

Sustained tachycardias are an important clinical problem. They often present as an emergency and most are managed by relatively junior staff. Safety is of paramount concern, particularly as tragedies can easily occur. Patients with sustained tachycardias may be haemodynamically compromised and very intolerant of administered therapies that have even modest hypotensive effects. Figure 1 shows a management scheme for the acute treatment of sustained tachycardias.

Characterization of tachycardia is based largely on the duration of the QRS complex on an ECG (broad ≥120 ms; ≥3 small squares on ECG paper recorded at 25 mm/s) and whether the arrhythmia is regular or irregular. This identifies the admittedly relatively crude categories of 'supraventricular tachycardia' (SVT), atrial flutter, atrial fibrillation, ventricular tachycardia (VT), torsade de pointes and pre-excited atrial fibrillation. Figure 1 offers options for first-line therapies designed to

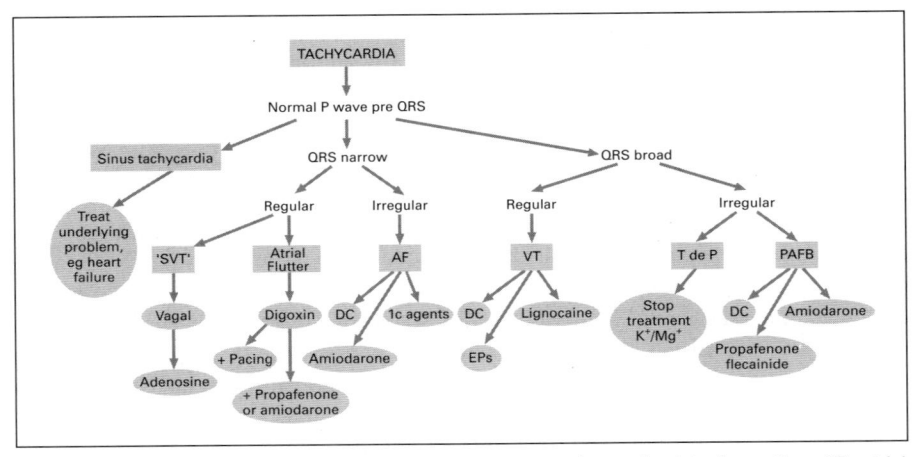

Fig. 1 A management scheme for the acute treatment of sustained tachycardias. AF, atrial fibrillation; VT, ventricular tachycardia; T de P, torsade de pointes; PAFB, pre-excited atrial fibrillation; EPs, electrophysiology study.

restore sinus rhythm or, in some cases where this is difficult, to control the ventricular rate. In situations where there is haemodynamic collapse, early recourse to DC version is appropriate. A glance at the suggested therapy shows that in fact relatively few anti-arrhythmic drugs feature within the scheme. Digoxin, adenosine, lignocaine, amiodarone and the class 1c agents (propafenone and flecainide) comprise the suggested therapies.

☐ ADENOSINE IN THE MANAGEMENT OF TACHYCARDIAS

Regular narrow QRS tachycardias

In the acute management of narrow regular QRS tachycardias adenosine is an important new therapy. Over 90% of regular narrow QRS tachycardias involve the atrioventricular (AV) node as part of the circuit. The two major contributing arrhythmias are reciprocating tachycardias involving accessory pathways (Wolff-Parkinson-White syndrome etc) and the para-AV nodal re-entry tachycardias. The inclusion of the AV node within the re-entrant circuit means that interventions that alter AV nodal electrophysiology may terminate the arrhythmia. This is the basis for the use of vagal manoeuvres. When these fail, adenosine is now the first-line choice. It is a short-acting intravenously administered muscarinic agent. It should be given in an escalating dose starting with 3 mg as an intravenous bolus progressing through doses of 6, 9 and 12 mg depending on response. Over 95% of regular narrow QRS tachycardias involving the AV node will terminate with this prescription (Fig. 2).

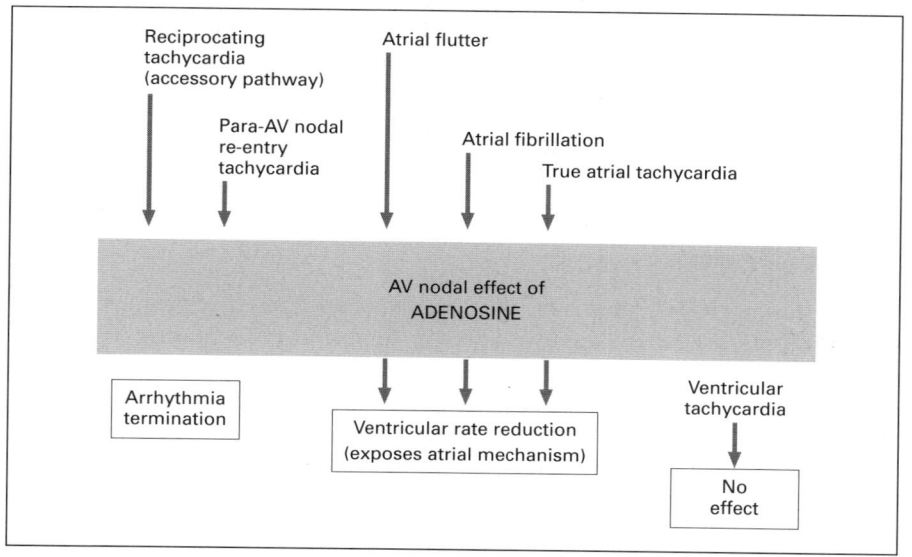

Fig. 2 Effects of adenosine on tachycardias.

Other atrial arrhythmias

Three atrial arrhythmias are transiently influenced by adenosine, but are unlikely to be terminated. They are atrial flutter, atrial fibrillation and the so-called true atrial tachycardias (whether due to re-entry or automaticity), which are contained within the atrial myocardium. The AV node is not directly involved in maintaining these arrhythmias; it only transmits impulses to the ventricle. The ventricular response rate in these arrhythmias is high and in many instances management of the arrhythmia may involve, at least initially, rate control. Adenosine administered during these arrhythmias will reduce the ventricular rate. This may be useful diagnostically as it will expose the atrial mechanism but, given the very short duration of action of adenosine, there is no therapeutic gain.

Broad QRS tachycardia – ventricular tachycardia

Ventricular tachycardia (VT) is contained within the ventricles and involves no part of the AV node. Adenosine therefore has no anti-arrhythmic effect. Any other action, particularly on blood pressure, is very transient and little, if any, harm is done. This is in marked contrast to the calcium antagonist drugs. Verapamil has been widely used for the acute termination of so-called 'supraventricular' arrhythmias. For this application it is safe and effective. Regrettably, however, there are many reports of verapamil being given in error to patients with VT. Deaths and serious complications have occurred [2]. Misdiagnosis of VT as 'SVT' should not happen – but it does. Any broad QRS tachycardia (QRS ≥ 120 ms) should be considered as VT until proven otherwise. 'SVT' with aberration that produces a broad QRS is uncommon, but even rarer is VT with a narrow QRS. Despite this simple QRS duration 'rule', mistakes still occur. Adenosine is an important new advance. It is much safer for acute arrhythmia control than verapamil if a totally reliable diagnosis of tachyarrhythmias cannot be made. Adenosine, however, is not without unwanted side effects. Patients feel uncomfortable for a few seconds after administration of the drug. They complain of nausea and flushing. There have been very rare reports of more serious reactions, including the precipitation of ventricular fibrillation and torsade de pointes.

☐ RADIOFREQUENCY ABLATION

Radiofrequency (RF) ablation is the most dramatic new advance in the management of arrhythmias. It offers curative therapy for an ever increasing variety of arrhythmias. As RF ablation involves highly trained personnel and sophisticated equipment, it is not widely available. This is unfortunate as the success rates of the technique are high, the complications are low and patients can usually return to a completely normal lifestyle without even the need for follow-up. RF ablation is so important that all physicians who have responsibilities for patients with arrhythmias must know something of the indications for RF ablation such that they seek appropriate help for their patients.

RF ablation involves the gentle heating of an intracardiac electrode catheter by radiofrequency energy. Cardiac tissue in contact with the heated tip is destroyed. The lesion created is controllable and small. Lesions are certainly less than 1 cm in diameter and probably most are no bigger than 0.5 cm. It is obvious then that RF ablation can apply only to the management of arrhythmias where the arrhythmia anatomy is understood and where critically placed small lesions can disrupt the arrhythmic process. Not surprisingly, accessory atrioventricular pathways were the first to be tackled. When these are capable of antegrade conduction, patients are at risk of re-entrant tachycardia and/or pre-excited atrial fibrillation. The surface ECG will show a delta wave (slurred QRS onset). When capable of only retrograde conduction, the risk of rapid response rates to atrial fibrillation is not present. RF ablation can be successfully applied to both types of pathway with success rates of 95% or better. Not surprisingly, RF ablation has completely supplanted surgery for accessory pathways and it is being used with increasing enthusiasm [3]. Already RF ablation is recommended first-line therapy for high-risk Wolff-Parkinson-White syndrome patients (Fig. 3), principally those at risk of very rapid response rates to atrial fibrillation.

Right ventricular outflow tract tachycardia or catecholamine-dependent tachycardia is an increasingly recognized entity. It can be very debilitating and is often difficult to control with drug therapy. This arrhythmia arises from a very small

```
RF ablation as          →  High-risk WPW syndrome
first-line therapy      ↗
                           Right ventricular
                        ↗  outflow tract tachycardia
RF ablation as          
second-line therapy     
after one drug failure  ↘  Symptomatic reciprocating tachycardia
                           Para-AV nodal re-entry tachycardia

RF ablation as             'True' atrial tachycardia
third-line therapy      →  Atrial flutter
after drug failure         Atrial fibrillation
                           (AV node ablation + pacemaker)
```

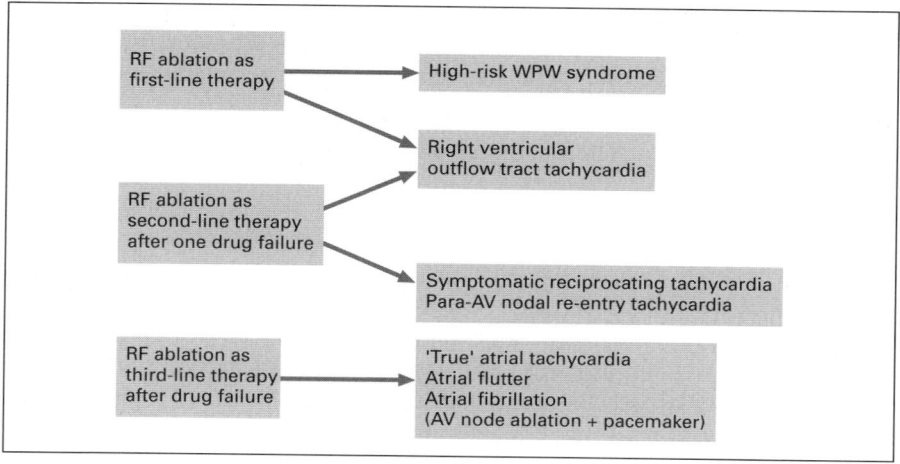

Fig. 3 Applications of radiofrequency (RF) ablation.

'focus' in the right ventricular outflow tract and it can be ablated by RF energy. Such is the success of the procedure that RF ablation is fast becoming first-line therapy for this condition [4].

The two major forms of regular narrow QRS tachycardia, reciprocating tachycardia using an accessory pathway and para-AV nodal re-entry, both involve accessible small conduction routes which can be destroyed by RF ablation. These arrhythmias are, however, common and it would be impractical to use RF energy as first-line therapy. Current strategies are to start management with a well chosen drug and, in the event of failure or non-tolerance of the therapy, then to resort to RF ablation. 'True' atrial tachycardia (an automatic focus or a re-entrant mechanism in the atrium), atrial flutter and atrial fibrillation can respond to RF ablation but are more difficult challenges when compared to the arrhythmias discussed thus far. For them, a thorough exploration of drug therapy is appropriate before considering RF ablation. In the case of true atrial tachycardia and atrial flutter, curative therapy is possible – in the former the complete arrhythmogenic site is destroyed while in the latter a series of RF lesions create lines of conduction block that prevent the circulation of re-entrant electrical activity that underlies atrial flutter. The RF management of atrial fibrillation is completely different. Curative RF approaches are being investigated but they are unreliable and there are few reported successes. The procedural time averages 12 h. This may change but for the present, in patients with atrial fibrillation who fail to respond to drug therapy, RF energy is used to destroy the AV node [5]. A pacemaker (usually a sophisticated rate-responsive variety) is then needed. This approach seems crude. It destroys a 'good' part of the heart; it leaves the atria fibrillating with the attendant risk of thromboembolism and it renders the patient pacemaker-dependent. Nonetheless, remarkable subjective and objective improvements are reported and, in my own experience, patients who reach the point of being considered for this approach are very debilitated by their uncontrolled atrial fibrillation. For them, even a crude procedure brings great benefit with a controlled and responsive ventricular response. An alternative to complete disruption of the AV node may lie with its RF modification to control the ventricular response rate [6]. For the moment, this approach remains experimental.

The risks

Apart from some very minor discomfort during the delivery of radiofrequency energy, the procedure is relatively innocuous. Cardiac perforation with or without tamponade has been reported in approximately 1 in 1000 procedures and there have been very occasional deaths [7]. No procedure involving intracardiac catheters and the delivery of destructive energy can be completely safe. For this reason RF ablation must not be used lightly. The risks and upset posed by the patient's arrhythmias must be balanced with the risks and benefits of curative therapy and with the risks and benefits of medical therapy. The indications for the procedure will develop but already the results are so dramatic that our approach to at least some arrhythmias must change.

REFERENCES

1. CAST: The Cardiac Arrhythmia Suppression Trial Investigators. Preliminary report: effect of encainide and flecainide on mortality in a randomised trial of arrhythmia suppression after myocardial infarction. *New Engl J Med* 1989; **321**: 406–12.
2. Rankin AC, Rae AP, Cobbe SM. Misuse of intravenous verapamil in patients with ventricular tachycardia. *Lancet* 1987; **2**: 472–4.
3. Jackman WM, Wang XZ, Friday KJ, *et al.* Catheter ablation of accessory atrioventricular pathways (Wolff–Parkinson–White syndrome) by radiofrequency current. *New Engl J Med* 1991; **324**: 1605–11.
4. Coggins DL, Lee RJ, Sweeney J, *et al.* Radiofrequency catheter ablation as a cure for idiopathic tachycardia of both left and right ventricular origin. *J Am Coll Cardiol* 1994; **23**: 1333–41.
5. Rodriguez LM, Smeets JL, Xie B, *et al.* Improvement in left ventricular function by ablation of atrioventricular nodal conduction in selected patients with lone atrial fibrillation. *Am J Cardiol* 1993; **72**: 1137–41.
6. Williamson BD, Man KC, Daoud E, Niebauer M, Strickberger SA, Morady F. Radiofrequency catheter modification of atrioventricular conduction to control the ventricular rate during atrial fibrillation. *New Engl J Med* 1994; **331**: 910–7.
7. Hindricks G. The Multicentre European Radiofrequency Survey (MERFS): complications of radiofrequency catheter ablation of arrhythmias. The Multicentre European Radiofrequency Survey (MERFS) investigators of the Working Group on Arrhythmias of the European Society of Cardiology. *Eur Heart J* 1993; **14**: 1644–53.

☐ MULTIPLE CHOICE QUESTIONS

1. Administration of adenosine:
    (a) Will stop reciprocating tachycardia
    (b) Will stop atrial fibrillation
    (c) Is recommended for VT
    (d) Can cause torsade de pointes
    (e) Is best given by the oral route

2 A broad QRS (≥120 ms) tachycardia:
   (a) Is always VT
   (b) Should be treated with intravenous verapamil
   (c) May respond to lignocaine
   (d) Is usually an atrial arrhythmia with aberrant conduction
   (e) Mandates anticoagulation

3 RF ablation:
   (a) Can cure accessory pathway arrhythmias
   (b) Can cure para-AV nodal re-entry tachycardia
   (c) Has a 1% rate for serious complications
   (d) Requires cardiopulmonary bypass
   (e) Is contraindicated for VT patients

ANSWERS

1a	True	2a	False	3a	True
b	False	b	False	b	True
c	False	c	True	c	False
d	True	d	False	d	False
e	False	e	False	e	False

Valve disease in the 1990s

R H Swanton

☐ INTRODUCTION

There have been many advances in the diagnosis and management of patients with valve disease over the past few years. Although the subjects discussed in this chapter outline some of these advances, there are still many problems to be solved, particularly in the search for the perfect prosthetic valve.

☐ TRANSOESOPHAGEAL ECHOCARDIOGRAPHY

Although two-dimensional transthoracic echocardiography equipment has become increasingly sophisticated, basic ultrasound principles still limit its value. Imaging structures at the back of the heart requires good ultrasound penetration (best with low-frequency transducers, eg 2–2.5 MHz). Good definition or resolution is better, however, with high-frequency transducers (5 MHz) but tissue attenuation means that these transducers are more use in paediatric than in adult patients. Adequate transthoracic echocardiographic images may be very difficult to obtain in obese or emphysematous patients and in those with chest deformities that result in the echo window being too narrow for the transducer.

As well as resolving these problems, transoesophageal echocardiography (TOE) can image cardiac structures virtually unseen on transthoracic imaging (Table 1). It is particularly valuable in the diagnosis of prosthetic valve regurgitation, and in patients with suspected infective endocarditis. Acoustic shadowing from prosthetic heart valves limits the use of transthoracic echocardiography in diagnosis. The back

Table 1 Cardiac structures best imaged by transoesophageal echocardiography.

Structure	Possible abnormality
Right atrium	Thrombus, myxoma, pacing wire, central lines
Left atrium	Spontaneous contrast, thrombus, myxoma
Left atrial appendage	Thrombus
Pulmonary veins	Anatomy, flow direction
Atrial septum	Patent foramen ovale, atrial septal defect, atrial septal aneurysms, shunts
Mitral valve	Anatomy, vegetations, strands, regurgitant jets
Mitral valve prosthesis	Prosthetic valve dysfunction
Aortic valve prosthesis	Posterior ring abscess, valve dysfunction
Ascending and descending aorta	Aortic dimensions, dissection, atheroma
Coarctation	Site, severity, gradient, possible post-dilatation aneurysms

of the mitral valve and left atrium are masked, particularly by mechanical mitral prostheses, and the posterior part of the aortic root by the mechanical aortic prosthesis. Low-intensity signals from left atrial thrombus can be detected and these may be missed by transthoracic imaging. The technique is superior in identifying any possible cardiac embolic source [1]. Disadvantages of the system are few (Table 2).

All mechanical valves have tiny puffs of regurgitation through the centre of the valve seen on colour Doppler as the ball or disc closes. These closing jets must be appreciated as part of normal valve function and not misinterpreted. Any regurgitant jet on the side of the valve is pathological. Valve dehiscence, thrombosis, paravalve abscess formation and paraprosthetic regurgitation are readily appreciated. The degree of stenosis or regurgitation through a deteriorating xenograft can be assessed just as readily.

Transoesophageal imaging is very important in the diagnosis and management of patients with infective endocarditis. With the higher resolution images, TOE will detect vegetations missed on transthoracic imaging. The presence of an abscess cavity, particularly around the aortic root, can be identified and with the addition of colour Doppler flow mapping the flow within the cavity can be seen. The site and severity of valve regurgitation and the degree of valve destruction can be assessed (see Plate 26). A negative test does not exclude infective endocarditis with either investigation. The two techniques complement each other and are not mutually exclusive. Patients with suspected infective endocarditis should have both investigations at the onset of treatment, regular monitoring at least weekly with transthoracic imaging, and repeat TOE if the patient deteriorates.

TOE can be performed easily in the ventilated patient in the intensive therapy unit (ITU) and the patient does not need to be rolled on to their left side (often necessary for transthoracic imaging). Nasogastric feeding should be discontinued for 4 h before the procedure. The technique is also of considerable value in the operating theatre, particularly during mitral valve repair surgery (see below).

Table 2 Disadvantages of transoesophageal echocardiography.

Cost: biplane probe £21 000; omniplane £28 000. Annual renewal in a busy unit
Doctor, nurse and technician required
Patient must be fasted and consented
Longer procedure
Patient may need sedation or even general anaesthetic
Cidex sterilization system needed for probe
Unsuitable patients:
    Chronic obstructive airways disease
    Severe pulmonary hypertension (hypoxic risk)
    Left ventricle failure: only if ventilated
    Oesophageal pathology
    Cervical spine pathology (eg rheumatoid arthritis)

☐ INFECTIVE ENDOCARDITIS

The disease changes, but the high mortality continues. Older patients, different organisms and increasing problems with antibiotic resistance have contributed to this. In addition, there are increasing numbers of patients with prosthetic valve endocarditis and more intravenous drug abusers with tricuspid valve endocarditis adding to the problem.

Surgery is an invaluable part in the management of patients with infective endocarditis and increasingly used early in the course of the disease with a short course of antibiotics prior to operation and a prolonged course of treatment afterwards. Typical indications for surgery are listed in Table 3. An example of large vegetations seen on echocardiography necessitating surgery is shown in Fig. 1.

Table 3 Indications for surgery in infective endocarditis.

Failure of antibiotics to control infection
Increasing valve regurgitation or destruction
Large fleshy vegetations, or increasing vegetation size on echo
Valve obstruction due to vegetations
Lengthening of the PR interval on ECG: septal abscess formation
Paravalve abscess on echo
Endocarditis due to *Staphylococcus aureus*, Q fever; most fungal cases
Systemic emboli
Most cases of prosthetic valve endocarditis
Relapse of infection after a full course of medical treatment

Patients who have an aortic root abscess (Fig. 2) may well need a further aortic valve replacement in the subsequent months as paraprosthetic regurgitation is common after the first operation [2].

Early in the course of treatment it is imperative to check the patient's dentition with radiological and clinical examinations. Extractions or a dental clearance should be performed early, with additional antibiotic cover prior to valve replacement if possible.

Prevention of a disease with a high mortality is vital. The subject has been reviewed by Prasad and Fraser [3]. All patients with valve disease should receive an antibiotic prophylaxis advisory booklet.

☐ VALVULOPLASTY

Balloon dilatation of all four valves is possible. The results with aortic valvuloplasty are poor, and the procedure is now only used in the very young with congenital aortic stenosis, or in the very old who are too infirm for an aortic valve replacement. Tricuspid valvuloplasty, while successful, is rarely needed. Pulmonary valvuloplasty is usually within the province of the paediatricians.

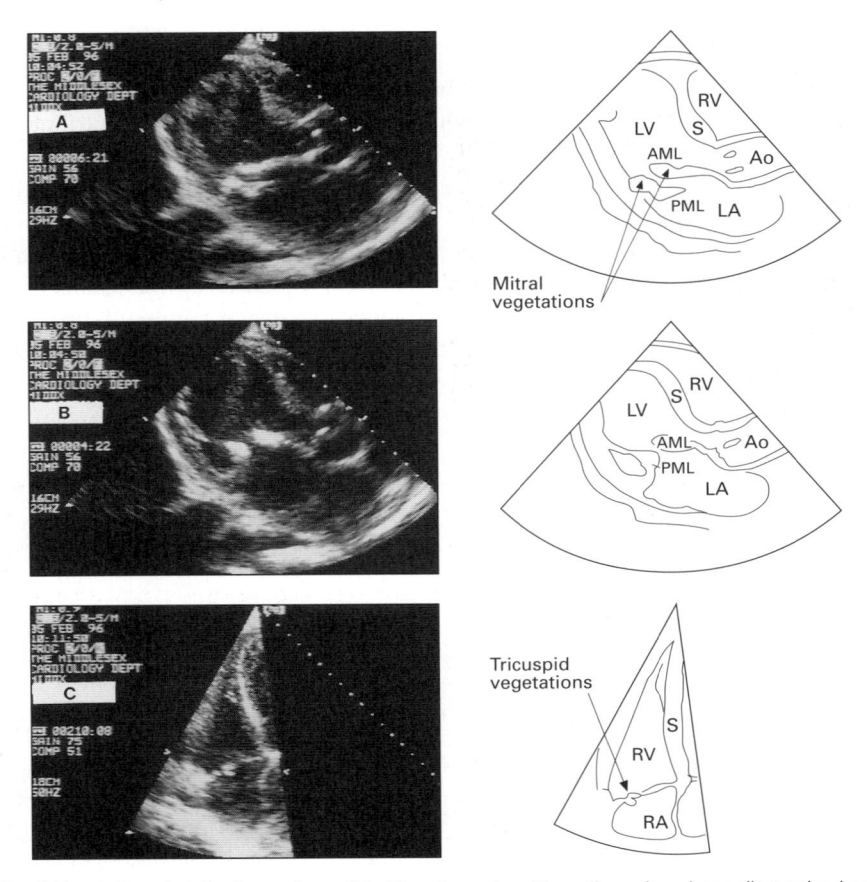

Fig. 1 Vegetations in infective endocarditis. Two-dimensional transthoracic echocardiography, long axis view. Large fleshy vegetations on both mitral leaflets. (A) Early systole showing flail posterior leaflet prolapsing behind anterior leaflet. (B) Diastolic image. (C) Coned four-chamber view in same patient showing smaller tricuspid vegetations. This patient had an urgent mitral and tricuspid valve replacement. LV, left ventricle; RV, right ventricle; LA, left atrium; S, interventricular septum; Ao, aortic root; AML, anterior mitral leaflet; PML, posterior mitral leaflet.

Balloon mitral valvuloplasty

Also known as percutaneous transvenous mitral commissurotomy (PTMC), balloon dilatation of the mitral valve has become a widely used procedure for the treatment of selected cases of mitral stenosis. The Inoue balloon has greatly improved the ease and safety of the procedure [4]. It can be performed in a routine cardiac catheter list, involves only a night's stay in hospital and can even be done as a day case. Balloon inflation is shown in Fig 3. Before PTMC, patients with non-calcific pure mitral stenosis were subjected to a closed mitral valvotomy: a left thoracotomy was required, a 10–14 day stay in hospital and 3 months off work. In contrast, patients who have had a PTMC can return to work in a day or two. About 450 of these procedures are performed annually in the UK. It is also making a large impact on the treatment of mitral stenosis in the third world, where the expensive balloons are re-used.

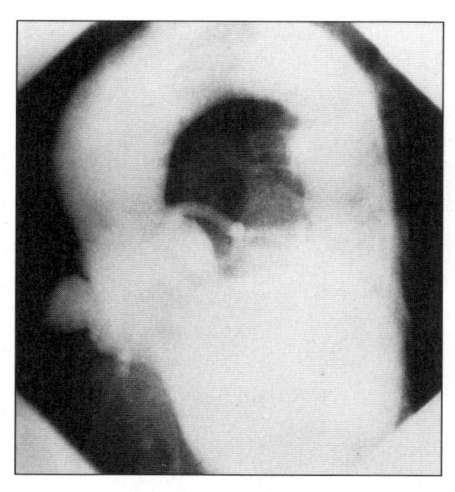

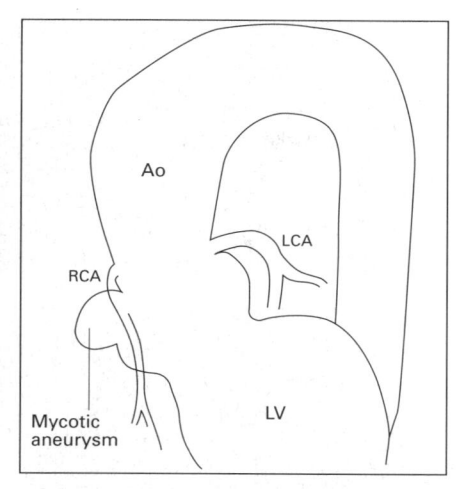

Fig. 2 Aortic root mycotic aneurysm (abscess). Aortography in a patient with aortic valve endocarditis. Left anterior oblique projection. There is severe aortic regurgitation into a dilated left ventricle (LV) with an anterior mycotic aneurysm (root abscess). Aortic valve replacement was needed. LCA, left coronary artery; RCA, right coronary artery. Aortography is less needed now with the advent of TOE but still may be useful before surgery.

The indications for a balloon mitral valvuloplasty are similar to those formerly used for a closed mitral valvotomy. However, since it is such a low-risk procedure with low morbidity, it can be used both in patients with less severe disease and also in those in whom surgical intervention was felt to be contraindicated because of poor lung or renal function, obesity, or age. Palliation of disease in quite heavily calcified valves can sometimes be achieved in high-risk surgical patients [5]. It can also be performed in the pregnant woman with much lower risk to the fetus than surgery [6].

The selection of a patient for balloon mitral valvuloplasty depends on the anatomy of the mitral valve, which is assessed by transthoracic and transoesophageal echocardiography. The ideal case is a young patient who has not had a previous closed mitral valvotomy, with a non-calcified mitral valve, mobile leaflets just with commissural fusion, no mitral regurgitation, no chordal fusion, good left ventricular function and no evidence of any intra-atrial thrombus.

The predictors of a good long-term outcome following PTMC have been described by Cohen *at al.* [7]. Multivariate analysis showed that independent predictors of a good long-term outcome in their 146 patients were a low echocardiographic score and a low left ventricular end-diastolic pressure (LVEDP). The echo score devised by Wilkins *et al.* [8] was used. Four features of the mitral valve anatomy were graded: mobility, thickening, calcification, and subvalvar chordal thickening. Each of these was graded 0–4 and the total was summated, the worst possible score being 16. Patients with echocardiographic scores of >8 and LVEDPs of >10 fared less well. They had a 23% event-free survival at 5 years compared with 84% in patients with echo scores <8 and LVEDPs <10.

Patients selected for balloon mitral valvuloplasty must have TOE before the

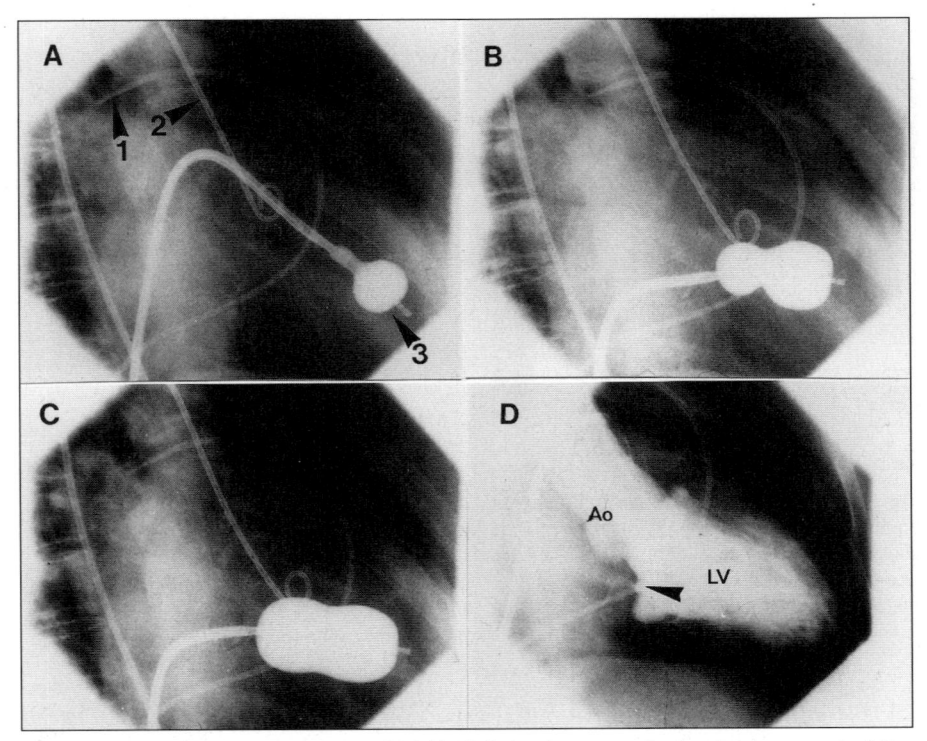

Fig. 3 Stages in mitral valvuloplasty. (A) Initial inflation just expands the distal segment of the balloon. 1, pulmonary artery catheter; 2, pigtail catheter in aortic root, positioned just above aortic valve; 3, Inoue balloon catheter advanced to apex of left ventricle via a trans-septal puncture. (B) The balloon is pulled back to the mitral valve and further inflation expands the proximal segment of the balloon producing an hour-glass shape. (C) The balloon is fully inflated. (D) Left ventricular angiography performed after balloon inflation. Systolic frame shows a small jet of mitral regurgitation. Ao, aortic root; LV, left ventricle.

procedure. Thrombus within the left atrium, particularly in the left atrial appendage is a contraindication to the procedure, as manipulation of the balloon or guide wire might easily dislodge friable thrombus. Patients with intra-atrial thrombus must have an open procedure on cardiopulmonary bypass: either an open mitral valvotomy or a valve replacement.

The mortality risk in experienced hands is <1%. The principal risks of the procedure are pericardial tamponade due to perforation of the left atrium with the trans-septal needle or catheter, the dislodgement of undetected thrombus-causing systemic emboli, the induction of ventricular arrhythmias by the balloon catheter, and the production of significant mitral regurgitation following mitral balloon dilatation. Acute tamponade due to perforation of the left atrium can be relieved by immediate pericardial aspiration but just occasionally needs formal surgical drainage. The production of moderate or severe mitral regurgitation necessitates mitral valve replacement though this is not usually an emergency.

In most patients the mitral valve area is doubled to >2.0 sq cm following balloon dilatation. The left atrial pressure drops sharply following the initial inflation (Fig. 4). Pulmonary artery pressure gradually falls and exercise tolerance improves. Re-stenosis has been reported in 15–50% of patients at 2 years though most patients maintain their clinical improvement much longer [9]. Many patients in time will need a mitral valve replacement, but balloon dilatation may delay the need for this and avoids the need for a closed mitral valvotomy.

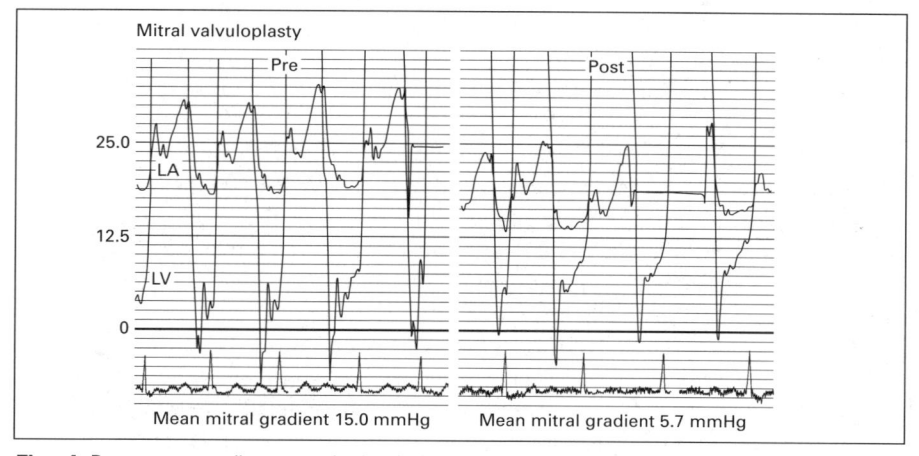

Fig. 4 Pressure recordings at mitral valvuloplasty. Direct left atrial (LA) pressure against left ventricular (LV) pressure in a patient with mitral stenosis pre- and post-valvuloplasty. The left atrial pressure drops after the initial inflation and the mean mitral gradient is reduced.

☐ MITRAL VALVE REPAIR

There is increasing interest in mitral valve repair as an alternative to mitral valve replacement, particularly in patients with mitral regurgitation due to myxomatous degeneration of the valve (floppy valve) causing severe mitral regurgitation. Although conventional valve replacement using a mechanical valve has the advantage of durability, the patient is committed to a lifetime on anticoagulants.

Mitral valve repair avoids the thrombotic risk of the mechanical valve and, to some extent, the degenerative risks of the xenograft. It also preserves the integrity of the valve itself, as excision of the subvalve apparatus in mitral valve replacement is known to cause a deterioration in left ventricular function.

A variety of surgical options are available and considerable surgical skill is required. Intraoperative TOE is valuable in assessing residual mitral regurgitation following a repair and before closing the chest. The mitral chordae can be shortened, or transferred to the other leaflet or substituted with Teflon filament sutures. The prolapsed leaflet (usually posterior) can be advanced, partially resected or repaired. A perforated leaflet can be patched using autologous pericardium. Stenosis of a rheumatic valve can be relieved by a commissurotomy and/or by fenestrating a fused subvalve apparatus. A variety of annuloplasty techniques are available to attempt to reduce the size of a dilated annulus.

☐ CHOICE OF PROSTHETIC VALVE

Mechanical prosthetic valves require warfarin treatment for life, and consequent bleeding or thrombotic risks with inadequate anticoagulant control. In addition, they are noisy. Xenografts are silent, and in the aortic position warfarin is unnecessary. However, they degenerate, with redo surgery becoming necessary after about 7 years in the mitral position and 10 years in the aortic. Xenograft degeneration occurs more quickly in the younger patient and rapid degeneration may occur during pregnancy. Xenografts may last only 3 to 4 years in children. Two randomized studies have confirmed a higher redo operation rate for porcine xenografts than a mechanical Bjork-Shiley valve, with a trend to a higher mortality in the xenograft groups in both trials [10,11].

The search for the perfect xenograft continues. We have been through the use of fascia lata, dura mater and bovine pericardium, all of which have failed. The porcine bioprosthesis is the most reliable xenograft presently available. There is now the possibility of using autologous pericardium with the valve manufactured in the operating theatre at the time of surgery using specially designed stents. Durability tests are awaited.

Xenografts must be reserved for patients for whom anticoagulation is contraindicated. They are also a useful alternative to a mechanical aortic valve in the elderly. They are not generally an alternative to a mechanical mitral valve as these patients are usually in atrial fibrillation and will need warfarin anyway.

Women of child-bearing age should, if possible, have their children before valve replacement, with valvuloplasty or valve repair a possible interim measure. If valve replacement is necessary, a mechanical valve should be used with careful anticoagulant control. The risk of warfarin-induced embryopathy is small (<10%). The mortality risk of a redo mitral valve replacement for a failed xenograft, however, is approximately 10%.

Antibiotic-treated cadaveric aortic homografts are a useful alternative to the porcine xenograft for an aortic valve replacement. Durability is better than the xenograft but valve failure does occur in time. Supplies are limited. Homografts are particularly valuable in replacing infected aortic valves (native or prosthetic) as they seem to have some resistance to reinfection.

Tricuspid valve replacement is most commonly needed for severe tricuspid regurgitation due to dilatation of the tricuspid annulus in patients with pulmonary hypertension. Valve replacement is also needed in drug abusers with a destroyed valve due to endocarditis or those who have had a valvulectomy. A tricuspid annuloplasty or xenograft valve replacement are of only temporary benefit. A mechanical Starr-Edwards valve is the valve of choice. Permanent pacing may be necessary postoperatively and can be a major problem [12].

REFERENCES

1. Daniel WG, Mugge A. Transesophageal echocardiography. *New Engl J Med* 1995; **332**: 1268–78.
2. John RM, Pugsley W, Treasure T, Sturridge MF, Swanton RH. Aortic root complications of infective endocarditis: influence on surgical outcome. *Eur Heart J* 1991; **12**: 241–8.

3   Prasad A, Fraser AG. Prevention of infective endocarditis: enthusiasm tempered by realism. *Brit J Hosp Med* 1995; **54:** 341–7
4   Inoue K. Percutaneous transvenous mitral commissurotomy using the Inoue balloon. *Eur Heart J* 1991; **12** (Suppl B): 99–108.
5   Lefevre T, Bonan R, Serra A, Cretlan J, Dyrda I, Teticlerc R. Percutaneous mitral valvuloplasty in surgical high risk patients. *J Am Coll Cardiol* 1991; **17:** 348–54.
6   Iung B, Cornier B, Elias J, *et al.* Usefulness of percutaneous balloon commissurotomy for mitral stenosis during pregnancy. *Am J Cardiol* 1994; **73:** 398–400.
7   Cohen DJ, Kuntz RE, Gordon SPF, *et al.* Predictors of long term outcome after percutaneous balloon mitral valvuloplasty. *New Engl J Med* 1992; **327:** 1329–35.
8   Wilkins GT, Weyman AE, Abascal VM, Block PC, Palacios IF. Percutaneous balloon dilatation of the mitral valve: an analysis of echocardiographic variables related to outcome and the mechanism of dilatation. *Brit Heart J* 1988; **60:** 299–308.
9   Block PC, Palacios IF, Block EH, Tuzcu EM, Griffin B. Late (two year) follow-up after percutaneous balloon mitral valvotomy. *Am J Cardiol* 1992; **69:** 537–41.
10 Bloomfield P, Wheatley DJ, Prescott RJ, Miller HC. Twelve-year comparison of a Bjork-Shiley mechanical heart valve with porcine bioprostheses. *New Engl J Med* 1991; **324:** 573–9.
11 Hammermeister KE, Sethi GK, Henderson WG, Oprian C, Tai K, Rahimtoola S. A comparison of outcomes in men 11 years after heart valve replacement with a mechanical valve or bioprosthesis. *New Engl J Med* 1993; **328:** 1289–96.
12 Cooper JP, Jayawickreme SR, Swanton RH. Permanent pacing in patients with tricuspid valve replacements. *Brit Heart J* 1995: **73:** 169–72.

☐ MULTIPLE CHOICE QUESTIONS

1   Contraindications to mitral valvuloplasty:
    (a) Moderate mitral regurgitation
    (b) Loud opening snap
    (c) Thrombus seen in atrial appendage on transoesophageal echocardiography
    (d) Age over 70
    (e) Pregnancy

2   A woman of 30 with a floppy mitral valve has severe mitral regurgitation. She would be best advised to have:
    (a) A mitral valvuloplasty
    (b) A homograft valve replacement
    (c) A mitral valve repair
    (d) A porcine xenograft valve replacement
    (e) A mechanical valve replacement

3   A man of 78 presents with effort syncope due to tight calcific aortic valve stenosis. He has a history of recurrent epistaxes and has had several nasal cauteries in the past. Left ventricular function is still good and his coronary arteries are normal on angiography. He is generally otherwise fit. The most appropriate recommendation is that he should have:
    (a) A porcine xenograft valve replacement
    (b) An aortic valvuloplasty
    (c) An aortic Starr-Edwards valve replacement

(d) A dual chamber pacemaker
(e) Medical management with beta-blockade

4   A 65 year old man has aortic valve endocarditis due to a penicillin-sensitive *Streptococcus viridans* group organism. His few remaining teeth are in poor condition. He is afebrile after two weeks iv penicillin but he has severe aortic regurgitation, due to a flail aortic leaflet confirmed on transthoracic echocardiography. Good views of the mitral valve are obtained and are normal. ECG is normal. His left ventricular function is good and he is not in left ventricular failure. His management should now be:
   (a) Continue medical treatment for 4 weeks then stop iv penicillin and monitor his progress
   (b) Dental clearance under additional iv antibiotic cover, then proceed a few days later to an aortic valve replacement using a homograft or mechanical valve
   (c) Proceed to a porcine xenograft replacement and then remove his teeth
   (d) Dental clearance under additional antibiotic cover and then continue medical treatment
   (e) Switch to oral antibiotics for a further two months

5   Transoesophageal echocardiography:
   (a) Is mandatory prior to balloon mitral valvuloplasty
   (b) Gives better images of the atrial septum than transthoracic echocardiography
   (c) Is contraindicated in patients with oesophageal varices
   (d) Is better than transthoracic echocardiography at detecting apical LV thrombus following myocardial infarction
   (e) Is the best way of imaging mitral vegetations

ANSWERS

1a	True	2a	False	3a	True	4a	False	5a	True
b	False	b	False	b	False	b	True	b	True
c	True	c	True	c	False	c	False	c	True
d	False	d	False	d	False	d	False	d	False
e	False	e	False	e	False	e	False	e	True

Chest pain in women

P Collins

☐ PRESENTATION OF SYMPTOMS

Coronary heart disease remains the most common cause of death in women. The main difference between men and women is the age at presentation of the disease. Women present at an older age probably because of the protection afforded by premenopausal oestrogen. The presentation of coronary heart disease in women can be more complicated. Difficulties arise in the differentiation between typical and atypical chest pain in women. Atypical chest pain is more common in women than in men and the reasons for this are not entirely clear. However, the condition syndrome X (anginal type chest pain, an exercise stress test that shows evidence of ST-segment depression on an electrocardiogram, and angiographically smooth coronary arteries) occurs more commonly in women than men. Within this group of patients there are a small number of subjects who have demonstrable evidence of true myocardial ischaemia but no evidence of epicardial coronary artery disease. These patients may have coronary microvascular abnormalities. Other syndromes of non-ischaemic chest pain, such as mitral valve prolapse, are more common in women. All types of chest pain, including typical anginal pain, are associated with a lower prevalence of angiographically confirmed coronary heart disease in women compared to men. Careful assessment of the nature of the pain is of particular importance in women. Coronary heart disease has been found in 62% of women with definite angina, 40% of women with probable angina and 4% with atypical non-ischaemic sounding chest pain. It is particularly important to realize that a pattern of non-ischaemic atypical chest pain is associated with a very low risk of coronary heart disease, although definite angina is still strongly suggestive of coronary heart disease.

Certain features of coronary heart disease presentation should be emphasized. A careful history is important in women. More women than men present with angina as their initial manifestation of coronary heart disease (65% *vs* 35%). Women with chronic stable angina are also more likely than men to have chest pain during inactivity, sleep or episodes of mental stress. Ischaemia seems to produce different patterns of chest pain in women with known coronary heart disease. Indeed women with neck and shoulder pain, fatigue, dyspnoea, nausea and vomiting in addition to chest pain are more likely to be undergoing an acute myocardial infarction.

Chest pain in women may be ignored by doctors, thereby delaying investigation. Conversely, fewer women than men initially present with myocardial infarction (29% *vs* 43%), but confounding this is the fact that the standard diagnostic tests are not as specific or as sensitive in women. Over 30% of women present with sudden cardiac death or fatal myocardial infarction.

☐ CORONARY HEART DISEASE

Risk factors

Risk factors for coronary heart disease should include menopausal status or hormonal status as, in the absence of known risk factors, coronary heart disease is unusual in women before the menopause. Surgical menopause in patients who have had oophorectomy carries a risk of coronary heart disease in excess of that associated with a natural menopause. The reasons for this are numerous, but include the fact that the menopause is associated with detrimental changes in lipid profile, such as an increase in low-density lipoprotein (LDL) cholesterol and a decrease in high-density lipoprotein (HDL) cholesterol [1].

A large number of observational studies suggest that postmenopausal women who use oestrogen have up to a 50% reduction in the risk of developing coronary heart disease and the risks associated with it [2]. The use of oral contraceptives in premenopausal women does not appear to increase their risk of atherosclerotic disease. Those women who develop myocardial infarction on oral contraceptives are more likely to be over 35 years of age and to smoke cigarettes.

Diabetes mellitus is a very powerful predictor of coronary heart disease in women and is associated with an adverse risk in terms of mortality and morbidity. Hypertension is an established risk factor for coronary heart disease, particularly in postmenopausal women of an older age. Among the elderly hypertension is a more powerful predictor of coronary heart disease in women than in men and is more common in women with coronary heart disease than in men with the disease. Cigarette smoking has been associated with a considerable number of coronary events in women and even in those women who smoke a relatively small number of cigarettes the risk of coronary heart disease is elevated. Other risk factors for coronary heart disease include age, obesity, a positive family history and psychosocial factors such as stress. All of these features therefore have to be taken into account with women presenting with chest pain, and chest pain associated with any number of these risk factors makes the diagnosis of coronary heart disease more likely.

Epidemiology

Women appear to be protected against coronary heart disease until the age of the menopause which in western countries occurs at approximately 51 years. It seems that, in women, the relationship between death from coronary heart disease and age is shifted to the right by about 10 years compared with men. By the age of 70 to 80 years, however, mortality from coronary heart disease is similar in men and women. It is believed that ovarian steroids may be protective in women, and a large number of observational epidemiological studies have shown that postmenopausal women who receive oestrogen therapy appear to have reduced risk of coronary heart disease. The effect of added progestin is not yet fully understood, although the available data also suggest a protective effect.

Disease severity and pathology

The manifestations of coronary heart disease in particular, but also of other heart diseases, are different in women, but is this because of variables relating to anatomy or physiology? To date, it has proved extremely difficult to determine whether these differing manifestations are due to the size of a myocardial infarction or to the sex of the patients. The coronary arteries are often smaller and narrower in women than in men, and there has been a suggestion that infarct size and outcome may differ. A few clinical studies suggest that women, in contrast to men, have a lower incidence of coronary artery stenosis and a higher incidence of acute coronary syndromes, resulting in adverse outcomes due to lack of a compensatory collateral circulation that could reduce infarct size and thus improve outcome. Moreover, once women have been diagnosed as having coronary heart disease, they do less well than men. This may be either because of delay in diagnosis, resulting from poor recognition of the different signs and symptoms that women present, or because the severity of disease is greater in women with milder symptomatology. Women are less likely than men to undergo invasive diagnostic procedures, for example coronary angiography and transluminal coronary angioplasty. Also, they are initially less likely to receive thrombolytic therapy.

There is evidence to suggest that oestrogen has both direct and indirect vaso-relaxing properties in the coronary arteries and other vascular beds. This has led to the belief that oestrogen improves blood flow in a number of organs, including the heart, although this depends to some extent on the sex hormone milieu present at the time. Overall, oestrogen appears to have a direct relaxing effect on vascular smooth muscle, possibly involving calcium antagonism, an effect via endothelium-derived vasorelaxing mediators, and effects on nuclear and non-nuclear oestrogen receptors.

Diagnosis in women

The standard tests for diagnostic obstructive coronary heart disease centre around exercise stress testing. Women with chest pain syndromes have a much higher incidence of positive exercise tests, ie exertion-induced depression of the ST segment in electrocardiograms in the absence of obstructive, atherosclerotic lesions of the coronary arteries. Indeed, up to 50% of women who undergo exercise testing may have positive results in the apparent absence of coronary artery disease, whereas the rate in men is about 10%. In addition, false negative results, ie no exertion-induced ST-segment depression in the presence of coronary heart disease, are more common. Exercise testing is thus not a particularly effective method of diagnosing coronary heart disease in women and should not be used as a screening test.

Other cardiac tests, particularly thallium stress testing and echocardiography, are also more difficult to evaluate in women. This is because the presence of breast tissue can attenuate the radioactive signal, making it more difficult to interpret, and can also reduce the access window size in echocardiography.

Some of these issues can be resolved by being clear about the clinical problem being addressed. The question is not whether diagnostic tests should be different for women, but rather how good the test is for diagnosing that disease entity in a particular individual. It is very important that physicians realize the use(s) of each test, and thus avoid making an incorrect diagnosis or using tests inappropriately, in either men or women.

Prognosis

Once coronary heart disease is diagnosed in women, mortality rates exceed those of men. For example, one-year mortality rate for first myocardial infarction in women is 39% against 31% for men, while their mortality rate for repeat myocardial infarction is 20% against 15% in men. This may reflect the fact that women suffer myocardial infarction at a later age; age is an independent risk factor for prognosis. However, despite the age effect, the risk of reinfarction and subsequent mortality at second infarction is greater in women.

Treatment

Conventional medical treatment for acute myocardial infarction – analgesics, aspirin and thrombolytics – is not fundamentally different in men and women, although women are, as mentioned above, less likely to receive thrombolytic therapy. Equally, the treatment of women with chronic angina pectoris is not greatly different in respect of use of nitrates, β-blockers and calcium antagonists. Issues arise, however, with regard to three treatments: coronary artery surgery, angioplasty and hormone replacement therapy.

Coronary artery bypass graft surgery in women appears to be associated with an increased risk of morbidity and mortality compared with men. Women have smaller coronary arteries, and tend to be older at the time of surgery; the increased risk after surgery is still present 5 and 10 years later. For angioplasty, however, the long-term outlook appears to be very similar in both men and women, though the number of procedures per 1000 population is greater in men.

Traditionally, hormone replacement therapy has been relatively contra-indicated in high-risk patients, including post-infarction cases and those with established coronary heart disease or heart failure. Recent evidence, however, suggests that oestrogens are not harmful to these groups of patients [3]. In particular, oestrogens appear to have vasodilator rather than vasoconstrictor properties; in one study in women with established coronary heart disease, oestrogen therapy improved both exercise time and time to myocardial ischaemia when compared with placebo [4].

The difficulty arises when progestin is added, and here the evidence is conflicting. At present, it is not possible to say with any certainty whether the acute effects of a combined hormone replacement therapy preparation are beneficial in women with myocardial ischaemia, although a recent Finnish study in post-menopausal women suggests a protective effect following myocardial infarction, despite added progestin [5]. A recent large study has reported no detrimental effect of progestin on long-term mortality [6].

Women in clinical trials

The issue of including women in clinical trials has been widely debated, and there are differing views. One is that clinical trials should include a substantial proportion of women, but this approach has considerable problems. Disease may be more common in men, particularly when specific age ranges are used. Also, analysing female subgroups may significantly reduce the power of a study, and failure to find a statistical difference between men and women does not prove that no difference exists. The alternative view is that there should be separate trials for men and women. This would provide clear answers, and our feeling is that the issues will only be resolved when good quality data are available from studies in women alone.

Problem of syndrome X in women

Angina pectoris is usually caused by atheromatous coronary artery disease and occurs predominantly in males. Normal or nearly normal coronary arteries are found in approximately 20% of patients who undergo coronary angiography. The majority of these patients are women. The triad of angina pectoris, a positive exercise test and angiographically smooth coronary arteries is commonly referred to as syndrome X, a term first used by Kemp in 1973. The pathophysiology of the troublesome chest pain in syndrome X is poorly understood, but there are many suggested mechanisms. Most of the women with syndrome X are postmenopausal. Indeed, oestrogen deficiency is associated with vasomotor instability and decreased arterial blood flow velocity in humans. Acute administration of oestradiol-17β improves myocardial ischaemia in female patients with coronary artery disease [4]. It has also been shown to increase peripheral blood flow in postmenopausal women [7].

A recent study has investigated the clinical and gynaecological features of female patients with syndrome X in order to ascertain whether ovarian hormone deficiency plays a role in unmasking the syndrome in female patients [8]. Another study has investigated the possibility of oestrogen being helpful in the treatment of this condition [9]. Imipramine, known to have visceral analgesic properties, has also been shown to be helpful in some patients [10].

☐ GENERAL CONCLUSIONS

The diagnosis of chest pain in women can pose problems for the physician because of a number of confounding factors. The high incidence of atypical chest pain makes conventional exercise stress testing misleading in the diagnosis of coronary heart disease. The risk factors for coronary heart disease in women are essentially similar to those in men, apart from oestrogen deficiency associated with the menopause. Oestrogen replacement may therefore retard the development of coronary heart disease and reduce myocardial events associated with it. Typical anginal chest pain is more likely to be associated with coronary heart disease and therefore a careful clinical history is important.

Cardiological syndrome X is more common in postmenopausal women;

oestrogen deficiency may be a trigger and oestrogen replacement may be a useful adjunctive therapy.

REFERENCES

1. Wenger NK, Speroff L, Packard B. Cardiovascular health and disease in women. *New Engl J Med* 1993; **329**: 247–56.
2. Stampfer MJ, Colditz GA. Estrogen replacement therapy and coronary heart disease: a quantitative assessment of the epidemiologic evidence. *Prev Med* 1991; **20**: 47–63.
3. Ettinger B, Friedman GD, Bush T, Quesenberry CP. Reduced mortality associated with long-term postmenopausal estrogen therapy. *Obstet Gynecol* 1996; **87**: 6–12.
4. Rosano GMC, Sarrel PM, Poole-Wilson PA, Collins P. Beneficial effect of oestrogen on exercise-induced myocardial ischaemia in women with coronary artery disease. *Lancet* 1993; **342**: 133–6.
5. Falkeborn M, Persson I, Adami HO, Bergstrom R, Eaker E, Lithell H, Mohsen R, Naessen T. The risk of acute myocardial infarction after oestrogen and oestrogen-progestogen replacement. *Brit J Obstet Gynaecol* 1992; **99**: 821–8.
6. Grodstein F, Stampfer MJ, Manson JE, Colditz GA, Willett WC, Rosner B, Speizer FE, Hennekens CH. Postmenopausal estrogen and progestin use and the risk of cardiovascular disease. *New Engl J Med* 1996; **335**: 453–61.
7. Volterrani M, Rosano GMC, Coats A, Beale C, Collins P. Estrogen acutely increases peripheral blood flow in postmenopausal women. *Am J Med* 1995; **99**: 119–22.
8. Rosano GMC, Collins P, Kaski JC, Lindsay DC, Sarrel PM, Poole-Wilson PA. Syndrome X in women is associated with estrogen deficiency. *Eur Heart J* 1995; **16**: 610–4.
9. Rosano GMC, Peters NS, Lefroy DC, Lindsay DC, Sarrel PM, Collins P, Poole-Wilson PA. 17-beta-estradiol therapy lessens angina in postmenopausal women with syndrome X. *J Am Coll Cardiol* 1996; **28**: 1500–5.
10. Cannon RO, III, Quyyumi AA, Mincemoyer R, Stine AM, Gracely RH, Smith WH, Geraci MF, Black BC, Uhde TW, Waclawiw MA, Maher K, Benjamin SB. Imipramine in patients with chest pain despite normal coronary angiograms. *New Engl J Med* 1994; **330**: 1411–7.

☐ MULTIPLE CHOICE QUESTIONS

1. Oestrogen:
   (a) Can cause coronary vasodilation
   (b) Is naturally derived from testosterone
   (c) Decreases the incidence of carcinoma of the uterus
   (d) Stimulates inducible nitric oxide synthase
   (e) Increases osteoblast activity
   (f) Decreases the frequency of supraventricular tachycardia in women
   (g) Decreases insulin sensitivity

2. Concerning women and chest pain:
   (a) More women than men with CHD present with angina
   (b) The one-year mortality after myocardial infarction is greater in women than in men
   (c) Diabetes carries a greater risk of CHD in women than in men
   (d) HDL levels fall after the menopause
   (e) Hormone therapy has been proven to cause weight gain in postmenopausal women

ANSWERS

1a	True	1e	True	2a	True	2d	True
b	True	f	True	b	True	e	False
c	False	g	False	c	True		
d	True						